ANNUAL REVIEW OF MEDICINE:
Selected Topics in
the Clinical Sciences

ANNUAL REVIEW OF MEDICINE:

Selected Topics in
the Clinical Sciences

VOLUME 34, 1983

WILLIAM P. CREGER, *Editor*
Stanford University School of Medicine

CECIL H. COGGINS, *Associate Editor*
Harvard Medical School

E. WILLIAM HANCOCK, *Associate Editor*
Stanford University School of Medicine

ANNUAL REVIEWS INC.   4139 EL CAMINO WAY   PALO ALTO, CALIFORNIA 94306   USA

ANNUAL REVIEWS INC.
Palo Alto, California, USA

International Standard Serial Number: 0066-4219
International Standard Book Number: 0-8243-0534-5
Library of Congress Catalog Card Number: A51-1659

Annual Review and publication titles are registered trademarks of Annual
Reviews Inc.

Annual Reviews Inc. and the Editors of its publications assume no responsibility
for the statements expressed by the contributors to this *Review*.

PRINTED AND BOUND IN THE UNITED STATES OF AMERICA

Annual Review of Medicine
Volume 34, 1983

CONTENTS

(*continued*)

CONTENTS *(continued)*

(continued)

CONTENTS *(continued)*

SOME RELATED ARTICLES IN OTHER *ANNUAL REVIEWS*

From the *Annual Review of Immunology,* Volume 1 (1983):

Autoimmunity—A Perspective, Howard R. Smith and Alfred D. Steinberg

The Role of Cell-Mediated Immune Responses in Resistance to Malaria, with Special Reference to Oxidant Stress, Anthony C. Allison and Elsie M. Eugui

T Cell and B Cell Responses to Viral Antigens at the Clonal Level, L. A. Sherman, A. Vitiello, and N. R. Klinman

Immunobiology of Tissue Transplantation: A Return to the Passenger Leucocyte Concept, Kevin J. Lafferty, Stephen J. Prowse, Charmaine J. Simeonovic, and Hilary S. Warren

From the *Annual Review of Neuroscience,* Volume 6 (1983):

Positron Emission Tomography, Marcus E. Raichle

From the *Annual Review of Nutrition,* Volume 3 (1983):

Nutrition in Renal Failure, Mackenzie Walser

From the *Annual Review of Pharmacology and Toxicology,* Volume 22 (1982):

Pharmacokinetics in the Ovine Maternal-Fetal Unit, H. H. Szeto

Evaluation of Platelet-Inhibiting Drugs in Models of Atherosclerosis, R. N. Saunders

From the *Annual Review of Physiology,* Volume 44 (1982):

Physiological Regulation of the Hepatic Circulation, Peter D. I. Richardson and Peter G. Withrington

Mechanisms of Cardiac Arrhythmias, Joseph F. Spear and E. Neil Moore

Bacterial Chemotaxis, Alan Boyd and Melvin Simon

Leukocyte Chemotaxis, Elliott Shiffmann

From the *Annual Review of Public Health,* Volume 4 (1983):

Critical Issues in the Conduct and Interpretation of Clinical Trials, Thomas A. Louis and Stanley H. Shapiro

Self-Care in Health, Lowell S. Levin and Ellen L. Idler

Nonpharmacologic Approaches to the Treatment of Hypertension, Alvin P. Shapiro and Rolf G. Jacob

Improving the Health of Children: Must the Children Be Involved?, Charles E. Lewis and Mary Ann Lewis

Ann. Rev. Med. 1983. 34:1–12

PROSTAGLANDINS, GLUCOSE HOMEOSTASIS, AND DIABETES MELLITUS

R. Paul Robertson, M.D.

Department of Medicine, University of Washington, Seattle, Washington 98195

ABSTRACT

Prostaglandins of the E series are implicated as regulators of glucose homeostasis because of their effects on glucose production and secretion of insulin and glucagon. PGE is postulated to play a role in the pathophysiology of insulin secretion in adult-onset (Type II) diabetes mellitus. Evidence supporting this hypothesis includes the demonstration that PGE inhibits glucose-induced acute insulin responses in normal humans. Moreover, drugs that inhibit synthesis of PGE improve abnormal insulin secretion in human subjects with Type II diabetes mellitus.

INTRODUCTION

A clear understanding of the role that prostaglandins may play in the pathogenesis of abnormal glucose homeostasis in diabetes mellitus requires an appreciation of two basic concepts. The first is that diabetes mellitus is more accurately described as a syndrome than as a disease. If asked, a group of clinicians will provide as many different definitions of diabetes as there are clinicians in the group—and all of the definitions will probably have merit. The reason for this is that diabetes mellitus in humans encompasses a wide range of findings starting with subtle changes in circulating glucose levels and ending with profound disturbances of organ function that result in tragedies such as blindness, renal failure, and limb amputation. The current view among most investigators in the area of diabetes mellitus allows for multiple etiologies for this disease such as viral infection, autoimmune processes, and abnormal hormonal interactions.

The second basic concept that is central to an understanding of the material in this chapter is that, despite the heterogeneity of this syndrome,

1

0066-4219/83/0401-0001$02.00

patients with diabetes mellitus and fasting hyperglycemia exhibit at least one metabolic phenomenon in common that reflects the functional status of the pancreatic islet. This phenomenon involves the acute insulin response, also known as first-phase insulin secretion. This response is a normal outpouring of insulin from the pancreatic islet in response to a sudden increment in glucose concentration in the blood reaching the pancreatic beta cells. The acute insulin response is quantified by measuring peripheral venous insulin levels at 3, 4, and 5 minutes after an intravenous injection of 5–20 grams of glucose. The fasting insulin level before the injection of the intravenous glucose pulse is subtracted from the average of the three levels obtained after glucose injection; the resultant number is used as a measure of the acute insulin response. This parameter of pancreatic beta-cell function is emphasized in this chapter for four reasons. The acute insulin response is invariably absent in patients with hyperglycemia (1); this absence results in a deterioration of glucose tolerance (1); prostaglandins of the E series inhibit the acute insulin response (11, 19, 20) and cause deterioration of glucose tolerance (8, 11, 19, 20); and drugs that inhibit synthesis of prostaglandins tend to restore the acute insulin response (13, 18) and improve carbohydrate tolerance in diabetics (14, 19).

PHARMACOLOGY: ARACHIDONIC ACID METABOLISM

The general scheme for the biochemical synthesis of prostaglandins and the pharmacologic effects of commonly used drugs on this pathway are given in Figure 1. Prostaglandins comprise a large family of closely related fatty acids. The compounds that are most relevant to human physiology and pathophysiology are derived from arachidonic acid. Arachidonic acid is incorporated in phospholipids, which are fundamental components of the plasma membrane of all cells. Cleavage of arachidonic acid from phospholipids is promoted by stimulating the enzyme phospholipase. This results in the formation of cyclic endoperoxides, which are pivotal intermediates in prostaglandin synthesis. From these intermediates can be formed the classical prostaglandins (PGD_2, PGE_2, $PGF_{2\alpha}$), prostacyclin (PGI_2), and thromboxane A_2. Not all of these prostaglandins can be made by every tissue, but all tissues have the ability to synthesize at least one and usually many of them. The prostaglandins and thromboxanes are referred to as products of the cyclooxygenase pathway. The alternate pathway for arachidonic acid metabolism is the lipoxygenase pathway. Although the products of this pathway are not considered in this chapter, it should be noted that the most important products of this pathway appear to be the leukotrienes. This group of compounds includes leukotriene C-D, which was formally known as SRSA or slow-reacting substance of anaphylaxis.

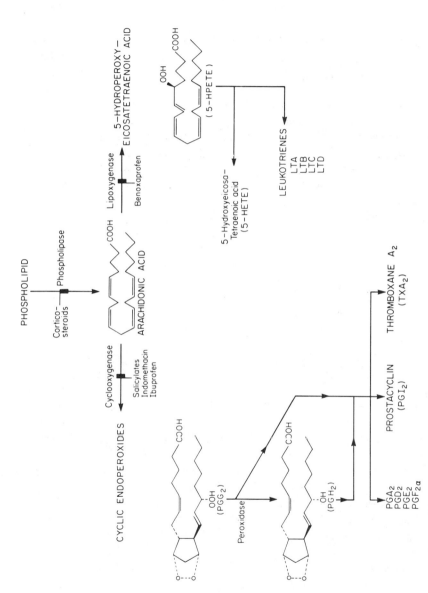

Figure 1 Arachidonic acid metabolism. See text for details. Note that prostaglandin E is formed through the cyclooxygenase pathway, which can be inhibited by nonsteroidal antiinflammatory drugs.

4 ROBERTSON

Current research suggests a stimulatory role in insulin secretion for the lipoxygenase pathway, but this area of investigation is too new to allow definite statements.

There are two important classes of drugs that are commonly used clinically and have a major impact on prostaglandin synthesis. Glucocorticoids inhibit activation of phospholipase and thereby prevent cleavage of arachidonic acid from phospholipids. Consequently, exposure of cells to these drugs inhibits the formation of all products of the cyclooxygenase and lipoxygenase pathways. The group of drugs referred to as nonsteroidal antiinflammatory drugs (NSAID) inhibits cyclooxygenase from converting arachidonic acid to cyclic endoperoxides. Consequently, this group of drugs inhibits formation of all prostaglandins and thromboxanes. It is important to emphasize that the drugs in both of these groups are global inhibitors of arachidonic acid metabolism rather than inhibitors of synthesis of specific prostaglandins or thromboxanes. Consequently, when interpreting the effects of these drugs, one must allow for the possibility that the decreased availability of one or more arachidonic acid products may be involved. It should also be noted that there are no receptor antagonists to any of the prostaglandins or thromboxanes that can be used in humans and that glucocorticoids and NSAID also have effects on biochemical processes unrelated to arachidonic acid synthesis.

PHYSIOLOGY: PROSTAGLANDINS AND GLUCOSE HOMEOSTASIS

A full appreciation of prostaglandins' effects on glucose homeostasis requires an understanding of the effects that these compounds have on circulating glucose, glucose production, insulin secretion, and glucagon secretion. The vast majority of reported data was collected in experiments that used PGE. Consequently, this chapter is limited to a consideration of prostaglandins of the E series (PGE). Other prostaglandins and thromboxanes either have had few effects on glucose homeostasis or have had effects that have not excited a great deal of scientific interest.

Circulating glucose levels in humans are generally increased by PGE (8, 20) and decreased by NSAID (3, 5, 6, 16, 18, 19, 25, 27). There have been no reports that PGE decreases circulating glucose. An increase in circulating glucose levels has rarely been found in patients receiving NSAID. The single exception to this generalization is indomethacin, which has discordant effects when compared to the other drugs in the NSAID group, i.e. indomethacin increases circulating glucose (3, 23, 24). Although the mechanism of this effect is not known, it presumably is not related to inhibition of cyclooxygenase.

There have not been many reports of experiments in which the effects of PGE and NSAID on endogenous glucose production were examined. However, it has been observed that PGE increases hepatic glucose production (7, 21). It is not possible to provide a valid generalization about the effects of NSAID on endogenous glucose production because of the paucity of reported studies and the contradictory results reported by these studies (26). It should be noted that none of these studies have been performed in humans. Virtually all information about endogenous glucose production has been derived from in vitro studies and in vivo experiments in animals.

The work in the area of pancreatic beta-cell function has dealt with the effects of PGE and NSAID on insulin secretion both in vitro and in vivo. This is a somewhat controversial area because different investigators have sometimes formed opposite conclusions. The controversy probably arises from an imprecise terminology used to describe insulin secretion and a failure to appreciate that indomethacin has discordant effects on insulin secretion when it is compared to the effects of other drugs in the NSAID group. When these two considerations are kept in mind, the data are reasonably consistent.

It is clear that PGE itself can stimulate insulin secretion (9, 15) and that this effect is probably mediated by cyclic-AMP (9). However, PGE has also been found by many to inhibit primary stimuli of insulin secretion such as glucose. An illustration of this can be found in the work of Metz et al (13) in which sodium salicylate decreased PGE production by pancreatic islet-cell cultures, a phenomenon accompanied by augmented insulin secretion (Figure 2). Moreover, the augmentation of insulin secretion caused by sodium salicylate was reversed by exposing the cultures to exogenous PGE_1 (Figure 3).

When one considers only those experiments in which glucose rather than PGE itself was used as the stimulus for insulin secretion, a consistent trend in the data is found. Inhibition of acute insulin responses has always been observed when stimulation was provided by a sudden increment in glucose concentration (2, 11, 19, 20). It is interesting to note that in one instance the inhibitory effect of PGE on glucose-induced insulin secretion was present only when high glucose concentrations were presented to the pancreatic islet; low glucose concentrations allowed the stimulatory effect of PGE on insulin secretion to be observed (2). More germane to human physiology and pathophysiology, all experiments in normal humans confirm that PGE inhibits glucose-induced acute insulin responses (11, 19; Figure 4), and that inhibitors of PGE synthesis with the exception of indomethacin uniformly augment glucose-induced insulin responses (3, 6, 14, 16, 19). The reason for this discordant effect of indomethacin (3, 24) is not yet clear, but it may involve one or more of the effects that indomethacin is known to have on biochemical processes other than the cyclooxygenase

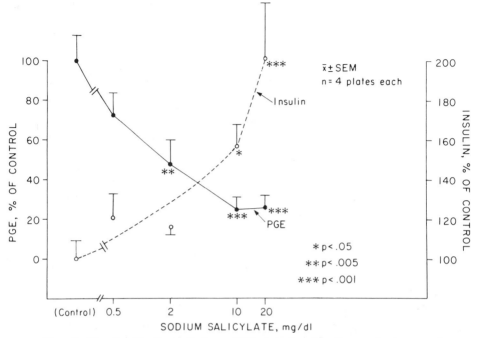

Figure 2 The effect of sodium salicylate on PGE synthesis and insulin secretion in neonatal rat pancreatic cell culture. Sodium salicylate caused a dose-response-related decrease in PGE synthesis and a concomitant increase in insulin secretion in the presence of 16.7 mM glucose. Data are from Reference 13.

reaction, such as interruption of calcium flux across membranes (17) and inhibition of cyclic-AMP-dependent protein kinase (10). Processes such as these are required for normal insulin secretion and interruption of them could lead to the hyperglycemia associated with the use of indomethacin in humans.

Glucagon potently stimulates endogenous glucose production and thereby causes hyperglycemia. Although much less work examining the effects of PGE and NSAID on glucagon secretion has been performed, it is clear that PGE stimulates glucagon secretion in laboratory animals and in humans (8, 15, 22). This stimulatory effect appears to be independent of the adrenergic nervous system in animals, but may be preventable by beta-adrenergic blockade in humans (8, 22). The effects of NSAID on glucagon secretion are inconsistent (12, 14, 16, 25). Here again whatever confusion exists with regard to the effects of NSAID on pancreatic alpha-cell function may be due to the failure to distinguish glucagon secretion as a general phenomenon from glucagon secretion stimulated by glucose signals, in this case hypoglycemia. This consideration parallels the necessity to distinguish insulin secretion as a general phenomenon from glucose-induced acute

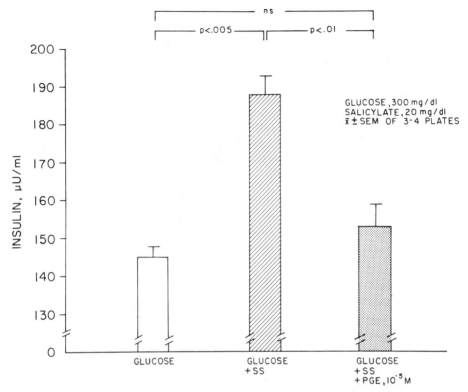

Figure 3   Reversal by PGE$_1$ of the augmenting effect of sodium salicylate on insulin secretion in neonatal rat pancreatic cell culture. Data are from Reference 13.

insulin responses when interpreting the effects of PGE and NSAID on pancreatic beta-cell function.

PATHOPHYSIOLOGY: PROSTAGLANDINS AND DIABETES MELLITUS

The rationale for postulating a role for PGE in the pathophysiology of abnormal insulin secretion in patients with diabetes mellitus stems from the observation that PGE inhibits glucose-induced acute insulin responses in normal human subjects (11, 19; Figure 4). These studies were performed because similar observations had previously been made in vivo in dogs (20) and in rats (4). The inhibitory effect of PGE on glucose-induced insulin secretion appears to be relatively specific since insulin responses to arginine and isoproterenol are not inhibited by PGE (19). This observation led to experimentation with intravenous infusions of sodium salicylate (19) in normal subjects and with oral administration of NSAID including sodium salicylate, acetylsalicylic acid, and ibuprofen in normal subjects (3, 14). All of these drugs enhanced glucose-induced insulin secretion. As mentioned before, indomethacin (3, 24) given orally had the opposite effect and thus acted unlike the other NSAID.

Subsequently, sodium salicylate infusions were administered to adult-onset diabetic subjects (Type II) who were hyperglycemic and lacked glucose-induced acute insulin responses (Figure 5). Although these subjects as a group had no acute insulin responses to intravenous glucose, a repeat glucose challenge elicited a response after a one-hour infusion of sodium salicylate. It should be noted that this response was not complete, yet no other drug is known to promote even this small a degree of restoration. Control experiments in which two sequential pulses of intravenous glucose were given did not succeed in restoring responses to the second glucose pulse. Hence, it was concluded that the improvement observed with the sodium salicylate infusion was directly attributable to the effects of the drug

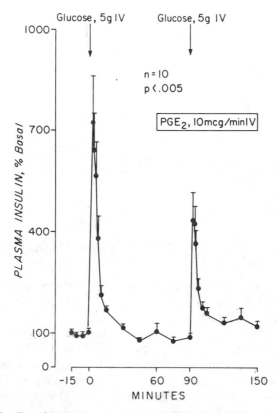

Figure 4   The effect of PGE_2 intravenous infusion on acute insulin responses to intravenous glucose in ten normal subjects. Note that the insulin response to glucose was significantly diminished during the infusion of PGE_2. Data are from Reference 19.

and not to a nonspecific effect of challenging the pancreatic beta cells sequentially with glucose.

It is an interesting historical fact that NSAID were used to improve glucose tolerance in diabetes mellitus over 100 years ago. In 1876 Ebstein (5) used oral sodium salicylate to treat diabetic subjects and observed that this treatment resulted in less glucosuria. Thereafter, several other early investigators made similar observations with salicylates. An example of the effect of acetylsalicylic acid on circulating glucose in diabetics is provided by the work of Reid et al (18; Figure 6). However, the doses of aspirin used in this study were so great that they caused symptoms of salicylism; consequently, aspirin should not be considered as conventional treatment for hyperglycemia in patients with diabetes. Rather, this trial with salicylates offers interesting retrospective evidence that endogenous prostaglandins, presumably PGE, may play a role in abnormal glucose homeostasis in diabetics. It is interesting to note that this trial was performed 15 years

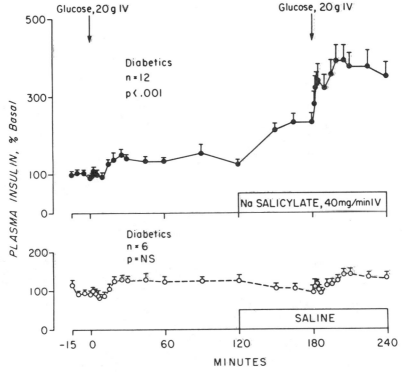

Figure 5 The effect of an intravenous sodium salicylate infusion on glucose-induced acute insulin responses in adult-onset (Type II) diabetics. Note the absence of the acute insulin response to glucose that was partially restored by the infusion of sodium salicylate. This restoration did not occur during control experiments when saline rather than sodium salicylate was infused. Data are from Reference 19.

before it was known that salicylates inhibit prostaglandin synthesis and that Ebstein's initial observation with sodium salicylate was made 50 years before prostaglandins had been discovered.

More recently, the effects on glucose tolerance of intravenous sodium salicylate infusion over a short period of time have been assessed. For example, during the experiments shown in Figure 5, glucose levels were used to calculate glucose disappearance rates (Figure 7). After the first intravenous glucose pulse was given to diabetics, glucose disappearance rates were abnormally depressed. After the one-hour infusion with sodium salicylate, ten of twelve patients had an improved rate of glucose disappearance after an intravenous glucose pulse, and four patients even had normal values. Thus, sodium salicylate, which decreases PGE synthesis and augments insulin secretion in pancreatic islet cultures (13), has been demonstrated in normal humans to augment glucose-induced acute insulin responses and in diabetic humans to partially restore absent glucose-

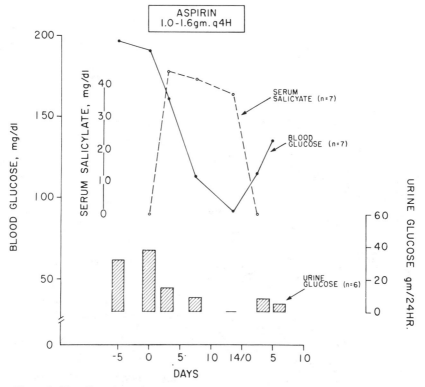

Figure 6   The effect of acetylsalicylic acid given orally on blood glucose levels and urine glucose excretion in seven diabetic subjects. During aspirin therapy there was an increase in serum salicylate and a corresponding decrease in both blood glucose levels and urinary glucose excretion. Data are from Reference 18.

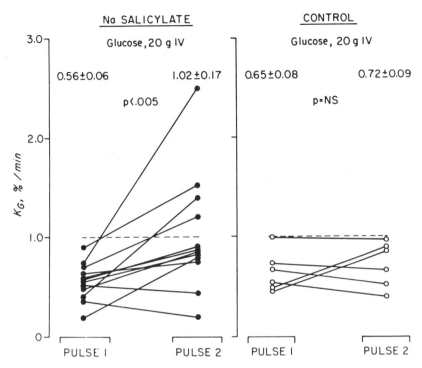

Figure 7 The effect of sodium salicylate on intravenous glucose tolerance in the subjects whose insulin responses are shown in Figure 5. Pulse one refers to the glucose disappearance rate following the first glucose injection; pulse two refers to the rate observed after the second glucose injection. Note that glucose tolerance improved during infusion of sodium salicylate but not during the control infusions of saline. Data are from Reference 19.

induced insulin responses and to improve intravenous glucose intolerance. Observations such as these form the basis for postulating a role for endogenous PGE in the pathogenesis of abnormal insulin secretion and glucose intolerance in adult-onset diabetics.

Literature Cited

1. Brunzell, J. D., Robertson, R. P., Lerner, R. L., Hazzard, W. R., Ensinck, J. W., Bierman, E. L., Porte, D. Jr. 1976. Relationships between fasting plasma glucose levels and insulin secretion during intravenous glucose tolerance tests. *J. Clin. Endocrinol. Metab.* 42(2):222–29

2. Burr, I. M., Sharp, R. 1974. Effects of prostaglandin E₁ and of epinephrine on the dynamics of insulin release in vitro. *Endocrinology* 94:835–39

3. Chen, M., Robertson, R. P. 1979. Effects of prostaglandin synthesis inhibitors on human insulin secretion and carbohydrate tolerance. *Prostaglandins.* 18(4):557–67

4. Dodi, G., Santoro, M. G., Jaffe, B. M. 1978. Effect of a synthetic analogue of PGE₂ on exocrine and endocrine pancreatic function in the rat. *Surgery* 83(2):206–13

5. Ebstein, N. 1876. Zur therapie des dia-

betes mellitus, insbesondere uber die anwendung des salicylsauren natrons bei demselben. Berl. Klin. Woschenschr. 13:337–40

6. Field, J. B., Boyle, C., Remer, A. 1967. Effect of salicylate infusion on plasma-insulin and glucose tolerance in healthy persons and mild diabetics. *Lancet* 1:1191–94

7. Ganguli, S., Sperling, M. A., Frame, E., et al. 1979. Inhibition of glucagon-induced hepatic glucose production by indomethacin. *Am. J. Physiol.* 236 (4):E358–65

8. Giugliano, D., Torella, R., Sgambato, S., D'Onofrio, F. 1979. Effects of α- and β-adrenergic inhibition and somatostatin on plasma glucose, free fatty acids, insulin, glucagon, and growth hormone responses to prostaglandin E_1 in man. *J. Clin. Endocrinol. Metab.* 48(2):302–8

9. Johnson, D. F., Fujimoto, W. F., Williams, R. H. 1973. Enhanced release of insulin by prostaglandins in isolated pancreatic islets. *Diabetes* 22(9):658–63

10. Kantor, H. S., Hampton, M. 1978. Indomethacin in submicromolar concentrations inhibits cyclic AMP-dependent protein kinase. *Nature* 276:841–43

11. Konturek, S. J., Mikós, E. M., Król, R., Wierzbicki, Z., Dobrzanska, M. 1978. Effect of methylated prostaglandin E_2 analogue on insulin secretion in man. *Prostaglandins* 15(4): 591–602

12. Luyckx, A. S., Deliege, M., Jardon-Jeghers, C., Lefebvre, P. J. 1981. Insulin, prostaglandin E_2 and glucagon release by human insulinoma tissue incubated *in vitro*. Influence of indomethacin. *Diabete Metab.* 7:13–17

13. Metz, S. A., Robertson, R. P., Fujimoto, W. Y. 1981. Inhibition of prostaglandin E synthesis augments glucose-induced insulin secretion in cultured pancreas. *Diabetes* 30(7):551–57

14. Micossi, P., Pontiroli, A. E., Baron, S. J., Tamayo, R. C., Lengel, F., Bevilacqua, M., Raggi, U., Norbiato, G., Foa, P. P. 1978. Aspirin stimulates insulin and glucagon secretion and increases glucose tolerance in normal and diabetic subjects. *Diabetes* 27(12):1196–1204

15. Pek, S., Tai, T.-Y., Elster, A., Fajans, S. S. 1975. Stimulation by prostaglandin E_2 of glucagon and insulin release from isolated rat pancreas. *Prostaglandins* 10(3):493–502

16. Prince, R. L., Larkins, R. G., Alford, F. P. 1981. The effect of acetylsalicylic acid on plasma glucose and the response of glucose regulatory hormones to intravenous glucose and arginine in insulin treated diabetics and normal subjects. *Metabolism* 30(3):293–98

17. Radomirov, R., Petkov, V. 1977. Indomethacin and aspirin influences on the contractile effects of prostaglandin E_1 on guinea pig ileum at different Ca^{++} concentration. *Med. Pharmacol.* 30: 775–77

18. Reid, J., MacDougall, A., Andrews, M. M. 1957. Aspirin and diabetes mellitus. *Br. Med. J.* 2:1071–74

19. Robertson, R. P., Chen, M. 1977. A role for prostaglandin E in defective insulin secretion and carbohydrate intolerance in diabetes mellitus. *J. Clin. Invest.* 60:747–53

20. Robertson, R. P., Gavareski, D. J., Porte, D., Bierman, E. L. 1974. Inhibition of *in vivo* insulin secretion by prostaglandin E_1. *J. Clin. Invest.* 54(2): 310–15

21. Sacca, L., Perez, G. 1976. Influence of prostaglandins on plasma glucagon levels in the rat. *Metabolism* 25:127–30

22. Sacca, L., Perez, G., Rengo, F. et al. 1974. Effects of different prostaglandins on glucose kinetics in the rat. *Diabetes* 23:532–35

23. Syvalahti, E. K. G. 1974. The effect of indomethacin on serum growth hormone, immunoreactive insulin, and blood glucose levels of young adult males. *Int. J. Clin. Pharmacol.* 10(2): 111–16

24. Topol, E., Brodows, R. G. 1980. Effects of indomethacin on acute insulin release in man. *Diabetes* 29:379–82

25. Torella, R., Giugliano, D., Siniscalchio, N., Sgambato, S., D'Onofrio, D. 1979. Influence of acetylsalicylic acid on plasma glucose, insulin, glucagon, and growth hormone levels following tolbutamide stimulation in man. *Metabolism* 28(9):887–89

26. Wheeler, G. E., Epand, R. M. 1975. Prostaglandin E_1: anomalous effects on glucose production in rat liver. *Mol. Pharmacol.* 11:335–39

27. Williamson, R. T. 1901. On the treatment of glycosuria and diabetes mellitus with sodium salicylate. *Br. Med. J.* 1:760–62

Ann. Rev. Med. 1983. 34:013–20

ETIOLOGY OF TYPE I DIABETES MELLITUS: Heterogeneity and Immunological Events Leading to Clinical Onset

D. Doniach, M.D., F.R.C.P., G. F. Bottazzo, M.D., M.R.C.Path., and A. G. Cudworth, M.D., Ph.D., F.R.C.P. ‡

Department of Immunology. The Middlesex Hospital Medical School, and Department of Diabetes, Medical Unit, St. Bartholomew's Hospital, London, United Kingdom

ABSTRACT

Type I diabetes is a heterogeneous disorder and the causes of pancreatic beta-cell destruction are unknown. In 1–2% of all cases, viruses (e.g. coxsackie, rubella, mumps, or beta-cell poisons) have been implicated. Twin studies suggest at most 50% of genetic predisposition.

In this review we describe the autoimmune components which, in association with inheritance of HLA-haplotypes in susceptible families, allow the future selection of predisposed sibs for possible preventive therapy to retard loss of insulin secretion. The known association of the endocrine autoimmune organ-specific disorders in 10% of Type I diabetics is the extreme expression of the other main genetic ingredient in the development of insulitis in this disease, irrespective of the triggering environmental components. In this "polyendocrine" subgroup and in the "juvenile-onset" cases there is a prolonged latency period during which pancreatic autoimmunity markers are present before clinical expression of the disease.

Introduction

The remarkable advances of the past 10 years in HLA tissue typing, immunohistochemistry, and pancreatic autoimmunity have at last led to one clear separation in the heterogenous collection of disorders of diabetes

‡ It is with great regret that we note the death of Dr. A. G. Cudworth shortly after the proofs for this review were received.

13

mellitus (DM). Everyone now agrees on Type I and Type II, which correspond roughly to insulin dependency and nondependency (1). The essential character of the Type I DM syndrome is in the gradual loss of insulin-secreting beta cells in the pancreas, mostly from unknown causes (2). In the 1970s we tried to separate the "polyendocrine-autoimmune" from the "early onset" cases (3). While it is true that islet-cell antibodies (ICA) are markers for both extremes of a spectrum in the autoimmune ingredient of idiopathic Type I diabetes, they are also found in the rare instances where known viruses are responsible for beta-cell destruction (4), and islet-cell surface antibodies (ICSA) have been detected in the insuloprivic rat-poison-diabetes, which can be likened to streptozotocin beta-cell toxicity in several animal models (5). These facts make it unlikely that a specific environmental attack can be totally dissociated from autoimmune responses to the beta cells.

There is general agreement that about 10% of Type I diabetics present many of the characteristics of "primary" endocrine autoimmune disorders (6). In the other 90% of insulin-dependent diabetics, often starting in childhood, with a 12–20% male excess and seasonal variations (7) as well as considerable ethnic differences (8), we are still puzzled at the disappearance of the pancreatic autoimmune phenomena within a relatively short time after clinical onset. These now include all the varieties of islet-cell antibodies, the cell-mediated immunity (CMI) to pancreas, and some of the abnormalities of the T-lymphocyte subsets including Ia-positive activated T cells (9). It is possible that insulitis in the two subtypes is triggered by as yet unidentified combinations and permutations of environmental agents, with genetic predisposition to organ-specific autoimmunity centered on the endocrine pancreas.

The connections of Type I diabetes with the HLA-DR region, the human equivalent of the immune response (Ir) genetic code, together with prospective investigations in susceptible families (10), will help to unravel the complex interactions of immune responses provoked initially against insulo-tropic viruses or poisons and the autoimmune manifestations that are intertwined with the various lymphocyte networks, including idiotype-anti-idiotype controls operating in our recognition of self from nonself (11).

Humoral Autoimmune Responses

Islet-cell antibodies are organ specific for endocrine pancreas, they cross react with other species, and they are of IgG class. Several antigens, including some that are only present in beta cells, can now be envisaged in what is basically a polyclonal autoimmune response with curious subclass restrictions (12) and complement-fixing (CF-ICA) as well as noncomplement-fixing variants (ICA-IgG). As the islet antigens have not yet been isolated, cytoplasmic ICA are detected by standard immunofluorescence (IFL), and unfixed group O human pancreas is still the substrate of choice (13). Fixed pancreas substrates give controversial readings, especially in complement-fixation immunofluorescence tests used to detect CF-ICA.

In the screening test ICA-IgG reacts with all four endocrine cells (14). This "shared" autoantigen is not represented on the cell surface and therefore cannot be in direct contact with sensitized lymphocytes in the living gland. Since circulating antibodies exert cytotoxic effects through complement-dependent mechanisms, extensive parallel tests for ICA-IgG and CF-ICA revealed that in all diabetic groups tested, only half the islet-cell antibodies fixed complement (15). Most significantly, this was also found in genetically predisposed first-degree relatives and in endocrine patients who later became diabetic. This led to the conclusion that CF-ICA reactions include the beta-cell-specific autoantibodies that are the most relevant markers for ongoing insulitis. We now know that some CF-ICA selectively stain beta cells (16). We also found some sera containing CF antibodies specific for glucagon or somatostatin cells that were known to exist in some diabetic sera (17).

Islet-cell surface antibodies (ICSA) are detected on viable cultured human fetal (18) or adult animal pancreas (19) and here also, separate specificities exist for alpha and beta cells respectively (19a). By analogy with the surface expression of other organ-specific "microsomal" systems such as the thyroid, gastric, or adrenal systems (20), it is probable that some "selective" CF-ICA represent the cytoplasmic expression of those ICSAs that react with beta cells and are therefore cytotoxic to cultured animal islets, or interfere with glucose-stimulated insulin secretion in these cultures (21). However, surface islet-cell staining is quite often obtained with sera that give negative results on sections. This suggests an additional antigen that is expressed entirely on the plasma membrane. These data support the existence of multiple antibodies specific to different islet antigens, and it is only when the antigens are isolated and characterized that we will be in a position to study their effects separately. The "monoclonal revolution" has already produced hybrid clones that permit the analysis of human polyclonal antibody mixtures in diseases such as myasthenia gravis and thyrotoxicosis (22).

Cell-Mediated Immune Mechanisms

It is likely that cell-mediated immune (CMI) mechanisms are as important for the initiation of insulitis as the humoral responses described above. Leucocyte migration inhibition and lymphocyte transformation tests have been shown to be positive using islet-enriched pancreatic antigens (23).

Lymphocyte adherence tests have also been employed with islet cells in culture (24). Peripheral lymphocytes from Type I DM produced cytotoxic effects. K cells are increased in newly diagnosed Type I DM (25) and antibody-dependent cell-mediated cytotoxicity (ADCC) experiments have also been performed (26). All these CMI reactions are also demonstrable in a proportion of "healthy" relatives who share HLA haplotypes with the diabetic proband in affected families, and they usually do not parallel the circulating antibody results (27).

Prolonged Latency Period in Prospective Family Studies

Because Type I diabetes often starts as an abrupt illness, it was a surprise to discover, by regular testing of "unaffected" relatives of diabetic children, that autoimmune phenomena exist for years in those who inherit the diabetogenic genes as identified by selecting sibs who are HLA-identical or haploidentical with the proband and who possess CF-ICA during the latency period (28). These sibs proved to be the most vulnerable for future diabetes.

In the Barts-Windsor study, 13 of 700 relatives had persistent CF-ICA and 7 of these became diabetic over a follow-up period of 4 years. There are still 6 sibs who have these features and are as yet euglycemic. It is of interest that "conversion" to CF-ICA (i.e. the antibody mixture that contains the putative beta-cell-specific, complement-fixing antibody) has not been observed only once in the follow-up studies.

Other Endocrine Glands and Pathogenesis

Diabetologists noticed for some years that prepubertal boys were too tall for their age when they presented with diabetes (29). This prompted a search for evidence of pituitary involvement. Previous studies showed anterior pituitary antibodies in about 7% of Type I adult diabetics who also suffered from "polyendocrine" autoimmunity, and most of these appeared to react with prolactin cells. In the family studies, predisposed relatives having CF-ICA proved to have, in addition, antibodies reacting with several pituitary cell types (30). The highest prevalence was in those who became diabetic during the follow-up: 4/7. In the prediabetic latency period, 36% of ICA-positive relatives had these antibodies; in newly diagnosed DM, 16% were positive by IFL on pituitary; and in old-standing DM, only 2% were positive. This suggests either that similar viruses may infect pituicytes and beta cells (31), or that the antibodies detected are markers of some as yet unknown stimulating immunoglobulins akin to those found in thyrotoxicosis but acting on the pituitary receptors either directly or through increased secretion of as yet uncharacterized hypothalamic hormones that affect insulin secretion (32). In this context it is of interest that some

HLA-identical relatives in other prospective studies have increased insulin responses to arginine (33), suggesting that something stimulates the pancreas to "regenerate" its beta cells, which we know from the presence of CF-ICA are gradually being damaged. In polyendocrine patients who have similar long latency periods, there is usually a decreased insulin production (34).

Gut-Endocrine-Related Antibodies

Because some diabetics showed diminished responses of gastric inhibitory peptide (GIP) to protein test meals, the IFL tests were carried out on human duodenum. A small proportion of Type II diabetics proved to have antibodies to the GIP-secreting cells, and, when Type I diabetic sera were applied to gut sections, 12 of 28 of the sera were positive on GIP and/or secretin cells (35). The significance of these unexpected organ-specific reactions either indicates further heterogeneity in this complex syndrome or it suggests that in some cases the enteroinsular axis is also involved in the final development of the diabetic syndromes.

Future Prospects

It is well established that a prolonged autoimmune process underlies certain endocrine diseases such as myxedema and Addison's disease, and the thyroid or adrenal antibodies are usually present for many years before organ failure supervenes (36). A similar slow time course has been demonstrated in nondiabetic adults in whom islet-cell antibodies are found when they come to hospital for thyrotoxicosis or one of the other autoimmune endocrine conditions. We have found the same prolonged pre-diabetic stage in selected sibs of diabetic children. The question now remains as to whether or not the pathogenic mechanisms operating in the "polyendocrine" are similar to those in the "early-onset" disease. Although the most vulnerable sibs of diabetic children (those 2% of all relatives who had CF-ICA in their sera), turned out to belong to "autoimmune" families, the diabetic children themselves showed only a slightly increased prevalence of thyroid antibodies in the absence of other endocrine insufficiencies. There was the usual excess of males and the probands were very young. It looks as though at least two sets of genes predispose certain families to Type I DM. In our family studies the distribution of thyroid, gastric, pituitary, and ICA-IgG reactions did not correspond to that of the diabetogenic HLA haplotypes inherited by the sibs from both parents. Only the CF-ICA seemed to occur more often in HLA identical sibs. Epidemiological studies tell us that 10–20% of such sibs can be expected to get diabetes. However, when two markers were employed, half of those who had CF-ICA became diabetic; hence the genes connected with autoimmunity are heavily skewed toward the pancreas, just as in thyroiditis families the autoimmunity is predominantly skewed toward the thyroid gland and pernicious anemia relatives have an excess of gastric autoimmunity. As in Type I diabetes, only the beta cells are destroyed; it must be presumed that some of the CF-ICA are beta-cell specific. Recent biochemical analysis of pancreatic antigens reacting with the islet-cell antibodies detected by various methods confirm the multiplicity of autoantigens (37).

Identification of beta-cell specific CF-ICAs will prove of great help when preventive measures become available so that a predisposed sib can be treated well before 90% of his beta cells are injured, i.e. years before the onset of clinical diabetes. It even looks as though in some cases, CF-ICA may appear soon after birth since nearly all those relatives with the marker were positive from the time they joined the prospective study. One of these was only 2 years old and developed his diabetes at the age of 5. Recent studies on the persistent diarrhea syndrome of babies (38) have shown that some of these babies may have Type I diabetes at 6 months and myxedema almost from birth with high autoantibody levels to the relevant affected organs.

ACKNOWLEDGMENTS

This work was made possible by the continuous interaction between the autoimmunity and the immunogenetic teams of our laboratories. We also acknowledge the inspiration provided by Professor I. M. Roitt over the years.

We thank Miss Queenie Jayawardena for her excellent editorial assistance. Our research was supported by the Medical Research Council, the British Diabetic Association, and the Juvenile Diabetes Foundations (USA).

Literature Cited

1. Cudworth, A. G. 1980. Current concepts of aetiology. Type I (insulin-dependent) diabetes mellitus. *Adv. Med.* 16:123–35
2. Gepts, W. 1981. Changes in islets in diabetes. In *The Islets of Langerhans,* ed. S. J. Cooperstein, D. Watkins, pp. 321–56. New York: Academic
3. Bottazzo, G. F., Doniach, D. 1976. Pancreatic autoimmunity and HLA antigens. *Lancet* 2:800 (Lett.)
4. Bottazzo, G. F., Pujol-Borrel, R., Doniach, D. 1981. Humoral and cellular immunity in diabetes mellitus. *Clin. Immunol. Allergy* 1:63–80
5. Karam, J. H., Lewitt, P. A., Young, C. W., Nowlain, R. E., Frankek, B. J., Fu-

jiya, H., Freedman, Z. R., Grodsky, G. M. 1980. Insulinopenic diabetes after rhodenticide (Vacor) ingestion. A unique model of acquired diabetes in man. *Diabetes* 29:971–78
6. Volpe, R. 1981. *Autoimmunity in the Endocrine System, Springer Monographs on Endocrinology,* Vol. 20. Berlin: Springer-Verlag
7. Gamble, D. R. 1980. An epidemiological study of childhood DM affecting two or more sibs. *Diabetologia* 19: 341–44
8. Reitnauer, P. J., Go, R. C. P., Acton, R. T., Murphy, C. C., Budowle, B., Barger, B. O., Roseman, J. M. 1982. Evidence for genetic admixture as a determinant

in the occurrence of insulin-dependent diabetes millitus in U.S. blacks. *Diabetes* 31:532–37
9. Jackson, R. A., Morris, M. A., Haynes, B. F., Eisenbarth, G. S. 1982. Increased circulating Ia-antigen bearing T-cells in Type I diabetes mellitus. *N. Engl. J. Med.* 306:785–88
10. Cudworth, A. G., Wolf, E. 1982. The genetic susceptibility to Type I (insulin-dependent) diabetes mellitus. *Clin. Endocrinol. Metab.* 11:389–406
11. Roitt, I. M., De Carvalho, L. C. 1982. The immunological basis of autoimmune diseases. In *Receptor Antibodies and Disease, Ciba Symp. No. 90.* London: Pitman Medical, pp. 22–34
12. Dean, B. M., McNally, J. M., Doniach, D. 1980. IgG subclass distribution in islet-cell and other organ-specific autoantibodies. *Diabetologia* 19:268 (Abstr.)
13. Bottazzo, G. F., Florin-Christensen, A., Doniach, D. 1974. Islet-cell antibodies in diabetes mellitus with autoimmune polyendocrine deficiencies. *Lancet* 2: 1279–83
14. Bottazzo, G. F., Doniach, D. 1978. Islet-cell antibodies in DM: evidence of an autoantigen common to all cells in the islets of Langerhans. *Ric. Clin. Lab.* 8:29–38
15. Bottazzo, G. F., Dean, B. M., Gorsuch, A. N., Cudworth, A. G., Doniach, D. 1980. Complement-fixing islet-cell antibodies in Type I diabetes: possible monitors of active beta cell damage. *Lancet* 1:668–72
16. Bottazzo, G. F., Mirakian, R., Dean, B. M., McNally, J. M., Doniach, D. 1982. How immunology helps to define heterogeneity in diabetes mellitus. In *Genetics of Diabetes Mellitus* ed. R. B. Tattersall, J. K. Koberling, pp. 79–90. London: Academic. 2nd ed.
17. Bottazzo, G. F., Lendrum, R. 1976. Separate autoantibodies to human pancreatic glucagon and somatostatin cells. *Lancet* 2:873–76
18. Pujol-Borrell, R., Khoury, E. L., Bottazzo, G. F. 1982. Islet cell surface antibodies in Type I (insulin-dependent) diabetes mellitus: use of human fetal pancreas cultures as substrate. *Diabetologia* 22:89–95
19. Lernmark, A., Freedman, S. F., Kanatsuna, T., Patzelt, C., Rubenstein, A. H., Steiner, D. F. 1980. Islet cell surface antibodies and diabetes mellitus. In *Immunology of Diabetes* ed. W. J. Irvine, pp. 155–67. Edinburgh: Teviot Sci.
19a. Van De Winkel, M., Smets, G., Gepts, W., Pipeleers, D. 1982. Islet cell surface antibodies from insulin-dependent diabetics bind specifically to pancratic B cells. *J. Clin. Invest.* 70:41–49
20. Doniach, D., Cudworth, A. G., Khoury, E. L., Bottazzo, G. F. 1982. Autoimmunity and the HLA-system in endocrine diseases. *Recent Prog. Endocrinol.* 2:99–132
21. Sai, P., Boitard C., Debray-Sachs, M., Pouplard, A., Assan, R. Hamburger, J. 1981. Complement-fixing islet cell antibodies from some diabetic patients alter insulin release in vitro. *Diabetes* 30: 1051–57
22. Kohn, L. D., Aloj, S. M., Beguinot, F., Vitti, P., Yavin, E., Yavin, Z., Laccetti, P., Grollman, E. F., Valente, W. A. 1982. Molecular interactions at the cell surface: role of glycoconjugates and membrane lipids in receptor recognition processes. In *Human Genetics and Membrane Biology, Dight Found. Symp.* New York: Academic
23. Nerup, J., Anderson, O. O., Bendixen, G., Egeberg, J., Gunnarsson, R., Kromann, G., Poulsen, J. E. 1974. Cell mediated immunity in diabetes mellitus. *Proc. R. Soc. Med.* 67:506–13
24. Huang, S. W. MacLaren, N. K. 1976. Insulin-dependent diabetes: a disease of autoaggression. *Science* 192:64–66
25. Pozzilli, P., Sensi, M., Gorsuch, A., Bottazzo, G. F. Cudworth, A. G. 1979. Evidence for raised K-cell levels in Type I diabetes. *Lancet* 2:173–75
26. Sensi, M., Pozzilli, P., Gorsuch, A., Bottazzo, G. F., Cudworth, A. G. 1981. Increased killer cell activity in insulin dependent (Type I) diabetes. *Diabetologia* 20:106–9
27. Pozzilli, P., Sensi, M., Cudworth, A. G. 1980. Identification of high risk subjects for Type I diabetes by means of HLA family studies and leucocyte migration tests. *Diabetologia Croatica IX Suppl.* 1:132–35
28. Gorsuch, A. N., Spencer, K. M., Lister, J., McNally, J. M., Dean, B. M., Bottazzo, G. F., Cudworth, A. G. 1981. The natural history of Type I (insulin-dependent) diabetes mellitus: evidence for a long pre-diabetic period. *Lancet* 2:1363–65
29. Edelsten, A. D. Hughes, I. A., Oakes, S., Gordon, I. R. S., Savage, D.C.L. 1981. Height and skeletal maturity in children with newly diagnosed juvenile-onset diabetes. *Arch. Dis. Child.* 56:40–44

30. Mirakian, R., Cudworth, A. G., Bottazzo, G. F., Richardson, C. A., Doniach, D. 1982. Autoimmunity to anterior pituitary cells and the pathogenesis of Type I (insulin-dependent) diabetes mellitus. *Lancet* 1: 755–59
31. Rayfield, E. J., Yoon, J. W. 1981. Role of viruses in diabetes. See Ref. 2, pp. 427–45
32. Bobbioni, E., Jeanrenaud, B. 1982. Effect of rat hypothalamic extract administration on insulin secretion in vivo. *Endocrinology* 110:631–36
33. Hollander, P. H., Asplin, C. M., Kniaz, D., Hansen, J. A., Palmer, J. P. 1982. Beta-cell dysfunction in nondiabetic HLA-identical siblings of insulin-dependent diabetics. *Diabetes* 31: 149–53
34. Irvine, W. J., Gray, R. S., Steel, J. M. 1980. Islet-cell antibody as a marker for early stage Type I diabetes mellitus. See Ref. 19, pp. 117–54
35. Mirakian, R., Richardson, C. A., Bottazzo, G. F., Doniach, D. 1981. Humoral autoimmunity to gut-related endocrine cells. *Clin. Immunol. Newslett.* 2:161–67
36. Doniach, D., Bottazzo, G. F. 1981. Polyendocrine autoimmunity. In *Clinical Immunology Update*, ed. E. C. Franklin, 2:95–121. New York: Elsevier
37. Baekkeskov, S., Nielsen, J. H., Marner, B., Bilde, T., Ludvigsson, J., Lernmark, A. 1982. Autoantibodies in newly diagnosed diabetic children immunoprecipitate human pancreatic islet cell proteins. *Nature* 298:167–69
38. Savage, M. O. Mirakian, R., Harries, J. T., Bottazzo, G. F. 1982. Could protracted diarrhoea of infancy have an autoimmune pathogenesis? *Lancet* 1: 966–67 (Lett.)

Ann. Rev. Med. 1983. 34:21–34
Copyright © 1983 by Annual Reviews Inc. All rights reserved

MANAGEMENT OF CHILDREN WITH PROGRESSIVE RENAL FAILURE

John T. Herrin, M.B.B.S., F.R.A.C.P.

Pediatric Nephrology, Massachusetts General Hospital, Boston, Massachusetts 02114; and Department of Pediatrics, Harvard Medical School, Cambridge, Massachusetts 02138

ABSTRACT

The strategy of management in childhood renal failure is to integrate available therapeutic modalities with the natural history of the disease in such a manner that linear growth is preserved. Attention to psychosocial growth is necessary for full rehabilitation. Treatment is ordered to provide hope and confidence to family and patient. Conservative medical therapy provides chemical stabilization and prophylaxis against bone disease and growth retardation. Planned progression to replacement of renal function by dialysis or renal transplant is made when growth or control of bone disease is no longer possible, but before complications occur. Therapy is effective; 90% of patients survive 5–10 years with 65% retaining a functioning allograft. Full rehabilitation is attained in 85–90% of post-transplant and 50% of dialysis patients. Technical advances now allow safe dialysis for all age groups. Although growth maintenance remains a major problem, it is possible that earlier metabolic control and transplantation to protect growth in the critical early years, together with improved control of rejection, may allow close approximation to optimal growth potential.

INTRODUCTION

To maintain maximal growth and maturation, the care of any child with renal failure requires integration of available resources and techniques with the natural history of the underlying disease. Age and statural growth of

21

0066-4219/83/0401-0021$02.00

the child influence timing more than biochemical indices. Children differ from adults in the capacity for growth and maturation. A series of coordinated events leads gradually to increase in stature, neurological, and motor development. Progress to a functioning social being requires continuing interaction with family, peers, and school; thus treatment must aim at integration of therapy with schooling and family support.

Knowledge of the changing physiological spectrum is helpful in planning health care. (a) An infant or child shows a larger ratio of surface area to mass, hence has a higher water and electrolyte turnover (1, 2). Changes in hydration are more rapid and electrolyte losses are as important as in adults, but must be balanced with the higher obligatory intake, i.e. the very young child or infant with gastrointestinal illness is at risk both from increased losses and decreased intake, (b) Total body water and extracellular water spaces are relatively increased per unit of mass at younger ages, slowly decreasing with age. This provides a larger distribution volume for electrolytes and drugs. (c) Caloric need in the younger child is increased by the need for the linear and mass increase (growth). An infant requires as many as 120 calories per kilogram of body weight compared to 45 calories per kilogram in the adult. Once the child is able to eat an adult diet (at approximately the age of 2 years), the relative loads of acid, phosphate, potassium, and protein are increased if adequate calories are provided, and restriction to produce metabolic control provides a major problem (3). (d) The younger child is in a relatively anabolic state and is able to maintain homeostasis with a lower urine volume and glomerular clearance. Hence even in renal failure, if sufficient caloric intake can be attained, rises in BUN, creatinine, phosphate, potassium, and magnesium are all blunted (4). It is this potential for anabolic growth that allows the treatment of the very young infant by conservative measures rather than early dialysis. It is imperative to press for metabolic control and full caloric intake, and to pay attention to bone growth (calcium-phosphorus balance and prophylaxis against hyperparathyroidism), at an early stage in renal failure. (e) Psychological needs vary with age and supportive intervention can best be provided by coordinating therapy with the child's normal development pattern (6).

With regard to this latter point, psychological needs, the younger infant gains gratification from feeding, sucking, and holding. Isolation and restrictive diets produce marked interference with normal lifestyle in this group. The school child has developed peer and parental relationships, curiosity, and an understanding of "tomorrow." Now cognitive explanation and empathy are most important. Teenagers are a special problem, their exaggerated investment in freedom and body image and their well-developed sense of time, together with the need for "limit testing," produce embarrassment, decreased self image, and often deeply felt frustration and depression. Full explanations with a sympathetic, firm, consistent approach are necessary (7). In general terms a methodical, firm, and practical approach works at all ages. Quiet and efficient work allow both child and parents to develop confidence and trust.

AIMS OF TREATMENT

The aim of treatment in progressive renal failure in childhood is maintenance of growth and maturation. An outline of philosophy of treatment and a discussion of present and potential therapies to replace renal function gradually educates the family and patient while allowing development of a coordinated approach with a sense of hope and confidence.

Using clinical and chemical criteria, standard therapies are applied in sequence to allow the minimum interruption to growth, schooling, and normal lifestyle (Table 1).

MODES OF THERAPY

Metabolic Control

Correction of acidosis, caloric and/or protein supplementation, and maintenance of the calcium-phosphorus balance are generally similar to adult schemes.

Growth requirements necessitate greater calorie and protein intake, together with "nonessential" amino acids as well as "essential" amino acid nitrogen in the diet (8). Caloric intake is monitored and appropriate adjustment made. Supplementation in early stages is maintained using a base of normal food selection and, if necessary, adding "empty supplements" as fat and carbohydrates (9). Excessive protein intake can produce nausea, anorexia, and vomiting as well as potentially increasing potassium loading. Skilled dietary assistance is necessary to provide an interesting, satisfying, and yet restricted diet. Peer pressure and mobility of the child within school groups make education of parents and patient to the importance of dietary restriction and constant monitoring necessary. Manipulation within dietary

Table 1 Treatment modalities

Metabolic control	Dialysis
acidosis	peritoneal
calories-protein	hemodialysis
calcium-phosphorus	Renal transplant
salt, water, potassium	living, related donor
	cadaver donor

limits is both possible and desirable so that the child may maintain normal social interaction.

Modulation of calcium and phosphorus balance is important to maximize growth (10) while protecting against hyperparathyroidism and "renal rickets." Vitamin D supplementation is introduced early in the course of renal insufficiency (5, 11).

Hyperphosphatemia is treated with aluminum binding gel in a fashion similar to that used with adults. It is necessary, however, to provide phosphorus for bone growth in the child, hence close chemical monitoring is required (to keep phosphorus in the 4–6 mg% range). In general those patients with glomerular lesions show phosphate retention earlier than children with tubular disorders or obstructive uropathy, where significant phosphate losses may be present.

Sodium, potassium, and fluid intake are adjusted to balance growth requirements (12) and excess losses from underlying tubular disease. Monitoring of growth parameters—weight and height as well as chemistries— to check adjustment is appropriate. The diet should be as flexible as possible while maintaining hydration and normal blood pressure. High-protein foods are generally high in potassium content so that potassium-binding resins (sodium polystyrene sulfonate) may be required to attain potassium balance if adequate calories and protein for growth requirements are met. Sodium restriction may be necessary in the face of fluid overload or if hypertension (12, 13) is present, particularly in those patients requiring correction of acidosis, one of the most potent forces in growth arrest.

Dialysis and Transplant

When renal function reaches a level where growth and/or metabolic control is no longer possible, dialysis is instituted as a rehabilitative measure prior to renal transplantation.

The choice of dialysis mode depends on geographic location, age, size, and unit preference (14). All modalities—hemodialysis (15), intermittent peritoneal (16), continuous ambulatory peritoneal dialysis (CAPD) (17), and continuous cycling peritoneal dialysis (CCPD) (18)—have been used and may have advantages and disadvantages to a particular patient.

At Massachusetts General Hospital (MGH) we prefer hemodialysis shunt access for the patient less than 15 kg and a fistula for the child greater than 15 kg (19). Tolerance for the repetitive needling of a fistula requires appreciation of the advantages of less restricted activity and relative freedom from infection compared with a shunt.

Experience with CAPD and CCPD is expanding and a number of children treated show significant metabolic control (20), greater mobility, and less need for a restrictive diet. Choice of CAPD versus CCPD depends on patient or parent work patterns to integrate treatment with family commitment.

Most pediatric nephrology units still believe dialysis is best used as a preparation for renal transplant or as a "back-up" treatment in the event of graft failure (19, 21–23). An increasing number of patients require long-term dialysis while awaiting a second transplant, e.g. those with high degrees of sensitization or recurrent disease in the transplanted kidney, which both provide relative contraindications to future transplantation. Survival in this group of long-term dialysis patients has been good enough to make reassessment necessary.

There is little doubt that a well-functioning renal transplant is more consistent with full rehabilitation; hence the search for safer, more specific, and less toxic immunosuppression is necessary to produce the optimal situation for graft survival with less risk to the recipient (26).

PROBLEMS IN THERAPY

The following outline of the general problems in end-stage renal disease therapy in childhood emphasizes timing in application of standard measures. The aim of this review is to discuss planning for treatment rather than exploring the more technical aspects of dialysis and transplantation in childhood.

Four major problem sets occur in end-stage renal disease (ESRD) therapy in the pediatric patient: (a) ethical; (b) technical; (c) immunological; and (d) growth and maturation. These are discussed separately for convenience.

Ethical

Renal dialysis and transplantation are complex procedures, time consuming, often painful, and very expensive (27). The child further requires special diet and frequent hospitalization. He or she constantly faces an increased risk of pain, infection, and death (19, 22, 23). Such treatment isolates and characterizes the child as different from his or her peers and stresses the family emotionally and financially, which hinders integration with normal family lifestyle.

In larger pediatric renal disease treatment centers, patients have an excellent chance for 90%, 5–10-year survival with dialysis/transplantation (21). Approximately 65% will have a functioning allograft. Fifty percent of children on dialysis and 85–90% of successful transplant patients are fully rehabilitated (19, 21–23). Strict conservative medical therapy is less likely to produce rehabilitation. Extended medical therapy may be associated with malnutrition (28), severe and painful bone disease (29), vessel disease, neuropathy (30), and ultimately death with uremic symptoms (31). Movement to dialysis and transplant should be made before such complications occur (32). In this manner the financial and emotional cost of prolonged conservative therapy is minimized. Conservative therapy provides initial stabilization, and well-planned movement to dialysis and transplant provides hope, support, and rehabilitation to patient and family.

Further ethical problems are raised if living, related-kidney donation is considered. Superior results are obtained from serologically defined HLA-identical siblings and well-matched parent-to-sibling pairs. Living, related-kidney donation is possible since the normal individual has two kidneys, each with a functional reserve of 4–5 times minimal necessary function. Morbidity and mortality incurred by a healthy kidney donor is small (mortality risk is less than 0.1%) (33). The courts have ruled in favor of donation, even by a minor, on the grounds that the donor may benefit psychologically or even be harmed if prevented from donating (34). Care, however, must be taken to present the benefit versus the risk of donation in such a manner that it does not threaten or pressure a potential donor.

Technical Problems

Technical problems include (a) access to circulation for dialysis, (b) fluid volume shifts, (c) need for scaled dialysis equipment—coil, plate, fiber, (d) greater mobility of child between dialysis treatments, and (e) technical problems associated with kidney size and placement during transplantation.

Over the past decade, new shunt materials and appropriately sized dialysis equipment have become available (35). Surgical techniques for creating access have improved and accurate weight monitoring is possible, which makes hemodialysis possible even in very small infants. Some units prefer to use peritoneal dialysis for the smaller patient (19) or for patients whose families live a significant distance from a center where pediatric dialysis can be performed (17, 36).

Specially trained nursing and ancillary personnel are necessary to integrate diet, schooling, and emotional needs of the child while minimizing family stress. A supportive social worker well versed in the complex legislative health resources and with knowledge of other support systems is necessary to minimize financial load from the time of metabolic supplementation to functioning transplant.

Transplantation using an adult kidney is possible in an infant over 9.5–10 kg (28, 37). In small children, an infant kidney is preferred to allow retroperitoneal placement (19). Intraperitoneal placement of renal grafts have been used, so that size of the graft is not a limitation (38). An adult-sized kidney will take a large proportion of the small infant's circulating blood volume, thus it is necessary to expand the infant's blood volume to allow for the increased blood flow through the transplanted organ intraoperatively. Early perfusion may be impaired, sometimes to sufficient degree to produce parenchymal damage if this is not done.

Increased glomerular clearances are present over the first few days, leading to large fluid diuresis that may jeopardize circulatory stability. This increased functional reserve often delays the diagnosis of acute rejection (19, 22).

Immunological Problems

Prevention and control of rejection without producing unacceptable side effects remains a major problem in pediatric renal transplantation.

To minimize the effects of immunotherapy, measures are taken to reduce the antigenic differences by using a well-matched sibling or parent donor and, in less favorable parent-to-child and cadaver matches, modifying antirejection therapy (37). Occasionally, well-matched and even HLA-identical recipients experience significant rejection episodes (39). The place of more extensive matching for B lymphocytes, monocytes, and DR antigens awaits fuller evaluation (40).

Prednisone and azathioprine remain the basis of antirejection therapy. Modulation of steroid dosage to prevent rejection while maintaining growth and minimizing other side effects requires experience. Using monoclonal antibodies to monitor for rejection is one method of titrating more closely immunosuppression to specific antirejection needs (41).

Antilymphocyte globulin is effective in controlling rejection without the need for marked increase in steroid dosage; this minimizes early steroid toxicity and infection (42). At least one study in childhood demonstrates that prolonged administration of rabbit antilymphocyte serum is associated with prolonged graft survival (37).

Criteria for diagnosis of rejection may differ in the smaller infant, where smaller absolute changes in serum creatinine are important (19, 22): greater functional reserve is present in an adult organ transplanted into a child. In those cases of intraperitoneal positioning of the renal allograft, difficulties in physical examination of the graft may further delay the diagnosis of rejection.

Growth

Restoration of growth remains the major problem in ESRD therapy in childhood. Pre-transplant growth requires attention to detail in metabolic therapy, while post-transplant integration of immunosuppressive therapy with prophylaxis of rejection and growth is necessary. Attention to psychosocial growth is necessary for full rehabilitation.

Pre-transplant metabolic control and dialysis, if necessary, aim at the restoration of normal growth and the prevention of hyperparathyroidism and rickets. This may allow normalization of lifestyle. If growth is not restored on optimal conservative therapy, early transplant should be considered (28). Recent graft survival rates in the very young child (1–7 years) are as good as in older children and adults, while growth is improved, even accelerated (24, 28). Transplantation in infants less than one year of age remains experimental without acceptable survival rates (20, 28). Dialysis (hemodialysis, CAPD, and intermittent peritoneal dialysis) have been used in some centers to sustain life and push for growth to a more suitable age and size (20).

Children with bone age over 12 years at the time of transplant grow poorly post-transplant, and growth potential (which depends on bone age, stature, and chronologic age) at the time of transplant affects subsequent linear growth. Early transplant as definitive therapy should be considered to preserve linear growth (22). Subsequent dialysis may be considered for later rejection episodes or if sensitization makes further transplant impractical.

Other factors that influence post-transplant growth include adequacy of renal function, control of rejection, and necessary steroid dosage. Attempts to balance steroid therapy and growth are necessary, and other means of controlling rejection and renal functional impairment from rejection can retard growth, which provides a dilemma. Rejection should be controlled and then a low dose of daily prednisone (0.2 mg/kg/day) or alternate day therapy (1.2 mg/kg/alternate days) should be used to restore a more normal growth pattern (43, 44).

TIMING OF TREATMENT

To maintain growth potential, timing in the application of different treatment modalities is important. Linear growth rather than biochemical normality is the symptom that signals introduction of metabolic control, supplemental Vitamin D, and correction of acidosis. These may be necessary at a much earlier stage than in the adult, when comparison is based on glomerular filtration rate alone.

Prophylactic care and education require early identification of potential renal failure based upon diagnosis. Parent, pediatrician, and nephrologist then discuss the need for monitoring chemical and growth parameters as a means of minimizing stress and keeping growth and development as normal as possible. Plans for future review and monitoring potential therapy, including the possible need for replacement of renal function, are fully discussed. Potential allograft donors are identified at this early stage to prevent pressures present when a child is in obvious symptomatic renal failure. Development of trust and confidence in medical support allows a smooth transition to the complex treatment phase of end-stage renal failure therapy.

Chemical and hormonal abnormalities—particularly acid-base abnormalities, calcium-phosphorus balance, parathyroid hormone, and Vitamin D levels—are monitored at intervals coordinated with growth rate. Growth and stage of nutrition are assessed by standard pediatric measurements of height, weight, skin fold thickness, and general habitus. Growth ideally will follow normal growth percentile channels. If growth rate is significantly impaired, even with renal function biochemically marginal, ESRD therapy is instituted (Table 2).

Marginal renal failure with biochemical bone disease that does not respond to dietary phosphate restriction, phosphate binding, correction of acidosis, and Vitamin D supplementation is an indication for transplantation and/or parathyroidectomy. Chemical correction should return the parathyroid hormone level to normal. If this does not occur, parathyroidectomy is advisable if renal function is moderately well maintained. If renal functional deterioration is advanced, renal transplantation is more appropriate.

Severe anemia limits exercise tolerance and there may be need for recurrent transfusion. Although recent data suggest that transfusions may be helpful in the selection and stabilization of transplant candidates (45), programmed administration rather than an indiscriminate use of transfusions is to be preferred. Transfusion may produce sensitization, which reduces the chance of future transplantation and also exposes the child to the risk of hepatitis (46). Frequent transfusion may lead to iron overload syndrome in the patient with severe renal failure (47).

Early interference with lifestyle from symptomatic renal failure with lethargy and fatigue, rather than the later symptoms of azotemia, is an indication for earlier transplant. Evaluation requires a fine balance since lethargy and fatigue may be present at certain stages of growth or associated peer and social pressures, particularly in a child with chronic illness that may produce depression.

Pure chemical reasons for transfer to end-stage renal failure therapy are the consequences of low glomerular clearance rates. Serum creatinine level is determined by the renal clearance and muscle mass. A younger or mal-

Table 2   Timing for ESRD therapy

1. Marginal renal function with growth retardation
2. Marginal renal function with bone disease
3. Severe anemia
4. Symptomatic renal failure interfering with lifestyle
5. Biochemical criteria—creatinine clearance of 10 ml/min/1.73 M^2

nourished infant with lower muscle mass will demonstrate a much lower serum creatinine level than an adult. For example, the 12-month-old infant in end-stage renal failure has a creatinine of 4 mg%. An 8-year-old child with serum creatinine 8–10 mg% and an adult with 20 mg% show similar clearance levels, thus serum creatinine and clinical course should be integrated with muscle mass to interpret chemical results.

INSTITUTION OF THERAPEUTIC REGIME

We now review prior discussions of potential ESRD therapy. Indications and prognosis are also reviewed and the timing for replacement of renal function is explained.

A review of family dynamics and a reevaluation of donor status, general health, and finances provide the necessary background both medical and social. Evaluation of the child's maturation, level of school achievement, and present school commitments is made. A plan to minimize loss of school time, implement tutorial services, and adjust possible elective school time and vacation is undertaken so that dialysis and transplantation become the most effective means of rehabilitation.

A family group meeting with the "transplant team" is arranged to review results of living related and cadaver renal allografts as applied to age group and potential biological donors. Our practice at Massachusetts General Hospital is to have the family, recipient if appropriate (older child or adolescent), transplant surgeons, psychiatrist, nursing, social service, dialysis physician, pediatric nephrologist, and family pediatrician at a common conference to discuss potential modes of therapy. Preparation for transplantation is reviewed, general contingency plans are discussed including studies proceeding in the unit aimed at control of rejection, and plans for support after graft failure are outlined.

The potential for greater graft survival and necessity for low immunosuppression in living, related-donor grafts is emphasized, and the relation to fuller growth and rehabilitation of the child on lower immunosuppression is discussed.

Tissue typing of recipient and potential donors is performed and medical work-up of potential donor initiated if possible before commencement of dialysis. This minimizes the pressure on a potential donor as refusal to donate is then not an immediate threat to the potential recipient's life. Such timing allows time for unforeseen biological problems to be reviewed and managed, e.g. unrecognized medical problems or blood group incompatibility.

Intentional blood transfusion and donor-specific transfusion protocols are now being carried out in a number of transplant centers (48, 49). Such transfusion therapy can be initiated and carried through while the child is prepared metabolically and psychologically for transplantation. Preparatory dialysis may be necessary.

Prior nephrectomy may be necessary in the presence of prior obstructive lesions or infective lesions or large polycystic kidneys, the removal of which would otherwise prolong the actual transplant operation. Bilateral nephrectomy at the time of transplant is reserved for patients with intractable hypertension or certain uncorrected anatomical lesions, e.g. vesico-ureteric reflux or megaureter.

Dialysis has been used as a primary mode of therapy in few pediatric centers (24, 25). Transplantation and dialysis in childhood are truly complementary modes of therapy to be used to the best possible rehabilitation of the child. Special technical problems with fluid and osmolar balance may be encountered during dialysis and in the perioperative transplant period. Miniaturization of equipment and smaller volume dialyzers and lines have made it practical to hold extracorporeal volume to 10% of the infants' blood volume, which thereby reduces the chances of acute volume shift. By varying dialyzer efficiency, control of rate of change in BUN, and osmolality decreases risk of intradialysis osmolar shifts. Postoperative fluid management is closely monitored, anticipating large urine volumes and matching replacement.

After transplantation, impairment to growth rate remains a major problem. With (a) allograft function, (b) growth rate prior to transplant, and (c) steroid dosage as the important variables to promoting growth posttransplant, attention focuses on these factors. Optimizing the kidney match or modifying antirejection therapy to reduce steroid dose can minimize the effects of immunotherapy on growth while protecting allograft function. Early transplant, before marked bone changes or growth retardation, is necessary to allow full growth potential.

It is possible that growth maintenance can be attained with early metabolic control and early transplantation, when growth slows or arrests, despite optimal medical regimes. In this fashion the greater growth potential post-transplant in the younger patient may be realized. Long-term dialysis may be necessary if immunological failure of the graft occurs, but this dialysis is at a stage where greater growth has been realized.

Standard azathioprine/prednisone regimes are likely to be modified in the future when further evaluation of antilymphocyte serum, antithymocyte globulin, monoclonal antibodies to "T lymphocyte" subsets, cyclosporin A, and retroplacental globulin defines proper usage of these agents. It is hoped that some combination of these or other agents will modify the rejection process with greater specificity and safety. Certain patients are highly immunoreactive and rapidly reject an allograft. In this group, thoracic duct drainage (50) and total lymph node irradiation (51) are presently being evaluated in an effort to modify the immune response to allow the allograft to function.

REHABILITATION

Rehabilitation is necessary whether the allograft is functioning well or is rejected and the child needs to return to dialysis. Integrating alternating visits with pediatrician and transplant team, returning to school, and planning for appropriate exercise and sporting activity are all necessary to simplify rehabilitation.

The only restrictions to lifestyle in a patient with a well-functioning renal allograft are exclusion from contact sports and the necessity for constant maintenance antirejection drugs. Education, however, is necessary to overcome the community bias that a transplant or dialysis patient is unable to function normally or requires major protection.

Literature Cited

1. Friis-Hansen, B. 1961. Body compartments in children: changes during growth and related changes in body composition. *Pediatrics* 28:169–81
2. Friis-Hansen, B. 1957. Changes in body compartments during growth. *Acta Pediatr. Scand. Suppl.* 46:110
3. Lewy, J. E., New, M. I. 1975. Growth in children with renal failure. *Am. J. Med.* 58:65–68
4. Williams, G. S., Klenk, E. L., Winters, R. W. 1973. Acute renal failure in pediatrics. In *The Body Fluids in Pediatrics,* ed. R. W. Winters, pp. 523–57. Boston: Little, Brown
5. Chan, J. C. M., Goplerud, J. M., Papadopoulou, Z. K., Novello, A. C. 1981. Kidney failure in childhood. *Int. J. Pediatr. Nephrol.* 2:201–22
6. Korsch, B. M., Negrete, V. F., Gardner, J. E., Weinstock, C. L., Mercer, A. S., Grushkin, C. M., Fine, R. N. 1973. Kidney transplantation in children: psycho-social follow up study on child and family. *J. Pediatr.* 83:399–408
7. Simmons, J. M., Wilson, C. J., Potter, D. E., Holliday, M. A. 1971. Relation of caloric deficiency to growth failure in children on hemodialysis and the growth response to calorie supplementation. *N. Engl. J. Med.* 285:653–56
8. Holliday, M. A. 1975. Calorie intake and growth in uremia. *Kidney Int.* 2:S73–78
9. Broyer, M. 1974. Renal failure and arterial hypertension. In *Pediatric Nephrology,* ed. R. Royer, R. Habib, H. Mathieu, M. Broyer. Philadelphia: Saunders. 373 pp.
10. Chan, J. C., Hsu, A. C. 1980. Vitamin D and renal diseases. *Adv. Pediatr.* 27:117–62
11. Chesney, R. W., Moorthy, A. V., Eisman, J. A., Jox, D. K., Mazess, R. B., DeLuca, H. F. 1978. Increased growth after long term oral 1-α-25-Vitamin D$_3$ in childhood renal osteodystrophy. *N. Engl. J. Med.* 298:238–42
12. Committee on Nutrition American Academy of Pediatrics. 1974. Salt intake and eating patterns of infants and children in relation to blood pressure. *Pediatrics* 53:115–21
13. Blumbert, A., Nelp, W. B., Hegstrom, R. M., Scribner, B. H. 1967. Extracellular volume in patients with chronic renal disease treated for hypertension by sodium restriction. *Lancet* 2:69–73
14. Feldman, W., Baliah, T., Drummond, K. N. 1968. Intermittent peritoneal dialysis in the management of chronic renal failure in children. *Am. J. Dis. Child.* 116:30–36
15. Potter, E. D., Larsen, D., Lenmann, E., Perin, D., Simmons, J., Piel, C. F., Holliday, M. A. 1970. Treatment of chronic uremia in children. II. Hemodialysis. *Pediatrics* 46:678–89
16. Counts, S., Hickman, R., Garbaccio, A., Tenckhoff, H. 1973. Chronic home peritoneal dialysis in children. *Trans.*

Am. Soc. Artif. Intern. Organs 19: 157–63

17. Alexander, S. R., Tseng, C. H., Maksym, K. S., Campbell, R. A., Talwalker, Y. B., Kohant, E. C. 1981. Clinical parameters in continuous ambulatory peritoneal dialysis for infants and children. In *C.A.P.D. Update: Continuous Ambulatory Peritoneal Dialysis,* ed. J. W. Moncrief, R. P. Popovich. New York/Paris/Barcelona/Milan/Mexico City/Rio de Janeiro: Masson

18. Lastar, J. M. 1981. An overview of a CCPD training program. *Contemp. Dialysis* (March), pp. 40–49

19. Herrin, J. T. 1980. Pediatric renal transplantation. *Kidney Int.* 18:519–29

20. Nolph, K. D., Popovich, R. P., Moncrief, J. W. 1978. Theoretical and practical implications of continuous ambulatory peritoneal dialysis. *Nephron* 21:117–22

21. Avner, E. D., Harmon, W. E., Grupe, W. E., Ingelfinger, J. R., Eraklis, A. J., Lever, R. H. 1981. Mortality of chronic hemodialysis and renal transplantation in pediatric end-stage renal disease. *Pediatrics* 67:412–16

22. Fine, R. N., Malekzadah, M. H., Pennsi, A. H., Ettenger, R. B., Uittenbogaart, C. H., Negrete, V. F., Korsch, B. M. 1978. Long-term results of renal transplant in children. *Pediatrics* 61: 641–50

23. DeShazo, C. V., Simmonds, R. L., Bernstein, D. M., DeShazo, M. M., Wilmet, J., Kjellstrand, C. M., Najarian, J. S. 1974. Results of renal transplant. *Surgery* 76:461–68

24. Avner, E. D., Harmon, W. E., Ingelfinger, J. R., Levey, R. H., Grupe, W. E. 1980. Mortality of chronic dialysis comparable to that of renal transplantation in pediatric end-stage renal disease. *Clin. Dialysis Transplant Forum* 9:1–4

25. Fine, R. N. 1975. Renal transplantation in children. In *Advances in Nephrology,* ed. J. Hamburger, J. Crosnier, M. H. Maxwell, 5:201–28. Chicago: Year Book

26. Russell, P. S. 1981. Monoclonal antibodies in renal transplantation: preliminary results. *Kidney Int.* 20:530–37

27. Barratt, T. M. 1974. Chronic renal failure in children. In *Urology in Childhood,* ed. D. I. Williams, pp. 24–33. New York/Heidelberg/Berlin: Springer-Verlag

28. Hodson, E. M., Najarian, J. S., Kjellstrand, C. M., Simmons, M. D., Maner, S. M. 1978. Renal transplantation in children ages 1–5 years. *Pediatrics* 61: 458–64

29. Potter, D. E., Wilson, C. J., Oxonoff, M. B. 1974. Hyperparathyroid bone disease in children undergoing long-term hemodialysis. Treatment with Vitamin D. *J. Pediatr.* 85:60–66

30. Jebsen, R. H., Tenckhoff, H., Honet, J. C. 1967. Natural history of uremic polyneuropathy and effect of dialysis. *N. Engl. J. Med.* 277:327–33

31. Knochel, J. P. 1981. The pathophysiology of uremia. *Hosp. Pract.* 16:65–76

32. Lazarus, J. M. 1981. Hemodialysis in chronic renal failure. In *Contemporary Issues in Nephrology,* ed. B. M. Brenner, J. Stein, 7:153–92. New York: Churchill Livingstone

33. Cosimi, A. B. 1979. *The Donor and Donor Nephrectomy in Kidney Transplantation—Principles and Practice,* ed. P. J. Morris, pp. 69–87. New York: Grune & Stratton

34. Masden *vs* Harrison. 1957. *Mass. Supreme Judicial Court, Equity Number 68651*

35. Mauer, S. M., Lynch, R. E. 1976. Hemodialysis techniques for infants and children. *Pediatr. Clin. North Am.* 23:843–56

36. Oreopoulos, D. G. 1977. The coming of age of home peritoneal dialysis. *Can. Med. Assoc. J.* 116:232

37. Levey, R. H., Ingelfinger, J., Grupe, W. E., Toper, M., Eraklis, A. J. 1978. Unique surgical and immunologic features of renal transplantation in children. *J. Pediatr. Surg.* 13:576–80

38. Starzl, T. E., Marchioro, T. L., Morgan, W. M., Waddell, W. R. 1964. A technique for use of adult renal homgrafts in children. *Surg. Gynecol. Obstet.* 119: 106–8

39. Carpenter, C. B. 1978. Transplant rejection in HLA-identical recipients. *Kidney Int.* 14:283–91

40. Persijn, G. G., Gabb, B. W., Van Laeuwen, A., Nagtegaal, A., Hoodgebram, J., Van Rodd, J. J. 1978. Matching for HLA antigens of A, B, and DR loci in renal transplantation by Eurotransplant. *Lancet* 1:1278–81

41. Colvin, R. B., Cosimi, A. B., Burton, R. C., Goldstein, G., Kung, P. C., Rubin, R. H., Herrin, J. T., Fuller, T. C., Delmonico, R. E., Russell, P. S. 1981. Immunologic monitoring and therapy with monoclonal antibodies to t-lymphocytes in renal allograft recipients. *Proc. 8th Int. Congr. Nephrol.,* pp. 990–96

42. Shield, C. F., Cosimi, A. B., Tolkoff-Rubin, N., Rubin, R. H., Herrin, J., Russell, P. S. 1979. Use of antithymocyte globulin for reversal of acute allograft rejection. *Transplantation* 28:461–62

43. McEnery, P., Gonzalez, L. L., Martin, L. W., West, C. D. 1973. Growth and development of children with renal transplants. Use of alternate-day steroid therapy. *J. Pediatr.* 83:806–14

44. Travis, L. B., Chesney, R., McEnery, P., Model, D., Pennsi, A., Potter, D., Talwalkar, Y. B., Wolff, E. 1978. Growth and glucocorticoids in children with kidney disease. *Kidney Int.* 14: 365–68

45. Opelz, G., Terasaki, P. I. 1980. Dominant effect of transfusion on kidney graft survival. *Transplantation* 29: 153–58

46. Russell, P. S. 1977. Steps toward immediate progress in clinical transplantation. *Transplant. Proc.* 9:1327–33

47. Eschbach, J. W., Cook, J. D., Scribner, B. H., Finch, C. A. 1977. Iron balance in hemodialysis patients. *Am. Intern.* *Med.* 87:710–13

48. Fuller, T. C., Delmonico, F. L., Cosimi, B., Huggins, C. E., King, M., Russell, P. S. 1978. Impact of blood transfusion on transplantation. *Am. Surg.* 187: 211–18

49. Salvatierra, O. Jr., Amend, W., Vincenti, F., Potter, D., Steney, R., Duca, R., Feduska, N. 1981. 1,500 Renal transplants at one center: evolution of a strategy for optimal success. *Am. J. Surg.* 142:14–20

50. Touraine, J. L., Laville, M., Malik, M. C., Dubernard, J. M., Betuel, H., Revillard, J. P., Archimbaud, J. P., Traeger, J. 1981. Thoracic duct drainage in renal transplantation. *Proc. 8th Int. Congr. Nephrol., Athens*, pp. 997–1004

51. Najarian, J. S., Sutherland, D. E. R., Fergnson, R. M., Simmons, R. L., Kersey, J., Mauer, S. M., Salvin, S., Kim, T. H. 1981. Total lymphoid irradiation and kidney transplantation. A clinical experience. *Transplant. Proc.* 13:417–24

Ann. Rev. Med. 1983. 34:35–46

CHEMOTHERAPY AND COGNITIVE DEFECTS IN CANCER PATIENTS

Peter M. Silberfarb, M.D.

Departments of Psychiatry and Medicine, Dartmouth Medical School and the Norris Cotton Cancer Center, Hanover, New Hampshire 03756

ABSTRACT

The cognitive functions are defined and discussed. Factors that place cancer patients at high risk for disorders of cognition are presented along with the problem of semantic confusion in this area. The cognitive impairment found in cancer patients receiving chemotherapy is reviewed, as is the importance of the mental status examination and the treatment of delirium in cancer patients. Several illustrative case reports are presented.

Introduction

During the past two decades, the use of cancer chemotherapeutic agents has become widespread. Patients now receive cancer chemotherapy as both curative and adjuvant treatments for many different types of cancer. Medical centers have joined cooperative oncology groups to conduct clinical trials of cancer chemotherapeutic agents and, recently, community hospitals have also been included in clinical trials of cancer chemotherapy (1) further disseminating the use of chemotherapeutic agents. In 1973, the American Board of Internal Medicine recognized the need to train physicians in the use of chemotherapeutic agents and established the subspecialty of clinical oncology with board certification requirements for medical oncologists.

With the increased and widespread use of chemotherapy to treat cancer patients alone or in combination with surgery and radiotherapy, increasing attention has been paid to the neurotoxic effects of these agents. The first exhaustive review of this subject was published by Weiss and colleagues in

35

1974 (2). Other reviews followed (3–6) as the increased use of antineoplastic medications brought further understanding of these agents.

Unfortunately, most authors do not distinguish the various types of neuropsychiatric effects and often refer to them in vague terms such as neurotoxicity, psychiatric toxicity, mental confusion, etc. Recently, Peterson & Popkin (7) reviewed the neuropsychiatric effects of chemotherapeutic agents but also were hampered by the varied terminology used in the case reports they reviewed. Silberfarb and colleagues (8, 9) investigated specific psychiatric effects—both cognitive and noncognitive—of hospitalized medical oncology patients who were receiving chemotherapy. They found cognitive deficits to be quite common in this population (8), but in a later study, where age was controlled, the deficiencies were less apparent (9).

Cognitive defects imply impaired cerebral functioning. They are found in those psychiatric disorders, such as delirium and dementia, that are physiological effects of physical illness and are not psychological responses to the meaning of the illness. Cognitive disorders are the psychopathologic manifestation of cerebral damage or dysfunction. In this context, cognitive defects in cancer patients refer to the cerebral effects of cancer and not to the reactive or functional disorders.

Cancer patients, because of the systemic nature of their illness, are at a high risk for cognitive impairment. People are living longer even though the maximum life span has not increased (10). They are, therefore, predisposed by age to cognitive impairment. In addition, cancer patients are living longer so are also apt to reach an age where they are more susceptible to cognitive impairment if challenged by chemotherapeutic agents. These factors plus the increase in use and wider distribution of the chemotherapeutic agents point to an emerging problem in patient care.

Cognitive functioning, which is synonymous with "thinking" or intellectual functioning, involves the higher attributes of humankind. These are memory, orientation, awareness, attention, comprehension, and perception. They are the higher integrative functions of the brain—the phases of information processing. The cognitive functions comprise the objective parts of the mental status examination. They can be formally measured and, while they often affect behavior, are distinct from the more descriptive and subjective aspects of a person's mental status, such as mood. The cognitive functions can be measured clinically with the same objectivity usually reserved for heart sounds (11). Unfortunately, few physicians do so.

Disorders of Cognitive Function

In 1980, a new psychiatric nomenclature was adopted. It is referred to as the Diagnostic and Statistical Manual III (DSM III) and lists delirium and dementia as organic mental disorders (organic brain syndromes in the old terminology) characterized by some degree of global cognitive impairment (12).

The key criteria for the diagnosis of delirium according to DSM III are a reduction in the clarity of awareness of the environment (which is usually of relatively rapid onset, brief duration, and manifested by impairment of ability to sustain attention), an impairment of orientation, and an impairment of memory. Typically, this decrease in level of awareness is accompanied by relative slowing of the electroencephalogram (11). In addition, there is usually disturbance of the sleep-wakefulness cycle with insomnia or daytime drowsiness; change in usual psychomotor activity (either increased or decreased); occasionally perceptual disturbances, which may take the form of misinterpretations, illusions, or hallucinations; and often decrease in clarity of thinking. Emotional, i.e. behavioral, disturbances are very common and prominent, often overshadowing the organic disturbance in delirium. Depression, irritability, anger, fear, anxiety, apathetic withdrawal, plus the associated behavior of crying, laughing, and angry outbursts are common. All symptoms tend to fluctuate over the course of the day often becoming more apparent at night. Neurologic signs on physical examination are usually absent unless the delirium is caused by a specific organic problem; asterixis, for example, may be present in hepatic encephalopathy.

Dementia is the other major cognitive disorder listed in DSM III that is frequently associated with clinical cognitive impairment. The key criterion in the diagnosis of dementia is "the loss of intellectual abilities of sufficient severity to interfere with social or occupational functioning." In contrast to delirium, however, there is no reduced awareness of the environment. There are memory impairment, impairment of ability to think abstractly, and impairment of judgement, which is usually evident from the history. Although the new DSM III deals mostly with descriptive syndromes and does not focus on prognosis, dementia is usually progressive and irreversible while delirium is reversible.

In summary, cognitive disorders are those in which there is relatively global impairment of memory and thinking. Clinically, the two major disorders of cognition are delirium and dementia. The main difference between delirium and dementia is that the former is usually acute in onset, relatively brief in duration, and reversible, while dementia denotes intellectual deterioration of a protracted and usually irreversible nature. Except for the long-term cognitive effects of some chemotherapeutic agents (e.g. intrathecal methotrexate as used to treat acute leukemias in childhood), most patients with cognitive impairment that the internist sees suffer from the syndrome of delirium. Only recently has dementia in previously treated childhood leukemics emerged as a problem for the internist (13).

Delirium in the Cancer Patient

The cancer patient is often subject to both the predisposing factors and the facilitating factors of delirium. The predisposing factors of delirium are age 65 years or greater, a history of alcohol or drug abuse or both, and preexisting cerebral damage (14). Factors that facilitate the occurrence of delirium if an organic etiology is present are psychological stress, sleep deprivation, sensory deprivation or sensory overload, and immobilization (14). Immobilization as occurs during bed rest is a frequently overlooked facilitating factor. Common knowledge and personal experience indicate how exceptionally difficult it is to perform intellectual work (i.e. the cognitive functions) while bedridden.

In reviewing the literature, it is apparent that there is a long-standing semantic confusion in the nosology of neuropsychiatric disorders and specifically in disorders of cognition. Only a few investigators (15, 16) have utilized DSM III in studies of cancer patients, and the prior literature does not reflect the new DSM III classification. Clarity of thinking has not found its way into the current literature where descriptions of higher cerebral functions are in question. Confusion, mental changes, toxic psychosis, neurotoxicity, neuropsychiatric side effects, and irritability are terms used to indicate delirium. The literature, therefore, has to be reviewed without benefit of the new classification. Judgements of incidence and prevalence of cognitive disorders in cancer patients receiving chemotherapy have to be made from the evidence supplied in clinical reports; more often than not, insufficient data are given to make this judgement.

In the oncology literature, psychiatric side-effects are often submerged into the category of central nervous system (CNS) side-effects or combined with behavioral disorders such as depression and anxiety. It is only recently that studies have addressed the psychiatric side-effects—both behavioral and cognitive (7, 8).

The problem is made more vexing because of the often subtle and "mild" presentation of delirium. The subtle decrease in comprehension of complex material, the subtle loss of ability to think abstractly, and the subtle loss of cognitive flexibility, such as being able to sequentially order alternating numbers and letters (e.g. as measured by the Trials B Test), are often missed by the examining physician. Other common symptoms are difficulty finding the correct word when talking, slight forgetfulness, complaints of "mental fatigue," difficulty concentrating, and complaints of irritability. These often go unnoticed or are attributed solely to "depression" or "anxiety." These mild prodromata of delirium (14) often can be overcome by heightened effort on the part of the patient (11). They may go undetected by the physician until the delirium resolves spontaneously or until major challenges to the patient's cognition promote more obvious evidence of behavioral disturbance. Delirium was found to be the most frequently missed diagnosis in psychiatric consultation referrals of 100 consecutive cancer patients (17).

The delirium found in cancer patients is often multifactorial in etiology. Medications, fever, infections, side-effects of therapy, plus nutritional, metabolic, or endocrine disorders, either alone or in combination, are all possible causes of delirium. Primary CNS tumors or cerebral metastasis from other sites need not be present for defects in cognition to occur. However, when metastasis to the CNS has occurred, cognitive defects are common. Wasserstrom and colleagues reported "mental changes" to be the commonest sign and second most frequent symptom in patients with leptomeningeal metastases from solid tumors (18).

Cognitive impairment found in cancer patients receiving chemotherapy can be conveniently organized into three categories [adapted from Stewart & Benjamin (5)]: cognitive impairment related directly to chemotherapy, cognitive impairment as a result of the cancer itself, and cognitive impairment resulting from concurrently administered medications.

Cognitive Impairment Related to Chemotherapy

Many chemotherapeutic agents have been implicated in causing cognitive impairment. However, since most of these medications are given in combinations or with radiotherapy, it is often difficult to identify a single agent. Methotrexate is one that is often implicated and one about which we know the most. Chronic methotrexate neurotoxicity is usually related to prolonged therapy by the intrathecal route. The cognitive impairment, which seems to become more frequent when cranial irradiation and intravenous methotrexate are combined with intrathecal methotrexate (19), frequently follows the treatment of childhood leukemias (20–25). Leukoencephalopathy with cognitive deficits following intrathecal methotrexate has also been reported in adults (26). Intravenous vincristine increases central spinal fluid levels of methotrexate (27), but much more needs to be learned about this interaction before it is implicated as the cause of cognitive impairment. The vinca alkaloids by themselves reportedly cause "mental changes," "hallucinations," "confusion," and delirium (28, 29). Combinations of chemotherapeutic agents such as vincristine, methotrexate, and cyclophosphamide may cause a fatigue syndrome (30) and even the newer vinca alkaloids such as vindesine have been reported to cause hallucinations and confusion (31).

Adrenal steroids, especially prednisone, are frequently used as a chemotherapeutic agent in the treatment of various cancers or to relieve the side-effects caused by the cancer or its treatment. Steroids have a long history of causing mental changes and these are frequently reported in the literature. Many excellent reviews deal with this phenomenon (32–34).

Hexamethylmelamine, a chemotherapeutic agent reviewed by Legha et al (35), causes "mental depression," "hallucinations," and sleep disturbance. Fluorouracil causes "mental changes" typical of delirium with disorientation and diffuse slowing of the electroencephalogram (36). Ftorafur, which is an analog of five-fluorouracil, reportedly caused "forgetfulness," "confusion," and "nervousness" (37) although in this report it was combined with methyl CCNU. L-asparaginase has frequently been reported to cause cognitive impairment described as "confusion," "disorientation," "somnolence" (28), and typical delirium (38).

Other chemotherapeutic agents reported as causing "confusion," "psychosis," "disorientation," or "altered levels of consciousness" are procarbazine (2), nitrogen mustard (28), and BCNU (39). CCNU in combination with brain irradiation caused global cognitive impairment (40). Several newer chemotherapeutic agents that may also cause cognitive impairment, as inferred from the clinical case reports, are DTIC (41), 5-azacytidine (42), and cytosine arabinoside (ARA-C) (43). In addition, isophosphamide reportedly caused "disorientation," "visual hallucinations," and "somnolence" (44). Recently, Heim and colleagues (45) reported "psychopathological symptoms" in 7 of 10 patients with renal carcinoma treated with this agent. Interferon has also been reported to cause "confusion" (46).

In addition to the direct effects of chemotherapeutic agents on cognitive functioning, chemotherapy can damage organs, which, theoretically at least, may secondarily result in cognitive defects. The azotemia following renal damage from cis-platinum (47); respiratory insufficiency from bleomycin (48), BCNU (49), or cyclophosphamide (50); and congestive heart failure from adriamycin and daunorubicin (51) are all clinical conditions where delirium commonly occurs.

It is fair to say that there is often gross evidence of cognitive impairment sporadically reported for almost all of the commonly used chemotherapeutic agents. It is this author's view that if the subtle and mild evidence of cognitive impairment is sought, symptoms of delirium have a very high prevalence in patients receiving chemotherapy.

Cognitive Impairment as a Result of Cancer Itself

A second cause of cognitive impairment in cancer patients is the effect of the malignancy itself. Central nervous system tumors (whether primary or metastatic), the remote effects of neoplastic lesions, endocrine changes in the paraneoplastic syndromes, and metabolic or toxic encephalopathies induced by the cancer are all possible and frequent causes of cognitive impairment. Elevated blood urea nitrogen, hypercalcemia, or altered blood gases are also common causes of the syndrome of delirium. Infections secondary to immunosuppression are another common cause of delirium.

Cognitive Impairment Resulting from Concurrently Administered Medications

The cognitive impairment in cancer patients can be related to medications administered to control the side effects of chemotherapy or of the cancer itself. Narcotic analgesics prescribed for pain, hypnosedatives prescribed for insomnia, or antiemetics prescribed for nausea and vomiting are all classes of medications commonly associated with cognitive impairment. Rarely, even psychotropic medications given to cancer patients, such as tricyclic antidepressants for treatment of depression or lithium for its white-blood-cell-stimulating effect, can cause delirium.

The Importance of the Mental Status Examination

Why is it important to diagnose the subtle manifestations of delirium? Why is it important for oncologists and internists to recognize the frequency of subtle impaired cognition in patients? Since delirium can be treated, the relief of suffering is one obvious response. Improved compliance with therapy is another practical reason. Since delirium is often subtle in its presentation, a thorough mental status examination where cognitive functions are objectively measured is important. Ideally, tests should be done at baseline prior to beginning chemotherapy and periodically throughout the course of treatment, just as one would monitor blood pressure or heart sounds.

The mental status examination can most conveniently be divided into two components, the noncognitive and the cognitive. The noncognitive or emotional aspects of the patient, such as anxiety, depression, fear, anger, and other observable behaviors (52), are easily and quickly assessed. Changes here can be quite subtle and can be a reflection of cognitive deficits as the patient realizes at some level that they are impaired. Alternately, they may be present without any defects in cognition and, as such, need to be assessed for further supportive, psychotherapeutic, or psychopharmacological treatment. However, the examiner needs to go beyond these obvious behavioral responses on the part of the patient and to move to the second part of the mental status examination—the test of cognitive functioning.

There are several brief standardized screening tests for cognitive function that are useful and can be administered by a nonphysician. The Mini Mental State (53, 54) and the Cognitive Capacity Screening Examination (55) are two standardized measures of cognitive function. Alternately, the physician can incorporate five simple measurements of cognitive functioning in his or her examination without lengthening the examination substantially. Impairment of attention can be quickly measured by digit span, asking the patient to spell the word "world" backwards, or serial subtractions of threes or sevens depending on the patient's education. These simple tests assess a patient's ability to maintain attention, shift attention, process information, and receive selective inputs of information. Disorders of thinking can be easily measured by asking a patient to interpret a simple proverb. This gives information as to the organization of the patient's thought, ability to think abstractly, and whether thought content is impoverished or deluded. Disorders of orientation are easily assessed by questioning the patient as to time and place. Finally, disorders of memory, that is, registration, retention, and retrieval of memory, can be assessed by asking a patient to remember three objects immediately and five minutes later. Digit span is another measurement of memory.

Treatment of Delirium

The treatment of cancer patients who have impaired cognition can be divided into two basic categories: specific treatment and nonspecific treatment. The specific treatment is simply directed at identifying and correcting the underlying cause of the delirium. Treating hypercalcemia, decreasing fever, treating infection, relieving cerebral edema, and discontinuing a chemotherapeutic agent found to be deliriogenic are all simple maneuvers that can return cognitive function to normal.

Nonspecific treatment is directed toward relieving anguish by reducing to a minimum the causes of psychological stress so that the patient's remaining cognitive abilities can be facilitated. If this is not followed, the resulting increase in anxiety or increase in depression or disorganization of ego functioning can cause a vicious cycle with further cognitive impairment. Avoiding unfamiliar surroundings, encouraging frequent orienting interactions on the part of the nursing and housestaff, attempts to limit sensory impairment by placing a large calendar in the room, leaving a light on in the evening, having sitters stay with the patient to reorient them when they become confused, and avoiding confronting a patient with a cognitive task that is beyond his or her capabilities are additional treatment strategies.

Medications to relieve the painful effects of depression or anxiety that frequently accompany impairment of cognition may be helpful. Antidepressant medications and benzodiazepines have been found useful. Finally, medications may be needed to control a patient's behavior if it becomes unmanageable and to prevent the complications of delirium such as falls, injuries, assaults on staff, and compliance problems (e.g. pulling out IV needles). In this regard, sedation is an important immediate goal. A commonly used and effective medication is the neuroleptic haloperidol, but other neuroleptics or even the benzodiazepines have been used successfully.

Brief Illustrative Case Reports

CASE ONE   A 31-year-old mother of two children was diagnosed as having localized small-cell carcinoma of the lung. She was started on a chemotherapy protocol consisting of vincristine, cyclophosphamide, and etoposide (VP-16). Three months later, she was readmitted to the hospital with fatigue, daytime somnolence, nighttime insomnia, and nausea. Physical examination and complete medical workup were unchanged from the time of diagnosis. Mental status examination revealed anxiety and depressive affect plus difficulty with serial subtraction of threes, prolonged hesitation in answering questions, inability to abstract simple proverbs, impaired digit span (only able to retain four digits forward and three backwards), and subtle disorientation (missed day of week by one day). The patient had been a straight-A student in high school. During mental status examination she consistently tried to change the subject and engage the examiner in another topic. Her anxiety and depression responded to the simple reassurance that she was not "losing her mind." Several weeks later, after the course of chemotherapy was stopped, her sleep-wakefulness cycle returned to normal as did her attention span, orientation, memory, ability to subtract numbers, and ability to think abstractly.

This patient most likely experienced a delirium caused by the chemotherapeutic agents. This was mild and discovered early so that her emotional symptoms (depression and anxiety), which were secondary to her perceived cognitive deficit, responded to simple reassurance. Her attempt to dissuade the examiner from asking the substantive questions pertaining to cognitive function is a common maneuver of the cognitively impaired. Patients who are cognitively impaired seldom volunteer their cognitive disabilities.

CASE TWO   A 41-year-old woman was admitted to the hospital with pneumonia and adenocarcinoma of the lung involving the external chest wall. Her temperature remained 38.6°C despite antibiotic therapy for four days following admission. At this time an intern's note describes the patient as being very withdrawn and depressed. Amitriptyline was begun. Two days later a psychiatric consultation revealed that she could recall only three digits forward and could remember none of three objects after five minutes. Amitriptyline was stopped. Her temperature eventually returned to normal over the next few days, her mood improved, she became more alert, and revealed an improvement in her memory and ability to retain digits.

In this case, the patient's delirium was manifested as the behavioral response of depression. Substantive cognitive testing, however, revealed definite impairment in attention and memory. As fever lessened so did her delirium and depression. There was no need for amitriptyline; the diagnosis of depression was an error and led to the use of an anticholinergic medication, amitriptyline, which could have worsened delirium. Withdrawal and depressive affect are compatible with the diagnosis of delirium; not all depressive affect is "depressive disorder."

CASE THREE   A previously oriented 70-year-old widow hospitalized with advanced breast cancer suddenly had unexpected episodes of weeping in the evenings. This was assumed by nurses and housestaff to be appropriate to her illness. However, as days passed, she became argumentative with nurses and demanded to return to her home in a nearby town. Further history from the family indicated that the patient had not lived in the nearby town since the death of her husband 15 years ago. Mental status examination revealed that she was disoriented to time and place and that her cooperativeness fluctuated with the time of day.

A search for an etiology of her delirium revealed severe hypercalcemia. This was treated, and her disorientation cleared and mood fluctuations ceased. Weeping was a manifestation of delirium and not a depressive disorder, nor was it "appropriate" to her illness.

ACKNOWLEDGMENTS

The author wishes to thank Drs. Z. J. Lipowski and Charles Solow for helpful editorial advice and Mrs. Cynthia Hewitt for editorial assistance.

Literature Cited

1. Begg, C. B., Carbone, P. P., Elson, P. J., Zelen, M. 1982. Participation of community hospitals in clinical trials. *N. Engl. J. Med.* 306:1076–80
2. Weiss, H. D., Walker, M. D., Wiernik, P. H. 1974. Neurotoxicity of commonly used antineoplastic agents. *N. Engl. J. Med.* 291:75–81, 127–33
3. Pochedly, C. 1977. Neurotoxicity due to CNS therapy for leukemia. *Med. Pediatr. Oncol.* 3:101–15
4. Allen, J. C. 1978. The effects of cancer therapy on the nervous system. *J. Pediat.* 93:903–9
5. Stewart, D. J., Benjamin, R. S. 1979. Cancer chemotherapeutic agents. In *Neuropsychiatric Side Effects of Drugs in the Elderly,* ed. A. J. Levenson, 9:191–224. New York: Raven
6. Kaplan, R. S., Wiernik, P. H. 1982. Neurotoxicity of antineoplastic drugs. *Semin. Oncol.* 9:103–30
7. Peterson, L. G., Popkin, M. K. 1980. Neuropsychiatric effects of chemo-therapeutic agents for cancer. *Psychosomatics* 21:141–53
8. Silberfarb, P. M., Philibert, D., Levine, P. M. 1980. Psychosocial aspects of neoplastic disease II. Affective and cognitive effects of chemotherapy in cancer patients. *Am. J. Psychiatry* 137:597–601
9. Oxman, T. E., Silberfarb, P. M. 1980. Serial cognitive testing in patients receiving cancer chemotherapy. *Am. J. Psychiatry* 137:1263–65
10. Fries, J. F. 1980. Aging, natural death, and the compression of morbidity. *N. Engl. J. Med.* 303:130–35
11. Engel, G. L., Romano, J. 1959. Delirium, a syndrome of cerebral insufficiency. *J. Chron. Dis.* 9:260–77
12. *Diagnostic and Statistical Manual of Mental Disorders.* Third Edition (DSM-III). 1980. Washington, DC: Am. Psychiatr. Assoc. 494 pp.
13. D'Angio, G. J. 1982. The child cured of cancer: a problem for the internist. *Semin. Oncol* 9:143–49

14. Lipowski, Z. J. 1980. *Delirium: Acute Brain Failure in Man.* Springfield, Ill: Thomas. 567 pp.
15. Derogatis, L. R., Morrow, G. R., Fetting, J. H., Schmale, A. H., Hendrichs, M. H., Holland, J. C., Penman, D., Gorzinski, J. G., Melisaratos, N., Carnrike, C. L. 1982. The prevalence of psychiatric disorders among cancer patients: a multi hospital study. *Proc. Am. Soc. Clin. Oncol.* 1:48 (Abstr.)
16. Fetting, J.H., Sitley, K. N., Capozzoli, K. D. 1982. Psychiatry consultation in a cancer center. *Proc. Am. Soc. Clin. Oncol.* 1:46 (Abstr.)
17. Levine, P. M., Silberfarb, P. M., Lipowski, Z. J. 1978. Mental disorders in cancer patients: a study of 100 psychiatric referrals. *Cancer* 43:1385–91
18. Wasserstrom, W. R., Glass, J. P., Posner, J. B. 1982. Diagnosis and treatment of leptomeningeal metastases from solid tumors: experience with 90 patients. *Cancer* 49:759–72
19. Bleyer, W. A., Griffin, T. W. 1980. White matter necrosis, mineralizing microangiopathy, and intellectual abilities in survivors of childhood leukemia: associations with central nervous system irradiation and methotrexate therapy. In *Radiation Damage to the Nervous System,* ed. H. A. Gilbert, A. R. Kagan, pp. 155–74. New York: Raven
20. Meadows, A. T., Evans, A. E. 1976. Effects of chemotherapy on the central nervous system. *Cancer* 37:1079–85
21. Pizzo, P. A., Bleyer, W. A., Poplack, D. G., Leventhal, B. G. 1976. Reversible dementia temporally associated with intraventricular therapy with methotrexate in a child with acute myelogenous leukemia. *J. Pediatr.* 88:131–33
22. Crosley, C. J., Rorke, L. B., Evans, A., Nigro, M. 1978. Central nervous system lesions in childhood leukemia. *Neurology* 28:678–85
23. Goff, J. R., Anderson, H. R., Cooper, P. F. 1980. Distractibility and memory deficits in long-term survivors of acute lymphoblastic leukemia. *J. Dev. Behav. Pediatr.* 1:158–63
24. Wimmer, R. S., Hill, W. B., Baird, H. W. 1981. Neurometric and psychometric evaluation of long-term survivors of childhood acute lymphocytic leukemia. *Proc. Am. Assoc. Cancer Res. Am. Soc. Clin. Oncol.* 22:398 (Abstr.)
25. Robison, L., Nesbit, M., Sather, H., Meadows, A., Ortega, J., Hammond, D. 1982. Intellectual function in long-term survivors of childhood acute lymphoblastic leukemia. *Proc. Am. Soc. Clin. Oncol.* 1:46 (Abstr.)
26. Bjorgen, J. E., Gold, L. H. A. 1977. Computed tomographic appearance of methotrexate induced necrotizing leukoencephalopathy. *Radiology* 122:377–78
27. Tejada, F., Zubrod, C. G. 1979. Vincristine effect on methotrexate cerebrospinal fluid concentration. *Cancer Treat. Rep.* 63:143–45
28. Hildebrand, J. 1978. *Lesions of the Nervous System in Cancer Patients.* New York: Raven. 150 pp.
29. Rosenthal, S., Kaufman, S. 1974. Vincristine neurotoxicity. *Ann. Intern. Med.* 80:733–37
30. Taylor, S. G., Desai, S. A., DeWys, W. D. 1978. Phase II trial of a combination of cyclophosphamide, vincristine, and methotrexate in advanced colorectal cancer. *Cancer Treat. Rep.* 62:1203–5
31. Ohnuma, T., Greenspan, E. M., Holland, J. F. 1980. Initial clinical study with vindesine: tolerance to weekly I. V. bolus and 24-hour infusion. *Cancer Treat. Rep.* 64:25–30
32. Quarton, G. C., Clark, L. D., Cobb, S., Bauer, W. 1955. Mental disturbances associated with ACTH and cortisone: a review of explanatory hypotheses. *Medicine* 34:13–50
33. Carpenter, W. T., Bunney, W. E. Jr. 1971. Behavioral effects of cortisol in man. *Semin. Psychiatry* 3:421–34
34. Whybrow, P. C., Hurwitz, T. 1976. Psychological disturbances associated with endocrine disease and hormone therapy. In *Hormones, Behavior, and Psychopathology,* ed. E. H. Sachar, pp. 125–43. New York: Raven
35. Legha, S. S., Slavik, M., Carter, S. K. 1976. Hexamethylmelamine—an evaluation of its role in the therapy of cancer. *Cancer* 38:27–35
36. Greenwald, E. S. 1976. Organic mental changes with fluoruracil. *J. Am. Med. Assoc.* 235:248–49
37. Belt, R. J., Stephens, R. 1979. Phase I-II study of ftorafur and methyl-CCNU in advanced colorectal cancer. *Cancer* 44:869–72
38. Holland, J., Fasanello, S., Ohnuma, T. 1974. Psychiatric symptoms associated with L-asparaginase administration. *J. Psychiatr. Res.* 10:105–13
39. Madajewicz, S., West, C. R., Park, H. C., Ghoorah, J., Avellanosa, A. M., Takita, H., Karakousis, C., Vincent, R., Caracandas, J., Jennings, E. 1981. Phase II study—intra-arterial BCNU

therapy for metastatic brain tumor. *Cancer* 47:653–57

40. Hochberg, F. H., Slotnick, B. 1980. Neuropsychiatric impairment in astrocytoma survivors. *Neurology* 30: 172–77
41. Paterson, A. H. G., McPherson, T. A. 1977. A possible neurologic complication of DTIC. *Cancer Treat. Rep.* 61: 105–6
42. Levi, J. A., Wiernik, P. H. 1976. A comparative clinical trial of 5-azacytidine and guanazole in previously treated adults with acute nonlymphocytic leukemia. *Cancer* 38:36–41
43. Lazarus, H. M., Herzig, R. H., Herzig, G. P., Phillips, G. L., Roessmann, U., Fishman, D. J. 1981. Central nervous system toxicity of high-dose systemic cytosine arabinoside. *Cancer* 48: 2577–82
44. Kovach, J. S., Schutt, A. J., Hahn, R. G., Reitemeier, R. J., Moertel, C. G. 1974. A phase-2 study of intermittent high-dose isophosphamide therapy of advanced colorectal cancer. *Oncology* 29:34–39
45. Heim, M. E., Feine, R., Schick, E., Wolpert, E., Queisser, W. 1981. Central nervous side effects following ifosfamide monotherapy of advanced renal carcinoma. *J. Cancer Res. Clin. Oncol.* 100:113–16

46. Priestman, T. J. 1980. Initial evaluation of human lymphoblastoid interferon in patients with advanced malignant disease. *Lancet* 2:113–18
47. Rozencweig, M., VonHoff, D. D., Slavik, M., Muggia, F. M. 1977. *Cis*-diamminedichloroplatinum (II). *Ann. Intern. Med.* 86:803–12
48. Bennett, J. M., Reich, S. D. 1979. Bleomycin. *Ann. Intern. Med.* 90:945–48
49. Holoye, P. Y., Jenkins, D. E., Greenberg, S. D. 1976. Pulmonary toxicity in long-term administration of BCNU. *Cancer Treat. Rep.* 60:1691–94
50. Whitcomb, M. D. 1973. Drug-induced lung disease. *Chest* 63:418–22
51. Yates, J. W. 1979. Anthracycline antibiotics—adriamycin and daunorubicin. *Hosp. Formulary* 14:987–93
52. Silberfarb, P. M., Greer, S. 1982. Psychological concomitants of cancer: clinical aspects. *Am. J. Psychother.* In press
53. Folstein, M. F., Folstein, S. E., McHugh, P. R. 1975. Mini-mental state. *J. Psychiatr. Res.* 12:189–98
54. Anthony, J. C., LeResche, L., Niaz, U., vonKorff, M. D., Folstein, M. F. 1982. Limits of the 'mini-mental state' as a screening test for dementia and delirium among hospital patients. *Psychol. Med.* 12:397–408
55. Jacobs, J. W., Bernhard, M. R., Delgado, A., Strain, J. J. 1977. Screening for organic mental syndromes in medically ill. *Ann. Intern. Med.* 86:40–46

Ann. Rev. Med. 1983. 34:47–53

INFECTIONS AND HYPOCOMPLEMENTEMIA

Ira M. Goldstein, M.D., and Shelley R. Marder, M.D.

Rosalind Russell Arthritis Research Laboratory, Department of Medicine, University of California, San Francisco, Medical Service, San Francisco General Hospital, San Francisco, California 94110

ABSTRACT

The complement system, phagocytic leukocytes, and antibodies constitute the "department of defense" in the battle against infections caused by pyogenic microorganisms. Complement components are capable of directly killing (by lysis) certain susceptible bacteria and are the source of chemotactic peptides and heat-labile opsonin, which facilitate recognition and killing of microbes by phagocytic cells. When these vital functions are compromised, as in individuals with inherited deficiencies of complement components, the result is unusual susceptibility to severe infections.

INTRODUCTION

Humoral factors as well as leukocytes are essential for maintaining normal host defenses against infections caused by pyogenic bacteria and fungi. Whereas phagocytic leukocytes (particularly polymorphonuclear leukocytes) are the major combatants in the battle that follows microbial invasion, these cells would be unable to effectively seek out, recognize, ingest, and kill invading microorganisms if it were not for the two additional "lines of defense" provided by specific antibodies and the complement system. In fact, if it were not for antibodies and complement, odds would be greatly in favor of invading microbes.

The purpose of this review is to illustrate the essential roles played by complement components in the maintenance of normal host defenses and to describe some inherited hypocomplementemic states that are associated with unusual susceptibility to severe, recurrent infections.

47

0066-4219/83/0401-0047$02.00

PATHWAYS OF COMPLEMENT ACTIVATION

The complement system in man can be activated by two major pathways (1). The classical pathway is typically initiated by the union of antibody with antigen. As a consequence of this reaction, a site on the Fc (nonantigen-binding) portion of the antibody molecule becomes capable of binding and activating the first component of complement, a multimolecular complex of three proteins (C1q, C1r, and C1s). Activated C1 then cleaves (by limited proteolytic reactions) its natural substrates, C4 and C2, to yield a complex (C4b2a or "C3 convertase"), which transiently possesses enzymatic activity capable of cleaving C3. Cleavage of C3 (by limited proteolysis) initiates a series of reactions leading to cleavage of C5 (the final proteolytic reaction) and ultimately to assembly of another multimolecular complex (C5b–C9), which possesses membranolytic activity.

The alternative pathway (or properdin system) bypasses the early-acting components (C1, C4, and C2) of the classical pathway and leads directly to cleavage of C3. The known components of the alternative pathway include factor A (C3b), factor B, factor D, and properdin. These components interact sequentially in a fashion somewhat analogous to the classical pathway to yield an enzyme (alternative pathway "C3 convertase") that is capable of cleaving C3 and of activating the terminal "attack" sequence, C5–C9. The alternative pathway may be activated by the introduction into serum of a variety of substances, including complex polysaccharides, bacterial lipopolysaccharides or endotoxins, and some immune complexes. Many intact, viable bacteria (both Gram-positive and Gram-negative) also are capable of activating the alternative complement pathway. In doing so, these microorganisms can become opsonized (see below) in the absence of specific antibody. Thus, the alternative complement pathway can be considered as the "first line of defense" against some infections.

BIOLOGICALLY ACTIVE PRODUCTS OF COMPLEMENT ACTIVATION

The major biologically active products of complement activation, by either the classical or alternative pathways, include C5a, C3a, and C3b. The low-molecular-weight peptides, C3a and C5a, possess anaphylatoxin activity; i.e. they provoke release of histamine from mast cells and basophils, contraction of smooth muscle, and increased capillary permeability (2). In addition, human C5a mediates several important functions of phagocytic leukocytes (3). For example, C5a is a potent chemotactic factor and stimulates polymorphonuclear leukocytes to increase their oxidative metabolism (i.e. generate superoxide anion radicals) as well as to discharge a portion of their lysosomal contents (i.e. degranulate). C5a also augments the adhesiveness of polymorphonuclear leukocytes and provokes aggregation of these cells in suspension.

C3b: Heat-Labile Opsonin

Although all of the products of complement activation participate in protecting the host from severe infection, it is appropriate to emphasize the very important role played by C3b. Many investigators have observed that fresh (but not heated) human serum greatly enhances ingestion and killing of bacteria by human peripheral blood polymorphonuclear leukocytes. The term "opsonize," meaning (from the Greek) "to prepare for dining," has been used to describe the action of serum components (opsonins) that act upon certain bacteria and other particles to increase their palatability. There are two major constituents of serum that act in this fashion. Heat-stable opsonins are immunoglobulins (antibodies), particularly those of the IgG class. As a consequence of reacting with antigens, these molecules or, more specifically, their Fc portions can bind to specific receptors ("Fc receptors") on the surfaces of phagocytic cells (4). Thus, phagocytes "recognize" particles (including bacteria and fungi) coated with IgG antibody.

Heat-labile opsonin, i.e. C3b, binds to a variety of particles (including bacteria and fungi) as a consequence of activation of either the classical or alternative complement pathways. C3b renders particles to which it is attached recognizable by phagocytic leukocytes (through "C3b receptors") and mediates firm particle-cell adherence (4).

Whereas phagocytic cells, such as polymorphonuclear leukocytes, appear capable of ingesting certain particles (e.g. polystyrene latex beads) in the absence of serum components, opsonins such as C3b and IgG clearly increase the rate of particle uptake. C3b receptors of polymorphonuclear leukocytes are involved primarily in recognition and attachment, while particle binding to Fc receptors is necessary for the induction of optimal phagocytosis (4).

COMPLEMENT AND HOST DEFENSES

Components of the complement system protect against overwhelming infections in a variety of ways. For example, some microorganisms call initial attention to themselves as a consequence of activating the alternative complement pathway. In the presence of specific antibodies, activation of the classical pathway also may occur. Following either or both of these events, chemotaxins (e.g. C5a) are generated that attract phagocytic cells (primarily polymorphonuclear leukocytes) to sites of microbial invasion. These cells then recognize (through their C3b receptors), ingest, and kill the invaders. In some instances, killing may not require phagocytes. For example, certain bacteria (e.g. gonococci, meningococci) may be killed by the action of complement alone (see below). These bacteria are susceptible to lysis by the terminal "attack" sequence C5–C9 (activated by either the classical or alternative pathways).

Considering the information summarized above, it should not be surprising that host defenses are compromised severely in individuals with inherited deficiencies of complement components. Examples of deficiency states that are associated with altered susceptibility to infections are discussed in the next section.

COMPLEMENT DEFICIENCIES

Deficiency of C2

The majority of individuals with inherited deficiencies of the early-acting components of the classical complement pathway (i.e. C1, C4, and C2) are not unusually susceptible to either recurrent or severe infections. An intact alternative complement pathway apparently enables these individuals to opsonize pathogenic microorganisms and to generate chemotaxins. Nevertheless, reports have appeared recently describing patients with inherited absence of C2 who have suffered from episodes of septicemia, meningitis, pneumonia, sinusitis, and arthritis caused by either *Streptococcus pneumoniae, Hemophilus influenzae,* or *Salmonella typhi* (5, 6). One explanation of these findings is that some pyogenic bacteria do not activate the alternative pathway and, consequently, may not be opsonized adequately in C2-deficient serum (7). Another explanation relates to the fact that some patients with C2 deficiency exhibit other immunologic abnormalities that may affect host defenses adversely. For example, some individuals with inherited deficiency of C2 also suffer from a deficiency of factor B (the genes that code for C2 and factor B are closely linked). As expected, alternative complement pathway activity in serum from these individuals is abnormal (8). Hypogammaglobulinemia and neutropenia also have been observed in association with inherited absence of C2 (5).

Deficiency of C3

Considering the fact that C3 is the source of heat-labile opsonic activity, it is not surprising that the most severe abnormalities of host defenses occur in individuals with deficiencies of this complement component. At least six patients with homozygous deficiency of C3 have been described (9–13). All but one of these patients suffered from recurrent infections (e.g. pneumonia, meningitis, otitis media, pharyngitis, furunculosis, arthritis) caused by *S. pneumoniae, S. pyogenes, H. influenzae, Klebsiella aerogenes,* and *Sta-*

phylococcus aureus. As a result of the absence of C3, sera from these patients failed to yield heat-labile opsonic activity (C3b), chemotactic activity (C5a), and complement-mediated bactericidal activity (C5b–C9).

Deficiency of C5

The first human kindred with hereditary deficiency of C5 was described in 1976 (14). The proband, a young woman with systemic lupus erythematosus, lacked detectable C5 and suffered from severe, recurrent bacterial infections caused by staphylococci, streptococci, and various species of *Proteus, Pseudomonas,* and *Enterobacteriacae.* Serum from this patient lacked bactericidal activity and failed to yield chemotactic activity after incubation with either aggregated IgG or bacterial endotoxin. Deficiency of C5 has been reported in other families. In one report, the proband had complete absence of C5 and had suffered from nine episodes of disseminated gonococcal infection (15). Other patients with C5 deficiency have had meningococcal meningitis and/or the gonococcal arthritis-dermatitis syndrome (16). As discussed below, it is now established that the terminal complement components (C5–C8) are required for normal host defenses against infections caused by *Neisseria gonorrhoeae* and *N. meningitidis.*

Deficiencies of C6, C7, and C8

As indicated above, the complement system not only provides the chemotactic peptides and heat-labile opsonin that facilitate killing of microbes by phagocytic cells, but also can cause direct lysis of certain susceptible bacteria. As expected, patients with inherited deficiencies of the late-acting complement components (i.e. C6, C7, C8), which comprise the lytic "attack" sequence, are unable to kill certain microbes by complement-mediated lysis. Sera from these patients yield normal amounts of chemotactic activity and facilitate ingestion of microorganisms, but completely lack bactericidal activity against *N. meningitidis, N. gonorrhoeae, H. influenzae* type b, *S. typhi,* and some strains of *Escherichia coli* (17–19). More than half of the patients with deficiencies of either C6, C7, or C8 that have been reported to date have had one or more episodes of disseminated *Neisserial* infections (20).

COMPLEMENT MEASUREMENTS

When one encounters a patient with either a history of recurrent infections or an unusual manifestation of a common infection (e.g. disseminated gonococcemia), a search for a complement deficiency state is warranted. The classical method for quantifying serum complement entails measuring the degree of hemolysis of antibody-sensitized sheep erythrocytes that have been incubated with serial dilutions of a test serum. Results of such determinations, which are dependent upon serum levels of all nine complement components (of the classical pathway), are referred to as "total hemolytic complement" and are most often expressed as CH_{50} units (calculated from the serum dilution yielding 50% hemolysis). This is an efficient method for detecting complement deficiency states since absence of any of the classical pathway components (C1 through C9) will result in the CH_{50} being zero. In fact, measurement of "total hemolytic complement" is the only method available to most clinicians for the detection of congenital deficiencies of C2, C6, C7, and C8. Routine immunochemical determinations of C3 are satisfactory for detecting complete absence of this complement component.

CONCLUSIONS

The proteins comprising the complement system of man, as well as the mechanisms bringing about their activation, can no longer be considered subjects of interest only to immunologists and biochemists. Whereas complement activity is still tested for and measured by its capacity to lyse antibody-sensitized sheep erythrocytes, there are many biologically important phenomena in which the same or related complement activity is involved. In this review, we have attempted to illustrate how some of these phenomena are essential for the maintenance of normal host defenses against infection.

Literature Cited

1. Müller-Eberhard, H. J. 1975. Complement. *Ann. Rev. Biochem.* 44:697–724
2. Hugli, T. E., Müller-Eberhard, H. J. 1978. Anaphylatoxins: C3a and C5a. *Adv. Immunol.* 26:1–53
3. Goldstein, I. M., Perez, H. D. 1980. Biologically active peptides derived from the fifth component of complement. In *Progress in Hemostasis and Thrombosis*, ed. T. H. Spaet, 5:41–79. New York: Grune & Stratton
4. Ehlenberger, A. G., Nussenzweig, V. 1977. The role of membrane receptors for C3b and C3d in phagocytosis, *J. Exp. Med.* 145:357–71
5. Sampson, H. A., Walchner, A. M., Baker, P. J. 1982. Recurrent pyogenic infections in individuals with absence of the second component of complement. *J. Clin. Immunol.* 2:39–45
6. Agnello, V. 1978. Complement deficiency states. *Medicine* 57:1–23
7. Repine, J. E., Clawson, C. C., Friend, P. S. 1977. Influence of a deficiency of the second component of complement on the bactericidal activity of neutrophils in vitro. *J. Clin. Invest.* 59:802–9
8. Newman, S. L., Vogler, L. B., Feigin, R. D., Johnston, R. B. Jr. 1978. Recurrent septicemia associated with congenital deficiency of C2 and partial deficiency of factor B and the alternative complement pathway. *N. Engl. J. Med.* 299:290–92
9. Alper, C. A., Colten, H. R., Gear, J. S. S., Rabson, A. R., Rosen, F. S. 1976. Homozygous human C3 deficiency. The role of C3 in antibody production, C1s-induced vasopermeability, and cobra-venom-induced passive hemolysis. *J. Clin. Invest.* 57:222–29
10. Alper, C. A., Colten, H. R., Rosen, F. S., Rabson, A. R., Macnab, G. M., Gear, J. S. S. 1972. Homozygous deficiency of C3 in a patient with repeated infections. *Lancet* 2:1179–81
11. Ballow, M., Shira, J. E., Harden, L., Yang, S. Y., Day, N. K. 1975. Complete absence of the third component of com-

plement in man. *J. Clin. Invest.* 56:703–10

12. Grace, H. J., Brereton-Stiles, G. G., Vos, G. H., Schonland, M. 1976. A family with total and partial deficiency of complement C3. *S. Afr. Med. J.* 50: 139–40

13. Hsieh, K-H., Lyn, C.-Y., Lee, T.-C. 1981. Complete absence of the third component of complement in a patient with repeated infections. 1981. *Clin. Immunol. Immunopathol.* 20:305–12

14. Rosenfeld, S. I., Baum, J., Steigbigel, R. T., Leddy, J. P. 1976. Hereditary deficiency of the fifth component of complement in man. II. Biological properties of C5-deficient human serum. *J. Clin. Invest.* 57:1635–43

15. Snyderman, R., Durack, D. T., McCarty, G. A., Ward, F. E., Meadows, L. 1979. Deficiency of the fifth component of complement in human subjects. Clinical, genetic, and immunological studies in a large kindred. *Am. J. Med.* 67:638–45

16. Peter, G., Weigert, M. B., Bissel, A. R., Gold, R., Kreutzer, D. McLean, R. H. 1981. Meningococcal meningitis in familial deficiency of the fifth component of complement. *Pediatrics* 67: 882–86

17. Leddy, J. P., Frank, M. M., Gaither, T., Baum, J., Klemperer, M. R. 1974. Hereditary deficiency of the sixth component of complement in man. I. Immunochemical, biologic, and family studies. *J. Clin. Invest.* 53:544–53

18. Petersen, B. H., Graham, J. A., Brooks, G. F. 1976. Human deficiency of the eighth component of complement. The requirement of C8 for serum *Neisseria gonorrhoeae* bactericidal activity. *J. Clin. Invest.* 57:283–90

19. Lee, T. J., Utsinger, P. D., Snyderman, R., Yount, W. J., Sparling, P. F. 1978. Familial deficiency of the seventh component of complement associated with recurrent bacteremic infections due to *Neisseria. J. Infect. Dis.* 138:359–68

20. Petersen, B. H., Lee, T. J., Snyderman, R., Brooks, G. F. 1979. *Neisseria meningitidis* and *Neisseria gonorrhoeae* bacteremia associated with C6, C7, or C8 deficiency. *Ann. Int. Med.* 90: 917–20

Ann. Rev. Med. 1983. 34:55–68

IRON ABSORPTION[1]

Robert W. Charlton, M.D., F.R.C.P., and Thomas H. Bothwell, M.D., D.Sc., F.R.C.P., F.A.C.P. (Hon.)

Joint University/Medical Research Council Iron and Red Cell Metabolism Unit, Department of Medicine, University of the Witwatersrand Medical School, Hospital Street, Johannesburg 2001, South Africa

ABSTRACT

The rate of absorption of iron is adjusted according to body iron requirements, but the virtual absence of heme and the poor bioavailability of the nonheme iron in the diets of many people, especially in developing countries, means that the amount that can be absorbed is limited. Those whose requirements are increased by growth, menstruation, or pregnancy frequently cannot absorb enough. Sufficient is now known about the factors in food that increase or diminish the bioavailability of nonheme iron to permit the effective fortification of dietary staples, although the application of this information has proved difficult particularly in the Third World where nutritional iron deficiency is most prevalent. Effective fortification may lead to iron overload in those whose control of iron absorption is genetically defective, and recent evidence that the HLA-linked recessive gene for idiopathic hemochromatosis may occur much more commonly than hitherto suspected makes it imperative that an effective monitoring system should form a part of every fortification program.

INTRODUCTION

Iron absorption is a complex process beginning with the intake of food and ending with the entry of iron into the plasma. The dietary iron must first be made available for absorption by the processes of digestion. It must then be taken up from the lumen of the gastrointestinal tract by the absorbing epithelial cells, and finally transferred to the plasma. There is a progressive

[1]This work was supported by a grant from the South African Atomic Energy Board.

55

0066-4219/83/0401-0055$02.00

reduction in quantity at each stage: of the approximately 15 mg in the average daily American diet, perhaps half is processed into a soluble form, 3 mg is taken up by the mucosal cells, and 0.9 mg transferred into the plasma by healthy adult males (1). Although small in relation to the total body iron content of 4–5 g, this is sufficient to replace what is lost in exfoliated cells from the skin, the gastrointestinal and urinary tracts. Women need to absorb more iron than men in order to meet the requirements associated with menstruation and childbearing. The median menstrual loss is such that about 1.4 mg per day is required, but in many women it is 2 mg or more (2). During the second and third trimesters of pregnancy the daily requirement is 4–6 mg. Phases of rapid growth and pathologic blood loss also increase the amount that must be absorbed. The absorptive behavior of the intestinal mucosa changes in an attempt to maintain the body iron content at optimal levels, but only a limited proportion of the iron in the diet can be absorbed because of its restricted bioavailability. Absorption from a mixed Western type diet rises to a maximum of 3–4 mg daily when the body is depleted of iron, and falls to less than 0.5 mg daily when iron overload is present (1). In countries such as India, the iron in the average diet is even less bioavailable and the body's ability to step up absorption is thus even more restricted.

When the physiologic needs cannot be met the result is nutritional iron deficiency; it affects particularly the women and children because not only are their requirements greater but their intake of food, and thus of absorbable iron, is less. It is the poor bioavailability of the iron in their diets that is largely responsible for the iron deficiency that afflicts such a large proportion of the world's population. In contrast, ferrous sulfate and other medicinal iron preparations are well absorbed in the fasting state, and indeed acute iron poisoning follows the ingestion of an overdose. When medicinal iron is taken with food, however, its bioavailability is restricted by a variety of ligands that render it unavailable to the receptors in the mucous membrane.

BIOAVAILABILITY OF FOOD IRON

Absorption of iron can be demonstrated to occur in the stomach, the ileum, and the colon, but to only a slight extent in comparison with the duodenum and upper jejunum (3). It follows that if dietary iron is to be absorbed efficiently, it must be in an absorbable form when it passes through the proximal part of the gastrointestinal tract. There is a great deal of variation in the extent to which this can be achieved. A well-absorbed iron compound is heme, present in meat in the form of hemoglobin, myoglobin, and heme enzymes. Heme is absorbed as such, and the iron is freed from the porphyrin ring after it has been taken up from the lumen into the mucosal cell (4). The iron in all the other chemical forms found in food is available for absorption only to the extent to which it ionizes within the lumen. While the bioavailability of the iron in some vegetable foods such as tomato and cauliflower is high, that in important staples such as rice, sorghum, wheat, maize and legumes is poor. It has become clear that a variety of ligands for iron are responsible for these differences in bioavailability. Moreover, the influence of the ligands present in a particular foodstuff is not limited to the iron in that food, but extends to all the nonheme iron that happens to be present at the same time within the lumen of the gastrointestinal tract, whatever its origin. In other words, it is the composition of the meal rather than the chemical nature of the iron within a particular dietary ingredient that determines how much iron can be absorbed. For example, if a rice meal contains sufficient ascorbic acid, perhaps in orange juice drunk during the meal, a much higher proportion of the rice iron can be absorbed; in contrast, if tea is drunk instead of orange juice, the amount of iron absorbed will be even lower than would be the case if the rice were eaten alone (1).

The Common Intraluminal Iron Pools

The development of the concept of intraluminal iron pools has aided understanding (5). Isotopic labeling of food iron has established that, with certain exceptions, all the nonheme iron in a meal exchanges with a common pool of ionized iron, and it is from this pool that absorption takes place. The known exceptions are certain insoluble inorganic compounds such as ferric orthophosphate and ferric oxide that may be present in contaminating dirt, and ferritin, the biological iron storage complex, that only exchanges partially (1, 5). The size of the intraluminal nonheme pool, and hence the quantity of bioavailable nonheme iron, is determined by many factors, including the amount of nonheme iron in the meal, manufacturing processes, cooking, the processes of digestion, and the relative proportions of the diverse iron ligands competing for the ionic iron. The role of some of the more important of these factors has been firmly established. The heme iron in the meal also forms a common pool, but this is not susceptible to ligand binding and is well absorbed, irrespective of the other constituents of the meal.

If the composition of the meal is constant, it is obvious that the size of the pool of ionized iron depends on how much food is eaten. While the iron content of different foods does vary considerably, that of the average mixed Western diet is remarkably constant at about 6 mg iron per 1000 kcal (6). However, significant amounts may be added if iron utensils are used for cooking (7). The iron content of typical diets in other parts of the world may differ significantly from this; nevertheless, it is crucial to appreciate that the composition of the meal is of far greater significance for iron nutrition than the amount of iron. Thus a fourfold variation in the amount of iron absorbed can be achieved without altering the total iron, protein, or calorie content of the meal (8). Relatively little is known about the effects of food processing and cooking on the bioavailability of the iron, but such information as is available suggests that the effects can be considerable. For example, the bioavailability of the iron in rice and in wheat is increased by milling, since factors that inhibit absorption are removed with the husks (5). During the preparation of the indigenous beer of southern Africa, which is made from fermented maize and sorghum, the bioavailability of the iron increases twelvefold (9); this is due to a combination of factors including the elimination of solids, a drop in pH, and the formation of ethanol and lactic acid. If this brewing is done in iron containers, the amount of absorbable iron is increased still further by the very considerable quantities of absorbable iron that may be solubilized as the pH falls (1). On the other hand, processes that reduce the ascorbic acid content, such as baking, significantly diminish the bioavailability (1).

Digestion of the food in the stomach and duodenum clearly plays a vital part in the liberation of ionized iron, and of the diverse ligands for iron in the meal. It is reasonable to suppose that the various digestive enzymes will be significant in this regard, but in fact the only component of the gastrointestinal secretions that has been unequivocally shown to be important is the hydrochloric acid in the gastric juice (10, 11). Various foods have been incubated with gastric juice in vitro; and it has been established that the proportion of nonheme iron solubilized depends on the pH. The proportion solubilized correlates in turn with the amount of iron absorbed when the food is consumed by that individual. Since the ionization of ferric iron in particular is critically dependent on the pH, this relationship is hardly surprising. Achlorhydria therefore has an adverse effect on the bioavailability of the nonheme iron in the diet. The pH of the luminal contents rises with progression from stomach to jejunum, and the absorption rate declines in parallel. The bicarbonate in the duodenal juice is responsible for this rise in pH, so it is obviously a factor also, although direct evidence of this is sparse.

Of crucial importance is the balance between inhibitory and promotory exogenous ligands in determining the bioavailability of the nonheme iron in a meal. This first became apparent when different isotopes were used to label the iron in two foods eaten together. For example, about 20% of the nonheme iron in veal was found to be absorbed when it was consumed alone, but when maize was eaten with the veal, this figure fell to about 10%. In contrast, the absorption of the maize iron, which had been low when it was the only food eaten, doubled to about the same figure as the veal iron (12). As such observations accumulated, it became apparent that the nonheme iron in each dietary ingredient entered a common pool from which absorption took place, and that the iron in this pool was susceptible to inhibitory or promotory influences originating from other foodstuffs (1, 5). Moreover, adding inorganic iron to the meal, for example in the form of ferrous sulfate, resulted in its being absorbed to exactly the same extent as the nonheme food iron in the meal (5, 13). Its bioavailability was clearly also determined by the balance between the various ligands present, and the implications for food fortification programs were immediately apparent.

Effects of Ligands

Some of the ligands in foods have been identified (1, 5). An important promotor of iron absorption is ascorbic acid, which probably acts in two ways: by reducing ferric ions to ferrous ions that are not so vulnerable to a rise in pH, and by forming an absorbable small molecular complex with ferric iron. Other organic acids, such as lactic acid (9), citric, malic, and tartaric (but not oxalic) acids (M. Gillooly, T. H., Bothwell, and R. W. Charlton, in preparation), have a similar effect, and it is their presence in vegetables such as broccoli, beetroot, pumpkin, cauliflower, cabbage, sauerkraut, tomato, and turnip that is responsible for the high bioavailability of the iron in such foods. Another promoting ligand(s) is present in meat and fish, but it is still not entirely clear exactly what it is (5). An amino acid that does promote iron absorption is cysteine, but since it is oxidized to cystine during cooking, it is not certain whether this can be the promotory factor (5, 14).

The iron in many vegetable foods, including cereals, is generally less well absorbed than that in animal foods, and there is mounting evidence that tannins or polyphenols are important in this regard. Tannins form large molecular colored complexes with iron. The absorption of the nonheme iron in soup made from rice, potato, and onion is inhibited when a cup of Indian tea is drunk with it (15). Tea reduces the absorption of iron from a breakfast meal by more than half, whereas orange juice increases it two and a half times (16). Many vegetable foodstuffs contain polyphenols in significant quantities, and it is hardly surprising that only a small fraction of the iron in them is ionizable (17). Such foods as lentils, eggplant, and spinach have a high polyphenol content and their iron is poorly bioavailable (M. Gillooly, T. H. Bothwell, and R. W. Charlton, in preparation). Polyphenol binding of iron can, however, be overcome partially by a promotor of absorption such as ascorbic acid (16).

Another potent inhibitor of nonheme iron absorption is bran (18) and it has been suggested that some factor or factors present in vegetable fiber may have an inhibitory effect on nonheme iron absorption. In this regard it has been shown that the fiber of wheat and maize binds iron (19). However, absorption studies with specific constituents of dietary fiber such as cellulose and pectin yielded negative results (M. Gillooly, T. H., Bothwell, and R. W. Charlton, in preparation) and bran maintains its capacity to inhibit iron absorption even after removal of its phytate content (20, 21). This latter finding is in accord with the observation that monoferric phytate, the major form of iron in bran, is as well absorbed from a mixed meal as ferrous sulfate (22). There is still, however, reason to believe that phytates do exert an inhibitory effect on iron absorption. Both diferric and tetraferric phytate are poorly bioavailable (23), as is the iron in various vegetables with high phytate contents such as wheatgerm, butterbeans, and lentils (M. Gillooly, T. H. Bothwell, and R. W. Charlton, in preparation). A variety of soy products also inhibit the absorption of nonheme iron but whether this is owing to their phytate content is not known (24).

The phosphoprotein in egg yolk is another inhibitor of iron absorption, but the effect of including an egg in the meal is negligible because this is balanced by the increase in the amount of iron ingested (16). Finally, a food additive that reduces the bioavailability of iron is ethylenediamine tetra-acetic acid (EDTA), which is present in significant quantities in a number of foodstuffs as a preservative (25).

It is possible to measure the absorption of heme iron from a meal by adding a small amount of radioactive hemoglobin to label the common pool (26). If a second radioactive isotope of iron is used to tag the nonheme iron in the meal, the total absorption of iron can be assessed. In a six-week study of a group of young men, 17.4 mg of iron were present in the food consumed each day, and only 1 mg of this was in the form of heme (27). Nevertheless, as much as 0.37 mg of the average of 1.16 mg absorbed each day came from the heme fraction of the food iron. In another study, 33% of the iron was in heme, and it contributed 74% of the amount of iron absorbed (28). It is therefore apparent that meat products are of critical importance for iron nutrition even when they form only a small part of the diet: to the highly bioavailable heme they contain must be added their promotory effect on the bioavailability of the nonheme iron in the meal, and the virtual disappearance of meat from the diet of most of the world's population is a major cause of nutritional iron deficiency.

MUCOSAL TRANSPORT OF IRON

The most active site of iron absorption is the duodenum and upper jejunum (3). An important reason for this is the pH of the luminal contents, which rises progressively from about 1 in the stomach to the small intestinal figure of about 8. Very little ferric iron remains once it has risen above 5, and, even if there are no exogenous inhibitory ligands present, the polymeric hydroxides that form render the iron inaccessible to the mucosal cells. In contrast, ferrous ions abound at higher pH values, even up to pH 8, and this is why at a dosage of 30 mg of iron, absorption from a solution of a ferrous salt is about three times that from a solution of a ferric salt (29). However, the luminal pH is not the only reason why the upper small intestine is the major site of iron absorption. Experiments with everted animal gut pouches indicate that duodenal mucous membrane absorbs iron more rapidly than ileal mucous membrane under identical luminal conditions (1), so it is apparent that the mucosal cells in the proximal intestine are partially specialized in this direction.

The absorption of iron by the cells of the intestinal mucosa consists of at least two distinct phases, namely the *uptake* of iron from the lumen into the cells and its *transfer* across the cell into the circulation. In animal experiments, the uptake of iron has been shown to be more rapid than its transfer, and less affected by the amount of absorbable iron ingested and by the body's need for iron (1). That at least two separate and specific processes are involved is confirmed by the existence of two mutant strains of mice, one known as *mk* in which uptake is defective but transfer normal, and the other, *sla,* in which the reverse is the case (30, 31).

The uptake of iron from the lumen into the cells is diminished by anoxia and by a number of metabolic inhibitors (32). The first step is a process of binding to specific receptors on the brush borders of mucosal cells from the proximal (but not the distal) small intestine. Iron is bound preferentially over metals such as cobalt and manganese (33), and, although the process is temperature dependent, it is not affected by anoxia (34). It therefore seems that it is the movement of iron across the cell membrane rather than the initial binding that requires metabolic energy.

Uptake can be varied according to the body's need for iron. This has been shown in animal studies both in vivo and in vitro, and also with specimens of human duodenal mucosa obtained by biopsy (35), and there is evidence that the adjustment is achieved at least partly by altering the number of the specific iron receptors (34).

A proportion of the iron entering the mucosal cells is transferred to the portal circulation within minutes. Transfer continues at a much slower rate for 12 to 24 hours, but some of the iron is stored as ferritin and is eventually discarded when the mucosal cell exfoliates (36, 37). The relative proportions following these alternative pathways depend on the requirement for iron, transfer being enhanced when iron deficiency is present and ferritin formation being maximal when the body is replete with iron. The carrier transporting iron through mucosal cells has been identified as a protein similar to, but not identical with, plasma transferrin (38), and the ratio between this transport protein and the storage protein ferritin alters according to whether more iron is to be transferred or excluded (39).

CONTROL OF IRON ABSORPTION

The amount of iron absorbed at any one time is dependent on the amount of bioavailable iron ingested. However, it is also influenced to a considerable extent by the body's need for iron. If the body iron content is diminished, a high percentage of the available dietary iron is absorbed, and as the content rises the percentage absorption falls. This has been firmly established in a number of human as well as animal studies (1, 40–42). If the body iron content falls to the point where the synthesis of functional iron-containing compounds such as hemoglobin is compromised, the percentage absorption rises further in proportion to the severity of the anemia (43).

In acute experiments in animals it has also been possible to show a direct relationship between iron absorption and the rate of erythropoiesis (44), but in chronic hemolytic states in man the absorption rate is usually normal (1). However, in those anemias, such as thalassemia major, in which erythropoiesis is markedly ineffective, iron absorption is inappropriately high (45). Why this should be so is not known.

While the rate of absorption has been shown to vary predictably in certain circumstances, the way in which the alteration in mucosal behavior is induced has not been elucidated. Attempts to demonstrate that the plasma iron transport system regulates iron absorption have been unsuccessful, as have those involving a search for some humoral controlling mechanism (46). Perhaps the most plausible of current hypotheses is that the iron content of individual tissues is itself a regulating factor (47). A labile pool of iron available to transferrin is assumed to be present in all body tissues, the size of the pool in each tissue being proportional to that tissue's iron stores. Iron uptake from transferrin is determined by the requirements of the erythroid marrow, and each tissue supplies iron to transferrin in proportion to its iron pool. Thus a decrease in tissue iron content results in an increased entrance of iron from the gut, while an acute rise in plasma iron turnover due to enhanced erythropoietic activity also results in increased iron absorption. Recent experimental evidence supporting the hypothesis has been obtained in rats (47, 48). When the requirement for transferrin iron was increased by the exchange transfusion of blood containing many reticulocytes, there was a rapid increase in the rate of delivery of iron from the tissues including the intestinal mucosa. The increase in iron absorption was not mediated by a decrease in plasma iron or an increase in the unsaturated iron binding capacity of transferrin. These findings suggest that iron turnover through the plasma is primarily determined by the number of tissue receptors for transferrin iron, and that the amount of iron supplied by each donor tissue, including the intestinal mucosa, is dependent on the output from other donor tissues. While the nature of the mechanism by

which donor tissue output of iron is regulated to match changing requirements is not known, it has been proposed that the donation of iron by
transferrin in some way immediately facilitates its procurement of more
iron (48).

DISTURBANCES OF IRON BALANCE

Iron Deficiency

In spite of the capacity of the specialized absorption apparatus for adaptive
expansion, the poor bioavailability of the iron in most diets limits the
amount that can be obtained so that by far the commonest disturbance of
iron balance is iron deficiency (49).

Infancy is a stage of life during which rapid growth creates a considerable
need for iron that cannot be met from the unsupplemented diet (1). Normally enough iron has been transferred from the mother to the fetus to last
until the infant is weaned, but the premature neonate starts out with an
undersupply and the increase in his body mass is greater; without supplementation, iron deficiency is inevitable. After weaning, the nature of the
diet is critical, but it is seldom that an unsupplemented diet will be adequate
up to the age of two years. The requirements created by the subsequent
slower rate of growth can usually be met, and the next phase of risk is
adolescence, particularly in girls where the growth spurt is accompanied by
the menarche. After menstruation is established the median loss expressed
in terms of daily iron balance is about 0.45 mg, and to this must be added
the 0.8–0.9 mg obligatory loss from skin, gastrointestinal and urinary tracts
(50) and then up to 0.45 mg for growth. The normally healthy appetite of
adolescence increases the food and thus the iron intake, and should permit
the absorption of this amount from a good mixed diet, but figure-conscious-
ness and faddish food selection may make it impossible.

Once adulthood is reached, most *women* can absorb enough from a diet
that is moderately good in iron nutritional terms not to develop iron deficiency anemia, although they will have only a small reserve of iron stored
in the tissues. The average in American women is about 300 mg (51). In
many women menstrual losses are naturally greater than the median, and
the daily iron requirement is more than 2 mg in over 10% of subjects (2);
only an optimal unsupplemented diet can permit the absorption of these
larger amounts, and in most developing countries the predominantly cereal
food intake and the resultant poor bioavailability of the dietary iron proves
inadequate. Nutritional iron deficiency is thus much commoner than in the
industrialized countries. The prevention of iron deficiency in such communities by iron fortification is not easy, since the added iron is as poorly
absorbed as the intrinsic iron present in the diet (49).

Pregnancy creates an additional iron requirement (1). Not only must obligatory daily losses be met, but about 500 mg must be found for the fetus and placenta and for blood loss at delivery, and a further 450 mg must be deployed in expanding the maternal red cell mass. The main burden is felt during the second and third trimesters, when 4–6 mg per day must be absorbed, and this cannot be done unless the diet is supplemented. Even if there is some reserve of iron to be mobilized, anemia usually develops if extra iron is not given.

In contrast, the healthy adult *male* needs to absorb only 0.9 mg per day to stay in balance, and can probably achieve this even if his diet contains little bioavailable iron. The situation in *women after the menopause* is similar. It follows that iron deficiency in such subjects is nearly always of pathologic rather than nutritional origin, and a search must be made for the cause (1). An increased requirement for iron due to blood loss is by far the commonest reason, and if there has been no overt hemorrhage or blood donation, occult bleeding from the gastrointestinal tract due to lesions such as peptic ulceration or carcinoma, or to the chronic use of drugs such as aspirin, is usually responsible. In tropical countries, hookworm infestation is an important cause. Malabsorption of iron can also lead to iron deficiency, but it is much less commonly encountered than hemorrhage. It may follow subtotal gastrectomy, which interferes with food iron absorption because of accelerated passage past the optimal area for iron uptake and because of the reduction in HCl secretion, although in some patients bleeding from stomal ulceration is the main factor. Iron absorption is also impaired in gluten-induced enteropathy and in tropical sprue, because the total absorbing area is reduced by the stunting of the villi.

Iron Overload

The opposite disturbance of iron balance, iron overload, is very much rarer than iron deficiency. It may be due to excessive amounts of absorbable iron in the diet, to disordered control of iron absorption, or to the repeated transfusion of blood for nonhemorrhagic anemias (1). Sometimes the iron has entered by both routes, as may be the case in thalassemia major. In southern Africa, moderate to severe iron overload due solely to the prolonged consumption of a home-brewed beer containing amounts of iron several-fold greater than that in normal diets occurs commonly (52). This unique form of iron overload is not due only to the increased dietary iron content, but also to the fact that it is highly bioavailable. This can be ascribed to the low pH of the drink, its lactic acid and alcohol contents, and to the reduction in solids that occurs during brewing (9). Diets containing the 50–150 mg of absorbable iron needed to cause significant iron loading in subjects with normal control of the absorptive rate are seldom, if ever, encountered elsewhere.

The genetic disease idiopathic hemochromatosis results from inappropriately increased iron absorption from a diet of normal iron content. The tendency to absorb excessive iron is transmitted by an autosomal recessive gene located in close proximity to the super-gene for HLA on the short arm of chromosome 6 (53, 54). Its expression in homozygous individuals depends on the amount of bioavailable iron in the habitual diet, since it is only if enough iron can be absorbed that the disease is recognized. The amount of iron lost from the body is clearly also relevant, and females are thus relatively protected by menstruation; if they develop the pathologic and clinical consequences, it is at a later average age than men do. Even in men the full-blown clinical disease is one of middle age, because the net iron gain in subjects consuming the average Western diet is only about 1–2 mg per day. Many years must therefore elapse before the 15–30 g of iron found in the tissues of symptomatic individuals has been accumulated.

The fact that only a proportion of homozygous individuals develop severe iron overload means that estimates of the frequency of the HLA-linked iron-loading gene based solely on the prevalence of the clinical disease are misleadingly low. In studies carried out in Brittany (55) and in Utah (56) the heterozygote carriers of the iron-loading gene were identified by combining the HLA typing of relatives of fully affected subjects with evidence of abnormal iron metabolism obtained by measuring their plasma iron and ferritin concentrations. As many as 8.4% and 10% were considered to be heterozygote carriers, yielding calculated homozygote frequencies of 1 in 319 and 1 in 400. While these figures may be falsely high because of biased ascertainment, they are strikingly similar, and certainly suggest that the gene occurs much more commonly than has hitherto been suspected. If this is indeed the case, it has implications for proposals to combat nutritional iron deficiency by dietary fortification, or by increasing the level of fortification in countries such as the USA that already have fortified flour (49, 57). Any such move must lead to the earlier presentation of the clinical disease in some homozygotes, and to its development in others who would not otherwise have accumulated toxic levels of iron (57). The possibility that some heterozygotes might also absorb enough unneeded iron to produce adverse effects has been raised, but the available evidence suggests that this is unlikely (56, 58).

In attempting to assess the seriousness of the danger it should be noted that significant iron overload is currently only seldom seen in the United States. None of the plasma ferritin concentrations of more than 3000 apparently normal individuals in the Seattle, Washington, area was anywhere near the values found in symptomatic hemochromatosis (59). In a comprehensive review the prevalence of the fully developed disease was estimated to be 1 in 20,000 hospital admissons and 1 in 7000 deaths (1). If the bioavailable iron content of the diet were increased, however, it would clearly be essential to monitor on a continuing basis the plasma ferritin and plasma iron concentrations of a selection of subjects shown by HLA typing to be homozygous for the iron-loading gene, and a group of heterozygous carriers, as well as an adequate sample of the population at large. It is to be hoped that such information will become available before long from Sweden, which for a number of years has had the highest level of iron fortification in the world and where ascorbic acid and iron tablets are consumed widely (47).

Literature Cited

1. Bothwell, T. H., Charlton, R. W., Cook, J. D., Finch, C. A. 1979. *Iron Metabolism in Man,* Oxford, England: Blackwell. 576 pp.
2. Hallberg, L., Hogdahl., A.-M., Nilsson, L., Rybo, G. 1966. Menstrual blood loss —a population study. Variation at different ages and attempts to define normality. *Acta Obstet. Gynecol. Scand.* 45:320–51
3. Wheby, M. S. 1970. Site of iron absorption in man. *Scand. J. Haematol.* 7:56–62
4. Raffin, S. B., Woo, C. H., Roost, K. T., Price, D. C., Schmid, R. 1974. Intestinal absorption of hemoglobin iron-heme cleavage by mucosal heme oxygenase. *J. Clin. Invest.* 54:1344–52
5. Hallberg, L. 1981. Bioavailability of dietary iron in man. *Ann. Rev. Nutr.* 1:123–47
6. US Dept. Health, Educ., Welfare Publ. No. 72–8131. 1972. *Ten States Nutrition Survey.* Washington, DC: GPO
7. Moore, C. F. 1965. Iron nutrition and requirements. *Scand. J. Haematol. Ser. Haematol.* 6:1–14
8. Monsen, E. R., Hallberg, L., Layrisse, M., Hegsted, D. M., Cook, J. D., Mertz, W., Finch, C. A. 1978. Estimation of available dietary iron. *Am. J. Clin. Nutr.* 31:134–41
9. Derman, D. P., Bothwell, T. H., Torrance, J. D., Bezwoda, W. R., MacPhail, A. P., Kew, M. C., Sayers, M. H., Disler, P. B., Charlton, R. W. 1980. Iron absorption from maize (*Zea mays*) and sorghum (*Sorghum vulgare*) beer. *Br. J. Nutr.* 43:271–79
10. Bezwoda, W., Charlton, R., Bothwell, T., Torrance, J., Mayet, F. 1978. The importance of gastric hydrochloric acid

in the absorption of non-heme food iron. *J. Lab. Clin. Med.* 92:108–16
11. Lock, S., Bender, A. E. 1980. Measurement of chemically-available iron in foods by incubation with human gastric juice in vitro. *Br. J. Nutr.* 43:413–20
12. Layrisse, M., Martinez-Torres, C., Roche, M. 1968. The effect of interaction of various foods on iron absorption. *Am. J. Clin. Nutr.* 21:1175–83
13. Cook, J. D., Minnich, V., Moore, C. V., Rasmussen, A., Bradley, W. B., Finch, C. A. 1973. Absorption of fortification iron in bread. *Am. J. Clin. Nutr.* 26:861–72
14. Martinez-Torres, C., Romano, E., Layrisse, M. 1981. Effect of cysteine on iron absorption in man. *Am. J. Clin. Nutr.* 34:322–27
15. Disler, P. B., Lynch, S. R., Charlton, R. W., Torrance, J. D., Bothwell, T. H. 1975. The effect of tea on iron absorption. *Gut* 16:193–200
16. Rossander, L., Hallberg, L., Björn-Rasmussen, E. 1979. Absorption of iron from breakfast meals. *Am. J. Clin. Nutr.* 32:2482–89
17. Narasinga Rao, B. S., Prabharathi, T. 1982. Tannin content of foods commonly consumed in India and its influence on ionisable iron. *J. Sci. Food Agric.* 33: In press
18. Björn-Rasmussen, E. 1974. Iron absorption from wheat bread. Influence of various amounts of bran. *Nutr. Metabol.* 16:101–10
19. Rheinhold, J. G., Garcia, J. S., Garzon, P. 1981. Binding of iron by fiber of wheat and maize. *Am. J. Clin. Nutr.* 34:1384–91
20. Morris, E. R., Simpson, K. M., Cook, J. D. 1980. Dephytinized vs. non dephyti-

nized wheat bran and iron absorption in man. *Am. J. Clin. Nutr.* 33:941

21. Simpson, K. M., Morris, E. R., Cook, J. D. 1981. The inhibitory effect of bran on iron absorption in man. *Am. J. Clin. Nutr.* 34:1469–78

22. Lipschitz, D. A., Simpson, K. M., Cook, J. D., Morris, E. R. 1979. Absorption of mono-ferric phytate by dogs. *J. Nutr.* 109:1154–60

23. Ellis, R., Morris, E. R. 1979. Effect of sodium phytate on stability of monoferric phytate complex and the bioavailability of the iron to rats. *Nutr. Rep. Int.* 20:739–47

24. Cook, J. D., Morck, T. A., Lynch, S. R. 1981. The inhibitory effect of soy products on non-heme iron absorption in man. *Am. J. Clin. Nutr.* 34:2622–29

25. Cook, J. D., Monsen, E. F. 1976. Food iron absorption in man. II. The effect of EDTA on absorption of dietary nonheme iron. *Am. J. Clin. Nutr.* 29:614–20

26. Martinez-Torres, C., Layrisse, M. 1971. Iron absorption from veal muscle. *Am. J. Clin. Nutr.* 24:531–40

27. Björn-Rasmussen, E., Hallberg, L., Isaksson, B., Arvidsson, B. 1974. Food iron absorption in man. Applications of the two-pool extrinsic tag method to measure heme and non-heme iron absorption from the whole diet. *J. Clin. Invest.* 53:247–55

28. Layrisse, M., Martinez-Torres, C. 1972. Model for measuring dietary absorption of heme iron: test with a complete meal. *Am. J. Clin. Nutr.* 25:401–11

29. Brise, H., Hallberg, L. 1962. Absorbability of different iron compounds. *Acta Med. Scand.* 171(Suppl. 376):23–38

30. Edwards, J. A., Hoke, J. E. 1972. Defect of intestinal mucosal iron uptake in mice with hereditary microcytic anemia. *Proc. Soc. Exp. Biol. Med.* 141:81–84

31. Edwards, J. A., Bannerman, R. M. 1970. Hereditary defect of intestinal iron transport in mice with sex-linked anemia. *J. Clin. Invest.* 49:1869–71

32. Dowdle, E. B., Schachter, D., Shenker, H. 1960. Active transport of ^{59}Fe by everted segments of rat duodenum. *Am. J. Physiol.* 198:609–13

33. Huebers, H., Huebers, E., Forth, W., Leopold, G., Rummel, W. 1971. Binding of iron and other metals in brush borders of jejunum and ileum of the rat in vitro. *Acta Pharm. Toxicol.* 29(Suppl. 4):22–27

34. Greenberger, N. J., Balcerzak, S. P., Ackerman, G. A. 1969. Iron uptake by isolated brush borders: changes induced by alterations in iron stores. *J. Lab. Clin. Med.* 73:711–21

35. Cox, T. M., Peters, T. J. 1980. Cellular mechanisms in the regulation of iron absorption by the human intestine: studies in patients with iron deficiency before and after treatment. *Br. J. Haematol.* 44:75–86

36. Conrad, M. E., Crosby, W. H. 1963. Intestinal mucosal mechanisms controlling iron absorption. *Blood* 22:406–15

37. Charlton, R. W., Jacobs, P., Torrance, J. D., Bothwell, T. H. 1962. The role of ferritin in iron absorption. *Lancet* 2:762–64

38. Pollack, S., Lasky, F. D. 1976. A new iron-binding protein isolated from intestinal mucosa. *J. Lab. Clin. Med.* 87:670–79

39. Savin, M. A., Cook, J. D. 1980. Mucosal iron transport by rat intestine. *Blood* 56:1029–35

40. Pirzio-Biroli, G., Finch, C. A. 1960. Iron absorption. III. The influence of the iron stores on iron absorption in the normal subject. *J. Lab. Clin. Med.* 55:216–20

41. Bezwoda, W. R., Bothwell, T. H., Torrance, J. D., MacPhail, A. P., Charlton, R. W., Kay, B., Levin, J. 1979. The relationship between marrow iron stores, plasma ferritin concentrations and iron absorption. *Scand. J. Haematol.* 22:113–20

42. Cook, J. D., Lipschitz, D. A., Miles, L. E. M., Finch, C. A. 1974. Serum ferritin as a measure of iron stores in normal subjects. *Am. J. Clin. Nutr.* 27:681–87

43. Norrby, A., Solvell, L. 1974. Iron absorption and haemoglobin regeneration in posthaemorrhagic anaemia—studies on the absorption pattern during oral iron therapy. *Scand. J. Haematol. Suppl.* 20:75–106

44. Bothwell, T. H., Pirzio-Biroli, G., Finch, C. A. 1958. Iron absorption. I. Factors influencing absorption. *J. Lab. Clin. Med.* 51:24–36

45. Heinrich, H. C., Gabbe, E. E., Oppitz, K. H., Whang, D. H., Gotze, Ch. B., Schafer, K. H., Schroter, W., Pfau, A. A. 1973. Absorption of inorganic and food iron in children with heterozygous and homozygous beta thalassemia. *Z. Kinderheilkd.* 115:1–22

46. Rosenmund, A., Gerber, S., Huebers, H., Finch, C. 1980. Regulation of iron absorption and storage iron turnover. *Blood* 56:30–37

47. Cavill, I., Worwood, M., Jacobs, A.

68   CHARLTON & BOTHWELL

1975. Internal regulation of iron absorption. *Nature* 256:328–29
48. Finch, C. A., Huebers, H., Eng, M., Miller, L. 1982. Effect of transfused reticulocytes on iron exchange. *Blood* 59:364–69
49. Bothwell, T. H., Charlton, R. W. 1982. A general approach to the problems of iron deficiency and iron overload in the population at large. *Semin. Haematol.* 19:54–67
50. Green, R., Charlton, R. W., Seftel, H., Bothwell, T., Mayet, F., Adams, B., Finch, C., Layrisse, M. 1968. Body iron excretion in man. A collaborative study. *Am. J. Med.* 45:336–53
51. Finch, C. A., Monsen, E. R. 1972. Iron nutrition and the fortification of food with iron. *J. Am. Med. Assoc.* 219:1462–65
52. Charlton, R. W., Bothwell, T. H., Seftel, H. C. 1973. Dietary iron overload. In *Clinics in Haematology,* ed. S. T. Callender. London: Saunders
53. Simon, M., Bourel, M., Genetet, B., Fauchet, R. 1977. Idiopathic hemochromatosis. Demonstration of recessive transmission and early detection by family HLA typing. *N. Engl. J. Med.* 297:1017–21
54. Kravitz, K., Skolnick, M., Cannings, C., Carmelli, D., Baty, B., Amos, B.,

Johnson, A., Mendel, N., Edwards, C., Cartwright, G. 1979. Genetic linkage between hereditary hemochromatosis and HLA. *Am. J. Hum. Genet.* 31:601–19
55. Beaumont, C., Simon, M., Fauchet, R., Hespel, J. P., Brissot, P., Benet, B., Bourel, M. 1979. Serum ferritin as a possible marker of the hemochromatosis allele. *N. Engl. J. Med.* 301:169–79
56. Cartwright, G. E., Edwards, C. Q., Kravitz, K., Skolnick, M., Amos, D. B., Johnson, A., Buskjaer, L. 1979. Hereditary hemochromatosis. Phenotypic expression of the disease. *N. Engl. J. Med.* 301:175–79
57. Bothwell, T. H., Derman, D., Bezwoda, W. R., Torrance, J. D., Charlton, R. W. 1978. Can iron fortification of flour cause damage to genetic susceptibles (idiopathic haemochromatosis and β-thalassaemia major)? *Human Gen. Suppl.* 1:403–10
58. Bassett, M. L., Halliday, J. W., Powell, L. W. 1981. HLA typing in idiopathic hemochromatosis: distinction between homozygotes and heterozygotes with biochemical expression. *Hepatology* 1:120–26
59. Cook, J. D., Finch, C. A., Smith, N. 1976. Evaluation of the iron status of a population. *Blood* 48:449–55

Ann. Rev. Med. 1983. 34:69–89
Copyright © 1983 by Annual Reviews Inc. All rights reserved

APPLICATIONS AND LIMITATIONS OF HEMAPHERESIS

Arthur J. Silvergleid, M.D.

Blood Bank of San Bernardino-Riverside Counties, PO Box 5729, San Bernardino, California 92412-5729; and Department of Medicine, University of California School of Medicine, 10833 Le Conte, Los Angeles, California 90024

ABSTRACT

Hemapheresis is the selective collection of any blood component. With the use of automated equipment, hemapheresis has become practical both for procuring specific components for transfusion and for removing specific components considered pathogenic factors in clinical disease. This review considers all aspects of hemapheresis, including its role in blood component procurement and its potential therapeutic applications. Attention is focused on the clinical indications for the use of apheresis-harvested components, and on the rationale for the effectiveness of therapeutic cytapheresis and plasma exchange.

INTRODUCTION

Clinical support for patients requiring blood products has improved dramatically over the past 40 years. Although large-scale blood banking really only began in the 1940s, in response to the increased need for plasma and whole blood occasioned by the second world war, significant technological advances characterize each of the succeeding decades. In the 1950s, blood component therapy became practical, as a result of the development of plastic blood containers; in the 1960s, wide-scale availability of such components as cryoprecipitate and platelet concentrates enabled clinicians to expand therapeutic horizons for patients with hemostatic disturbances and malignant disease; and in the 1970s large-scale collection of single donor platelets, granulocytes, and plasma became technically feasible. The technology of the 1970s, developed primarily for blood component procurement, may well provide the most significant contribution of blood banking to the 1980s as well. For already, blood bankers have begun en masse to

69

take their hemapheresis equipment out of the blood bank and into the hospital, to the bedside of patients with a myriad of diseases, aggressively to "treat" such patients via a wholesale removal (and/or partial exchange) of presumptive etiologic factors, including pathologic cells, antibody, or immune complexes. Unfortunately, much of this has been done without the kind of rigorous controls that are necessary in order most accurately to assess this new treatment modality. Thus, although the list of conditions treated by hemapheresis is prodigious, the list of conditions that are clearly responsive to this kind of therapeutic maneuver is considerably smaller. Although the bulk of the recent literature concerns itself with hemapheresis as a therapeutic maneuver, this review concentrates on all aspects of hemapheresis, including its role in blood component procurement and its potential therapeutic applications.

TERMINOLOGY

The most appropriate general term for the process of selective collection of any blood component is "hemapheresis." This may be shortened to "apheresis," which most closely resembles the Greek "apairesos" and the Latin "aphairesis" (meaning "to take away") from which it derives. Use of the term "pheresis" is discouraged. When a particular cellular constituent is harvested by apheresis, the procedure is named accordingly; i.e. "lymphocytapheresis" (or "lymphapheresis"), "leukapheresis" (or "granulocytapheresis"), and "erythrocytapheresis." Unfortunately "plateletpheresis" has been in common usage for so long that it is unlikely that "thrombocytapheresis," or "plateletapheresis" will ever succeed in replacing it. Plasma procurement via apheresis is most properly referred to as "plasmapheresis." This term is also quite commonly applied to the therapeutic removal of large volumes of plasma, although "plasma exchange" much more accurately reflects the intent and result of such therapeutic intervention.

TECHNOLOGY

In mid 1982, as this is written, there are three different pieces of equipment designed for on-line cell and/or plasma separation, procurement or removal: Haemonetics' Model 30 (Haemonetics Corp., Braintree, Mass.), IBM's 2997 (IBM Biomedical Systems, Princeton, New Jersey), and Fenwal's CS3000 (Fenwal Laboratories, Deerfield, Illinois). All three are designed to create an interface between different constituents of the blood based on the differential effect of centrifugation, and to effect collection and/or removal of the desired component based on harvesting at that interface, but the technology, advantages, and disadvantages of each are sufficiently unique so as to deserve a brief review.

The Haemonetics Model 30, the first heavily marketed cell separator, relies on a disposable (Latham) bowl in which separation occurs, and component harvesting is an operator-dependent function, based on visual appraisal of the interface level. It is also a discontinuous, or intermittent, procedure that depends upon a certain number of passes, or runs, during which blood is withdrawn, separated, and the desired component harvested. After each pass, residual plasma and red blood cells are combined and returned to the donor. The advantages of the Model 30 are the relatively low initial cost, its portability, the simplicity of the principle upon which it operates, and the fact that as a discontinuous procedure it can be performed entirely through one venipuncture, if necessary. The disadvantages have mainly to do with the discontinuous nature of the procedure, which necessitates larger extracorporeal volumes and a greater frequency of reactions to the rapid infusion of citrate and blood cooled to ambient temperature.

Both the IBM 2997 and the Fenwal CS3000 are based on continuous flow, which gives them the advantage of requiring a much smaller and better tolerated extracorporeal volume. In addition, the IBM is partially, and the Fenwal almost completely, automated and therefore less dependent upon operator judgment. One further advantage for the Fenwal CS3000 is the fact that it does not rely upon a rotating seal and is, in effect, a closed collection system. This may ultimately impact on the storage duration (currently limited to 24 hours) of components harvested with it. Neither machine is easily transportable (from blood center to hospital), and two venipunctures are mandated by the continuous nature of the procedure.

APHERESIS FOR COMPONENT PROCUREMENT

Cell separators were developed in the mid to late 1960s primarily to give clinicians access to large numbers of viable and functional granulocytes and platelets for the interim management of patients with chemotherapy- or radiotherapy-induced bone marrow hypoplasia and cytopenias. With currently available technology it is possible to collect single donor platelets, granulocytes, lymphocytes, young erythrocytes ("neocytes"), and hyperimmune plasma.

Platelets

Single donor platelets are primarily indicated for the thrombocytopenic patient who has become allosensitized and, as a consequence, refractory to random donor platelets. HLA-compatible donors can, in the course of a 1½–2-hour run on a cell separator donate approximately 4–6 $\times$ 10^{11} platelets, which is roughly equivalent to six to eight platelet concentrates. Numerous studies document the value of apheresis-harvested platelets in this setting (1). In addition, allosensitized (refractory) patients who undergo a clinical remission associated with normalization of hematologic parameters may donate platelets via apheresis so that they may be frozen for future autologous use when their almost inevitable relapse occurs.

In isoimmune neonatal thrombocytopenic purpura, an infant is thrombocytopenic because of the presence in its bloodstream of maternal IgG antibodies directed against a very common platelet antigen (e.g. Pl[A1]) present on the infant's but lacking on the mother's platelets. In this setting, it is possible to combine an exchange transfusion on the infant (to lower the antibody titer) with a transfusion of washed, apheresis-harvested Pl[A1]-negative maternal platelets, and effect a rapid cure of the thrombocytopenia. In some communities platelets are routinely collected via apheresis as a means of inventory management, although this may be a questionable indication for this procedure. Finally, there is support for the notion of transfusing chronically thrombocytopenic patients with only single donor platelets (ABO matched) from the outset of their support program, in an effort to decrease exposure to hepatitis, and possibly to delay a broad allosensitization, although the evidence for the latter is not very convincing at present.

Granulocytes

Large numbers ($1-3 \times 10^{10}$) of single donor granulocytes may be harvested via apheresis, in the presence of a rouleauxing agent (generally hydroxyethyl starch, HES), from a donor who has been premedicated with steroids. Such granulocyte concentrates are indicated for the management of patients who are severely neutropenic ($\leq$ 200 absolute PMNs/μl), septic (preferably with a documented organism), unresponsive to a 24–48-hour trial of appropriate antibiotics, and who, in addition, have a realistic opportunity for early return of bone marrow function. Granulocyte concentrates are generally given daily until there is clear-cut evidence of resolution of the infection, or a return of autologous granulocytes. Granulocyte transfusions are not without significant risk (or potential morbidity). It is primarily because of this risk, the expense, improvements in medical management of severe infections, and the fact that 60–80% of severely neutropenic, infected patients will survive without granulocytes that the indications for their use are becoming more circumscribed, and it is likely that this trend will continue.

Neocytes

In an effort to decrease the severity of the inevitable hemochromatosis and hemosiderosis that complicate the long-term management of patients with congenital transfusion-dependent anemias (e.g. thalassemia major, sickle cell anemia), techniques have been developed whereby reticulocyte-rich preparations of erythrocytes ("neocytes") might be harvested via apheresis (2). These longer-lived red blood cells may decrease the frequency of transfusions and thereby decrease the iron load the patient is required to handle. There is also the theoretical potential for performing apheresis in order to remove older erythrocytes ("gerocytes") from patients to whom neocytes are to be given. Neocytes have also been used therapeutically, when coupled with plasma exchange, for patients who have porphyria syndromes (see below). Although neocytes are theoretically useful, they are far too expensive when harvested via apheresis and it is likely that other less expensive techniques, some of which have already been described in preliminary fashion (3), will assume greater importance in the collection of neocytes in the next few years.

Lymphocytes

Lymphocytes may be harvested via apheresis, although as yet there is no clinical application for them. However, large numbers of lymphocytes may be useful for the elaboration of lymphokines, the generation of interferon, and possibly for hybridization to human myeloma cell lines for the production of monoclonal antibodies.

Stem Cells

Cytapheresis techniques can take advantage of the fact that pluri-potential stem cells are normally found in the peripheral blood, and therefore are available for harvesting. In CML patients, where granulocyte/monocyte precursors (CFU-c) occur in even greater than normal concentration, these cells were harvested from patients in the chronic phase of the disease, frozen, and stored until blast crisis supervened. At this point they were reinfused (after the patient had received marrow ablative chemotherapy) reestablishing the marrow pattern of the chronic phase of the disease once again (4). It is not clear, however, that this approach can delay the onset of another blastic phase, or whether it can be repeated. Of perhaps greater interest and significance is the potential harvesting of stem cells from patients with solid tumors, in whom the possibility of delivering more aggressive, potentially curative chemotherapy is enhanced by virtue of being able to reconstitute their bone marrows after chemotherapy with previously harvested and frozen, stored stem cells.

Plasma Products

Plasmapheresis is a useful and efficient method for generating large volumes of plasma, which may have value as diagnostic reagents (because of the presence of a useful antibody or other serologic marker) or as therapeutic reagents (as a source of hyperimmune plasma versus hepatitis virus, Vari-cella-Zoster virus, etc). Certainly the plasma fractionation industry relies heavily upon plasmapheresis for the generation of sufficient source plasma for production of gamma globulin, plasma protein fraction (PPF), albumin, and high-potency clotting concentrates.

THERAPEUTIC CYTAPHERESIS

Pathologic conditions associated with cellular proliferation (and/or pro-longed survival of abnormal cells) lend themselves well to therapeutic inter-vention via cytapheresis techniques. Rapid cytoreduction is easily achieved with cell separators, often alleviating potentially life-threatening situations either through the abrupt lowering of the cell count by itself, or by allowing for an exchange of abnormal cells for normal cells. While the efficacy of apheresis in achieving prompt cytoreduction is unquestioned, the evidence is less convincing that cytapheresis, by itself, represents adequate manage-ment of the more chronic myelo- or lymphoproliferative disorders. Cyta-pheresis has been attempted and reported on for all of the cell lines: platelets, leukocytes, lymphocytes, and erythrocytes, each of which is briefly discussed below.

Plateletpheresis

Therapeutic cytapheresis for thrombocytosis is indicated only in those situ-ations associated with potentially life-threatening thrombotic or hemor-rhagic complications. Cytapheresis can acutely decrease the platelet count by as much as 30–50%, depending upon the amount of blood processed. In one series of five patients, all of whom had platelet counts in excess of $1 \times 10^6/\mu l$, and all of whom were symptomatic (including symptoms of cerebral ischemia, pulmonary embolism, angina pectoris, and gastrointesti-nal bleeding), a mean reduction in platelet count of 52%, as well as prompt relief of symptoms, was achieved with a single cytapheresis procedure (5). In those patients, 2–6 procedures were required over approximately 1–3 weeks in order to keep the platelet counts low until cytotoxic chemotherapy began to have a noticeable impact.

Long-term plateletpheresis has had mixed results in several patients with chronic thrombocytosis (6). While an adequate response was obtained with each procedure, an unacceptably high frequency of procedures was required in order to maintain the platelet count at a safe level. It thus appears that patients with chronically elevated platelet counts are more efficiently managed with chemotherapy than with repeated cytapheresis.

In summary, plateletpheresis is an excellent approach for the patient symptomatic from thrombocytosis. It can abruptly lower the platelet count, relieve symptoms, and allow time for more definitive intervention (e.g. chemotherapy) to achieve a more sustained effect. Repeated plateletpheresis is not useful or indicated for patients who are chronically thrombocytotic, nor does it appear at present to be indicated prophylactically in patients who are thrombocytotic yet asymptomatic.

Leukapheresis

The role of leukapheresis in the management of patients with myeloproliferative diseases is analogous to that of plateletpheresis. There is good documentation of the beneficial effects of rapid cytoreduction (via apheresis) in symptomatic patients with acute (AML) or chronic (CML) myelogenous leukemia with hyperleukocytic leukostasis (7). This syndrome, a hyperviscosity syndrome caused by large numbers (usually $\geq$ 50,000) of poorly deformable blast cells in the circulation, which may present with papilledema, pulmonary edema, or other neurologic symptoms, has been quite responsive to intensive leukapheresis. Unfortunately, long-term management of patients with acute or chronic myeloproliferative diseases using cytapheresis as the sole modality of treatment has been neither successful, nor practical. Since cytapheresis cannot completely eliminate a malignant clone, it is easy to understand its failure to alter significantly the natural history of those myeloproliferative disorders in which it has been tried as the primary mode of therapy. Leukapheresis is successful at lowering white blood cell counts, and, when rouleauxing agents (HES) are used to increase the efficiency of the separation, one can achieve approximately a 30% reduction in granulocyte count after a single procedure. If repeated intensive procedures are performed, it is possible to achieve an 80% decrease in total white blood cell count, diminish organomegaly, decrease symptoms such as fever and malaise, and reduce the risk of uric-acid-related problems.

Several groups have reported treating patients with CML with repeated leukapheresis as the only mode of therapy (8, 9). Although these groups have reported comparable survival to patients treated with conventional chemotherapy, they were unable to obtain a bone marrow remission or to delay the onset of blast crisis. Thus, it is hard to justify the expense, as well as try to guarantee patient compliance, for repeated apheresis procedures for a disease in which conventional chemotherapy is so inexpensive, well-tolerated, and at least as successful. Nevertheless, certain patients with CML for whom chemotherapy is either contraindicated or likely to be too slowly acting to prevent a catastrophe (i.e. pregnant patients or patients with leukostasis, thrombocytopenia, or severe hyperuricemia) may well derive significant benefit from intensive therapeutic leukapheresis until such time as alternative therapy can be instituted.

In chronic lymphocytic leukemia (CLL), significant cytoreduction and a decrease in organomegaly can be achieved through cytapheresis, although because of the generally mild long-term course of this disease it is difficult to detect any substantial improvement over conventional management (10). Thus, considering the expense and inconvenience of repeated cytapheresis procedures, it is difficult to justify managing uncomplicated CLL patients with this modality. There remains, however, a role for cytapheresis for the CLL patient who is either severely thrombocytopenic or refractory to conventional therapy.

Other myeloproliferative and lymphoproliferative syndromes have also been approached with cytapheresis as a therapeutic tool. Among these are the hypereosinophilic syndromes (11), in which the results have been quite poor; hairy cell leukemia (leukemic reticuloendotheliosis) (12), in which several quite dramatic responses have been reported, and the Sézary syndrome (13), in which marked resolution of skin involvement was reported to occur as a direct result of intensive leukapheresis. Clearly these latter two findings are stimulating and need to be confirmed through careful study of additional patients.

Lymphocytapheresis

Based on early work demonstrating the efficacy of thoracic duct drainage as a means for inducing immunosuppression (14), primarily via lymphocyte depletion, and given the presumed immunological basis of a number of disease entities, including the collagen vascular diseases (rheumatoid arthritis, systemic lupus erythematosus) and several neurologic syndromes (multiple-sclerosis, Guillain-Barré), and the clear-cut immunological basis of transplant rejection, it is not suprising that a number of studies were done to evaluate the efficacy of lymphocytapheresis in modifying the immune response and the course of the diseases alluded to above. Lymphocytapheresis is easily accomplished, and it is indeed possible to alter the T-cell "helper/suppressor" ratio, which is abnormally elevated in some rheumatic diseases, although the results have not been very striking using lymphocytapheresis as the sole therapy. It is possible that as technology progresses sufficiently to allow for the removal of selected lymphoid subpopulations, which will enable us to alter the immune balance, we will be able to obtain profound and predictable responses to lymphocytapheresis. Currently, however, this technique appears to offer no substantial benefits as compared to plasmapheresis or lymphoplasmapheresis combined with immunosuppressive therapy.

Erythrocytapheresis

Partial exchange transfusion has, up until the present, been a theoretically attractive though technically difficult procedure for the management of selected patients with sickle cell disease (SCD). There is accumulating evidence that by increasing the percentage of hemoglobin A above 50% one can protect the microvasculature and avoid serious complications attributable to sludging and increased blood viscosity occasioned by irreversibly sickled cells. Partial exchange transfusions in adult patients with SCD represent a formidable technical achievement using standard blood bags, but automated procedures using cell separators are considerably easier to perform. In the past few years numerous case reports attest to the substantial improvement noted in SCD patients with priapism, pregnancy, exercise intolerance, or even those anticipating elective surgery, as a result of automated red blood cell exchange (15–17). It is possible, using a cell separator, to achieve a 50% exchange in less than two hours, and up to 90% hemoglobin-A levels have been reached after a 3½-hour exchange (16). Other conditions in which erythrocytapheresis or automated red blood cell exchange may have a role include neocyte-gerocyte exchange (as mentioned earlier); porphyria syndromes, for which one institution has reported remarkable improvement utilizing plasmapheresis combined with partial exchange with washed neocytes (18); polycythemia, as adjunctive therapy; paroxysmal nocturnal hemoglobinuria (PNH), in preparing a patient for surgery (19); and in overwhelming red blood cell parasitism, as in falciparum malaria (20) and babesiosis (21). In these conditions, as in sickle cell disease, automated red blood cell exchange is rapid, technically simple, and extremely efficient; it is ideally suited to the management of emergent medical conditions attributable to pathologic erythrocytes.

THERAPEUTIC PLASMA EXCHANGE

"It eliminates rheumatic ailments, warms the marrow, promotes digestion, cleans the mind, dries up the brain, cures various sicknesses, and makes the urine clean and clear" (22).

The above justification for performing therapeutic bloodletting in medieval England might very easily be applied to justify the increasing and all-encompassing indications for therapeutic plasma exchange in the present decade. Reports in the literature as of June 1982 document the use of plasma exchange in well over 60 different disease entities, embracing a wide spectrum of pathologic processes. For some of these, the rationale for the use and effectiveness of plasma exchange is understandable, and the results are clearly positive; for others, the rationale is less well defended, and the results are equivocal or even uninterpretable. Case reports submitted for publication rarely document therapeutic failures, which makes interpretation of the published literature difficult. In addition, few well-controlled studies (double-blind, including a sham exchange) have been attempted, a failure justified by allusions to the cost of the procedure or to the critical clinical status of the patient, either of which would make sham exchanges unethical. While this may well be the case in certain situations, such restricted evidence of efficacy with which we are left, based as it is on uncontrolled case studies, should be afforded no more than its appropriate significance; therapeutic plasma exchange, undeniably valuable as it is in certain selected situations, should still be considered largely an experimental technique.

Physiology of Plasma Exchange

While a complete discussion of the fluid kinetics of plasma exchange is beyond the scope of this review, a brief summary of some of the volume considerations is important so that the rationale for the various treatment schedules, intensity of individual treatments, and choice of replacement solutions may be better understood. Formulas have been developed to express the relationship between the amount of any particular substance left in the plasma and the volume of plasma exchanged with any inert (i.e. lacking the substance in question) material (23). In general, a plasma exchange equal to the patient's plasma volume (usually between three and four liters) should result in the reduction of the substance in question to approximately 30% of its original value. A two-plasma-volume exchange should result in an 85–90% reduction; and a three-volume exchange should result in almost a 95% reduction. These percentages are only approximations, and there are wide individual variations depending upon changes in blood volume, the synthetic rate of the substance in question, and the extent to which the substance may be mobilized from the extravascular to the intravascular space.

The intensity of plasma exchange does not affect just the abnormal plasma component; normal plasma constituents are also affected and to the same degree. After intensive plasma exchange, particularly when plasma is not used as a replacement fluid, there may be striking and clinically significant depression of plasma proteins and clotting factors that may persist for up to 24 hours (24). The choice of replacement solution is therefore quite important. In general, crystalloid solutions are adequate replacement fluids only when exchanges of less than 1000 ml are performed. Larger volume exchanges require protein replacement, for which 5% albumin or plasma protein fraction (PPF) are adequate. When exchanges in the range of a complete plasma volume are performed it is probably judicious to replace with at least some fresh frozen plasma (FFP), in spite of the hepatitis risk, in order to maintain adequate levels of clotting factors. For some (pathological) entities it is, in fact, not entirely clear whether it is the removal of pathologic plasma, or the infusion of normal plasma, that is the more important therapeutic maneuver.

Complications of Plasma Exchange

Plasma exchange performed with a cell separator is a relatively safe procedure. Nevertheless, there are a number of complications associated with the procedure, some of which are quite significant. Already alluded to was the reduction in normal plasma constituents that accompanies large volume exchanges (24); thus, hemostatic disturbances, thrombocytopenia, and impaired immunity have all been reported. Complications may also attend the infusion of plasma. Included here are citrate toxicity, cardiac arrhythmias, hepatitis, anaphylaxis, and hemolysis. Numerous problems related to vascular access, thromboembolism, and hypovolemia/hypotension have also been noted. Most significant, however, is the fact that approximately 24 deaths directly attributable to plasma exchange have been reported (25). Plasma exchange is an expensive procedure, associated with substantial morbidity. It should be reserved for patients with clear-cut indications for its use, sufficient to justify the risks involved.

Clinical Conditions Treatable by Plasma Exchange

In a review of this scope it would be impossible even simply to enumerate all of the diseases purportedly amenable to treatment via plasma exchange. Rather, it is more profitable to develop categories, based on mechanisms of disease, that could be discussed in a more general way in terms of the potential effectiveness of plasma exchange for diseases within that category. (Please refer to Table 1.)

I. Diseases associated with abnormal (or excess) plasma proteins, toxins, or metabolic products: This category is perhaps the most intellectually satisfying with regard to the theoretical and practical efficacy of plasma exchange. Diseases in this category, almost by definition, should show substantial improvement when managed by plasma exchange. In fact, the hyperviscosity syndrome, associated with macroglobulinemia and multiple myeloma, was the first disorder for which plasmapheresis was performed as a therapeutic maneuver (26). Plasma exchange has successfully been performed for patients with multiple myeloma, macroglobulinemia, light-chain disease, and cryoglobulinemia (27). A particularly interesting approach, "cryoglobulinpheresis," has been described for patients with cryoglobulinemia (28). For these patients, their own cryoglobulin-rich plasma, harvested at the time of plasma exchange, is stored in the cold,

Table 1   Diseases treated by plasma exchange

Category	Disease	Reference
I. Abnormal (excess):		
proteins	hyperviscosity syndrome	26
	multiple myeloma	27
	macroglobulinemia	27
	cryoglobulinemia	28
toxins	mushroom poisoning	29
poisons	paraquat	30
	methylparathion	31
metabolite	Refsum's disease	32
	familial hypercholesterolemia	33
	porphyria	18
II. Autoantibodies:	autoimmune hemolytic anemia	35, 36
	cold agglutinin disease	36, 37
	immune thrombocytopenic purpura	38, 39
	aplastic anemia	40
	pure red blood cell aplasia	41
	acquired inhibitors to Factor VIII	42
	myasthenia gravis	43, 44
	Guillain Barré syndrome	45
	multiple sclerosis	46
	diabetes mellitus	47
	Grave's disease	48
	pemphigus vulgaris	49
	Goodpasture's syndrome	34, 50
III. Alloantibodies:	Factor VIII, IX inhibitors	42, 51
	ABO incompatible transplantation	52
	alloantibodies to RBC antigens	53
	(Rh) hemolytic disease of the newborn	54, 55
	posttransfusion purpura	56, 57
	renal transplant rejection	58
IV. Immune complexes:	polyarteritis nodosa	59
	dermatomyositis	60
	rheumatoid arthritis	61–63
	systemic lupus erythematosus	64–66
V. Miscellaneous	metastatic cancer	67
	hereditary angioneurotic edema	68
	Crohn's disease	69
	Raynaud's syndrome	70
	hepatic encephalopathy	71
	psoriasis	72
	hemolytic uremic syndrome	73
	thrombotic thrombocytopenic purpura	74–76

which precipitates the cryoglobulins, after which the autologous cryoglobulin-poor plasma is returned to the patient at the next plasma exchange session. While plasma exchange cannot affect the basic malignant process in these disorders, it can provide substantial relief from complications attributable to excess plasma protein while the underlying disease is appropriately treated.

Syndromes associated with toxins, e.g. mushroom poisoning (29), or poisons, e.g. paraquat (30) or methylparathion (31), are essentially curable via plasma exchange provided end organ damage has not occurred. Other disorders are also responsive to plasma exchange, including those characterized by the accumulation of an abnormal metabolite, e.g. Refsum's disease (phytanic acid) (32) or an excess of a normal plasma constituent, e.g. familial hypercholesterolemia (cholesterol) (33), or a metabolic intermediary, e.g. porphyria syndromes (delta amino levulinic acid) (18).

II. Diseases associated with autoantibodies: Immune-mediated disorders, inasmuch as their pathogenesis is directly related to endogenous immune factors, would seem to be almost ideally suited to the kind of manipulation possible with plasma exchange or lymphoplasmapheresis. Thus it is not surprising that the earliest descriptions of successful intervention by plasma exchange were in patients with disorders having an immunological basis. Among the various immunological diseases are those that are caused by autoantibodies, alloantibodies, or that are related to the presence and tissue deposition of immune complexes. While it would be gratifying to be able to show a 100% correlation between the levels of each of these immune mediators and disease activity, this is generally only possible in the case of alloantibodies. For autoantibody or immune-complex-mediated diseases, the correlation is not absolute, and therefore the mechanism of action of plasma exchange, when there is therapeutic benefit, may include removal of antibody, removal of antigen, removal of immune complexes, elimination of blocking antibody, depletion of other immune mediators (e.g. complement components), removal of reticuloendothelial blockade, replacement of missing or depleted factors, or enhancement of the immunosuppressive effect of concomitantly administered immunosuppressive agents.

In considering the many different diseases associated with autoantibodies that have been treated with plasma exchange, it is possible to make a few generalizations regarding the effectiveness of plasma exchange and its most appropriate role in the overall management of patients with these disorders. Most of the autoantibodies responsible for clinical disease are of the IgG class. Since IgG antibodies are distributed in both the intravascular and extravascular spaces, the efficiency of plasma exchange in these disorders is somewhat less than that seen in the hyperviscosity syndrome or cold agglutinin disease (CAD), which are IgM-mediated disorders. In addition, rapid post-exchange equilibration of IgG from the extravascular to intravascular compartment would tend to dictate a rather short-lived response to a single plasma exchange. Where tissue-bound or cell-bound antibody is important pathogenetically, the response to plasma exchange will be slower and less complete than anticipated. It is therefore understandable that only those autoantibody-mediated disorders that may themselves be somewhat self-limited in duration [e.g. Goodpasture's syndrome (34)] are associated with some of the more dramatic, long-lasting, and occasionally permanent responses to intensive plasma exchange.

While removal of autoantibody is in most cases associated with clinical improvement, there is also accumulating evidence that rapid reduction in autoantibody levels may be associated (perhaps as a result of a diminished feedback inhibition) with a sudden, marked rise in antibody titer. Thus, for many of the disorders in this category, plasma exchange must be accompanied by active immunosuppression in order to achieve a sustained beneficial effect. Given all of the above considerations, it is clear that plasma exchange in autoimmune diseases may be a valuable adjunctive procedure, capable of producing dramatic temporary control of symptoms, while more definitive therapy is instituted and allowed to become effective. Chronic plasma exchange for these disorders, as the primary therapeutic modality, is almost certainly not indicated, as evidenced by the lack of any substantive data to support such a therapeutic maneuver.

A final caveat regarding the diseases treated by plasma exchange, in this category as well as in subsequent categories, is that many of them are subject to spontaneous exacerbations, remissions, and unpredictable changes in clinical course, which complicates our ability to ascribe direct benefit to any new therapeutic modality until it can be shown to be unequivocably successful on repeated occasions.

Hematologic autoimmune diseases for which plasma exchange has been used include autoimmune hemolytic anemia (warm type) (35, 36), in which results have been mixed and the procedure poorly tolerated; cold agglutinin disease (36, 37), in which, again, results have not been striking, and the procedure has proven technically quite difficult (specifically in developing methods for keeping the ex vivo plasma warm enough to prevent agglutination); autoimmune thrombocytopenic purpura (38, 39), in which some long-lasting results have been achieved in patients with acute disease, although given the generally good response to "conventional" immunosuppressive therapy in this syndrome plasma exchange may well be reserved for patients with particularly severe or refractory disease in whom conventional therapy is either ineffective or likely not to produce results within an adequate time frame; aplastic anemia (40) and pure red blood cell aplasia

(41), in which modest success has been achieved in the subgroup of patients with antibodies to erythropoietin or red blood cell precursors; and in the management of patients with inhibitors to Factor VIII (42) (spontaneously acquired anticoagulants), in whom antibody titers are successfully lowered, and hemostatic levels of Factor VIII achieved, through intensive plasma exchange.

Neurologic autoimmune disorders for which plasma exchange has been used include myasthenia gravis (43, 44), in which striking results have been reported in younger patients with disease of relatively short ($\leq$ 10 years) duration, particularly during crises and always when coupled with the use of immunosuppressive chemotherapy; acute Guillain-Barré syndrome (45) (demyelinating polyneuropathy), in which, although a few positive reports have been published, there simply is not enough data acquired in a controlled fashion upon which to base any recommendations whatsoever about the role of plasma exchange; and multiple sclerosis (46), in which, as in Guillain-Barré syndrome, a national cooperative trial to assess the role of plasma exchange in managing acute disease exacerbations is underway.

Other antibody-mediated autoimmune disorders that have been treated with plasma exchange include diabetes mellitus (47) (associated with antibodies to insulin receptors), Grave's disease (48) (with refractory exophthalmos), pemphigus vulgaris (49), and rapidly progressive glomerulonephritis associated with pulmonary hemorrhage (Goodpasture's syndrome) (34, 50). In this latter entity excellent results have been reported when intensive plasma exchange is combined with immunosuppression in patients who have residual renal function. Pulmonary hemmorrhage (secondary to antiglomerular basement membrane antibody) has been dramatically responsive to plasma exchange therapy, and because of the apparently self-limited nature of the pathogenetic process, long-lasting clinical remissions (cures) have been obtained when plasma exchange has been instituted prior to the development of irreversible renal lesions.

III. Diseases associated with alloantibodies: Alloantibodies are, by definition, directed against foreign antigens and are therefore generally not involved in the pathogenesis of immune disorders per se; but there are clinical situations in which removal of alloantibody may be an important therapeutic maneuver. Removal of Factor VIII or Factor IX inhibitors in hemophilic patients via plasma exchange has allowed for successful management of difficult clinical situations in these patients (42, 51). In addition, titers of ABO isohemagglutinins have been successfully lowered prior to performing ABO-incompatible bone marrow transplantation (52). Patients with antibodies to red blood cell antigens of high frequency, for whom, as a consequence, it has been difficult to provide compatible blood, have also benefited from intensive plasma exchange (53).

Two other situations in which alloantibodies are directly involved in disease pathogenesis and in which plasma exchange has successfully been employed are (Rh) hemolytic disease of the newborn (HDN) (54, 55) and posttransfusion purpura (PTP) (56, 57). In HDN, antibody titers have been lowered and fetal salvage rates improved, especially in patients in whom severe disease does not begin until after the 30th week of gestation; in PTP, as in isoimmune neonatal thrombocytopenic purpura, excellent results have been obtained, particularly when plasma exchange has been accompanied by infusion of washed, Pl^{A1}-negative platelets.

A final alloantibody-mediated condition for which plasma exchange has been proposed as a therapeutic maneuver is renal transplant rejection (58). In this condition, although HLA antibody titers have been lowered via plasma exchange, there are generally so many therapeutic maneuvers instituted simultaneously that it has been difficult precisely to assess the true value and/or role of plasma exchange.

IV. Diseases associated with immune complexes: The most important diseases in this category are rheumatoid arthritis (RA) and systemic lupus erythematosus (SLE). Although other vasculitides such as polyarteritis nodosa (59) and dermatomyositis (60) have also been treated with plasma exchange, these disorders are distinctly less common than RA or SLE. Unlike many of the disorders in categories I, II, or III, in which disease activity could be directly related to abnormal levels of a pathologic factor (e.g. toxin, autoantibody, alloantibody), RA and SLE both defy attempts at simple categorization. While immune complexes are clearly implicated in certain manifestations of these disorders, they are by no means exclusive etiologic factors. In addition, complicating our ability to quantify the role of plasma exchange in the management of patients with RA or SLE is the unpredictable clinical course of both disorders; remissions and exacerbations are part of the natural history of both RA and SLE, a fact that must be carefully considered when evaluating any new therapeutic maneuver. Lastly, one must also take into account the tremendous susceptibility of patients afflicted with RA or SLE to a placebo effect. The very nature of plasma exchange—the time involved, the direct personal attention required, the high technology utilized, and the investigative enthusiasm associated with new techniques—contributes to generate a profound placebo effect.

While numerous reports of the beneficial effects of plasmapheresis, or lymphoplasmapheresis, in RA (61–63) and SLE (64–66) have been published, too few controlled studies (which include a sham procedure) with adequate numbers of patients have been performed to enable one to make anything more than a few generalizations regarding the effectiveness of plasma exchange in these disorders. It would seem, from published studies, that plasma exchange can occasionally lead to rather dramatic early responses, particularly in SLE, and when combined with immunosuppressive chemotherapy may provide a valuable adjunctive therapeutic modality in managing SLE patients with severe vasculitis, nephritis, or cerebritis. In RA, plasma exchange appears to have a similar adjunctive role for selected patients who are refractory to all conventional chemotherapy or who have life-threatening complications, including vasculitis, cryoglobulinemia, and severe pulmonary hypersensitivity reactions. In both disorders it is imperative that immunosuppressive drugs be administered simultaneously, both to prevent a rebound effect (e.g. a rapid rise in the level of circulating immune complexes) and to help produce a more sustained clinical remission. The precise mechanism of action of plasma exchange in RA and SLE is unknown and may include a decrease in the level of circulating immune complexes (CIC), an unblocking of receptors for CIC in the reticuloendothelial system, the stimulation and subsequent deletion of clones of antibody-producing B cells, or an alteration of the balance of helper and suppressor interactions (between lymphocytes) by removal of humoral factors. Because responsiveness of patients with these disorders to plasma exchange cannot be correlated directly with any specific parameter felt to be important pathogenetically, and because adequately controlled trials have not been performed, the use of plasma exchange in RA and SLE must perforce still be considered investigational, and limited either to highly selected patients with life-threatening complications or to patients participating in clinical trials.

V. Miscellaneous disorders: Numerous other disorders, which do not fit into the previous categories, have been the subject of case reports attesting to a positive response to intensive plasma exchange. These are enumerated in Table 1. Perhaps most striking in this group is thrombotic thrombocytopenic purpura (TTP) (74–76). This disorder, if untreated, carries approximately an 80% mortality, generally within two weeks of diagnosis. Recent reports, in which plasma exchange has been combined with antiplatelet agents, steroids, and occasionally splenectomy document survival rates of $\geq 70\%$. Because the precise etiology is unknown, and alternative hypotheses include the presence of a "toxic" (platelet-aggregating) factor and the absence of a normally present inhibitor of platelet aggregation, it is a matter of debate whether it is the removal of autologous plasma or the infusion of homologous plasma that is the more important therapeutic maneuver. In addition, the relative rarity of TTP makes it highly unlikely that controlled clinical trials can be efficiently accomplished. Thus, our ability to define the role of plasma exchange in TTP must await a more definitive understanding of the pathogenesis of the disorder.

FUTURE DIRECTIONS

Plasma exchange is an important application of an exciting technological development. There are disorders for which it can already be described as the treatment of choice; there are other disorders for which it appears to be a useful adjunct, in special situations, to more conventional management; and, finally, there are disorders for which its true role is still to be defined through controlled clinical trials. Nevertheless, plasma exchange as currently performed should still be viewed as only an intermediate technique, one that logically should be replaced by techniques capable of more selective removal of pathogenic factors. Some of these newer techniques have already been described, and include the removal of lipoproteins by circulating plasma over a column of heparin-treated agarose (77), the removal of bile acids by circulating plasma over charcoal-coated glass beads (78), the removal of toxic substances by circulating blood over amberlite resin columns (79), and the removal of immunoglobulins by circulating blood over columns to which protein A has been coupled (80). As important as plasma exchange is today, it is clear that this crude, expensive, and potentially hazardous procedure will ultimately be replaced by more limited and highly specific removal of pathogenic factors. The transition to these more optimal techniques will require not only additional technological advances but will be predicated on a substantial increase in our understanding of the basic pathophysiology of disorders amenable to such manipulation.

Literature Cited

1. Lohrmann, H., Bull, M. I., Decter, J. A., Yankee, R. A., Graw, R. G. 1974. Platelet transfusions from HL-A compatible unrelated donors to alloimmunized patients. *Ann. Intern. Med.* 80:9–14
2. Propper, R. D., Button, L. N., Nathan, D. G. 1980. New approaches to the transfusion management of thalassemia. *Blood* 55:55–60
3. Graziano, J. H., Piomelli, S., Seaman, C., Wang, T., Cohen, A. R., Kelleher, J. F. Jr., Schwartz, E. 1982. A simple technique for preparation of young red cells for transfusion from ordinary blood units. *Blood* 59:865–68
4. Goldman, J. M., Catovsky, D., Galton, D. A. G. 1978. Reversal of blast-cell crisis in C.G.L. by transfusion of stored autologous buffy-coat cells. *Lancet* 1:437–39
5. Taft, E. G., Babcock, R. B., Scharfman, W. B., Tartaglia, A. P. 1977. Plateletpheresis in the management of thrombocytosis. *Blood* 50:927–33
6. Goldfinger, D., Thompson, R., Lowe, C., Kurz, L., Belkin, G. 1979. Long-term plateletpheresis in the management of primary thrombocytosis. *Transfusion* 19:336–38
7. Eisenstadt, R. S., Berkman, E. M. 1978. Rapid cytoreduction in acute leukemia. Management of cerebral leukostasis by cell pheresis. *Transfusion* 18:113–15
8. Morse, E. E., Carbone, P. P., Freireich, E. J., Bronson, W., Kliman, A. 1966. Repeated leukapheresis of patients with chronic myelocytic leukemia. *Transfusion* 6:175–78
9. Vallejos, G. S., McCredie, K. B., Britten, G. M. 1973. Biological effects of repeated leukapheresis of patients with chronic myelogenous leukemia. *Blood* 42:925–33
10. Curtis, J. E., Hersh, E. M., Freireich, E. J. 1972. Leukapheresis therapy of chronic lymphocytic leukemia. *Blood* 39:163–75
11. Pineda, A. A., Brzica, S. M. Jr., Taswell, H. F. 1977. Continuous- and semi-

continuous-flow blood centrifuge systems: therapeutic applications, with plasma-, platelet-, lympha-, and eosinapheresis. *Transfusion* 17:407–16
12. Fay, J. W., Moore, J. O., Logue, G. L., Huang, A. T. 1979. Leukopheresis therapy of leukemic reticuloendotheliosis (hairy cell leukemia). *Blood* 54:747–49
13. Edelson, R., Facktor, M., Andrews, A., Lutzner, M., Schein, P. 1974. Successful management of the Sézary syndrome. *N. Engl. J. Med.* 291:293–94
14. Paulus, H. E., Machleder, H. I., Levine, S., Yu, D. T. Y., MacDonald, N. S. 1977. Lymphocyte involvement in rheumatoid arthritis: studies during thoracic duct drainage. *Arth. Rheum.* 20:1249–62
15. Morrison, J. C., Whybrew, W. D., Bucovaz, E. T. 1978. Use of partial exchange transfusion preoperatively in patients with sickle cell hemoglobinopathies. *Am. J. Obstet. Gynecol.* 132:59–63
16. Kernoff, L. M., Botha, M. C., Jacobs, P. 1977. Exchange transfusion in sickle cell disease using a continuous-flow blood cell separator. *Transfusion* 17:269–71
17. Morrison, J. C., Wiser, W. L. 1976. The use of prophylactic partial exchange transfusion in pregnancies associated with sickle cell hemoglobinopathies. *Obstet. Gynecol.* 48:516–20
18. Spiva, D. A., Lewis, C., Langley, J. W. 1981. New treatment for the porphyrias: porphyria (AIP) and variegate porphyria (VP). *Blood* 58(5):186a (Abstr.)
19. Cundall, J. R., Moore, W. H., Jenkins, D. E. 1978. Erythrocyte exchange in paroxysmal nocturnal hemoglobinuria prior to cardiac surgery. *Transfusion* 18:626 (Abstr.)
20. Yarrish, R. L., Janas, J. S., Nosanchuk, J. S., Steigbigel, R. T., Nusbacher, J. 1982. Transfusion malaria: treatment with exchange transfusion after delayed diagnosis. *Arch. Intern. Med.* 142:187–88
21. Jacoby, G. A., Hunt, J. V., Kosinski, K. S., Demirjian, Z. N., Huggins, C., Etkind, P., Marcus, L. C., Spielman, A. 1980. Treatment of transfusion-transmitted babesiosis by exchange transfusion. *N. Engl. J. Med.* 303:1098–1100
22. Talbot, C. H. 1967. *Medicine in Medieval England*, p. 131. London: Oldbourne
23. Collins, J. A. 1974. Problems associated with the massive transfusion of stored blood. *Surgery* 75:274–95
24. Flaum, M. A., Cuneo, R. A., Applebaum, F. R., Deisseroth, A. B., Engel, W. K., Gralnick, H. R. 1979. The hemostatic imbalance of plasma-exchange transfusion. *Blood* 54:694
25. Huestis, D. W. Personal communication, June 1982
26. Schwab, P. J., Fahey, J. F. 1960. Treatment of Waldenstrom's macroglobulinemia by plasmapheresis. *N. Engl. J. Med.* 263:574–79
27. Russell, J. A., Toy, J. L., Powles, R. L. 1977. Plasma exchange in malignant paraproteinemias. *Exp. Hematol.* 5:105–16 (Suppl.)
28. McLeod, B. C., Sassetti, R. J. 1980. Plasmapheresis with return of cryoglobulin-depleted autologous plasma (cryoglobulinpheresis) in cryoglobulinemia. *Blood* 55:866–70
29. Mercuriali, F., Sirchia, G. 1977. Plasma exchange for mushroom poisoning. *Transfusion* 17:644–46
30. Dearnaley, D. R., Martin, M. F. R. 1978. Plasmapheresis for paraquat poisoning. *Lancet* 1:162
31. Luzhnikov, E. A., Yaraslavsky, A. A., Molodenov, M. N. 1977. Plasma perfusion through charcoal in methylparathion poisoning. *Lancet* 1:38–39
32. Gibberg, F. B., Billimoria, J. D., Page, N. G. R. 1979. Heredopathia atactica polyneuritiformis (Refsum's disease) treated by diet and plasma exchange. *Lancet* 1:575–78
33. Thompson, G. R. 1981. Plasma exchange for hypercholesterolaemia. *Lancet* 1:1246–48
34. Lockwood, C. M., Boulton-Jones, J. M., Lowenthal, R. M. 1975. Recovery from Goodpasture's syndrome after immunosuppressive treatment and plasmapheresis. *Br. Med. J.* 2:252–54
35. Branda, R. F., Moldow, C. F., McCullough, J. J., Jacob, H. S. 1975. Plasma exchange in the treatment of immune disease. *Transfusion* 15:570–76
36. Petz, L. D., Garratty, G. 1980. *Acquired Immune Hemolytic Anemias,* pp. 418–20, 424–25. New York: Churchill Livingstone
37. Taft, E. G., Propp, R. P., Sullivan, S. A. 1977. Plasma exchange for cold agglutinin hemolytic anemia. *Transfusion* 17:173–76
38. Branda, R. F. 1979. Plasma exchange in the treatment of immune thrombocytopenia. *Plasma Therapy* 1:43–48
39. Marder, V. J., Nusbacher, J., Anderson, F. W. 1981. One-year follow-up of plasma exchange therapy in 14 patients

with idiopathic thrombocytopenic purpura. *Transfusion* 21:291–98

40. Abdou, N. I. 1982. *Plasma exchange in the treatment of aplastic anemia.* Presented at 3rd Natl. Conf. Therapeutic Apheresis, May 13, 1982, Dallas

41. Messner, H. A., Fauser, A. A., Curtis, J. E., Dotten, D. 1981. Control of antibody-mediated pure red-cell aplasia by plasmapheresis. *N. Engl. J. Med.* 304:1334–38

42. Slocombe, G. W., Newland, A. C., Colvin, M. P., Colvin, B. T. 1981. The role of intensive plasma exchange in the prevention and management of haemorrhage in patients with inhibitors to Factor VIII. *Br. J. Haematol.* 47:577–85

43. Dau, P. C., Lindstrom, J. M., Cassel, C. K., Denys, E. H., Shev, E. E., Spitler, L. E. 1977. Plasmapheresis and immunosuppressive drug therapy in myasthenia gravis. *N. Engl. J. Med.* 297:1134–40

44. Newsome-Davis, J., Wilson, S. G., Vincent, A. 1979. Long-term effects of repeated plasma exchange in myasthenia gravis. *Lancet* 1:464–68

45. Cook, J. D., Tindall, R. A. S., Walker, J. 1980. Plasma exchange as a treatment of acute and chronic idiopathic autoimmune polyneuropathy: limited success. *Neurology* 30:361–62

46. Hauser, S. 1982. *Plasmapheresis, lymphocytapheresis and immunosuppressive therapy in multiple sclerosis.* Presented at 3rd Natl. Conf. Therapeutic Apheresis, May 14, 1982, Dallas

47. Muggeo, M., Flier, J. S., Abrams, R. A. 1979. Treatment by plasma exchange of a patient with autoantibodies to the insulin receptor. *N. Engl. J. Med.* 300:477–80

48. Dandona, P., Marshall, N. J., Bidey, S. P. 1979. Successful treatment of exophthalmos and pretibial myxoedema with plasmapheresis. *Br. Med. J.* 1:374–76

49. Catterill, J. A., Basker, D. J., Millard, L. G. 1978. Plasma exchange in the treatment of pemphigus vulgaris. *Br. J. Dermatol.* 98:243

50. Rosenblatt, S. G., Knight, W., Bannayan, G. A., Wilson, C. B., Stein, J. 1979. Treatment of Goodpasture's syndrome with plasmapheresis. *Am. J. Med.* 66:689–96

51. Cobcroft, R. 1977. *Serial Plasmapheresis in a Hemophiliac with Antibodies to Factor VIII.* Proc. HRI Adv. Comp., Semin, London, England

52. Berkman, E. M., Caplan, S., Kim, G. S. 1978. ABO-incompatible bone marrow transplantation: preparation by plasma exchange and in vivo antibody absorption. *Transfusion* 18:504–8

53. Steane, E. A. 1982. *Therapeutic plasmapheresis in patients with antibodies to high frequency red cell antigens.* Presented at 3rd Natl. Conf. Therapeutic Apheresis, May 13, 1982, Dallas

54. James, V., Weston, J., Scott, I. V., Doughty, R., Tomlinson, J., Whitfield, M. 1979. Intensive plasma exchange in Rhesus isoimmunization. *Vox Sang.* 37:290–95

55. Fraser, I. D., Bennett, M. O., Bothamley, J. E., Airth, G. R. 1976. Intensive antenatal plasmapheresis in severe rhesus isoimmunization. *Lancet* 1:6–9

56. Cimo, P. L., Aster, R. H. 1972. Posttransfusion purpura. Successful treatment by exchange transfusion. *N. Engl. J. Med.* 287:290–92

57. Phadke, K. P., Isbister, J. P. 1980. Posttransfusion purpura. *Med. J. Aust.* 1:430–32

58. Rifle, G., Chalopin, J. M., Ture, J. M. 1979. Plasmapheresis in the treatment of renal allograft rejections. *Transplant. Proc.* 11:20–26

59. Chenais, F., Debru, J. L., Baret, L., Faure, J., Chalopin, J. M., Rifle, G. 1980. Plasma exchange in the treatment of polyarteritis nodosa. In *Plasma Exchange, Plasmapheresis-Plasmaseparation,* ed. H. G. Sieberth, pp. 285–88. Stuttgart: Schattauer

60. Dau, P. C., Bennington, J. 1981. Plasmapheresis in childhood dermatomyositis. *J. Pediatr.* 98:237–40

61. Rothwell, R. S., Davis, P., Gordon, P. A., Dasgupta, M. K., Johny, K. V., Russell, A. S., Percy, J. S. 1980. A controlled study of plasma exchange in the treatment of severe rheumatoid arthritis. *Arth. Rheum.* 23:785–89

62. Wallace, D. J., Goldfinger, D., Gatti, R., Lowe, C., Fan, P., Bluestone, R., Klinenberg, J. R. 1979. Plasmapheresis and lymphoplasmapheresis in the management of rheumatoid arthritis. *Arth. Rheum.* 22:703–10

63. Brubaker, D. B., Winkelstein, A. 1981. Plasma exchange in rheumatoid vasculitis. *Vox Sang.* 41:295–301

64. Jones, J. V., Cummings, C. H., Pacon, P. A. 1979. Evidence for a therapeutic effect of plasmapheresis in patients with systemic lupus erythematosus. *Q. J. Med.* 48:555–76

65. Schildermans, F., Dequeker, J., Van de Puthe, I. 1979. Plasmapheresis combined with corticosteroids and cyclophosphamide in uncontrolled active SLE. *J. Rheum.* 6:687

66. Schlansky, R., DeHoratius, R. J., Pincus, T., Tung, K. S. K. 1981. Plasmapheresis in systemic lupus erythematosus: a cautionary note. *Arth. Rheum.* 24:49–53
67. Israel, L., Edelstein, R., Mannoni, P. 1977. Plasmapheresis in patients with disseminated cancer: clinical results and correlation with changes in serum protein. *Cancer* 40:3146–54
68. Young, D. W., Thompson, R. A., Mackie, P. H. 1980. Plasmapheresis in hereditary angioneurotic edema and systemic lupus erythematosus. *Arch. Intern. Med.* 140:127–28
69. Holdstock, G. E., Fisher, J. A., Hamblin, T. J. 1979. Plasmapheresis in Crohn's disease. *Digestion* 19:197–201
70. Talpos, G., Horrocks, M., White, J. M. 1978. Plasmapheresis in Raynaud's disease. *Lancet* 1:416–17
71. Lepore, M. J., McKenna, P. J., Martinez, D. B. 1979. Fulminant hepatitis with coma successfully treated by plasmapheresis. *Plasma Ther.* 1:49–56
72. Dav, P. S. 1979. Resolution of psoriasis during plasmapheresis therapy. *Arch. Dermatol.* 115:1171
73. Beattie, T. J., Murphy, A. V., Willoughby, M. L. N., Machin, S. J., Defreyn, G. 1981. Plasmapheresis in the haemolytic-uraemic syndrome in children. *Br. Med. J.* 282:1667–68

74. Myers, T. J., Wakem, C. J., Ball, E. D., Tremont, S. J. 1980. Thrombotic thrombocytopenic purpura: combined treatment with plasmapheresis and antiplatelet agents. *Ann. Intern. Med.* 92(Part 1):149–55
75. Taft, E. G. 1979. Thrombotic thrombocytopenic purpura and dose of plasma exchange. *Blood* 54:842–49
76. McLeod, B. C., Wu, K. K., Knospe, W. H. 1980. Plasmapheresis in thrombotic thrombocytopenic purpura. *Arch. Intern. Med.* 140:1059–60
77. Burgstaler, E. A., Pineda, A. A., Ellefson, R. D. 1980. Laboratory study. Removal of plasma lipoproteins from circulating blood with a heparin-agarose column. *Mayo Clin. Proc.* 55:180–84
78. Lauterburg, B. H., Pineda, A. A., Dickson, E. R., Baldus, W. P., Taswell, H. F. 1978. Plasmaperfusion for the treatment of intractable pruritus of cholestasis. *Mayo Clin. Proc.* 53:403–7
79. Lynn, R. L., Honig, C. L., Jatlow, P. I., Kliger, A. S. 1979. Resin hemoperfusion for treatment of ethchlorvynol overdose. *Ann. Intern. Med.* 91:549–53
80. Pineda, A. A. 1980. Therapeutic plasmapheresis: new technics and applications. In *Therapeutic Hemapheresis*, ed. E. M. Berkman, J. Umlas, 9:139–50. Washington, DC: Am. Assoc. Blood Banks. 150 pp.

Ann. Rev. Med. 1983. 34:91–105

PATHOGENESIS OF THE POSTPHLEBITIC SYNDROME

Peter Jacobs, F.A.C.P., F.R.C.Path.

Department of Hematology, University of Cape Town, and Groote Schuur Hospital, Cape Town, South Africa

ABSTRACT

The dependent edema, skin pigmentation, local inflammation associated with subcutaneous fibrosis, chronic ulceration, and current infection are the hallmarks of postphlebitic syndrome. In one fifth of the patients there is no evidence of antecedent deep venous occlusion. Current emphasis is therefore on improvement in investigation and the use of treatment programs designed to return venous patency and valve function to normal. Modern management must also take into account local changes in capillary permeability and fibrinolytic activity in the pathogenesis of the venous ulceration.

INTRODUCTION

Traditionally, occlusion of the deep veins in the lower limbs has been exclusively incriminated in the pathogenesis of a unique clinical syndrome described as the postphlebitic syndrome. Characteristic symptoms are heaviness of the leg, fatigue, pain with dependent edema, skin pigmentation, varicose veins, and local inflammation associated with subcutaneous fibrosis, chronic ulceration, and recurrent infection. At least in some patients this is a misnomer since approximately 20% of individuals will have no history of either thrombophlebitis or conditions where this possibility might have been missed (1–3). Increasing awareness that preceding thrombosis does not occur in every instance has had two important consequences. First, greater emphasis has been given to the investigation of these patients in an attempt to recognize less obvious degrees of venous occlusion that may nevertheless play an important role in pathogenesis. Second, attention has been focussed, for the first time, on capillary permeability and fibrinolytic activity (4) in pathogenesis of the venous ulceration.

91

0066-4219/83/0401-0091$02.00

These recent advances, coupled with a better understanding of disturbances in the physiology of the venous circulation associated with this entity, are compelling reasons for re-examining the pathophysiology of a clinical syndrome that affects 0.5% of the population of Great Britain and the United States (4), causing substantial morbidity that is reflected in enormous loss of working time each year. Understanding and managing the postphlebitic syndrome, a term that remains acceptable as long as its limitations are recognized, is most likely to be optimal when approached by a team including physiologists, hematologists, radiologists, and surgeons working together in a single clinic. Only in this way will the patients' best interests be served while further clarification of the causative mechanism and alternative forms of therapy are objectively evaluated.

ANATOMY

The basis for understanding the characteristic varicosities and localization of skin changes is the distribution of the venous system in the lower limb. Of particular note is the applied or surgical anatomy of the superficial and the perforating veins. Based on a dissection study, Thomson (5) emphasized an essential difference between arteries and veins: veins include the longitudinally disposed saphenous system with its associated perforating vessels and system of valves which, under normal circumstances, direct venous return centripetally. In this meticulous study, the medial ankle perforators were demonstrated to be different from the rest, constituting a venous triangle where their course is short and poorly buttressed by surrounding tissues. The conclusion is that they may be damaged in their entire short length with incompetence of the valves resulting from either direct injury or extension of deep venous thrombosis.

PHYSIOLOGY

In the last decade, the simultaneous measurement of pressure and flow in the lower limbs has been carefully examined, both at rest and during exercise. This approach to understanding the physiology of hemodynamics is the result of painstaking work that goes back half a century (6) and has reached its present level of sophistication as a result of technical advances that include electromagnetic flow meters (7, 8) and direct reading electromanometers with photorecorders and treadmill to standardize stress (9, 10). It is in consequence of these changes that the anatomy of the vascular system of the lower limbs was brought to life by showing clearly what happens to blood flow (particularly in the complex venous system) at rest, in response to change in posture, and with exercise. Furthermore, this same approach was extended to diseases of the lower limb and plays a particularly important role both in the upright position and during variations associated with exercise.

Flow in the deep vessels with the subject in the supine position is toward the heart and varies physiologically with changes in intraabdominal pressure resulting from respiration. On standing, mean venous pressure at the ankle changes from 11.7 mmHg to 86.8 mmHg (9) with pressures in the superficial and deep veins being the same (12, 13). During exercise, flow varies according to the phase of walking (9, 14, 15). Flow is toward the heart in both superficial and deep veins under normal circumstances, and in an inward direction through the perforating veins except during muscular contraction when pressure in the deep veins reaches its maximum value (16, 17).

Pressure is also affected by the pumping action of the soleus and gastrocnemius muscles and, with exercise, mean pressure in both superficial and deep veins is below hydrostatic levels (13, 18, 19). These changes in the leg veins are but part of the wider reflex change in the venous system that accompanies exercise (11). Thus, there is associated dilatation of resistance vessels in the working muscles with accelerated flow which occurs without changes in systemic arterial blood pressure reflecting redistribution of blood volume with diminished supply to splanchnic area (20). Superimposed upon these changes are responses in the cutaneous veins where thermoregulatory mechanisms are of major importance.

THE HEMOSTATIC MECHANISM

There are three reasons for considering the hemostatic mechanism as well as rheology in the pathophysiology of the postphlebitic syndromes. First, changes in quantity and quality of the blood may predispose to venous occlusion. Second, therapy with antithrombotic agents necessitates a knowledge of the principles of hemostasis. Third, disturbances in the intrinsic properties of the vessel wall have been incriminated in at least the liposclerotic component of this syndrome (21).

Hemostasis is the physiologic process that repairs vascular injury while maintaining patency. In contrast, thrombosis is the pathological counterpart in which vascular obstruction occurs and may reflect inappropriate response to vascular injury or abnormalities in the blood, ranging from thrombocytosis through increased viscosity in the erythrocytoses to abnormalities in the clotting system, exemplified by deficiency of antithrombin III. In both hemostasis and thrombosis, the initial event is interaction between platelet and subendothelial tissues in which adhesion is followed by aggregation. Local release of vasoactive amines from the platelets results in vasospasm and further local platelet accumulation. This is followed by activation of the coagulation cascade via procoagulant plasma factors present on the surface of the platelets. Finally, there is local conversion of plasminogen to plasmin, which restricts excess fibrin formation, and eventually endothelial cell regrowth returns the vessel to normal.

The antithrombotic drugs are classified according to their site of action on this hemostatic mechanism. Anticoagulants interfere with fibrin formation, and of these heparin and coumarin are best known. Drugs that handicap platelet function diminish the initial interaction between platelet and vessel wall, mediating this by either decreased synthesis or impaired degradation of cyclic adenosine monophosphate (cAMP) with the ultimate mechanism being disturbances in calcium metabolism (22). The third major group of antithrombotic drugs arc those that lyse the fibrin and, while both streptokinase and urokinase are effective, they also destroy other essential clotting factors. In contrast the acyl-plasmin complexes have the advantage of a more localized activity (23).

THE CLINICAL SYNDROMES

The approach to the postphlebitic syndrome is logically considered in three steps. The first of these is recognition of the high-risk patient in whom preventive therapy may avoid later morbidity. The second is the appropriate investigation and treatment of the acute deep venous occlusion with the objective of returning total venous function to normal. Third is consideration of the established postphlebitic limb, where an awareness of the newer therapeutic options may lead to subjective and objective improvement.

There is no uniformity of opinion about the individual who will develop either the acute occlusion or the later consequences of chronic vascular insufficiency in the lower limb. There is, however, consensus about the high-risk patient. A congenital absence of iliofemoral valves is incriminated in the development of varicose veins (24), but there is no evidence that, in the absence of venous occlusion, this finding results in symptomatic venous insufficiency. Congenital disturbances in the hemostatic mechanism, notably deficiency of antithrombin III, predisposes affected individuals to venous occlusion, and long-term oral anticoagulant therapy is indicated.

Of greater importance numerically are acquired conditions predisposing to venous occlusion and having absolute or relative indications for prophylactic management. Previous proven deep vein thrombosis in the presence of persisting chronic illness is an absolute indication for antithrombic therapy unless precluded by poor patient compliance or a bleeding diathesis. Relative indications, which may often be short term, are seriously ill medical patients exemplified by those with acute myocardial infarction, congestive cardiac failure, and selected patients undergoing surgical procedures where short-term antithrombotic therapy may diminish the risk of deep vein thrombosis (25). Similarly, hyperviscosity syndromes including expanded red cell mass, as occurs with erythrocytosis, or raised platelet counts are reasonable indications for prophylactic antithrombic drug treatment until the hematologic abnormality has been reversed. Other predisposing factors are obesity, blood group (26), therapeutic estrogens, and geographical factors (27), but patients in the latter group are clearly unsuitable for prophylactic therapy with dangerous drugs unless a second factor is added, such as debilitating illness or surgery.

The clinical presentation of acute deep vein occlusion is local inflammation, pain, and distal edema occurring usually in the appropriate clinical setting. A multitude of additional clinical signs and bedside tests are described but modern practice, particularly in view of the increasingly recognized hazards of antithrombotic therapy, necessitates confirmation with venography. The latter procedure is necessary since pain occurs in only 50% of acute episodes and the remainder are silent.

Chronic changes that exemplify the postphlebitic syndrome characteristically arise in a leg that contains varicose veins and include edema, which is usually mild to moderate and is thought to result from a recirculating volume in the leg that has increased beyond the capacity of the remaining competent veins to maintain venous flow toward the heart (28). Pain is present, often described as heaviness or fullness, and recurrent thromboses are recognized sequelae. The hallmark of this syndrome is the extensive skin changes: pigmentation due to hemosiderin, ulceration occurring in the venous triangle above the inner malleolus, and the lipodermatosclerosis or simply liposclerosis (4).

PATHOPHYSIOLOGIC CONSIDERATIONS

Review of the now voluminous literature on the postphlebitic syndrome emphasizes the fact, increasingly acknowledged in clinical practice, that recognition and correction of a predisposing cause is optimal treatment or, stated more conventionally, prevention is better than cure. Accordingly, consideration is given to the prethrombotic, the acute thrombotic, and the chronic, established, or postphlebitic syndrome.

The pathophysiologic factors predisposing an individual to deep venous occlusion fall into two major categories. Of a general nature are gross obesity, smoking, and perhaps such less clearly defined factors as lifestyle and diet (27). In this group, commonsense measures will diminish the risk but, all too frequently, patients are seen for the first time with deep venous occlusion. Secondly, there is the high-risk group where rheology of the blood or the hemostatic mechanism are disturbed either chronically, as with erythrocytosis, thrombocytosis, chronic debility, and heart failure, or acutely, during admissions for medical or surgical reasons. In the majority of these patients, recognition of risk factors and appropriate prophylaxis should be standard practice.

The pathophysiology of the acute venous lesion emphasizes both the role of the hematologist and the importance of collaboration between disciplines in investigation and management. In contrast to hemostasis, which is the physiologic and extravascular process by which vascular integrity is maintained, thrombosis is an intravascular or occlusive phenomenon that may alter hemodynamics and lead to distal tissue injury. Furthermore, during hemostasis a balance is maintained between coagulation and fibrinolysis with the initiating event being involvement of platelets following exposure of subendothelial tissues. In thrombosis, the hemostatic mechanism is disturbed while the inciting event is not restricted to minor vascular injury with appropriate platelet response but may lie in quantitative or qualitative changes in other components of the blood. It follows that a number of different lesions may find common expression in venous occlusion and, since the time of Virchow, these have conveniently been considered as defects predominantly in blood, in venous flow, or the vessel wall.

In the blood, congenital deficiency of inhibitors is exemplified by antithrombin III deficiency although other less common abnormalities are described (29). Acquired defects in the coagulation system occur during pregnancy and following estrogen administration (30). In addition to situations that predispose to thrombosis, defective fibrinolysis resulting from alpha-2-plasmin inhibitor (31), alpha-1-antitrypsin, C1 inhibitor, and interalphatrypsin inhibitor may be involved in the pathogenesis of deep vein occlusion (32–35). Similarly, thrombocytosis, particularly in the myeloproliferative syndrome, is a risk factor.

Changes in the composition of the blood may profoundly alter the normal characteristics of blood flow or rheology and occur in heart failure and with low left ventricular output. In individuals otherwise normal, a similar situation may result following increased viscosity. This may be due to raised immunoglobulin concentration in the plasma (36) or may affect the whole blood. The latter situation is particularly dangerous in the myeloproliferative syndrome where both expanded red cell mass and thrombocytosis coexist.

Disturbances in the vessel wall have received more attention as understanding of prostacyclin metabolism has increased because, in the pathogenesis of venous occlusion, the primary event is interaction between platelet and vessel wall, although the role of fibrin is subsequently of major importance in clot propagation. It now appears clear that the critical balance between thromboxane from the platelet and prostacyclin from the endothelial cell may result in a local environment favorable to platelet deposition. Furthermore, it has long been recognized that veins are rich in a specific species of plasminogen activator, and disturbances in fibrinolytic function must be considered as an additional factor in acute venous occlusion. Furthermore, direct damage to vessels occurs by immune complex deposition in collagen-vascular disorders, as a result of rickettsial or viral infections and in septicemia, all of which result in sufficient local damage to favor thrombosis.

These three variables that make up the Virchow triad come together, to a variable degree depending upon the major physiologic disturbance, in thrombus formation. Nevertheless, the pathology is relatively clear cut in that a nidus for platelet deposition occurs, characteristically behind a valve cusp, and then local activation of the coagulation cascade results in fibrin generation. There follows the addition of successive layers of fibrin and platelets, flow decreases, and retrograde extension occurs with venous occlusion. The structure of the thrombi, identification of primary sites of venous occlusion, and the consequential thrombogenic effects of venous stasis are well recognized (27).

The development of the postphlebitic syndrome follows most commonly on failure to recognize and adequately treat venous thrombosis. Traditionally, attention is focused primarily on flow and pressure changes. However, more recent studies (4) have emphasized the role of fibrinolysis and capillary permeability in the pathogenesis of skin change and ulceration.

Despite recanalization of occluded segments, valve damage is permanent (13, 36–38) and dynamics altered. The net shift of blood between the deep, superficial, and perforating vessels varies with valve competence. At rest, there is little flow in the deep veins, and during muscular contraction this is toward the heart but retrograde during relaxation (16, 17). Valve competence results in blood entering the long saphenous vein through the perforating system but when this mechanism is destroyed, reflux results in extremely poor efficiency in the system. These findings may be summarized by stating that during exercise flow is bidirectional in deep and superficial systems but valvular incompetence has a resultant mean flow through the perforating system from deep to superficial veins (8).

Pressure patterns vary depending upon the presence of occlusion, adequacy of collateral circulation, and in response to exercise. In the presence of iliofemoral thrombosis, pressures are raised during the period of obstruction but diminish with the development of collateral circulation (39). Furthermore, at rest, there is no significant difference between normal limbs and those where recanalization of the deep veins has occurred (9). However, during exercise, incompetent deep veins result in marked venous pressure fluctuation in the long saphenous vein at the ankle, being between two and three times greater than that found in normal limbs. Furthermore, the rate at which pressures return to resting levels is 30 seconds in the normal limb and is as short as 1.5 seconds in diseased limbs (15, 40, 41). These data have been assembled with the summary (42) that hemodynamic changes in the presence of deep venous insufficiency result in failure to physiologically decrease pressure at the ankles which may, on occasions, exceed resting levels. Typically, venous claudication occurs when ambulatory pressures exceed those found during systole, but it may also arise, particularly during exercise, in patients with deep venous valvular incompetence without associated increase in venous pressure.

Turning away from purely mechanical considerations to changes that underlie the development of venous ulceration, researchers observed that carefully planned surgery may nevertheless be associated with recurrence of ulcer and that, in these patients, there was extensive phlebographic evidence of deep vein damage (43). Burnand and his co-workers emphasized the essential difference between the previously incorrect use of the term fat necrosis and lipodermatosclerosis or liposclerosis and questioned rupture of small venules as the explanation for the development of pigmentation with hemosiderin deposit in the affected area of the limb. In an elegant series of studies, they correlated significant reduction in blood and tissue fibrinolytic activity (44) with changes in capillary permeability and enunciated their concept of perivascular tissue clearance (4), stating "that the principal physiologic function of tissue fibrinolysis is to keep the pericapillary spaces clear, therefore acting as a perivascular clearing mechanism." The relationship of this hypothesis to altered hemodynamics is through the failure of the calf muscle pump mechanism with failure of venous pressure to approximate normal during exercise. The resultant venous hypertension is associated with the development of multiple small new capillaries in the dermis from whose wide intracellular pores leak large molecules from the blood into the vascular space including fibrinogen, which is then converted to fibrin. In patients with liposclerosis, inadequacy of fibrinolysis is reflected in the skin changes where impaired nutrition and poor oxygenation result ultimately in necrosis and ulceration (4).

INVESTIGATION

A convenient approach, as with the description of the clinical syndrome and pathophysiologic considerations, is investigation of the high-risk patient, proof of acute deep vein thrombosis, and demonstration of venous insufficiency.

It is not practical to extensively investigate (45) all patients considered to be at risk (46); studies in this group are best limited to those where confirmation is needed for suspected deficiency of inhibitors such as antithrombin III. The numbers of patients at risk make it logistically impractical to invest large amounts of time and effort in any but a minute, highly selected subpopulation.

By way of contrast, patients considered on clinical grounds to have a deep venous thrombosis justify thorough study to define the extent of the lesion and also to provide a basis for confirming the adequacy of subsequent treatment. Venography (42) has been available for over half a century and now enjoys preeminence in the study of the veins, largely as a result of continuing improvement in the contrast medium and more sophisticated radiographic techniques. Indications vary between institutions (47) and in our experience (48) venography remains the single investigation on which we base therapeutic decisions. While this procedure does have limitations in being uncomfortable and an invasive procedure, adverse side effects are related to hypersensitivity reactions to the dye and are comparable to intravenous pyelography.

Radioisotopic studies originally employed the ^{125}I-fibrinogen test, which remains a useful research tool, contributes to an understanding of the pathogenesis in natural history of the venous occlusion, is helpful for studying prophylactic measures, and can be applied to monitoring lysis or extension of established clot. Largely, as the limitations of radioactive fibrinogen studies became recognized, attempts were made to label plasminogen, streptokinase, or urokinase, but use of human substrate was only partially successful. Porcine plasmin labelled with technetium, while limited by the same false-positive results as fibrinogen, has now been relatively well established and provides information within an hour of injection (49).

The noninvasive tests have increased rapidly, including Doppler ultrasound, impedance plethysmography, thermography, and phleborheography (50). Thus, Doppler ultrasound is rapid, safe, and may be repeated; it is most useful for thrombosis proximal to the calf, where a sensitivity of 96% and a specificity of 86% have been documented. Impedance plethysmography is both sensitive and specific for clot above the calf. Currently, these two methods may be combined, and it has been suggested that when a third test, ^{125}I-fibrinogen test, is added venography will become unnecessary in the majority of the patients (50).

The crucial objective of therapy is to ensure venous patency and preservation of valve function. In this regard there is as yet insufficient evidence that any method can replace venography, particularly when the latter is combined with cinematographic studies of valve function (51).

The investigation of the patient with established venous insufficiency has traditionally concentrated on pathophysiologic changes in the venous circulation. Pressure measurements are invasive and, while they remain the reference standard, are being increasingly replaced by noninvasive techniques including Doppler ultrasound, calf volume plethysmography, photoplethysmography, and foot volumetry (52). In a recent extensive review of the investigation of vascular disorders (53), the importance of accurate history and careful clinical examination were emphasized. Furthermore, the routine application of the tourniquet test and Doppler ultrasound examination established the correct diagnosis and enabled the planning of appropriate therapy in 92% of patients. It was only in the remaining 8% that other investigations were needed.

However, it is no longer appropriate to restrict investigations to altered hemodynamics; the adequate investigation of these patients must now include studies of fibrinolysis and capillary permeability (4). The latter approach is long overdue and, coupled with ever-improving sophistication in the investigation and diagnosis of venous thrombosis and its late sequelae, marks an important change in the philosophy and investigation of these patients.

MANAGEMENT

Prophylaxis rests upon recognition of the high-risk patient (46) and is largely common sense: weight loss, discontinuation of smoking, maintenance of adequate hydration, mechanically assisted movement of the legs where the patient is ill, and prophylactic antithrombotic drugs in selected groups (54–58), although controversy still attends this practice (48). Dextran has also been studied as a form of prophylaxis for venous thromboembolism (59) as well as oral anticoagulants and antiplatelet drugs (60), and intermittent compression of the legs (61). There is a large literature which is, as yet, controversial. Protagonists for different mechanical or systemic methods have brought impressive evidence to bear in favor of prophylactic techniques. However, more critical analysis of the data and the experience with further studies have not resolved the role of prophylaxis, and the widely recognized importance of this possibility is a strong stimulus for continued work in this area. Nevertheless, there remains a subgroup of high-risk patients who can be clearly identified and here the risk of hemorrhage, particularly in the intraoperative and postoperative periods, must be balanced against the benefits of prophylactic measures.

Management of the patients with established deep vein thrombosis now rests upon proof of venous thrombosis. Two problems require consideration. The first is the return of venous patency and valve preservation. The second is the prevention and treatment of pulmonary embolism.

For a long period of time patients were treated with therapeutic doses of heparin, but this is not ideal since it does not induce thrombolysis (62). As a result, thrombolytic therapy followed by anticoagulation has been increasingly employed (63). Our own studies have demonstrated that thrombolytic therapy can result in maintenance of valve function (51). It remains to be shown that this approach will also uniformly leave the patients symptom free.

In patients with thromboembolism, data come from one controlled study (64). However, recent critical review of all the available literature (65) casts considerable doubt on the adequacy of this data and not only emphasizes the hazards of anticoagulation but clarifies the need for urgent research in this area, particularly a comparison between treatment and conservative management.

Management of the patient with the postphlebitic syndrome is testimony to the inadequacy of prophylactic therapy and the improper management of the acute predisposing thrombotic event. However, when faced with the patient having venous insufficiency of the lower limb, conservative, medical, and surgical possibilities exist. The former (66) recommends that this be on an outpatient basis and anticipates excellent to good results in 85% of the patients with this syndrome. Medical management, based on the work of Burnand & Browse (4) suggests a place for the anabolic androgen, Stanozolol, 5 mg twice daily, an opinion confirmed subsequently by Hobbs (67). Surgical treatment (28) focuses attention primarily on the Linton procedure (68). In addition, a series of much more extensive procedures including cross-over grafting for iliofemoral venous occlusion, venous thrombectomy, and direct venous reconstruction are described; these fall within the ambit of specialized vascular surgical units.

SUMMARY AND CONCLUSIONS

The indolent but relentlessly progressive clinical syndrome that occurs in the lower limbs of humans, characterized by pain, edema, pigmentation, liposclerosis, and refractory ulceration, is known as the postphlebitic syndrome. In the majority of patients, a well-recognized episode of acute venous occlusion can usually be identified, but in the remainder no such precipitating event is documented.

The pathogenesis is of particular importance. Thus, the development of this entity remains an indictment of medical care, which, in the majority of patients, is the consequence of unrecognized or inadequately treated deep vein thrombosis. The latter results in disruption of venous anatomy of the lower limb, incompetence of valves, and altered hemodynamics. There follows venous hypertension that fails to return to normal following exercise and is associated with increased volume in the leg. Final expression is the venous blow-out syndrome where liposclerosis and refractory ulceration occur classically in the venous triangle above the medial malleolus.

Not unreasonably, major attention has in the past been given to the way in which blood flow and pressure deviate from normal at rest and in response to exercise so that medical management and vascular reconstruction have long been the mainstay of treatment.

Two important concluding comments are necessary.

The first of these is that anticoagulant therapy with heparin or warfarin does not enhance clot lysis and, therefore, even if venous channels are reestablished, valve dysfunction will persist. Consequently, it is essential that high-risk patients be recognized and given appropriate prophylaxis to prevent venous thrombosis. In addition, patients with established venous occlusion should have the lesion accurately defined with venography and, unless contraindications are present, treated with thrombolytic agents; this should then be followed by prolonged anticoagulation. Subsequent or follow-up studies are essential to confirm the adequate resolution of clot and reconstitution of valve function, and to correlate these observations with the duration of symptomatic improvement.

Secondly, it should be appreciated that disturbances of flow and pressure, while often initiating events that can be easily studied, can no longer overshadow the importance of associated changes that include alterations in local and systemic fibrinolytic activity, new vessel formation, and capillary permeability in the pathogenesis of the pigmented liposclerotic lesion around the ankle. In this situation, therapy aimed at enhancing fibrin breakdown, and thereby facilitating clearance of large-molecular-weight molecules that may have leaked into the interstitium from the plasma, are promising new forms of treatment that may further decrease morbidity.

Finally, it is necessary to reflect on the enormous morbidity that attends the postphlebitic syndrome and to emphasize that its continued occurrence often reflects poor quality medical care, inadequate initial diagnosis, and inappropriate subsequent treatment. To this end, a team of interested and dedicated individuals are necessary for optimal management and should include a diagnostic radiologist, hematologist, physician, and surgeon.

ACKNOWLEDGMENTS

Supported by the University of Cape Town Leukemia Center and the Staff Research Fund, the Medical Research Council, the National Cancer Association, and the Kaliski and Chanani Bequests. I thank Jackie Davies for typing, Shelia Katcher for bibliographic assistance, and the Medical Superintendent of Groote Schuur Hospital for permission to publish.

It is a particular pleasure to be able to record my appreciation to Professor Norman L. Browse from the Department of Surgery at St. Thomas's Hospital Medical School for his advice in preparation of the manuscript.

Literature Cited

1. Linton, R. R. 1953. The post-thrombotic ulceration of the lower extremity: its etiology and surgical treatment. *Ann. Surg.* 138:415–32
2. Bauer, G. 1955. Rationale and results of popliteal vein division. *Angiology* 6:169–89
3. Owens, J. C., Anderson, L. L. 1957. Indications for surgical treatment of the postphlebitic syndrome. *Surgery* 1:81
4. Browse, N. L., Burnand, K. G. 1978. The postphlebitic syndrome: a new look. In *Venous Problems,* ed. J. J. Bergan, J. S. T. Yao, pp. 395–404, Chicago: Year Book Medical
5. Thomson, H. 1979. The surgical anatomy of the superficial and perforating veins of the lower limb. *Ann. R. Coll. Surg. Engl.* 61:198–205
6. McPheeters, H. O., Rice, C. O. 1929. Varicose veins: circulation and direction of the venous flow: experimental proof. *Surg. Gynecol. Obstet.* 49:29–33
7. Bjordal, R. I. 1970. Simultaneous pressure and flow recordings in varicose veins of the lower extremity. *Acta Chir. Scand.* 136:309–17
8. Angelides, N. S. 1981. Venous hemodynamics of the lower limb. In *Investigation of Vascular Disorders,* ed. A. N. Nicolaides, J. S. T. Yao, pp. 452–40, New York: Churchill Livingstone
9. Pollack, A. A., Wood, E. H. 1949. Venous pressure in saphenous vein at the ankle in man during exercise and changes in posture. *J. Appl. Physiol.* 1:649–62
10. Kriessman, A. 1981. Ambulatory venous pressure measurements. See Ref. 8, pp. 461–77
11. Shepherd, J. T. 1978. Reflex control of the venous system. See Ref. 4, pp. 5–23
12. Hojensgard, I. C., Sturup, H. 1952. Static and dynamic pressures in superficial and deep veins of the lower extremity in man. *Acta Physiol. Scand.* 27:49
13. Ludbrook, J. 1966. The musculovenous pumps of the human lower limb. *Am. Heart J.* 71:635–41
14. Stegall, H. F. 1966. Muscle pumping in the dependent leg. *Circ. Res.* 19:180–90
15. Strandness, D. E. 1978. Applied venous physiology in normal subjects and venous insufficiency. See Ref. 4, pp. 25–45
16. Bjordal, R. I. 1971. Pressure patterns in the saphenous system in patients with venous leg ulcers. The proximal saphenous occlusion test as a guide to diagnosis, therapy and prognosis. *Acta Chir. Scand.* 137:495–501
17. Bjordal, R. I. 1972. Circulation patterns in incompetent perforating veins in the calf and in the saphenous system in primary varicose veins. *Acta Chir. Scand.* 138:251–61
18. Arnoldi, C. C., Greitz, T., Linderholm, H. 1966. Variations in cross sectional area and pressure in the veins of the normal human leg during rhythmic muscular exercise. *Acta Chir. Scand.* 132:507–22
19. Arnoldi, C. C., Linderholm, H. 1969. Venous blood pressures in the lower limb at rest and during exercise in patients with idiopathic dysfunction of the venous pump of the calf. *Acta Chir. Scand.* 135:601–9
20. Goodwin, G. M., McCloskey, D. I., Mitchell, J. H. 1972. Cardiovascular and respiratory responses to changes in central command during isometric exercise at constant muscle tension. *J. Physiol. (Lond.)* 226:173–90
21. Browse, N. L., Clemenson, G., Thomas, M. L. 1980. Is the postphlebitic leg always postphlebitic? Relation between phlebographic appearances of deep-vein thrombosis and late sequelae. *Br. Med. J.* 281:1167–70
22. Fuster, V., Chesebro, J. H. 1981. Antithrombic therapy: role of platelet-inhibitor drugs. *Mayo Clin. Proc.* 56:185–95
23. Smith, R. A. G., Dupe, R. J., English, P. D., Green, J. 1981. Fibrinolysis with acyl-enzymes: a new approach to thrombolytic therapy. *Nature* 290:505–8

24. Ludbrook, J., Beale, G. 1962. Femoral venous valves in relation to varicose veins. *Lancet* 1:79–81
25. Kakkar, V. V. 1981. Prevention of venous thromboembolism. *Clin. Haematol.* 10:543–82
26. Jick, H., Slone, D., Westerholm, B., et al. 1969. Venous thromboembolic disease and ABO blood type. *Lancet* 1:539–42
27. Sevitt, S. 1978. Pathology and pathogenesis of deep vein thrombi. See Ref. 4, pp. 257–79
28. Barker, W. F. 1978. The postphlebitic syndrome: management by surgical means. See Ref. 4, pp. 383–93
29. Hirsh, J. 1977. Hypercoagulability. *Semin. Hematol.* 14:409–25
30. Tooke, J. E., McNicol, G. P. 1981. Thrombotic disorders associated with pregnancy and the pill. *Clin. Haematol.* 10:613–30
31. Moroi, M., Aoki, N. 1976. Isolation and characterization of the alpha-2-plasmin inhibitor from human plasma. A novel proteinase inhibitor which inhibits activator-induced clot lysis. *J. Biol. Chem.* 251:5956–65
32. Schreiber, A. D., Kaplan, A. P., Austen, K. F. 1973. Inhibition of C1INH of Hageman factor fragment activation of coagulation, fibrinolysis, and kinin generation. *J. Clin. Invest.* 52:1402–9
33. Crawford, G. P., Ogston, D. 1974. The influence of alpha-1-antitrypsin on plasmin, urokinase and Hageman factor cofactor. *Biochim. Biophys. Acta* 354: 107–13
34. Harpel, P. C., Cooper, N. R. 1975. Studies on human plasma C1 inactivator-enzyme interactions. I. Mechanisms of interaction with C1s, plasmin, and trypsin. *J. Clin. Invest.* 55:593–604
35. Gallimore, M. J. 1975. Serum inhibitors of fibrinolysis. *Br. J. Haematol.* 31: 217–31
36. Bauer, G. 1942. Roentgenological and clinical study of the sequels of thrombosis. *Acta Chir. Scand.* 86(Suppl. 74):1–116
37. Barnes, R. W., Collicott, P. E., Mozersky, D. J., Sumner, D. S., Strandness, D. E. 1973. Noninvasive quantitation of venous reflux in the postphlebitic syndrome. *Surg. Gynecol. Obstet.* 136: 769–73
38. Barnes, R. W., Collicott, P. E., Sumner, D. S., Strandness, D. E. 1973. Noninvasive quantitation of venous hemodynamics in the postphlebitic syndrome. *Arch. Surg.* 107:807–14
39. Negus, D., Cockett, F. B. 1967. Femoral vein pressures in post-phlebitic iliac vein obstruction. *Br. J. Surg.* 54:522–25
40. Hjelmstedt, A. 1968. Pressure decrease in the dorsal pedal veins on walking in persons with and without thrombosis. *Acta Chir. Scand.* 134:531–39
41. Hjelmstedt, A. 1968. The pressure in the veins of the dorsum of the foot in quiet standing and during exercise in limbs without signs of venous disorder. *Acta Chir. Scand.* 134:135–44
42. Nicolaides, A. N. 1981. Venography: development and current status. See Ref. 8, pp. 354–68
43. Burnand, K., Thomas, M. L., O'Donnell, T. F., Browse, N. L. 1976. Relation between postphlebitic changes in the deep veins and results of surgical treatment of venous ulcers. *Lancet* 1:936–38
44. Browse, N. L., Gray, L., Jarrett, P. E. M., Morland, M. 1977. Blood and vein-wall fibrinolytic activity in health and vascular disease. *Br. Med. J.* 1:478–81
45. Lowe, G. D. O. 1981. Laboratory evaluation of hypercoagulability. *Clin. Haematol.* 10:407–42
46. Meade, T. W. 1981. Risk associations in the thrombotic disorders. *Clin. Haematol.* 10:391–405
47. Neiman, H. L. 1978. Phlebography in the diagnosis of venous thrombosis. See Ref. 4, pp. 111–40
48. Immelman, E. J., Jeffrey, P., Benatar, S. R., Elliott, M. S., Smith, J. A. 1979. Failure of low-dose heparin to prevent significant thromboembolic complications in high-risk surgical patients: interim report of prospective trial. *Br. Med. J.* 1:1447–50
49. Olsson, C.-G. 1981. ^{99m}Tc-plasmin: development and current status. See Ref. 8, pp. 443–51
50. Nicolaides, A. N., Yao, J. S. T. 1981. General considerations and conclusions. See Ref. 8, pp. 600–16
51. Elliott, M. S., Immelman, E. J., Jeffery, P., et al. 1979. A comparative randomized trial of heparin versus streptokinase in the treatment of acute proximal venous thrombosis: an interim report of a prospective trial. *Br. J. Surg.* 66: 838–43
52. Lawrence, D., Kakkar, V. V. 1980. Post-phlebitic syndrome—a functional assessment. *Br. J. Surg.* 67:686–69
53. Nicolaides, A. N., Yao, J. S. T., eds. 1978. *Investigation of Vascular Disorders.* New York: Churchill Livingstone. 635 pp.
54. Sharnoff, J. G., Bagg, J. F., Breen, S. R., Rogliano, A. G., Walsh, A. R., Scar-

dino, V. 1960. The possible indication of post-operative thromboembolism by platelet counts and blood coagulation studies in the patient undergoing extensive surgery. *Surg. Gynecol. Obstet.* 111:469–74

55. Sharnoff, J. G. 1966. Results in the prophylaxis of postoperative thromboembolism. *Surg. Gynecol. Obstet.* 123: 303–7

56. Sharnoff, J. G., De Blasio, G. 1970. Prevention of fatal postoperative thromboembolism by heparin prophylaxis. *Lancet* 2:1006–7

57. Kakkar, V. V., Field, E. S., Nicolaides, A. N., Flute, P. T., Wessler, S., Yin, E. T. 1971. Low doses of heparin in prevention of deep-vein thrombosis. *Lancet* 2:669–71

58. Kakkar, V. V., Corrigan, T., Spindler, J., et al. 1972. Efficacy of low doses of heparin in prevention of deep-vein thrombosis after major surgery. A double-blind, randomised trial. *Lancet* 2:101–6

59. Bergentz, S.-E. 1978. Dextran prophylaxis of venous thromboembolism. See Ref. 4, pp. 529–40

60. Salzman, E. W. 1978. Prevention of venous thromboembolism by oral anticoagulants and drugs affecting platelet function. See Ref. 4, pp. 545–51

61. Cotton, L. T., Roberts, V. C. 1978. The prevention of postoperative deep venous thrombosis by intermittent compression of the legs. See Ref. 4, pp. 553–57

62. Hull, R., Hirsh, J. 1982. Advances and controversies in the diagnosis and treatment of venous thromboembolism. *Prog. Hematol.* 13:73–123

63. Thrombolytic therapy in thrombosis: a National Institutes of Health Consensus Development Conference. 1980. *Ann. Intern. Med.* 93:141–44

64. Barritt, D. W., Jordan, S. C. 1960. Anticoagulant drugs in the treatment of pulmonary embolism. A controlled trial. *Lancet* 1:1309–12

65. Egermayer, P. 1981. Value of anticoagulants in the treatment of pulmonary embolism: a discussion paper. *J. R. Soc. Med.* 74:675

66. Owens, J. C. 1978. The postphlebitic syndrome: management by conservative means. See Ref. 4, p. 369–82

67. Hobbs, J. 1978. Discussion. See Ref. 4, pp. 407–8

68. Linton, R. R. 1938. Communicating veins of the lower leg and the operative technic for their ligation. *Ann. Surg.* 107:582–93

Ann. Rev. Med. 1983. 34:107–16

BIOLOGICAL AND CLINICAL IMPLICATIONS OF LYMPHOCYTE HYBRIDOMAS: Tumor Therapy with Monoclonal Antibodies

Ronald Levy, M.D., and Richard A. Miller, M.D.

Department of Medicine, Division of Oncology, Stanford University, Stanford, California 94305

ABSTRACT

Monoclonal antibodies of defined specificity can be produced using hybridoma technology. New attempts are being made to explore the potential of antibody therapy for cancer. Preliminary studies show that problems such as antigenic modulation, circulating free antigen, effector cell shortage, and host anti-mouse immunoglobulin response must be overcome. Uses of monoclonal antibodies in cancer treatment include the administration of unconjugated antibodies or of antibodies coupled to drugs, toxins, or radioisotopes, and the use of monoclonal antibodies in vitro to eradicate residual malignant cells.

Introduction

It has long been hoped that antibodies directed against tumor cell surfaces could be exploited for therapy (1). Because of their specificity and their cytotoxic effects, antibodies provide an appealing theoretical approach to cell destruction in vivo. Despite these hopes and extensive experimental attempts (2), antibodies are not as yet a part of the therapeutic armamentarium.

Until recently, the primary limitation on antibodies as therapeutic agents was their impurity and heterogeneity. Since the advent of hybridoma technology (3), unlimited quantities of pure, homogeneous antibodies of defined specificity can be easily produced, and new attempts are being made to explore the potential of antibody therapy.

Table 1 lists the problems that must be considered when attempting to treat tumors with antibodies. To begin with, there is the problem of anti-

107

0066-4219/83/0401-0107$02.00

body specificity. It is intuitively obvious that the goal is to use an antibody that recognizes a tumor-specific antigen and thus distinguishes absolutely between tumor cells and normal cells. However, with the notable exception of idiotypes on B-cell tumors, no such tumor-specific antigen has yet been found. Rather, a number of tumor-related antigens have been defined that are more or less restricted to tumor cells and their tissue of origin.

How specific must an antibody be to achieve a therapeutic effect? Bernstein and his colleagues (4) described an animal model in which a monoclonal antibody directed against a normal differentiation antigen was used to eliminate leukemia cells. This was true despite the fact that the antigen was simultaneously expressed by normal cells in the host.

A number of other important lessons have been learned from this and other animal models (2–11). The antibody, to be effective in eliminating tumor cells in vivo, must have the Fc portion. The most important mechanism of tumor-cell destruction by antibodies involves uptake of antibody-coated cells in the reticuloendothelial system or killing by macrophages in the local area. Antibodies of the IgM class are far less effective than those of the IgG class. Tumor cells can escape the effects of antibody by a number of mechanisms. These include (*a*) antigenic heterogeneity—some cells may lack the target for the antibody, (*b*) antigenic modulation (12–14)—the temporary disappearance of a cell surface antigen caused by the presence of antibody, and (*c*) an exhaustion of effector cells or reticuloendothelial system saturation (15).

Clinical Studies

Table 2 summarizes the available data from clinical trials with monoclonal antibodies. Most of these studies were conducted on patients with leukemia or lymphoma. All of the patients in these trials had advanced disease and had failed the conventional treatments. Collectively, these studies encountered most of the issues enumerated in Table 1. Antibodies with varying degrees of tumor specificity have been employed, ranging from individual tumor-specific antiidiotype antibodies to antibodies that react with normal as well as malignant T cells.

Table 1 Problems encountered in antitumor therapy with monoclonal antibodies

Specificity of the antibody	Circulating free antigen
Is there a human tumor-specific antigen?	Circulating host antibodies
How specific an antibody do we need?	Antigenic modulation
Fate of the antibody in vivo—pharma-	Antigen-negative tumor cells
cokinetics	Immune response of host against foreign
Antibody class	antibody
Antibody fragments	
Antibody coupled to drugs or toxin	

Table 2 Monoclonal antibody clinical trials

Disease[a]	Antibody/Class	Specificity	Patients (no.)	Maximum single dose (mg)	Toxicity	Effect	Reference
DLPD	89/IgG2	lymphoma	1	1500	Renal	Blocking of antibody by circulating antigen Transient reduction in circulating cells	16
CALL	J5/IgG2a	CALLA	4	170	None	Transient reduction in circulating cells Rapid escape of leukemia due to antigenic modulation	14
CTCL	L17F12/IgG2a	Leu–1	1	20	None	Partial remission lasting 10 weeks Escape of tumor in new sites due to effector-cell shortage	17
CTCL	L17F12/IgG2a	Leu–1	7	100	Cutaneous pain, one patient Dyspnea, one patient Hives, one patient	Partial remission in 5/7 patients Escape of tumor due to anti-mouse antibody	
T-ALL	L17F12/IgG2a 12E7/IgG1 4H9/IgG2a	Leu–1 T and B cells T cells	8	50	Sporadic coagulopathy, one Otherwise, none	Transient reduction in circulating cells in some, but not all, patients No lasting clinical benefit	
NLPD	4D6/IgG2b	idiotype	1	150	None	Complete remission lasting 15+ months	18
CLL	T101/IgG2a	Leu–1	2	12	Anaphylactoid reaction after rapid infusion	Transient reduction in circulating cells	19
GI cancer	171A/IgG2a	GI cancer	4	200	None	None	20

[a] DLPD: diffuse poorly differentiated lymphocytic lymphoma   NLPD: nodular poorly differentiated lymphocytic lymphoma
CALL: common acute lymphocytic leukemia of children   CLL: chronic lymphocytic leukemia
CTCL: cutaneous T-cell lymphoma   GI: gastrointestinal
T-ALL: T-cell acute lymphocytic leukemia

Toxicity

There has been very little toxicity of mouse monoclonal antibody administered to man. As can be seen from the table, mouse monoclonal antibodies
have been infused into patients in doses as high as 1500 mg. However, most
of the experience involved doses in the 1–100-mg range. In many of these
studies, repeated treatments were given, which, in some cases, extended
over several months. Rapid infusion rates can be associated with fever,
chills, dyspnea, and anaphylactoid reactions, especially in patients with
high numbers of circulating leukemia cells in the blood or with underlying
cardiopulmonary disease. Other toxicities have been rare, but have included
renal impairment in one patient with high levels of free antigen in the serum,
and a sporadic coagulation defect in one patient with T-cell acute lymphocytic leukemia (ALL). The lack of toxicity of monoclonal antibodies,
in contrast to that of other foreign globulin preparations used therapeutically, such as antithymocyte globulin (ATG), is undoubtedly due to their
purity and specificity.

Immunogenicity of Mouse Monoclonal Antibodies in Man

Most of the patients who have received monoclonal antibodies thus far have
had diseases or other treatments that could impair their immunocompe-
tence. Nevertheless, more than half of the patients who were properly
observed made significant antibody responses against the mouse Ig. In no
case has the antibody response resulted in allergy, serum sickness, immune
complex disease, or other evident toxicity. This has been true despite the
continued administration of the mouse monoclonal antibody in the face of
serum antibody against it. However, the antibody response against the
mouse Ig neutralizes the therapeutic effect of the monoclonal antibodies.
Serum from such a treated patient can block the binding of the monoclonal
antibody to target cells in vitro, and this blocking power increases with time
after the patient's initial exposure to mouse Ig.

It is important, at this point, to distinguish between antibody reacting
against the constant portions of the mouse Ig molecule and that reacting
with the combining site (idiotype). The major portion of the anti-mouse
antibody response of the lymphoma patients receiving anti-Leu-1 is directed
against common mouse Ig determinants, since unrelated mouse Ig can
remove approximately 95% of the binding activity in their serum. These
antibodies account for the rapid clearance eventually seen with the injected
monoclonal antibody. Colvin and his colleagues (21) report that renal transplant patients receiving the anti-T-cell monoclonal antibody OKT3 make
antiidiotype antibody. Antiidiotype antibodies are also produced by lymphoma patients receiving anti-Leu-1. Although this antiidiotype portion of
the immune response is only approximately 5% of the total response, it is

functionally important. Most of the blocking activity of immune serum is due to antiidiotype antibody, and cannot be removed by absorption of the serum with unrelated mouse Ig. It is clear, therefore, that the neutralizing effect of human anti-mouse antibody in vivo is due to a host immune response against both the constant region and the idiotype of the mouse monoclonal antibody. These conclusions have important implications for the eventual use of human monoclonal antibodies for therapy. Such human antibodies may likewise evoke an antiidiotypic immune response.

Antigenic Modulation, Free Antigen Blockade, and Immunoselection

The most dramatic example of antigenic modulation occurred in the study by Ritz and colleagues (14), who used the anti–common acute lymphocytic leukemia antigen (CALLA) monoclonal antibody in patients with common ALL. The CALLA antigen was subsequently shown to disappear totally from the surface of leukemic cells within minutes after their exposure to the antibody in vitro (22). In the clinical trial, escape of leukemic cells from the effects of antibody in vivo was completely explained by antigenic modulation. Cell surface antigens vary in their propensity to undergo antibody-induced antigenic modulation. For instance, the Leu-1 antigen only partially modulates in vitro, and, in the clinical trials with the anti-Leu-1 monoclonal antibody, some degree of modulation was observed but was easily overcome by intermittent dosing (17). Free antigen in the serum explained the ineffectiveness of the antilymphoma monoclonal antibody in the study of Nadler et al (16) as well as the renal toxicity of high doses. One patient with adult T-cell leukemia treated with the anti-Leu-1 antibody was documented to release free antigen into the serum upon destruction of leukemic cells, whereupon a subsequent dose of antibody was rendered ineffective (23). Low levels of free idiotype in the serum of a patient with B-cell lymphoma initially blocked the effect of antiidiotype monoclonal antibody, but this blockade was overcome with higher doses of antibody (18). No clinical examples of immunoselection are documented as yet since all relapses in antibody-treated patients occurred with antigen-positive cells. However, the true test of whether immunoselection will be an important problem will require larger numbers of patients achieving prolonged clinical remissions.

Therapeutic Effects

The primary purpose of all the initial clinical trials has been to define the toxicities and problems of monoclonal antibodies in humans. However, almost every case offered the opportunity to make some preliminary observations on therapeutic effects as well. In no instance has the maximum

tolerated dose or the optimum schedule of monochlonal antibody administration been determined. Yet, some positive results have been described.
Many of the studies showed that leukemia cells can be cleared from the
blood, at least temporarily (14, 16, 17, 19, 23). In one case evidence was
presented to argue that cells were actually destroyed and not just redis-
tributed (23). The first patient in whom a clinically significant response was
achieved had a T-cell lymphoma with disease in skin, lymph nodes, and
blood (17). He received 15 infusions of anti-Leu-1 antibody extending over
a period of ten weeks. Disease in all sites regressed after the first two weeks,
but, despite continued therapy, he never achieved a complete remission.
Histologic analysis of the regressing lesions disclosed fewer tumor cells but
no evidence of infiltration by other reactive lymphoreticular cells. Small
amounts of mouse antibody could be documented on the tumor cells in the
skin. The disease eventually recurred, largely in new lymph node and skin
sites, and the tumor cells that grew expressed the Leu-1 antigen. The most
likely explanation for tumor-cell resistance to therapy was a shortage of
effector cells in the local tumor sites. This patient produced no anti-mouse
antibody.

These observations on the anti-Leu-1 antibody have now been extended
to another seven patients with cutaneous T-cell lymphoma. The therapeutic
effects have been confirmed, with five of the seven patients achieving a
partial response that was clinically meaningful. None of these patients
achieved a complete response. Unlike the first patient, four of these subsequent patients have made significant anti-mouse Ig antibody responses, and
it is this response that led to the loss of clinical benefit.

Simultaneously, a series of eight patients with T-cell ALL, mostly children, were studied with anti-Leu-1 antibody infusions. In addition, many
of these same patients received one or more other antibodies that were
highly reactive with their leukemic cells. The other two antibodies studied,
12E7 (24) and 4H9, were of the IgG1 and IgG2a class, respectively, and,
unlike anti-Leu-1, neither induced antigenic modulation. Some of these
treatments included combinations of two or three antibodies. Many of these
infusions resulted in transient reductions of circulating leukemic cells, but
no lasting clinical benefit was achieved. In contrast to the patients with
cutaneous T-cell lymphoma, these patients with refractory T-cell ALL had
very rapidly progressive disease and were unstable clinically. For this reason, observations on the therapeutic effects were very limited and no conclusions can be drawn at this time about the relative effectiveness of the three
different antibodies, about the effects of multiple antibodies in comparison
to single antibodies, or about the therapeutic promise for monoclonal antibodies in general for this disease. For the time being, these studies in T-cell
ALL provide the phase I toxicity data to justify trials of antibody in patients
with more limited tumor burdens.

Antiidiotype Antibody

B-cell malignancies present a special opportunity to test the potential of antibody therapy. Each B-cell tumor expresses a unique cell surface Ig that is common to all the members of the malignant clone and different from virtually all normal B cells of the host. The idiotype of the tumor cell surface Ig represents the closest approximation of a tumor-specific antigen available (25). It is the nonsecreting B-cell malignancies that are the prime candidates for antiidiotype therapy, since they are not associated with high serum levels of idiotype protein, which could block the effects of antibody. Diseases in this category include follicular lymphoma, Burkitt's lymphoma, diffuse large-cell lymphoma, and chronic lymphocytic leukemia (CLL).

One report has appeared on the treatment of a patient with CLL with antiidiotype antibodies (26). In that study, transient effects on circulating leukemia cells were noted, but there was considerable toxicity. The antibody preparation used in that case was a globulin fraction of an antiserum prepared in sheep. By contrast, a dramatic clinical result was achieved in one patient with follicular lymphoma with a monoclonal antiidiotype antibody (18). This patient had failed other therapies and had growing disease in all lymph node sites, skin, liver, spleen, and bone marrow. He was treated with a monoclonal mouse IgG2b antibody in doses escalating from 1 to 150 mg. Low levels of serum idiotype initially blocked the antibody in vivo, but higher doses of antibody eventually reached tumor cells whereupon the tumor began to regress. After eight doses of antibody over four weeks the therapy was discontinued. The patient entered a complete remission that has continued now for over one year with no other therapy of any kind. There was no toxicity of therapy and the patient did not make an anti-mouse antibody response. The regressing lesions in this patient contained large numbers of macrophages and activated T cells. It is likely that such reactive cells were important in the antitumor effect of the antiidiotype antibody.

Monoclonal Antibodies in Autologous Bone Marrow Transplantation

Bone marrow toxicity represents the limiting factor in most of the effective therapies for leukemia and lymphoma. The patient's own bone marrow may be harvested prior to therapy, cryopreserved, and used to reconstitute hematopoietic function after supralethal therapy. Antibodies can be used to eliminate contaminating tumor cells from such bone marrow specimens. The use of antibodies to remove tumor cells from autologous bone marrow in vitro has many advantages over the use of antibodies for therapy in vivo. For instance, incubations can be performed under conditions that do not allow antigenic modulation, such as reduced temperature. Circulating blocking factors can be removed. Heterologous complement can be added to lyse antibody-coated cells. Multiple treatments can be used to enhance elimination of tumor cells. The requirements for specificity of the antibody are far fewer; it must react with all tumor cells and spare hematopoietic stem cells, but it may react with other normal cells that are irrelevant for marrow engraftment.

Preliminary results are available from two ongoing clinical trials using monoclonal antibodies for autologous bone marrow transplantation in acute lymphocytic leukemia. Ritz, Bast, Schlossman, and their colleagues (27) at the Sidney Farber Cancer Center used the anti-CALLA monoclonal antibody for patients with common ALL; and Kaizer, Santos, and co-workers (28) at Johns Hopkins Medical School used the anti-Leu-1 antibody for patients with T-cell ALL (28). The study designs are similar, in that patients who have relapsed at least once with the appropriate type of leukemia have been re-induced into remission with chemotherapy. At that point the bone marrow is harvested, treated with antibody and complement, and cryopreserved. The patients then receive supralethal radiotherapy and chemotherapy followed by infusion of the treated marrow. Both groups have established that marrow treated with antibody and complement in vitro and cryopreserved can successfully reconstitute hematopoietic function. At this point, it is too early to conclude whether or not the antibody treatment actually eliminated leukemia cells, which are presumed to have been present in the marrow.

Future Prospects

It is clear that monoclonal antibodies offer promise in the therapy of malignant disease. It is equally clear that their true role remains to be established and that they will certainly be used in conjunction with other effective modalities of treatment rather than as a substitute for them. Before that role can be found, their limitations, listed in Table 3, will have to be overcome.

Table 3 Monoclonal antibody therapy in humans

Limitations	Possible solutions
1. Finite capacity to eliminate antibody-coated cells	Improve schedule of antibody administration
Antibody-dependent cellular cytotoxicity (ADCC)	Augment effector cells
The reticuloendothelial system	Treat minimal residual disease
2. Immunogenicity of mouse antibody (chronic therapy is ineffective)	Induce tolerance to mouse Ig
	Use human antibodies
	Use antibody coupled to a cytotoxic agent

The most important limitation seems to be the finite capacity of the effector-cell system that eliminates antibody-coated cells in vivo. Perhaps methods will be found to enhance or augment this system. Alternatively, it may be possible to make the antibodies more toxic on their own, perhaps by arming them with radioactive or toxic substances. If antibodies were directly cytotoxic, the problem of their immunogenicity might disappear, since their toxicity would likely be expressed on the antibody-forming cell ("B-cell suicide") as well as on the tumor-cell target.

Solid tumors may not be as susceptible to the therapeutic effects of antibodies as are the leukemias and lymphomas, which, as single cells, are exposed to the vascular and reticuloendothelial effector systems. Ultimately, whether they are used for leukemias or for solid tumors, it seems likely that antibodies will have maximum effect when the number of target cells is low. It is for this reason that clinical trials of antibody therapy will eventually need to be done as properly randomized, controlled studies in patients who are in remission but who are at high risk for eventual relapse. The studies being conducted at the present time are addressing the issues of toxicity and mechanism of antitumor effect. It is hoped that they will lay the foundation for the definitive studies of the future.

Literature Cited

1. Ehrlich, P. 1906. *Collected Studies on Immunity,* 2:441–47. New York: Wiley
2. Wright, P. W., Bernstein, I. D. 1980. Serotherapy of malignant disease. *Prog. Exp. Tumor Res.* 25:140
3. Kohler, G., Milstein, C. 1975. Continuous cultures of fused cells secreting antibody of predefined specificity. *Nature* 256:495
4. Bernstein, I. D., Tam, M. R., Nowinski, R. C. 1980. Mouse leukemia: therapy with monoclonal antibodies against a thymus differentiation antigen. *Science* 207:68
5. Kirch, M. E., Hammerling, U. 1981. Immunotherapy of murine leukemias by monoclonal antibody. I. Effect of passively administered antibody on growth of transplanted tumor cells. *J. Immunol.* 127:805
6. Herlyn, D. M., Steplewski, Z., Herlyn, M.F., Koprowski, H. 1980. Inhibition of growth of colorectal carcinoma in nude mice by monoclonal antibody. *Cancer Res.* 40:717
7. Shin, H. S., Hayden, M., Langley, S., Kaliss, N., Smith, M. R. 1975. Antibody-mediated suppression of grafted lymphoma. III. Evaluation of the role of thymic function, non-thymus-derived lymphocytes, macrophages, platelets, and polymorphonuclear leukocytes in syngeneic and allogeneic hosts. *J. Immunol.* 114:1255
8. Lanier, L. L., Babcock, G. F., Raybourne, R. B., Arnold, L. W., Warner, N. L., Haughton, G. 1980. Mechanism of B-cell lymphoma immunotherapy with passive xenogeneic antiidiotype serum. *J. Immunol.* 125:1255
9. Langlois, A. J., Matthews, T., Roloson, G. J., Thiel, II. J., Collins, J. J., Bolognesi, D. P. 1981. Immunologic control of the ascites form of murine adenocarcinoma 755. V. Antibody-directed macrophages mediate tumor-cell destruction. *J. Immunol.* 126:2337–41
10. Shin, H. S., Economou, J. S., Pasternack, G. P., Johnson, R. G., Hayden, M. L. 1976. Antibody-mediated suppression of grafted lymphoma. IV. Influence of time of tumor residency in vivo and tumor size upon the effectiveness of suppression by syngeneic antibody. *J. Exp. Med.* 144:1274
11. Bernstein, I. D., Nowinski, R. C., Tam, M. R., McMaster, B., Houston, L. L., Clark, E. A. 1980. Monoclonal antibody therapy of mouse leukemia. In *Monoclonal Antibodies,* ed. R. H. Kennett, T. J. Mckearn, K. B. Bechtol, p. 275. New York: Plenum

116   LEVY & MILLER

12. Boyse, E. A., Stockert, E., Old, L. J. 1967. Modification of the antigenic structure of the cell membrane by thymus-leukemia (TL) antibody. *Proc. Natl. Acad. Sci.* 58:954
13. Stackpole, C. W., Jacobson, J. B. 1978. Antigenic modulation. In *The Handbook of Cancer Immunology,* ed. H. Waters, p. 55. New York: Garland STPM
14. Ritz, J., Pesando, J. M., Sallan, S. E., Clavell, L. A., Notis-McConarty, J., Rosenthal, P., Schlossman, S. F. 1981. Serotherapy of acute lymphoblastic leukemia with monoclonal antibody. *Blood* 58:141
15. Johnson, R. J., Siliciano, R. F., Shin, H. S. 1979. Suppression of antibody-sensitized cells by macrophages: insufficient supply or activation of macrophages within large tumors. *J. Immunol.* 122:379
16. Nadler, L. M., Stashenko, P., Hardy, R., Kaplan, W. D., Button, L. N., Kufe, D. W., Antman, K. H., Schlossman, S. T. 1980. Serotherapy of a patient with a monoclonal antibody directed against a human lymphoma-associated antigen. *Cancer Res.* 40:3147
17. Miller, R. A., Levy, R. 1981. Response of cutaneous T-cell lymphoma to therapy with hybridoma monoclonal antibody. *Lancet* 2:226
18. Miller, R. A., Maloney, D. G., Warnke, R., Levy, R. 1982. Treatment of B-cell lymphoma with monoclonal antiidiotype antibody. *N. Engl. J. Med.*
19. Dillman, R. O., Shawler, D. L., Sobol, R. E., Collins, H. A., Beauregard, J. C., Wormsley, S. B., Royston, I. 1982. Murine monoclonal antibody therapy in two patients with chronic lymphocytic leukemia. *Blood* 59:1036
20. Sears, H. F., Mattis, J., Herlyn, D., Hayry, P., Atkinson, B., Ernst, C., Steplewski, Z., Koprowski, H. 1982. Phase-I clinical trial of monoclonal antibody in treatment of gastrointestinal tumors. *Lancet*:762
21. Colvin, R. B., Cosimi, A. B., Burton, R. C., Kurnick, J. T., Struzziero, C., Goldstein, G., Russell, P. S. 1982. Antiidiotype antibodies in patients treated with murine monoclonal antibody, OKT3. *Fed. Proc.* 41:363
22. Pesando, J. M., Ritz, J., Lazarus, H., Tomaselli, K. J., Schlossman, S. F. 1981. Fate of a common acute lymphoblastic leukemia antigen during modulation by monoclonal antibody. *J. Immunol.* 126:540
23. Miller, R. A., Maloney, D. G., McKillop, J., Levy, R. 1981. In vivo effects of murine hybridoma monoclonal antibody in a patient with T-cell leukemia. *Blood* 58:78
24. Levy, R., Dilley, J., Fox, R. I., Warnke, R. 1979. A human thymus-leukemia antigen defined by hybridoma monoclonal antibodies. *Proc. Natl. Acad. Sci.* 76:6552
25. Stevenson, G. T., Elliot, E. V., Stevenson, F. K. 1977. Idiotypic determinants on the surface immunoglobulin of neoplastic lymphocytes: a therapeutic target. *Fed. Proc.* 36:228
26. Hamlin, T. J., Abdul-Ahad, A. K., Gordon, J., Stevenson, F. K., Stevenson, G. T. 1980. Preliminary experience in treating lymphocytic leukemia with antibody to immunoglobulin idiotypes on the cell surface. *Br. J. Cancer* 42:295
27. Ritz, J., Sallan, S. E., Bast, R. C., Lipton, J. M., Nathan, D. G., Schlossman, S. F. 1981. Autologous bone marrow transplantation in CALLA-positive ALL following in vitro treatment with J5 monoclonal antibody and complement. *Blood* 58:Suppl. 5, Abstract #612, p. 175a
28. Kaizer, H., Levy, R., Santos, G. 1982. Autologous bone marrow transplantation in T cell malignancies: Use of in vitro monoclonal antibody treatment of remission marrow to eliminate tumor cells. *J. Cell. Biochem.,* Suppl. 6, Absrt. #0114, p. 41

Ann. Rev. Med. 1983. 34:117–31

IDENTIFICATION AND SIGNIFICANCE OF CELL MARKERS IN LEUKEMIA AND LYMPHOMA[1]

Roger A. Warnke, M.D. and Michael P. Link, M.D.

Departments of Pathology and Pediatrics, Stanford University School of Medicine, Stanford, California 94305

ABSTRACT

The identification of markers of human hematopoietic cell differentiation and function has revealed the nature of the proliferating cell in many lymphoid neoplasms and demonstrated marked phenotypic heterogeneity in traditional subgroups. Selected markers are described that define common subgroups of lymphoid leukemia and non-Hodgkin's lymphoma. The identification of cell markers has significant implications for accuracy of diagnosis, for predicting clinical characteristics, and for understanding the biology of these diseases.

INTRODUCTION

Types of leukemia and lymphoma have traditionally been defined by morphologic features and/or enzyme histochemical profiles. Such characteristics have identified patient groups with certain common clinical features; but as advances have taken place in the staging and treatment of these diseases, traditional methods in many instances have proven inadequate for defining patient groups. These deficiencies, combined with a marked increase in the variety and quality of cell markers that are available, as well as in the methodology for their detection, led many investigators to apply new immunologic, functional, enzymatic, karyotypic, and cell culture

[1]Supported in part by grants AI11313 and CA 05838, CA 21223, and CA 21555 from the National Institutes of Health.

0066-4219/83/0401-0117$02.00

methods alone or in combination to define the nature of the proliferating cell in the hematopoietic neoplasms. The identification and significance of the myriad of markers in all of the leukemias and lymphomas cannot be addressed in this brief review. Since most studies attempting to assess the significance of phenotyping have been performed on lymphoproliferative disorders and because the authors are actively engaged in studying the lymphoid leukemias and lymphomas, we focus our discussion on these disorders.

SELECTED MARKERS OF HUMAN HEMATOPOIETIC CELL DIFFERENTIATION AND FUNCTION

Individual B lymphocytes produce surface and/or cytoplasmic immuno-globulin (Ig) of a single light-chain type (1). It appears that the majority of B lymphocytes possessing surface Ig lack readily detectable intracellular Ig (see Table 1). IgM represents the predominant immunoglobulin class on the vast majority of B cells, alone or in combination with IgD (2). A minority of B cells produce IgG or IgA. Pre-B cells are defined as lacking surface immunoglobulin but containing cytoplasmic mu chains ($C\mu$) without kappa or lambda light chains (3). Terminally differentiated B cells (plasma cells) usually contain abundant cytoplasmic Ig without surface Ig (2). Monoclonal antibodies are available that recognize antigens present on varying numbers of cells belonging to the B-cell lineage (4–6). It is likely that some of these antibodies will recognize cells committed to B-cell differentiation which lack immunoglobulin production. Other markers such as complement receptors (7) and Fc receptors (8) are useful in subdividing B-cell tumors but are not specific for cells of B-cell lineage.

Human T lymphocytes and the majority of their neoplastic counterparts bear receptors for unsensitized sheep erythrocytes (E) (9, 10). Monoclonal antibodies are available that recognize sheep erythrocyte receptors (11, 12), as well as other antigens that are widely distributed on T lymphocytes (13–15). One such antigen, Leu-1 and its equivalents, is also present on certain B-cell neoplasms (16, 17). Monoclonal antibodies are also available that recognize subpopulations of T lymphocytes [helper T cells, cytotoxic/suppressor T cells, and subpopulations of thymocytes (13, 14, 18)]. Some of the T-cell antigens are present on cells other than those of the T-cell lineage as in the case of Leu-1 on B-cell chronic lymphocytic leukemia (B CLL). Thus, it is often necessary to detect more than one T-cell marker to avoid erroneous interpretations. Other investigators have successfully used enzyme markers such as alpha-naphthyl acetate esterase to identify normal and neoplastic T cells (19).

Table 1 Selected markers of human hematopoietic cell differentiation and function

Marker	Common distribution
Intrinsic immunoglobulin (Ig)	
Cytoplasmic mu chains (Cμ) without light chains	Pre-B cells
Surface and/or cytoplasmic Ig of single light-chain type	B cells
Cytoplasmic Ig without surface Ig	Plasma cells
Complement receptors (C3)	
C3b	B cells, M cells[a], G cells[b], some thymic T-cell neoplasms
C3d	B cells
IgG Fc receptors	M cells, G cells, most B cells, some T cells
Sheep erythrocyte receptors (E)	T cells
Ia (HLA-DR) antigens	B cells, most M cells, G cells, some T cells
Pan B-cell antigens (B)	Varied spectrum of B lineage cells
Pan T-cell antigens (T)	T cells (Leu–1 and its equivalents on some B-cell neoplasms)
Helper T-cell antigens (Th)	Helper T cells, some M cells and their neoplasms
Cytotoxic/suppressor T-cell antigens (Tc/s)	Cytotoxic/suppressor T cells
Thymic T-cell antigens (Tthy)	Some (T–6 and its equivalents) present on thymic cortex cells and Langerhans cells, some (T–9 and its equivalents) represent a proliferation-associated transferrin receptor, some (T–10 and its equivalents) present on thymic T cells and their neoplasms but also on plasma cells and some B-cell and G-cell neoplasms
Leukocyte common antigens	Varied spectrum of B cells, T cells, M cells, some G cells
Common ALL antigens (CALLA)	Some B-cell and T-cell precursors and their neoplasms, germinal center B cells and some B-cell neoplasms, some M cells, certain non-hematopoietic cells (e.g. renal glomeruli and proximal tubules)
Deoxynucleotidyl terminal transferase (TdT)	Some B-cell and T-cell precursors and their neoplasms, thymic T cells and their neoplasms, rare myeloid leukemias
Alpha-naphthyl acetate esterase	M cells (diffuse), T cells (focal)

[a] Cells of monocyte/macrophage lineage.
[b] Cells of granulocyte lineage.

A number of other markers, although not lineage specific, may be extremely useful alone or in combination for identifying certain lymphoid lymphomas and leukemias. Deoxynucleotidyl terminal transferase (TdT) is useful in identifying lymphoblastic lymphomas and leukemias (20). The common acute lymphoblastic leukemia antigen (CALLA) (21, 22) is present on the blast cells of the majority of children with non-T, non-B acute lymphoblastic leukemia (ALL). While this antigen is present in small amounts on the blast cells from some patients with T-derived (23, 24) and B-cell neoplasms (24), as well as in some normal nonhematopoietic tissues (25), CALLA is a useful marker for diagnosis and immunophenotyping of lymphoid neoplasms. When CALLA is detected in combination with TdT, the common and relatively favorable form of ALL is identified (26).

Lymphomas that are difficult to differentiate histologically from non-hematopoietic neoplasms may be identified by the expression of one or more of a family of leukocyte-common antigens (27).

IDENTIFYING MARKERS OF CELLULAR DIFFERENTIATION AND FUNCTION

Types of Samples

The types of samples that are generally studied include cell suspensions, cell smears or cytospin preparations, or tissue sections of either fresh frozen tissue or tissue fixed in one of a variety of fixatives, dehydrated, and embedded in paraffin wax or resin. Each type of sample has inherent advantages and disadvantages, the details of which were previously reviewed (28, 29). Cell suspensions are excellent for studying lymphoid neoplasms in bone marrow, peripheral blood, and malignant effusions, particularly if the percentage of neoplastic cells relative to non-neoplastic cells recovered from such a sample is high. Cell smears or cytospin preparations are excellent for the identification of intracytoplasmic antigens such as mu chains in pre-B cells or intranuclear enzymes such as TdT. Tissue sections allow the identification of a minor neoplastic population, circumvent problems in recovering neoplastic populations that are fragile or adherent to stromal cells or connective tissue, and allow the appreciation of potentially important cell-to-cell interactions. Unfortunately, most of the markers we are considering, including most surface membrane antigens, are altered or destroyed by conventional fixation and processing procedures.

Reagents

Most markers are identified by erythrocyte rosettes, polyclonal antisera, monoclonal antibodies and enzyme assays. The development of erythrocyte rosette methods for cell receptor identification was a major advance in the study of leukemia and lymphoma (30). Nevertheless, numerous reagent variables and methodologic differences, for example in the E-rosette test, lead to difficulties in application and data interpretation. Furthermore, some B-cell tumors produce an Ig with anti-sheep erythrocyte activity, which results in a false-positive E-rosette test (31). It is likely that many laboratories will use monoclonal antibodies directed against the E-rosette receptor or directed against specific complement components in place of traditional rosetting assays. Four features of monoclonal antibodies make them extremely useful for identifying markers of cellular differentiation: (a) The homogeneity of the antigen-binding region of the antibody confers exquisite specificity, allowing single determinants on a given molecule to be recognized. (b) The absence of contaminating antibodies of unrelated specificity eliminates false-positive reactions and excessive background staining. (c) Antibody-producing hybridomas can be obtained that react with previously unrecognized antigens, including those that were impossible to purify or were relatively poor immunogens. (d) Monoclonal antibodies can be produced in potentially unlimited amounts allowing widespread distribution, standardization, and comparisons among investigators utilizing the same reagents. For example, a monoclonal antibody to TdT would allow many investigators to overcome the difficulties of the direct enzyme assay and the deficiencies of many of the available antisera.

Labeling and Analysis

The most widely used labeling procedures for many of the cell markers employ fluorochromes (usually fluorescein isothiocyanate or tetramethyl rhodamine isothiocyanate) or enzymes (usually horseradish peroxidase). The principal advantages of immunofluorescence are the ease with which such immunofluorescent staining can be performed and the fact that it is relatively simple to label pairs of antigens in contrasting colors. Increasingly sophisticated qualitative and quantitative analyses employ fluorescent labeling in combination with cytofluorography (see Figure 1). A major disadvantage of immunofluorescence for tissue section studies is that cytology and architecture cannot be visualized at the same time as the label; moreover, fluorescent-labeled sections fade with photography and storage, which precludes later examination. Immunoenzymatic labeling circumvents these problems and allows analysis with a relatively inexpensive light microscope (see Figure 2).

IMMUNOPHENOTYPES OF LYMPHOID LEUKEMIAS

Immune marker studies are particularly useful in dissecting the subsets of lymphoid leukemia. These studies detect a heterogeneity of these diseases not predictable from their morphology and histochemistry alone (see Table 2). The earliest marker studies of childhood ALL utilizing rosetting meth-

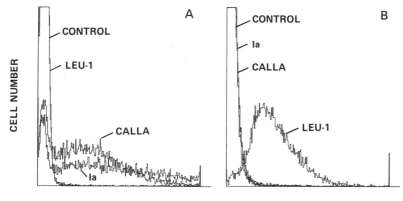

Figure 1 Flow cytometric analysis of fluorescence staining of blast cells from two children with acute lymphoblastic leukemia. Ten thousand cells were counted in each sample and the results presented as a histogram plotting the fraction of total cells versus the intensity of fluorescence. Reactivity with a nonreactive myeloma protein used as a negative control is also shown. (*a*) A case of common ALL. The blast cells are reactive with anti-Ia and anti-CALLA but are not reactive with anti-Leu-l (nor with several other T-specific antibodies). (*b*) A case of T-cell ALL. The blast cells are reactive with anti-Leu-l but demonstrate no reactivity with anti-Ia and anti-CALLA. Blast cells from this patient are reactive with other T-cell-specific monoclonal antibodies and demonstrate spontaneous rosette formation with sheep erythrocytes, which confirm the T-cell lineage of this leukemia.

ods and anti-immunoglobulin reagents identified approximately 20% of cases as T-lineage derived, 2% B-cell derived, and the remaining 75–80% as non-T, non-B ("null" ALL) (32–38). Additional marker studies led to the delineation of subclasses of non-T, non-B ALL. Approximately 75% of children with non-T, non-B ALL have blast cells bearing CALLA (designated "common ALL"), and almost all of these bear HLA-DR (Ia) antigens as well (Figure 1) (22, 33, 34, 37). Almost one quarter of children with non-T, non-B ALL have blast cells with cytoplasmic mu chains and have leukemia of pre-B type (39–41). Recent studies demonstrating immunoglobulin gene rearrangements in the blast cells of children with common ALL support the concept that most cases of common ALL are linked to the B-cell lineage (42).

The availability of monoclonal antibodies has been instrumental in dissecting the T ALLs, and significant heterogeneity of immunophenotype has been demonstrated within this subset of ALL (14, 23, 26, 43, 44). The majority of childhood T ALLs bear surface markers similar to those found on immature T cells (i.e. thymocytes in the earliest stages of differentiation) and most of the remaining cases have immunophenotypes similar to cortical thymocytes (see Table 2). However, other cases of T ALL have immuno-

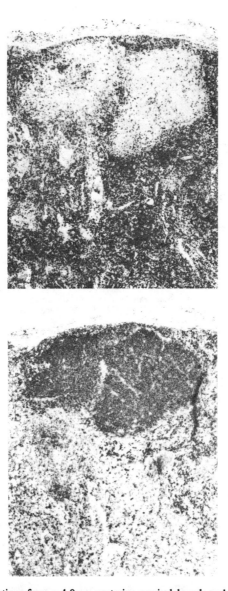

Figure 2 Frozen sections from a 1.0-cm posterior cervical lymph node removed from a 55-year-old man. This patient had undergone a previous biopsy of a lumbar vertebral lesion; routine paraffin sections of this bone lesion were variously interpreted by different pathologists as metastatic carcinoma or large-cell lymphoma. (*Top*) Staining for a T-cell antigen Leu-1 demonstrated two small neoplastic nodules that did not stain for this marker. (*Bottom*) Staining for Ia antigens demonstrated dark staining of the neoplastic nodules. Further studies demonstrated an IgM, kappa B-cell lymphoma.

egm

Table 2 Immunophenotypes of lymphoid leukemias

Designation	Common profile
B lineage related[a]	
Unclassified (null) ALL	T^- Ia^+ or Ia^- $CALLA^-$ sIg^- $C\mu^-$ TdT^+
Common ALL	T^- Ia^+ $CALLA^+$ sIg^- $C\mu^-$ TdT^+
Pre-B ALL	T^- Ia^+ $CALLA^+$ sIg^- $C\mu^+$ TdT^+
B-ALL	T^- Ia^+ $CALLA^+$ sIg^+ TdT^-
T lineage related[b]	
Immature T cell (T ALL)	
Early thymic	T^+ Ia^- $Tthy^+$ E^- Th^- Tc/s^- TdT^+
Cortical thymic	$\left\{\begin{array}{l} T^+\ Ia^-\ Tthy^+\ E^+\ Th^\pm\ Tc/s^\pm\ TdT^+ \\ T^+\ Ia^-\ Tthy^+\ E^+\ Th^+\ Tc/s^+\ TdT^+ \end{array}\right.$
Mature T cell	
T CLL "suppressor"	T^+ $Tthy^-$ E^+ Th^- Tc/s^+ TdT^-
T CLL "helper"⎫ PLL ⎬ Sezary ⎭	T^+ $Tthy^-$ E^+ Th^+ Tc/s^- TdT^-

[a] None of these leukemias express T-cell-specific antigens. Occasional cases may lack expression of TdT, Ia, or CALLA when the rest of the phenotype predicts such expression.

[b] None of these leukemias express B-cell-specific antigens. About 10% of cases of immature type may express CALLA. Occasional cases may lack TdT or a T-cell-specific antigen when the rest of the phenotype predicts its expression. Most do not express Ia antigens.

phenotypes that do not correspond to any seen in normal T-cell ontogeny. Even further heterogeneity of immunophenotype can be demonstrated within the subset of T ALL if different thymic T-cell antigens are analyzed separately, or if one considers that these cases show variable expression of common ALL antigens and that occasional cases lack TdT or particular T-cell-specific antigens (26).

By contrast, cases of T-cell chronic lymphocytic leukemia (T CLL) express phenotypes characteristic of mature T cells (either T helper or T cytotoxic/suppressor) and do not express thymic T-cell antigens or TdT (26, 44). These differences in immunophenotype between T CLL and T ALL can help in diagnosis, and they suggest different cellular origins for these neoplasms.

SELECTED PHENOTYPES OF NON-HODGKIN'S LYMPHOMA

Although the subclasses of ALL are defined based on immunologic markers, the designation of important groups of non-Hodgkin's lymphoma is based on architectural and/or cytological features. The morphologic designations used in Table 3 are derived from the recently published *Working*

Formulation for Non-Hodgkin's Lymphomas, which gives comparable terminology for the different classifications currently in use (45). In contrast to the rarity of B-cell ALL in children or adults, the majority of non-Hodgkin's lymphomas derive from the B-cell lineage (46–48). A number of the non-T, non-B lymphomas may derive from the B-cell lineage at a stage prior to Ig production since a number of these lymphomas express Ia antigens (31, 49), B-cell specific antigens, and/or common ALL antigens. A number of the small lymphocytic lymphomas like B CLL express Leu-1 antigens. A lesser number of B-cell lymphomas in the other morphologic

Table 3 Selected phenotypes of non-Hodgkin's lymphoma

Designation	Common antigenic profiles
Small lymphocytic (B-CLL)	$B^+ Ia^+ Ig^+ Leu-1^+$
	$B^+ Ia^+ Ig^+ Leu-1^-$
Follicular lymphoma types[a]	$B^+ Ia^+ Ig^+$
	$B^+ Ia^+ Ig^-$
Diffuse small cleaved cell[b]	$B^+ Ia^+ Ig^+$
	$B^+ Ia^+ Ig^-$
Diffuse mixed cell[c]	$B^+ Ia^+ Ig^+$
	$T^+ E^+ Th^+ Tc/s^-$
	$T^+ E^+ Th^- Tc/s^+$
Diffuse large cell[d]	$B^- Ia^- Ig^- T^- E^-$
	$B^- Ia^+ Ig^- T^- E^-$
	$B^+ Ia^+ Ig^-$
	$B^+ Ia^+ Ig^+$
	$T^+ E^+ Th^+ Tc/s^-$
	$T^+ E^+ Th^- Tc/s^+$
Lymphoblastic[e]	$T^+ E^- Tthy^+ Th^- Tc/s^-$
	$T^+ E^+ Tthy^+ Th^- Tc/s^-$
	$T^+ E^+ Tthy^+ Th^+ Tc/s^+$
	$B^+ Ia^+ CALLA^+ Ig^-$
	$B^+ Ia^+ CALLA^+ C\mu^+$
Burkitt's	$B^+ Ia^+ Ig^+$
Mycosis fungoides[f]	$T^+ E^+ Th^+ Tc/s^-$

[a] These lymphomas show variable expression of Leu-1, C3, and CALLA.
[b] Some of the Ig-bearing lymphomas may express Leu-1.
[c] The T-cell types generally lack thymic T-cell antigens and Ig antigens.
[d] An extremely heterogeneous group of lymphomas. Some of the Ig-bearing lymphomas may express Leu-1 or CALLA. The T-cell types may lack expression of one or more T-cell antigens when the rest of the phenotype predicts expression and commonly express Ia antigens.
[e] The T-cell types express thymic T-cell antigens and do not express Ia antigens.
[f] Occasional cases do not express Leu-1 and may express Ia antigens.

categories express Leu-1. A small number of follicular lymphomas do not express Ig but bear B-cell-specific and Ia antigens.

The T-cell lymphomas in the mixed and large-cell groups are generally of a mature nonthymic phenotype and may express Ia antigens. We have encountered lymphoblastic lymphomas corresponding to nearly all of the subclasses of lymphoblastic leukemia related to both the B-cell and T-cell lineages. For example, we have seen cases of lymphoblastic lymphoma of pre-B-cell type that presented in the skin without evidence of bone marrow involvement, and one case of common ALL type presenting in the testis without evidence of marrow involvement. All of the cases of cutaneous T-cell lymphoma (mycosis fungoides/Sezary's syndrome) have expressed the helper phenotype with occasional cases expressing Ia antigens or lacking expression of Leu-1 antigens (50).

SIGNIFICANCE OF CELL MARKER IDENTIFICATION

Biological Significance

Immunoglobulin light-chain restriction in the large number of B-cell lymphomas that have been studied confirms data from glucose-6-phosphate-dehydrogenase isoenzyme patterns and karyotypic analyses demonstrating that these lymphomas are monoclonal at the time of diagnosis (51). Whether these lymphomas arose from a single clone initially or arose in multiple clones with a single dominant clone outgrowing the others cannot be determined from these studies. In contrast to some of the myeloid leukemias, particularly chronic myeloid leukemia (52), no data exist to suggest that the lymphoid leukemias are stem cell disorders. A limited number of studies employing cell markers suggest that the phenotype of these diseases remains constant over time irrespective of intervening treatment, although some phenotypic "shifts" have been encountered at the time of relapse (53). The limited number of leukemia and lymphoma cell lines that have been studied generally show remarkable stability of phenotype despite maintenance in culture for more than a year (54).

Data based on the identification of cell markers in lymphomas and leukemias led a number of investigators to the conclusion that most of these lymphomas and leukemias represent a normal but arrested stage of cellular differentiation, with the corollary that a normal counterpart exists for each neoplastic phenotype (23, 26, 43, 44). While this concept may be generally correct, an increasing number of phenotypes are extremely difficult to reconcile with current concepts of differentiation and function. Nevertheless, cell markers serve as useful probes for exploring the origins of the various lymphoid neoplasms and dissecting the heterogeneity of these diseases.

Marker studies of neoplastic cells also help to elucidate the stages of normal cellular differentiation. Furthermore, improvements in techniques for identifying different populations with the advent of monoclonal antibodies allow an increased appreciation of cell-to-cell interactions and rekindle an awareness that many lymphoid tumors consist not only of tumor cells, but also contain a significant number of reactive host cells of varying type.

Finally, marker studies provide important data to correlate with biological and clinical parameters. Correlations between immunophenotype and clinical features have been best demonstrated in childhood leukemia (32–41) and lymphoma (55–58). The T ALL phenotype occurs more often in adolescents, especially in males. Children with T ALL often present with marked elevations of the leukocyte count, significant adenopathy and organomegaly, and the presence of a mediastinal mass. By contrast, common ALL usually occurs between the ages of two and six years with an equal incidence in males and females. Children with common ALL often present without marked organomegaly or elevations of the leukocyte count. In the childhood lymphomas, children with mediastinal or supradiaphragmatic lymph node primaries characteristically have T-cell markers, whereas children with abdominal tumors usually have B-cell neoplasms.

Diagnostic and Prognostic Significance

Cell markers are likely to play an increasingly important role in diagnosis (59). The identification of a single light-chain type of B cell in difficult follicular lesions or in small lymphocytic tumors, particularly in extranodal sites, strongly supports the diagnosis of lymphoma (60, 61). The anomalous expression of Leu-1 and its equivalents may also be of diagnostic import in such instances. A marked predominance of a single type of T lymphocyte can be used to support a diagnosis of a T-cell lymphoma, especially if the cells also lack expression of one or more normal T-cell antigens. A relatively common diagnostic problem in histopathology concerns differentiation between high-grade lymphoma and poorly differentiated carcinoma. Antibodies to B-cell antigens, T-cell antigens, common ALL antigens, or leukocyte common antigens will allow the identification of lymphoma in nearly all instances. The detection of the same markers may also be useful in identifying lymphoma or leukemia in a child who presents with a primitive small round cell tumor in an unusual site. Immune markers have already demonstrated their usefulness in the diagnosis of "undifferentiated" leukemias where the presence of CALLA or T-cell antigens suggests lymphoid rather than myeloid derivation.

Data regarding the relationship between immune markers and prognosis derive from studies of childhood ALL, although it has not yet been demonstrated that immune markers are of independent prognostic significance when other clinical features such as age and leukocyte count are considered (37, 62–65). Nevertheless, it appears that children with B-cell leukemia have a very adverse prognosis, and children with common ALL have a more favorable outlook. Children with T ALL and pre-B ALL have an intermediate prognosis. The data on markers and prognosis in adults with ALL and in non-Hodgkin's lymphoma are less clear. Such information is forthcoming from studies now in progress. These studies correlating the results of cell-marker studies, clinical features, histopathological features, and biologic behavior are likely to contribute significantly to our understanding of the lymphoid malignancies. They should also help to provide the clinician with more accurate diagnostic information and additional prognostic data with which to plan therapy for individual patients. In the future, cell-marker studies should be useful to identify homogeneous groups of patients for treatment protocols including experimental strategies employing appropriate monoclonal antibodies.

Literature Cited

1. Nisonoff, A., Hopper, J. E., Spring, S. B. 1975. *The Antibody Molecule.* New York: Academic
2. Pernis, P. 1978. Lymphocyte membrane immunoglobulins: an overview. In *Immunoglobulins,* ed. G. W. Litman, R. A. Good, pp. 359–72. New York: Plenum
3. Gathings, W. E., Lawton, A. R., Cooper, M. D. 1977. Immunofluorescent studies of the development of pre-B cells, B lymphocytes and immunoglobulin isotype diversity in humans. *Eur. J. Immunol.* 7:804–10
4. Abramson, C. S., Kersey, J. H., LeBien, T. W. 1981. A monoclonal antibody (BA-1) reactive with cells of human B lymphocyte lineage. *J. Immunol.* 126:83–88
5. Kersey, J. H., LeBien, T. W., Abramson, C. S., Newman, R., Sutherland, R., Greaves, M. 1981. p24: A human leukemia-associated and lymphohemopoietic progenitor cell surface structure identified with monoclonal antibody. *J. Exp. Med.* 153:726–31
6. Stashenko, P., Nadler, L. M., Hardy, R., Schlossman, S. F. 1980. Characterization of a human B lymphocyte alloantigen. *J. Immunol.* 125:1678–85
7. Frank, M. M., Jaffe, E. S., Green, I. 1976. Detection of specific mononuclear cell receptors in tissue sections. In *In Vitro Methods in Cell-Mediated and Tumor Immunity,* ed. B. R. Bloom, J. R. David, pp. 203–15. New York: Plenum

8. Winchester, R. J., Hoffman, T., Ferrarini, M., Ross, G. D., Kunkel, H. G. 1979. Comparison of various tests for Fc receptors on different human lymphocyte subpopulations. *Clin. Exp. Immunol.* 37:126–33
9. Jondal, M., Holm, G., Wigzell, H. 1972. Surface markers on human T and B lymphocytes. I. A large population of lymphocytes forming nonimmune rosettes with sheep red blood cells. *J. Exp. Med.* 136:207–15
10. Wybran, J., Carr, M. C., Fudenberg, H. H. 1972. The human rosette forming cell as a marker of a population of thymus-derived cells. *J. Clin. Invest.* 51:2537–43
11. Howard, F. D., Ledbetter, J. A., Wong, J., Bieber, C. P., Stinson, E. B., and Herzenberg, L. A. 1981. A human T lymphocyte differentiation marker defined by monoclonal antibodies that block E-rosette formation. *J. Immunol.* 126:2117–22
12. Kamoun, M., Martin, P. J., Hansen, J. A., Brown, M. A., Siadak, A. W., Nowinski, R. C. 1981. Identification of a human T lymphocyte surface protein associated with the E-rosette receptor. *J. Exp. Med.* 153:207–12
13. Kung, P. C., Goldstein, G., Reinherz, E. L., Schlossman, S. F. 1979. Monoclonal antibodies defining distinctive human T cell surface antigens. *Science* 206:347–49
14. Reinherz, E. L., Kung, P. C., Goldstein, G., Levey, R. H., Schlossman, S. F.

1980. Discrete stages of human intra-thymic differentiation: analysis of normal thymocytes and leukemic lymphoblasts of T lineage. *Proc. Natl. Acad. Sci. USA* 77:1588–92

15. Engleman, E. G., Warnke, R., Fox, R. I., Dilley, J., Benike, C. J., Levy, R. 1981. Immunologic studies of a human T lymphocyte antigen recognized by a monoclonal antibody. *Proc. Natl. Acad. Sci. USA* 78:1791–95

16. Wang, C. Y., Good, R. A., Ammirati, P., Dymbort, G., Evans, R. L. 1980. Identification of a p69, 71 complex expressed on human T cells sharing determinants with B-type chronic lymphatic leukemic cells. *J. Exp. Med.* 151:1539–44

17. Wormsley, S. B., Collins, M. L., Royston, I. 1981. Comparative density of the human T cell antigen T65 on normal peripheral blood T cells and chronic lymphocytic leukemia cells. *Blood* 57:657–62

18. Ledbetter, J. A., Evans, R. L., Lipinski, M., Cunningham-Rundles, C., Good, R. A., Herzenberg, L. A. 1981. Evolutionary conservation of surface molecules that distinguish T lymphocyte helper/inducer and cytotoxic/suppressor subpopulations in mouse and man. *J. Exp. Med.* 153:310–23

19. Knowles, D. M. II, Halper, J. P., Machin, G. A., Sherman, W. 1979. Acid alpha-naphthyl acetate esterase activity in human neoplastic lymphoid cells; usefulness as a T-cell marker. *Am. J. Pathol.* 96:257–78

20. McCaffrey, R., Lillquist, A., Sallan, S., Cohen, E., Osband, M. 1981. Clinical utility of leukemia cell terminal transferase measurements. *Cancer Res.* 41:4814–20

21. Greaves, M. F., Brown, G., Rapson, N. T., Lister, T. A. 1975. Antisera to acute lymphoblastic leukemia cells. *Clin. Immunol. Immunopathol.* 4:67–84

22. Pesando, J., Ritz, J., Lazarus, H., Costello, S., Sallan, S., Schlossman, S. 1979. Leukemia-associated antigens in ALL. *Blood* 54:1240–48

23. Bernard, A., Boumsell, L., Reinherz, E., Nadler, L., Ritz, J., Coppin, H., Richard, Y., Valensi, F., Dausset, J., Flandrin, G., Lemerle, J., Schlossman, S. 1981. Cell surface characterization of malignant T cells from lymphoblastic lymphoma using monoclonal antibodies: evidence for phenotypic differences between malignant T cells from patients with acute lymphoblastic leukemia and lymphoblastic lymphoma. *Blood* 57:1105–10

24. Ritz, J., Nadler, L., Bhan, A., Notis-McConarty, J., Pesando, J., Schlossman, S. 1981. Expression of common acute lymphoblastic leukemia antigen (CALLA) by lymphomas of B-cell and T-cell lineage. *Blood* 58:648–52

25. Metzgar, R., Borowitz, M., Jones, N., Dowell, B. 1981. Distribution of common acute lymphoblastic leukemia antigen in non-hematopoietic tissues. *J. Exp. Med.* 154:1249–54

26. Greaves, M. F. 1981. Analysis of the clinical and biological significance of lymphoid phenotypes in acute leukemia. *Cancer Res.* 41:4752–66

27. Pizzolo, G., Sloane, J., Beverly, P., Thomas, J. A., Bradstock, K. F., Mattingly, S., Janossy, G. 1980. Differential diagnosis of malignant lymphoma and nonlymphoid tumors using monoclonal anti-leukocyte antibody. *Cancer* 46:2640–47

28. Mason, D. Y., Biberfeld, P. 1980. Technical aspects of lymphoma immunohistology. *J. Histochem. Cytochem.* 28:731–45

29. Knowles, D. M. II. 1980. Non-Hodgkin's lymphomas. I. Immunologic and enzymatic markers useful in their evaluation. In *Progress in Surgical Pathology*, ed. C. Fenoglio, M. Wolff, pp. 71–105. New York: Masson

30. Jaffe, E. S., Shevach, E. M., Sussman, E. H., Frank, M., Green, I., Berard, C. W. 1975. Membrane receptor sites for the identification of lymphoreticular cells in benign and malignant situations. *Br. J. Cancer* 31:107–20

31. Halper, J. P., Knowles, D. M. II, Wang, C. Y. 1980. Ia antigen expression by human malignant lymphomas: correlation with conventional lymphoid markers. *Blood* 55:373–82

32. Brouet, J. C., Valensi, F., Daniel, M. T., Flandrin, G., Preud'homme, J. L., Seligmann, M. 1976. Immunological classification of acute lymphoblastic leukemias: Evaluation of its clinical significance in a hundred patients. *Br. J. Haematol.* 33:319–28

33. Chessels, J., Hardisty, R., Rapson, N. 1977. Acute lymphoblastic leukemia in children: classification and prognosis. *Lancet* 2:1307–9

34. Sallan, S. E., Ritz, J., Pesando, J., Gelber, R., O'Brien, C., Hitchcock, S., Coral, F., Schlossman, S. 1980. Cell surface antigens: prognostic implications in childhood acute lymphoblastic leukemia. *Blood* 55:395–402

35. Tsukimoto, I., Wong, H. Y., Lampkin, B. 1976. Surface markers and prognostic factors in acute lymphoblastic leukemia. *N. Engl. J. Med.* 294:245–48
36. Foon, K., Herzog, P., Billing, R., Terasaki, P., Feig, S. 1981. Immunologic classification of childhood acute lymphocytic leukemia. *Cancer* 47:280–84
37. Greaves, M., Janossy, G., Peto, J., Kay, H. 1981. Immunologically defined subclasses of acute lymphoblastic leukemia in children: their relationship to presentation features and prognosis. *Br. J. Haematol.* 48:179–97
38. Brouet, J. C., Seligmann, M. 1978. The immunological classification of acute lymphoblastic leukemias. *Cancer* 42:817–27
39. Vogler, L., Crist, W., Bockman, D., Pearl, E., Lawton, A., Cooper, M. 1978. Pre-B-cell leukemia: a new phenotype of childhood lymphoblastic leukemia. *N. Engl. J. Med.* 298:872–78
40. Vogler, L., Crist, W., Sarrif, A., Pullen, D. J., Bartolucci, A., Falletta, J., Dowell, B., Humphrey, G., Blackstock, R., van Eys, J., Metzgar, R., Cooper, M. 1981. An analysis of clinical and laboratory features of acute lymphocytic leukemias with emphasis on 35 children with pre-B leukemia. *Blood* 58:135–40
41. Brouet, J., Preud'homme, J., Penit, C., Valensi, F., Rouget, P., Seligmann, M. 1979. Acute lymphoblastic leukemia with pre-B-cell characteristics. *Blood* 54:269–73
42. Korsmeyer, S. J., Hieter, P. A., Ravetch, J. V., Poplack, D. G., Waldmann, T. A., Leder, P. 1981. Developmental hierarchy of immunoglobulin gene rearrangements in human leukemic pre-B cells. *Proc. Natl. Acad. Sci. USA* 78:7096–7100
43. Reinherz, E., Schlossman, S. 1981. Derivation of human T-cell leukemias. *Cancer Res.* 41:4767–70
44. Greaves, M., Rao, J., Hariri, G., Verbi, W., Catovsky, D., Kung, P., Goldstein, G. 1981. Phenotypic heterogeneity and cellular origins of T-cell malignancies. *Leuk. Res.* 5:281–99
45. The Non-Hodgkin's Lymphoma Pathologic Classification Project. 1982. National Cancer Institute sponsored study of classifications of non-Hodgkin's lymphomas: Summary and description of a working formulation for clinical usage. *Cancer* 49:2112–35
46. Lukes, R. J., Taylor, C. R., Parker, J. W., Lincoln, T. L., Pattingale, P. K., Tindle, B. H. 1978. A morphologic and

47. Mann, R. B., Jaffe, E. S., Berard, C. W. 1979. Malignant lymphomas—a conceptual understanding of morphologic diversity. *Am. J. Pathol.* 94:105–92
48. Aisenberg, A. C., Wilkes, B. M., Long, J. C., Harris, N. L. 1980. Cell surface phenotype in lymphoproliferative disease. *Am. J. Med.* 68:206–13
49. Warnke, R., Miller, R., Grogan, T., Pederson, M., Dilley, J., Levy, R. 1980. Immunologic phenotype in 30 patients with diffuse large-cell lymphoma. *N. Engl. J. Med.* 303:293–300
50. Wood, G. S., Deneau, D. G., Miller, R. A., Levy, R., Hoppe, R. T., Warnke, R. A. 1982. Subtypes of cutaneous T-cell lymphoma defined by expression of Leu-1 and Ia. *Blood* 59:876–82
51. Levy, R., Warnke, R., Dorfman, R. F., Haimovich, J. 1977. The monoclonality of human B-cell lymphomas. *J. Exp. Med.* 145:1014–28
52. Boggs, D. R. 1981. Clonal origin of leukemia: site of origin in the stem cell hierarchy and the significance of chromosomal changes. *Blood Cells* 7:205–15
53. Bernard, A., Raynal, B., Lemerle, J., Boumsell, L. 1982. Changes in surface antigens on malignant T cells from lymphoblastic lymphomas at relapse: An appraisal with monoclonal antibodies and microfluorometry. *Blood* 59:809–15
54. Minowada, J., Janossy, G., Greaves, M. F., Tsubota, T., Srivastava, B. I. S., Morikawa, S., Tatsumi, E. 1978. Expression of an antigen associated with acute lymphoblastic leukemia in human leukemia-lymphoma cell lines. *J. Natl. Cancer Inst.* 60:1269–77
55. Crist, W., Kelly, D., Ragab, A., Roper, M., Dearth, J., Castelberry, R., Flint, A. 1981. Predictive ability of Lukes-Collins classification for immunologic phenotypes of childhood non-Hodgkin's lymphoma. *Cancer* 48:2070–75
56. Bernard, A., Murphy, S., Melvin, S., Bowman, W., Caillaud, J., Lemerle, J., Boumsell, L. 1982. Non-T, non-B lymphomas are rare in childhood and associated with cutaneous tumor. *Blood* 59:549–54
57. Williams, A., Taylor, C., Higgins, G., Quinn, J., Schneider, B., Swanson, V., Parker, J., Pattengale, P., Chandor, S., Powars, D., Lincoln, T., Tindle, B., Lukes, R. 1978. Childhood lymphoma-

leukemia. I. Correlation of morphology and immunogical studies. *Cancer* 42: 171–81

58. Bloomfield, C., Gajl-Peczalska, K., Frizzera, G., Kersey, J., Goldman, A. Clinical utility of lymphocyte surface markers combined with the Lukes-Collins histologic classification in adult lymphoma. *N. Engl. J. Med.* 301: 512–18

59. Warnke, R. A., Gatter, K. C., Mason, D. Y. 1982. Monoclonal antibodies as diagnostic reagents. In *Recent Advances in Clinical Immunology,* ed. N. Rose, R. A. Thompson. Edinburgh: Churchill Livingstone. In press

60. Warnke, R., Levy, R. 1978. Immunopathology of follicular lymphomas. A model of B lymphocyte homing. *N. Engl. J. Med.* 298:481–86

61. Knowles, D. M. II, Jakobiec, R. A., Halper, J. P. 1979. Immunologic characterization of ten ocular lymphoid neoplasms. *Am. J. Ophthalmol.* 87:603–19

62. Simone, J., Verzosa, M., Rudy, J. 1975. Initial features and prognosis in 363 children with acute lymphocytic leukemia. *Cancer* 36:2099–2108

63. Heideman, R., Falletta, J., Mukhopadhyay, N., Fernbach, D. 1978. Lymphocytic leukemia in children: prognostic significance of clinical and laboratory findings at time of diagnosis. *J. Pediatr.* 92:540–45

64. Robinson, L., Sather, H., Coccia, P., Nesbit, M., Hammond, D. 1980. Assessment of the interrelationship of prognostic factors in childhood acute lymphoblastic leukemia. A report from the Children's Cancer Study Group. *Am. J. Pediatr. Hematol/Oncol.* 2:5–13

65. Hann, H. L., Lustbader, E., Evans, A., Toledano, S., Lillie, P., Jasko, L. 1981. Lack of influence of T-cell marker and importance of mediastinal mass on the prognosis of acute lymphocytic leukemias of childhood. *J. Natl. Cancer Inst.* 66:285–90

Ann. Rev. Med. 1983. 34:133–44

IMMUNOLOGICAL FACTORS INFLUENCING RENAL GRAFT SURVIVAL

G. Opelz, M.D., and V. Lenhard, M.D.

Institute of Immunology, University of Heidelberg, Im Neuenheimer Feld 305, D 6900 Heidelberg, West Germany

ABSTRACT

The results of clinical renal transplantation are determined mainly by immunological factors, the most important of which are compatibility for the HLA chromosomes and pretransplant blood transfusions. Other factors include HLA matching in cadaver transplantation, compatibility for the Lewis blood group system, and sensitization to lymphocyte panels or to endothelial-monocyte antigens. Performance of the previous graft is the most reliable predictor of success in recipients of retransplants. Because several immunological factors may interact, multiple variables must be considered simultaneously.

Introduction

Today, renal transplantation is the therapy of choice for patients with endstage renal disease whose age and background clinical condition permit this form of treatment. Current surgical and immunosuppressive methods are the result of some 25 years of clinical research. Great advances have been made in the clinical management of transplant patients and this is reflected primarily in improved patient survival rates. The improvement in the rate of successfully functioning grafts has been much less impressive. Graft rejection remains the primary obstacle.

Rejection of a kidney graft is caused by an immunological reaction of the recipient against the donor's "foreign" tissue antigens. The routine use of immunosuppressive drugs in transplanted patients, which reduces the recipient's ability to mount an immune response, allows the more or less successful transplantation of kidneys in spite of tissue incompatibility. Without the aid of immunosuppression, clinical transplantation would not be possible.

133

0066-4219/83/0401-0133$02.00

The use of immunosuppressive drugs (primarily corticosteroids, azathio-prine, and, more recently, cyclosporin) is limited by their side effects and by the danger that a dose sufficiently potent to reverse a severe rejection response may reduce the patient's ability to fight off bacterial or viral infection. Frequent fatal infections in the early transplantation experience led physicians to use immunosuppressives with moderation. The patient's life is preserved at the cost of losing the graft.

It has been the aim of transplantation immunologists to prevent or reduce rejection, either by selecting recipients and donors whose tissues would be compatible, or by using immunological means to eliminate the specific response against incompatible antigens of the grafted kidney. Although not yet entirely successful, immunological research has provided means for reducing the transplant immune reaction to a degree where immunosuppression by drugs becomes more effective.

The Major Histocompatibility Antigens—HLA

Kidney transplants between siblings who inherited identical HLA chromosomes from their parents (HLA-identical siblings) survive at a rate of approximately 90% at one year and 80% at five years. This fact, recognized 15 years ago (1) and firmly established in numerous subsequent studies, remains proof for the overriding role of HLA in renal transplantation. When recipient and donor share one HLA chromosome (haplotype), as in parent-to-child transplants or transplants from HLA one-haplotype-matched siblings, the one-year success rate is approximately 70%, whereas it is only about 50% if both HLA chromosomes are different, which usually is the case in cadaver transplants (Figure 1) (2). Even if recipient and donor are siblings, graft success is in the range of only 50% if they do not share an HLA chromosome (3). Thus, in clinical practice, whether recipient and donor are "matched" for their HLA chromosomes is more important than all other variables, such as age, sex, type of underlying disease, surgical technique, etc. Using this single criterion, HLA typing of families and selecting HLA-identical siblings, the very high 90% one-year success rate can be achieved. Naturally, and unfortunately, this selection criterion is limited to those who have healthy siblings willing to donate a kidney. Since the likelihood of two siblings being HLA identical is 25%, the trend towards smaller families sets a natural limit leaving most patients without this option.

The 10% one-year failure rate among HLA-identical siblings must be caused by incompatibilities for non-HLA antigens. (Among identical twins, because of their complete tissue identity, we would expect no rejections at all.) We must consider that this small 10% failure rate is achieved with the use of immunosuppressive drugs, even though they can be administered in

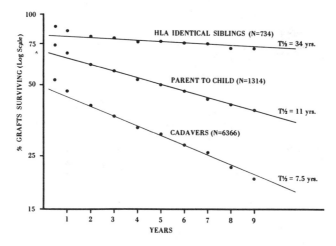

Figure 1 Long-term graft survival rates for cadaver, parent-to-child, and HLA-identical sibling transplants plotted on a log scale. For each category the risk after the second year is constant, as indicated by the straight lines. Half-life times ($T_{1/2}$) for the constant risk periods are given. From Opelz, Mickey, Terasaki (2).

much smaller doses than in HLA-mismatched situations. We may conclude that HLA is the major histocompatibility system and that, provided HLA is matched, additional incompatibilities for minor antigen systems can be controlled usually with small doses of immunosuppressive drugs.

Among transplants from cadaver donors it has been much more difficult to demonstrate a convincing HLA effect. The two largest representative series of North American and European data show nearly identical results (4, 5). A statistically highly significant improvement is obtained with HLA matching; however, the results of HLA-matched cadaver transplants are far inferior to those of HLA-identical sibling grafts (Figure 2).

An important difference between HLA-identical unrelated individuals and HLA-identical siblings lies in the fact that the former are identical only with respect to the HLA antigens that are typed in the laboratory, whereas the latter, by reason of their common ancestry and genetic inheritance, are identical even for other, hitherto unrecognized genetic loci in the HLA region. Indeed, the most plausible explanation for the difference in success rates between these two categories of HLA-identical grafts is that additional important transplantation loci exist in the HLA region.

New evidence in support of this contention was provided by reports that matching for antigens controlled by the more recently discovered HLA-DR locus was much more important than matching for the conventional A and B loci of HLA (6–9). The HLA-DR locus is linked closely to HLA-D, the locus that controls reactivity in the mixed leukocyte culture reaction, which

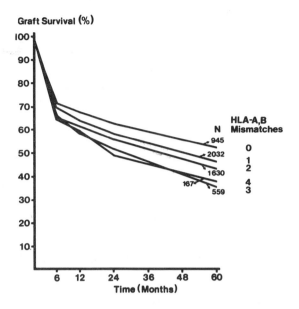

Figure 2 Eurotransplant data of correlation between cadaver kidney graft survival and matching for HLA-A and -B loci. Number of incompatible antigens is given at end of each curve. N = number of patients studied. From Van Rood et al (5).

is considered an in vitro correlate of the transplant immune reaction; therefore, such a development would appear attractive from an immunogenetic viewpoint. It has been difficult, however, to obtain proof in large patient series that HLA-DR matching indeed would provide the long awaited breakthrough. Whereas the Eurotransplant series showed a clear—albeit smaller than anticipated—effect (5), only a small improvement was attributed to HLA-DR matching in the recently completed collaborative International Workshop Study (10); in the latter series, a strong effect of HLA-DR was found only in second transplants (10). It is entirely possible that technical difficulties may have been responsible for the rather disappointing results of the International Workshop Study. HLA-DR typing was new at the time, the reagents were not very well characterized, and the actual typing procedure was not well standardized. Since HLA-DR antigens are typed on B lymphocytes (and not on T lymphocytes), the necessary B-cell enrichment procedures and the greater sensitivity of B cells to the rabbit complement used in the typing assay may have caused typing errors. New single- and multicenter studies are underway to reevaluate the role of HLA-DR matching in cadaver transplantation, now that much progress has been made in typing technology.

Generally, it is believed that matching of cadaver kidneys for HLA-DR will prove more effective than matching for HLA-A,B. An important question to answer will be whether matching for HLA-DR alone will prove sufficient or whether DR and A,B have additive effects. Because of the extreme polymorphism of the HLA-A and -B loci, in contrast to the limited polymorphism of the HLA-DR locus (11), matching for HLA-DR without consideration of HLA-A,B would be attractive logistically. It would be much easier to find a "perfect match" for a patient on the cadaver transplant waiting list. Currently ongoing studies must be completed before new selection criteria can be established.

With respect to matching of cadaver transplants for HLA-A and -B, interesting interactions have been noted that influence the correlation of matching with graft outcome. For example, the effect of matching is much stronger in male than in female recipients (12), in blood group A, B, or AB recipients than in recipients of blood group O (13), and it is stronger in relatively old recipients than in young ones (14). Perhaps not so surprising is the observation of a stronger effect of matching in "presensitized" recipients (those who had lymphocytotoxic antibodies in their serum prior to transplantation) as compared to patients without antibodies (15, 16) although this effect has not been consistently reproducible (4). Whether similar relationships exist with respect to HLA-DR antigens is unknown.

Non-HLA Histocompatibility Antigens

In independent studies, incompatibility for the Lewis blood group system was shown to decrease cadaver graft survival by approximately 10% (Figure 3) (17–19). An additive effect of Lewis and HLA incompatibilities was noted, with transplants incompatible for both antigen systems having the poorest outcome. Very few transplant centers have incorporated the Lewis antigens into their prospective selection routines. If additional studies confirm the Lewis effect, the Lewis antigens will have to be determined prior to transplantation and Lewis incompatible kidneys will have to be excluded. Since, in comparison to HLA typing, typing for Lewis is technically simpler and not as time consuming, this addition to the histocompatibility selection procedure should not pose a serious problem.

More difficult would be to prospectively utilize the finding of the International Workshop Study that incompatibilities for additional red cell antigens (D, C, c, E, e, Duffy, Kell, S, s, M, N were evaluated) have an additive effect; that is, if four or more antigens were mismatched simultaneously, graft survival was markedly decreased (20). It remains to be seen whether certain antigens will be shown to have a stronger influence than others, thus allowing a more selective approach. Because of the complexity involved in analyzing the effects of multiple separate markers, large series of transplants will have to be studied.

There is increasing evidence for a significant role of endothelial-monocyte antigens in the transplant rejection process. Cerilli et al (21) were the first

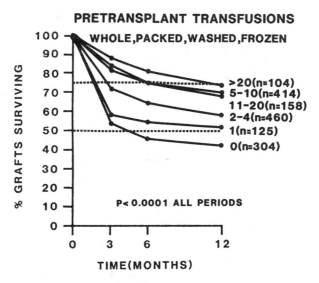

Figure 3 Actuarial survival rates of first cadaver donor transplants by the number of transfusions given to the recipients before transplantation. Whole blood, packed cells, washed cells, and frozen blood were combined. Numbers of units transfused are indicated at ends of curves and numbers of patients studied are given in parentheses. *P* values by weighted regression. From Opelz & Terasaki (10).

to show a relationship between anti-endothelial antibodies and graft rejection. Moraes & Stastny (22) identified a monocyte-specific antigen system with multiple alleles, independent of HLA. In a series of 97 transplants, Paul et al (23) were able to demonstrate that patients with antibodies directed against the kidney donor's endothelial monocytes nearly all went on to fail. The practical importance of this finding is limited by the fact that, at least with current testing procedures, only very few prospective recipients possess anti-endothelial antibodies. Nevertheless, the search for endothelium-specific antibodies using sensitive techniques and the improved characterization of the endothelial antigen polymorphism are promising research ventures.

Pretransplant Blood Transfusions

Some ten years have passed since it first was reported that previously nontransfused transplant recipients, contrary to the then common view, fared particularly poorly even though they had not been "sensitized" by transfusions (24). The initial scepticism toward this claim has given way to nearly universal acceptance, based on the confirmatory results of numerous independent investigations. Today it is mandatory in most transplant centers that prospective transplant recipients be transfused. Their chance for a successful graft outcome is improved by transfusions.

The clinical findings of a beneficial effect of pretransplant transfusions on graft survival were confirmed in monkeys (25), dogs (26, 27), rats (28), and mice (29). Yet, in spite of intensive clinical and experimental research, neither the underlying mechanism nor a transfusion protocol that reliably would prevent graft rejection in every recipient have been established. Rather, the improvement of graft outcome by transfusions remains a phenomenon that can be measured statistically. For the time being, it is impossible to predict whether a given patient who was transfused will accept his graft; just his odds of accepting the graft have been improved. Of course, the improved odds make transfusions no less important as a clinical tool. However, the current inability to measure in vitro whether the desired effect has been induced by a transfusion can be seen as the main reason for the controversies surrounding the transfusion issue: How many transfusions should be given? At what intervals? Which type of blood product is best? Does the HLA type of the blood donor matter?

It was shown in several large series that patients with many transfusions fared better than patients with only a few transfusions (Figure 3) (30). In contrast to these findings, Persijn et al (31) reported that one single transfusion already yielded the maximum benefit in a series of Dutch patients. Since it would be desirable to reduce the number of transfusions to the minimum necessary for induction of the transplant-protective effect, it is important to settle this issue. Prospective single- and multicenter trials are underway.

The more often a patient is transfused, the higher is the likelihood that lymphocytotoxic antibodies will develop. It can be estimated that approximately 10% of polytransfused patients will develop highly reactive antibodies (reactive with 90% or more of the random population) (32). Because one of the ground rules of renal transplantation is that the lymphocytotoxic crossmatch test must be negative prior to transplantation, patients with highly reactive antibodies are difficult to transplant—they react in the crossmatch assay against most potential donors. That crossmatch-positive transplants usually go on to fail acutely is an accepted fact (33). Because a negative crossmatch must be obtained, highly sensitized patients experience prolonged waiting times for a transplant. Thus, the side effect of lymphocytotoxic antibody production remains a risk that must be considered.

It has been argued that the entire transfusion effect could be explained by an exclusion of antibody-producing "responders" in the crossmatch test. Prospective data, however, indicate that, although this type of indirect selection may well play some role, it cannot account for the entire beneficial effect of transfusions on graft outcome (34).

Recently, Salvatierra et al (35) introduced transfusion from the actual kidney donor as a preconditioning regimen in HLA-mismatched related-donor transplants. By administering three transfusions and monitoring carefully the patient's antibody response, graft survival rates comparable to those of HLA-identical sibling transplants were achieved. Some 30% of the patients treated in this manner, however, developed cytotoxic antibodies against the donor (positive crossmatch) and were not transplanted (35). The short experience with donor specific transfusions does not yet permit a definite judgment of this procedure. It should be noted that transfusion of random (not donor-specific) blood also provides for improved related-donor graft survival rates, albeit to a somewhat lesser degree than transfusion from the specific kidney donor (36).

Most authors agree that blood depleted of white cells is not effective in inducing the beneficial transfusion effect. Surprisingly, it does not seem to matter a great deal whether the transfusions were given several months or just a few hours prior to transplantation (10, 37). Even transfusions given during transplantation surgery have been found effective by some (38, 39), although this could not be confirmed in large patient series (10, 40).

Aside from the "selection of responders" hypothesis mentioned above, the available data indicate that an additional induction of one or more immunological mechanisms must occur to account for the improved graft success rates following transfusions. Currently most favored are the possibilities that transfusions either induce suppressor cells (41–43) or anti-idiotypic antibodies (44). Both mechanisms are thought to improve graft outcome by abrogating the recipient's cellular immune response against the graft.

Retransplants

As the clinical transplantation programs at many centers enter their second decade, patients who return to dialysis after their graft has failed are becoming an increasingly important issue. In the United States alone, it can be estimated that some 2000 patients per year reject their transplant. The desire for a second (or third) graft is usually strong in these patients, who for some period of time have experienced the freedom of independence from the dialysis machine.

Overall success rates of second related transplants are essentially the same as for first related grafts (45). Even with cadaver donor grafts, second transplants do only slightly worse than first ones (45). Research into the factors that influence second transplant outcome has produced information that allows a differentiation of patients into those with good or poor chances of success.

The most important recognition was the statistical similarity between the duration of function of first and second grafts (46). Transplants that have functioned for prolonged periods the first time are more likely to be followed by well-functioning grafts the second time than transplants that lasted for only a few months. This relationship was found to hold true even for third transplants (47). A likely explanation is that different degrees of responsiveness exist and that patients with relatively low responses, as measured by their prolonged first graft duration, are likely to respond weakly even the second time.

Another important factor in evaluating whether a patient is a favorable candidate for a retransplant is whether lymphocytotoxic antibodies were formed following rejection of the first graft. Whereas the influence of preformed antibodies, given the current sensitive crossmatch techniques, is weak in first transplants, the influence is much more pronounced in second and third grafts (47). Since all transplants are done after specific anti-donor antibody reactivity has been excluded in the crossmatch test, the results indicate that antibodies identify the patients as strong responders. The data stress the need for cytotoxic antibody screenings in patients who rejected their kidney grafts. Because antibody levels fluctuate and frequently disappear completely within a few weeks or months, regular screening for lymphocytotoxins should be mandatory.

Additional factors may well be influential. However, because the number of retransplants available for analysis is relatively small, it has not been possible to carry out reliable detailed studies (for example, whether HLA matching would be more effective in the highly responsive rapid rejectors of first grafts than in the privileged slow rejectors). For practical purposes, combined consideration of first graft duration and post-rejection antibody status is the safest guide to evaluating a patient's chance for a successful retransplant.

Conclusions

Clinical renal transplantation is a multifactorial event. Aside from clinical factors, numerous immunological factors determine the outcome of a graft. The cadaver donor situation is particularly complex. With so many factors competing, each contributing a few percentage points depending on what other factors are present concurrently, it seems unlikely that a change in one single factor will solve the entire rejection problem. More promising seems a pragmatic approach, taking advantage of each piece of information and weighing the factors against each other, thereby working toward a stepwise improvement of transplant success rates. Because it is difficult to calculate the combined weight of all factors occurring simultaneously in each individual transplant, computers will be required to assist the physician. Usable computer models have been developed (48), but they need to be refined. Already it is possible to roughly predict the likelihood of success for a transplant prior to actually carrying it out. Improving the predicted value, for example by choosing a better-matched donor, will be the next logical step.

Very large numbers of transplants (thousands) are required in order to study the multiple ways in which the various factors interact, in which the weight of their individual influence changes depending on the profile of their occurrence. This complex picture is complicated further by the fact that the entire system is changing continuously. Refinements in tissue typing, improved immunosuppression, new immunological monitoring assays, etc call for a "fresh start" every time a new factor is introduced. For example, if the effect of matching for HLA-DR is to be evaluated, transplants performed as recently as two years ago cannot be included because of the rapid change in typing technology. This makes it all the more difficult to accumulate sufficient information for studies of interactions of new factors with other well-established ones. In turn, the importance ascribed to an established factor based on "old" data may well change once a new factor is added.

Studies of immunological factors influencing renal graft survival have contributed significantly to making renal transplantation more successful. One can be optimistic that further improvements will result from the intensive research efforts currently underway.

Literature Cited

1. Singal, D. P., Mickey, M. R., Terasaki, P. I. 1969. Serotyping for homotransplantation XXIII. Analysis of kidney transplants from parental versus sibling donors. *Transplantation* 7:246–50

2. Opelz, G., Mickey, M. R., Terasaki, P. I. 1977. Calculations on long-term graft and patient survival in human kidney transplantation. *Transplant. Proc.* 9:27–30

3. Opelz, G., Terasaki, P. I. 1977. Studies on the strength of HLA antigens in related-donor kidney transplantation. *Transplantation* 24:106–11

4. Opelz, G., Mickey, M. R., Terasaki, P. I. 1977. HLA matching and cadaver kidney transplant survival in North America: influence of center variation and presensitization. *Transplantation* 23:490–97

5. van Rood, J. J., Persijn, G. G., Cohen, B., Landsbergen, Q., Schuurman, R. K. B. 1981. *Eurotransplant-Report 1981.* Leiden: Eurotransplant Foundation

6. Ting, A., Morris, P. J. 1978. Matching for B-cell antigens of the HLA-DR series in cadaver renal transplantation. *Lancet* 1:575–77

7. Albrechtson, D., Flatmark, A., Jervell, J. 1978. HLA-DR matching in cadaver renal transplantation. *Lancet* 1:825

8. Martins da Silva, B., Vassalli, P., Jeannet, M. 1978. *Lancet* 1:1047

9. Persijn, G. G., Gabb, B. W., van Leeuwen, A., Nagtegaal, A., Hoogeboom, J., van Rood, J. J. 1978. Matching for HLA antigens of A,B, and DR loci in renal transplantation by Eurotransplant. *Lancet* 1:1278–81

10. Opelz, G., Terasaki, P. I. 1982. International study of histocompatibility in renal transplantation. *Transplantation* 33:87–95

11. Terasaki, P. I., ed. 1980. *Histocompatibility Testing 1980.* UCLA Los Angeles: Univ. Calif. Tissue Typing Laboratory

12. Opelz, G ., Terasaki, P. I. 1977. Influence of sex on histocompatibility matching in renal transplantation. *Lancet* 2:419–21

13. Opelz, G., Terasaki, P. I. 1977. Effect of blood-group on relation between HLA match and outcome of cadaver kidney transplants. *Lancet* 1:220–22

14. Oriol, R., Opelz, G., Chun, C., Terasaki, P. I. 1980. Combined effects

of HLA matching and age in renal transplantation. *Transplantation* 29: 125–26

15. Opelz, G., Terasaki, P. I. 1972. Histocompatibility matching utilizing responsiveness as a new dimension. *Transplant. Proc.* 4:433–37

16. van Hooff, J. P., Schippers, H. M. A., van der Steen, G. J., van Rood, J. J. 1972. Efficacy of HL-A matching in Eurotransplant. *Lancet* 2:1385–87

17. Oriol, R., Cartron, J., Yvart, J., Bedrossian, J., Deboust, A., Bariety, J., Gluckman, J. C., Gagnadoux, M. F. 1978. The Lewis system: new histocompatibility antigens in renal transplantation. *Lancet* 1:574–75

18. Lenhard, V., Roelcke, D., Dreikorn, K., Wernet, P., Müller, G., Bockhorn, H., Dorn-Zachertz, D., Fassbinder, W., Fetta, R. F., Jansen, A. M., Wilms, H., Halbfass, H. J., Gumbel, B., Albert, F. W., Ewald, R. W., Sprenger-Klasen, I., Fischer, M., Goldmann, S. F. 1981. *Transplant. Proc.* 13:930–33

19. Oriol, R., Opelz, G., Chun, C., Terasaki, P. I. 1980. The Lewis system and kidney transplantation. *Transplantation* 29:397–400

20. Opelz, G., Terasaki, P. I. 1980. International Histocompatibility Workshop study on renal transplantation. See Ref. 11, pp. 592–624

21. Cerilli, J., Holliday, J. E., Fesperman, D. P., Folger, M. R. 1977. Role of antivascular endothelial antibody in predicting renal allograft rejection. *Transpl. Proc.* 9:771–73

22. Moraes, J. R., Stastny, P. 1977. A new antigen system expressed in human endothelial cells. *J. Clin. Invest.* 60: 449–54

23. Paul, L. C., van Es, A. A., van Rood, J. J., Leeuwen, A., Brutel de la Riviere, B., de Graeff, J. 1979. Antibodies directed against antigens on the endothelium of peritubular capillaries in patients with rejecting renal allografts. *Transplantation* 27:175–79

24. Opelz, G., Sengar, D. P. S., Mickey, M. R., Terasaki, P. I. 1973. Effect of blood transfusions on subsequent kidney transplants. *Transplant. Proc.* 5:253–59

25. van Es, A. A., Marquet, R. L., van Rood, J. J., Kalff, M. W., Balner, H. 1977. Blood transfusions induce prolonged kidney allograft survival in rhesus monkeys. *Lancet* 1:506–8

26. Abouna, G. M., Barabas, A. Z., Pazderka, V., Boyd, N., Vetters, J. M., Kinniburgh, D. W., Lao, V. S., Schlaut, J., Kovithavongs, T., Dossetor, J. B. 1977.

Effect of pretreatment with multiple blood-transfusions and with skin grafts on the survival of renal allografts in mongrel dogs. *Transplant. Proc.* 9:265

27. Obertop, H., Bijnen, A. B., Vriesendorp, H. M., Westbroek, D. L. 1978. Prolongation of renal allograft survival in DLA tissue-typed beagles after third-party blood transfusions and immunosuppressive treatment. *Transplantation* 26:255–59

28. Martin, D. C., Hewitt, C. W., Osborne, J. G., Dowdy, S. F., Fristoe, T. L., Russell, L. A., Cote, J. 1982. Enhanced kidney graft survival in rats by single or multiple blood transfusion(s) and various blood products. *Transplant. Proc.* 14:407–9

29. Okazaki, H., Maki, T., Wood, M. L., Jones, S., Monaco, A. P. 1981. Prlongation of skin allograft survival in H-2 K and I region-incompatible mice by pretransplant blood transfusion. *Transplantation* 32:111–15

30. Opelz, G., Terasaki, P. I. 1980. Improvement of kidney graft survival with increased numbers of blood transfusions. *N. Engl. J. Med.* 299:799–803

31. Persijn, G. G., van Leeuwen, A., Aprlevliet, J., Cohen, B., Landsbergen, Q., D'Amaro, J., van Rood, J. J. 1981. Two major factors influencing kidney graft survival in Eurotransplant: HLA-DR matching and blood transfusion(s). *Transplant. Proc.* 150:150–54

32. Opelz, G., Graver, B., Mickey, M. R., Terasaki, P. I. 1982. Lymphocytotoxic antibody responses to transfusions in potential kidney transplant recipients. *Transplantation* 32:177–83

33. Patel, R., Terasaki, P. I., Mickey, M. R. 1968. Significance of the positive crossmatch test in kidney transplantation. *N. Engl. J. Med.* 280:735

34. Opelz, G., Graver, B., Terasaki, P. I. 1981. Induction of high kidney graft survival rate by multiple blood transfusion. *Lancet* 1:1223–25

35. Salvatierra, O., Vincenti, F., Amend, W., Potter, D., Iwaki, Y., Opelz, G., Terasaki, P., Duca, R., Cochrum, K., Hanes, D., Stoney, R. J., Feduska, N. J. 1980. Deliberate donor-specific blood transfusions prior to living related renal transplantation. *Ann. Surg.* 192:543–52

36. Opelz, G., Mickey, M. R., Terasaki, P. I. 1981. Blood transfusions and kidney transplants: remaining controversies. *Transplant. Proc.* 13:136–41

37. Fassbinder, W., Frei, U., Persijn, G., Bechstein, P. B., Schopow, K., Danthe, G., Jonas, D., Weber, W., Kuehnl, P.,

Schoeppe, W. 1982. Graft survival in renal allograft recipients transfused perioperatively only. *Transplant. Proc.* 14:164–67

38. Stiller, C. R., Sinclair, N. R., Sheppard, R. R., Lockwood, B. L., Sharpe, J. A., Hagman, P. 1978. Beneficial effect of operation-day blood-transfusions on human renal-allograft survival. *Lancet* 1:169–72

39. Williams, K. A., Ting, A., French, M. E., Oliver, D., Morris, P. J. 1980. Peroperative blood-transfusions improve cadaveric renal-allograft survival in non-transfused recipients. *Lancet* 1:1104–6

40. Opelz, G., Terasaki, P. I. 1981. Importance of preoperative (not peroperative) transfusions for cadaver kidney transplants. *Transplantation* 31:106–8

41. Fischer, E., Lenhard, V., Seifert, P., Kluge, A., Johannsen, R. 1980. Blood transfusion-induced suppression of cellular immunity in man. *Immunobiol.* 3:187–94

42. Smith, M. D., Williams, J. D., Coles, G. A., Salaman, J. R. 1981. The effect of blood transfusion on T-suppressor cells in renal dialysis patients. *Transplant.* Proc. 13:181–83

43. Lenhard, V., Seifert, P., Maassen, G., Grosse-Wilde, H., Johannsen, R., Geisen, H. P., Kluge, A. 1982. Blood transfusion-induced suppression of cellular immunity in prospective kidney-graft recipients. *Transplant. Proc.* 14:160–63

44. Singal, D. P., Joseph, S. 1982. Role of blood transfusions in the induction of antibodies against recognition sites on T lymphocytes in renal transplant recipients. *Hum. Immunol.* 4:93–108

45. Opelz, G., Terasaki, P. I. 1976. Recipient selection for renal retransplantation. *Transplantation* 21:483–88

46. Opelz, G., Mickey, M. R., Terasaki, P. I. 1972. Prolonged survival of second human kidney transplants. *Science* 178:617–19

47. Opelz, G., Terasaki, P. I. 1978. Absence of immunization effect in human kidney retransplantation. *N. Engl. J. Med.* 299:369–74

48. Mickey, M. R., Opelz, G., Terasaki, P. I. 1979. Prospective estimates of probability of success of kidney transplants: a basis for recipient selection. *Transplant. Proc.* 11:1914–15

Ann. Rev. Med. 1983. 34:145–60

INSULIN RECEPTORS AND INSULIN RESISTANCE

Jeffrey S. Flier, M.D.

The Charles A. Dana Research Institute and the Harvard-Thorndike
Laboratory of Beth Israel Hospital, Department of Medicine, Beth Israel
Hospital and Harvard Medical School, Boston, Massachusetts 02215

ABSTRACT

Resistance to the action of insulin plays a central role in many important
disease states, including diabetes and obesity. Many insights into the mechanism and significance of insulin resistance in these and other disorders have
followed upon our expanding knowledge regarding insulin receptors. In this
article, we review our current understanding of insulin receptors and their
regulation, and we assess the role of insulin receptor pathology in the
various syndromes characterized by insulin resistance.

INTRODUCTION

Insulin is a 6000 MW peptide secreted by the beta cell of the pancreas; it
plays a central role both in the regulation of metabolism and in the pathophysiology and treatment of the diabetic syndromes. Since its discovery,
considerable efforts have been directed toward determining the mechanism
of action of this hormone. Although much remains unknown, a great deal
has been learned about the first step in insulin action—the binding to
specific receptors in the plasma membrane of the cell (1, 2). The rapid
accumulation of information regarding insulin receptors has furthered our
understanding of disease mechanisms. This is especially true for diseases
characterized by insulin resistance.

Insulin resistance is a state in which a given concentration of insulin
produces a subnormal biologic response. Over the past 10 years, studies of
insulin receptors and of insulin-resistant disease states have advanced in
parallel. Thus, the direct measurement of insulin receptors on target tissues

145

0066-4219/83/0401-0145$02.00

has improved our understanding of the mechanism responsible for insulin resistance in a variety of diseases (2, 3). In a complementary fashion, studies of the manner in which insulin receptors may be altered in disease have led to many insights into the molecular mechanism of insulin action (4). In this review, I discuss the mechanisms of insulin resistance in the light of current knowledge of insulin action, and assess the clinical states of insulin resistance from the perspective of insulin receptor biology.

INSULIN ACTION—GENERAL CONSIDERATIONS

A complete understanding of the mechanism of insulin action at the cellular level has been difficult to obtain, for several reasons. Although insulin is best known for its promotion of glucose metabolism, it exerts a wide variety of effects at the cellular level (5). Thus, in addition to stimulating glucose and amino acid transport, insulin can also activate or inactivate cytoplasmic and membrane enzymes, alter the rate of synthesis of protein and DNA, and influence the processes of cell growth and differentiation. These multiple effects vary widely with respect to dose response and time course. Some effects, such as stimulation of glucose transport, occur within seconds at very low insulin concentrations (10^{-11}M). At the other extreme, actions on DNA synthesis and cell growth require hours and generally involve higher concentrations of the hormone (10^{-7}M). A recently recognized factor that further complicates the study of insulin action is the relationship between insulin and another family of peptides possessing a similar range of activities, the so-called insulin-like growth factors (IGFs) (6). These peptides (IGF I and II) have major structural homologies with insulin, but have little or no immunologic cross reactivity with the hormone (7). In general, they have more potent growth-promoting effects, but less potent metabolic actions when compared to insulin. Both IGF I and II have distinct receptors to which insulin is capable of binding with reduced affinity (8). Any discussion of insulin action must take account of these complexities.

Insulin Receptors

In order for insulin to act, it must first bind to specific receptors located on the plasma membranes of cells (1, 2). These receptors were first defined by virtue of their insulin-binding characteristics, which typically included high affinity for insulin, rapid and saturable binding, and specificity for insulin and related molecules in proportion to their biological activity (1, 2). These functional characteristics of the binding of insulin to its receptor have been highly conserved through evolution (9). In recent years, much has also been learned about the structure of the receptor molecule (4, 5, 10). The insulin receptor is now known to be a glycoprotein, composed of at least two distinct subunits referred to as α and β with MW of 135,000 and 95,000. Interchain disulfide bonds are present and the stoichiometry, although not known with certainty, may be $\alpha_2\beta_2$. A similar subunit composition has been found in receptors purified from a number of species and from a variety of target tissues. Subtle structural or organizational heterogeneity of insulin receptors from different tissues, or within a single tissue, may yet be found. The number of receptors expressed per cell varies considerably, from several hundred per mature erythrocyte, to several hundred thousand per adipocyte.

RECEPTOR REGULATION   A central feature of insulin receptor physiology is the fact that insulin receptors are not a static component of the cellular machinery; rather, they have a half-life measured in hours. In addition to this rapid turnover under basal conditions, the affinity and number of insulin receptors are subject to dynamic regulation by many signals emanating from inside and outside the cell (2, 11). A major factor now known to regulate the concentration of insulin receptors is insulin itself (12). Thus, when cells (including lymphocytes, hepatocytes, fibroblasts, and adipocytes) are cultured in media containing insulin, they exhibit a time- and temperature-dependent decrease in the concentration of insulin receptors, a phenomenon termed down regulation (12, 13). The mechanism for this phenomenon may be complex, but accelerated receptor degradation after exposure to insulin appears to be involved (14). In addition to this in vitro phenomenon of down regulation, the number of insulin receptors on cells acutely removed from patients with a variety of diseases correlated inversely with the concentration of insulin to which the cells are tonically exposed in vivo (11). This phenomenon, whereby the concentration of insulin receptors is regulated by ambient insulin levels, is believed to play a major role in the pathogenesis of insulin resistance in a variety of disease states. Many other modulators of receptor concentration or affinity have been described through in vivo or in vitro studies. These include dietary maneuvers such as fasting or high carbohydrate feeding; exercise; and the levels of specific molecules that can influence receptor expression such as hormones (cortisol, growth hormone), ions, nucleotides, ketones, and autoantibodies against the receptor (15–17). In many diseases, one or more of these receptor modulators may be responsible for insulin receptor alterations and clinical resistance to insulin.

POSTRECEPTOR MECHANISMS OF INSULIN ACTION   The mechanism (or mechanisms) by which the insulin-receptor complex generates a signal (or signals) to activate (or inactivate) cellular processes is largely unknown at this time. Potential mediators such as cyclic nucleotides and ions have been studied, but as yet none of the actions of insulin can be attributed to such known biochemical mediators (5). Several recent studies suggest that unique early events may be involved in insulin's signal to the cell. Several laboratories report the existence of an as yet poorly characterized small peptide that may be generated in plasma membranes subsequent to insulin binding (5, 18). This molecule has been claimed to act upon a variety of insulin-responsive enzymes, and to modify their activity by changing their state of phosphorylation. In this regard, it was also recently demonstrated that insulin receptors may themselves be rapidly phosphorylated after interaction with insulin (19). Given the diverse nature of insulin's effects on cellular function, it may be that no single early biochemical event will emerge as central to all of the actions of insulin. The limited state of our knowledge in this area increases the difficulty of defining molecular defects responsible for insulin resistance in disease.

INSULIN RESISTANCE—GENERAL CONSIDERATIONS

Insulin resistance may be defined as a state in which a given concentration of insulin produces less than the expected biologic effect. Clinically, this brings to mind the image of an insulin-treated patient who remains hyperglycemic while on large doses of exogenous insulin. Although such a patient certainly qualifies as being insulin resistant, the example ignores the many subtleties inherent in the concept of insulin resistance. To avoid confusion, a number of points should be clarified in any case of presumed insulin resistance. As discussed above, insulin has diverse cellular actions that may result from more than one biochemical mediator and that may even involve more than one receptor type (e.g. insulin action via IGF receptors). As a consequence, resistance to one action of insulin (e.g. its glucose-lowering effect) need not necessarily be associated with resistance to other important actions (i.e. antilipolysis, amino acid uptake, or growth stimulation). Discordance in the degree of resistance in various pathways may have great clinical importance. A second caveat relates to the level of organization at which the insulin resistance is being analyzed. Studies at the level of isolated cells may be expected to produce different data from that obtained with isolated organs or with the intact organism. Extrapolation of data from one level to another may not always be appropriate.

States of insulin resistance span a broad spectrum with respect to glucose homeostasis and, as a consequence, insulin resistance may be discovered by a variety of means. Thus, at one end of the spectrum patients with insulin resistance may be grossly diabetic despite large doses of insulin. At the other end of the clinical spectrum, patients may be normoglycemic through the effect of compensatory secretion of endogenous insulin. In the latter, very common situation (e.g. most patients with obesity), resistance to insulin is not clinically evident, but can be demonstrated by a variety of methods. A commonly employed indirect approach infers the degree of insulin resistance from the level of insulin in blood, most often the level of insulin after an overnight fast. In many situations the fasting insulin level was inversely related to the directly measured insulin sensitivity, but the approach is subject to error if the insulin measured by radioimmunoassay is not fully potent in a bioassay, as is the case in a syndrome involving a point mutation in the structure of the insulin molecule (20). Insulin sensitivity can also be assessed by measuring the response to direct infusion of insulin, usually by the intravenous route. Although useful information can be obtained by measuring the response to a bolus injection of insulin, the variable secretion of counter-insulin hormones in response to hypoglycemia makes mechanistic interpretation of data obtained with such a method difficult. To circumvent this problem, many investigators employ the euglycemic insulin clamp technique first used by Andres et al (21). With this technique, the response (i.e. glucose disposal, antilipolysis, etc) can be assessed at different steady-state insulin levels while plasma glucose levels are being held constant with a computer-assisted variable glucose infusion.

A quantitative analysis of insulin action also requires an assessment of dose response data, i.e. measurement of hormone action over a wide range of hormone concentrations. Two useful parameters that are easily measured with such an approach are (a) the hormone concentration that produces a half-maximal biological response and (b) the maximal biological response that the hormone is capable of producing. Kahn (22) proposed that an altered dose response curve due to a change in the concentration of hormone producing half-maximal activation be referred to as a change in hormone sensitivity, and that an altered dose response curve characterized by a change in the maximal response to the highest concentration of hormone be called a change in hormone responsiveness (22). Uniform use of this terminology may be expected to dispel controversies based solely on imperfect communication between investigators.

A key question to be addressed at this point is: How would we expect the insulin dose response curve to change with a change in the number of insulin receptors, or with changes in intracellular, postreceptor pathways in insulin action? This question cannot be answered without brief consideration of the subject of spare receptors (23). Most insulin-sensitive pathways are maximally activated at hormone concentrations that occupy less than the total number of available receptors. The receptors available for binding after the maximal bioeffect has been reached may be considered "spare." (Many lines of evidence show that all available receptors are potentially coupled to a biological response, and that which receptors become occupied and which are spare is simply a statistical matter.) After a certain number of receptors become occupied, subsequent steps in the biochemical sequence being measured may become rate limiting, and thus no further response is observed. In this context, a sequential reduction in the overall number of receptors would, by the law of mass action, be expected to progressively shift the biological dose response curve to the right, with decreased response at low hormone concentrations and normal insulin action at maximally effective concentrations. If receptor loss becomes so severe that "spare receptors" are no longer present and inadequate receptors are present to generate a maximal insulin response, then the dose response curve, in addition to being shifted to the right, becomes flattened as well. The effect of postreceptor alterations on insulin dose response curves is more ambiguous. Depending upon whether or not the defective step is rate limiting for a particular insulin action, a post-receptor abnormality could cause either pattern of dose response alteration (i.e. decreased sensitivity or responsiveness). Mechanistic interpretation of insulin dose response data is further complicated by the fact that the proportion of "spare receptors" varies with different cell types and is also a function of which particular bioeffect is being measured. Attempts to analyze in vivo dose response data according to this scheme are useful, but, because of the existence of many intervening variables, overinterpretation from a mechanistic point of view should be avoided.

CLINICAL STATES OF INSULIN RESISTANCE: ROLE OF THE INSULIN RECEPTOR

It is helpful to classify the clinical states of insulin resistance according to a pathophysiological scheme. One such scheme considers three general causes of insulin resistance: (a) certain abnormalities of the insulin molecule; (b) circulating antagonists of insulin action; and (c) target cell defects in the pathways for insulin action. I discuss the insulin-resistant states according to this scheme, bearing in mind the fact that overlap between these categories exists. Greatest attention is paid to those conditions in which receptor defects are important components of the insulin-resistant state.

Abnormal Insulin

According to receptor theory, an abnormal insulin molecule that had reduced intrinsic activity compared to receptor-binding ability would be expected to produce a state of hormone resistance, analogous to that produced by pharmacologic receptor antagonists, such as those that inhibit angiotensin action. Although suspected for years, it was recently demonstrated for the first time that a structurally abnormal insulin does exist, although at this point only in a single patient (20). The patient was a Type II diabetic with fasting hyperglycemia and hyperinsulinemia, but with surprisingly normal sensitivity to exogenous insulin. Insulin purified from this patient had a single leucine-phenylalanine substitution in the bioactive site of the insulin molecule, associated with a 60% reduction in binding affinity and an 85% reduction in bioactivity in isolated adipocytes. The prevalence of this disorder is probably low. Abnormalities at the level of the insulin receptor would not be expected in this disorder, and in limited studies receptor binding has been normal.

Circulating or Prereceptor Antagonists of Insulin Action

ANTIBODIES TO INSULIN   Virtually all patients treated with exogenous insulin (beef, pork, or even human) develop insulin-binding IgG antibodies within a few months. These antibodies have not proven significant in most patients; in a small minority (0.1%) antibody titers rise and clinically important insulin resistance ensues (24). This resistance is usually self-limited, but may be treated by substitution of less immunogenic forms of insulin (pork vs beef; sulfated) or by therapy aimed at the immune response itself (i.e. prednisone). These antibodies appear to limit the access of insulin to its receptors, and no receptor abnormalities have been described in this setting.

AUTOANTIBODIES TO THE INSULIN RECEPTOR   Although these antibodies are present in the circulation, the insulin resistance that they produce is more reasonably considered together with the target tissue defects in insulin action (see below).

HORMONAL ANTAGONISTS   Cortisol, growth hormone, glucagon, and catecholamines are each capable of producing states of insulin resistance (25). The phenomenon is relevant to the insulin resistance seen in clinical syndromes due to hypersecretion of these hormones (e.g. Cushings), as well as to the insulin resistance of stress, in which the hormones synergize to amplify their insulin antagonism (26). These hormones may produce insulin antagonism by a variety of mechanisms, including (a) actions on peripheral tissues to influence the levels of important substrates such as fatty acids, which may antagonize insulin action; (b) actions to stimulate hepatic enzymes that counter the action of insulin, such as those that mediate gluconeogenesis and glycogenolysis; (c) actions to influence insulin secretion by the beta cell; and (d) actions to directly impair insulin-sensitive processes in target tissues, including effects on the glucose transport system and on the expression of insulin receptors (25).

Because of the complexity of these mechanisms and the capacity for interaction between them, it is difficult to assess the role of insulin receptor changes in the insulin resistance due to an excess of these hormones. Two examples will suffice. Many studies of insulin binding and insulin action in response to glucocorticoid excess have now been carried out. In early studies, in vivo glucocorticoid excess reduced insulin binding to rat hepatocytes and fat cells, and this was predominantly due to a change in receptor affinity (27, 28). A major role for receptor alterations in the production of steroid-induced insulin resistance has been questioned, however. First, when cells are exposed to glucocorticoids in vitro, insulin receptor changes are found in some, but not all studies (29, 30). Second, in a large number of in vivo studies of insulin receptors on circulating monocytes or red cells, diverse and conflicting observations were made (31–33). Unexpected differences between different steroid preparations were also noted. Although a role for insulin receptor abnormalities in glucocorticoid-induced insulin resistance in man seems likely, more in vivo studies employing relevant target tissues such as liver, fat, and muscle are needed.

The insulin resistance due to growth hormone excess is less well studied, but current evidence does not support a major role for insulin receptor alterations in this situation. Thus, insulin binding over the physiologic range of insulin concentrations is normal in cells removed from man (monocytes) and rats (liver) with growth hormone excess, although subtle alterations of receptor affinity may be seen (27, 34). Exposure of adipocytes to growth hormone in vitro produces insulin resistance, but insulin receptors are unchanged (35). The nature of the postreceptor defect in insulin action induced by growth hormone has not been defined.

As discussed below, insulin itself may be considered to be a potent hormonal antagonist of insulin action, via the phenomenon of insulin-induced down regulation or desensitization of target cells (12).

Clinical States of Insulin Resistance with Target Cell Defects

INSULIN RESISTANCE AND OBESITY Following the development of the insulin radioimmunoassay, it became evident that nondiabetic obese individuals had high circulating levels of insulin both in the fasting and postprandial states (36, 37). This indirectly suggested that such individuals were resistant to the action of insulin. Subsequent studies in man and experimental animals confirmed these observations, and in vivo infusions of insulin were employed to directly demonstrate that tissues of obese individuals were resistant to the glucose-lowering effect of insulin (38). The clinical significance of insulin resistance in nondiabetic obese individuals has not been defined; however, many studies of this phenomenon were motivated by the knowledge that obesity is present in 80–90% of adults with Type II diabetes, a disorder characterized by insulin resistance as well (see below). Thus, it is hoped that insight into the mechanisms responsible for insulin resistance in obesity can be applied to our understanding of Type II diabetes.

Animal studies Insulin resistance has been demonstrated in a variety of animal models of obesity, including those that are genetic and acquired, with and without abnormal glucose tolerance (39). The insulin receptor was studied in many of these models, and, with one exception, insulin binding to plasma membrane receptors was reduced in the basal state (39). The reduction of insulin binding in obesity was shown to be due to a decrease in the number of available receptors, with all other binding parameters (e.g. affinity, temperature dependence) being normal (39). In addition, the receptor defect has been seen in all tissues studied, including muscle, liver, fat, and thymic lymphocytes (39). In most of these models, the extent of the decrease in insulin receptor concentration is proportional to the height of the basal insulin level (39). This relationship could be due to a primary receptor defect and compensatory hyperinsulinemia, but little evidence has accrued to support this thesis. Instead, the major factor regulating the concentration of receptors in obesity appears to be the circulating level of insulin. Thus, amelioration of the hyperinsulinemia through diet or streptozotocin treatment corrects the receptor defect (40, 41). It should be stressed that correction of the receptor defect can be seen even while obesity persists, which stresses that obesity per se is not the proximate cause of the observed receptor defect. The suggestion from these animal experiments that insulin regulates the expression of its own cellular receptors is consistent with the pioneering work of Roth and colleagues, who first demonstrated that insulin could directly regulate the concentration of its own receptors in vitro, a phenomenon that they termed down regulation (12). This phenomenon has been observed subsequently with insulin in adipocytes and fibroblasts in vitro, and it appears to be a general mechanism for hormonal regulation of target cell sensitivity (23).

Although the insulin receptor deficiency of obesity is indisputable, and its cellular mechanism is fairly well understood, the relationship between the receptor deficiency and the target cell resistance to insulin is not straightforward, at least in part because of the phenomenon of spare receptors. To probe this question, insulin binding to its receptor has been assessed over a wide range of insulin concentrations, and this has been compared with dose response curves for both early (glucose transport) and late (glucose oxidation) events in insulin action. The results obtained in studies with adipocytes from spontaneously obese rodents and muscles from ob/ob mice have been quite similar. In each case, the functional consequence of receptor loss was seen as a rightward shift in the insulin dose response curve for stimulation of glucose transport (42, 43). However, the predominant abnormality responsible for the cellular insulin resistance in both cases has proven to be a postreceptor defect in the intracellular pathway of glucose metabolism (42, 43). The precise biochemical locus of this intracellular abnormality is not known, but recent in vitro experiments suggest, at least for adipocytes, that prolonged exposure to high concentrations of insulin may induce resistance to insulin not only by causing loss of insulin receptors, but by impairing postreceptor steps as well (44). Thus, both receptor and postreceptor defects in obesity could be the consequence of hyperinsulinemia.

Human studies   Studies of insulin receptors and insulin action in obese humans strongly parallel those just described for obese rodents. Thus, the concentration of insulin receptors on freshly obtained monocytes, red blood cells, and adipocytes was reduced in the basal state in most studies (45, 46). The receptor deficiency is, in general, inversely related to the basal insulin level, and diet as well as diazoxide (a drug that inhibits insulin secretion) can restore insulin binding to or toward normal (45). As with obesity in rodent models, it appears most likely that the receptor impairment is secondary to the hyperinsulinemia, and this is most likely a consequence of hyperphagia.

A causal connection between receptor deficiency and the systemic resistance to insulin has been assessed by considering receptor status in the context of in vivo insulin dose response curves obtained by the euglycemic insulin clamp technique. It is concluded from these studies that the insulin receptor deficiency contributes to insulin resistance in all obese subjects (47). However, in those subjects with the most marked hyperinsulinemia and insulin resistance, a postreceptor abnormality is present as well (47). If the in vitro data discussed above can be extrapolated to these in vivo experiments, it may be postulated that the postreceptor defect is also a consequence of the hyperinsulinemia. Much further work is needed to substantiate this hypothesis.

INSULIN RESISTANCE AND TYPE II DIABETES   Insulin secretion and insulin sensitivity have been carefully studied in Type II, non-insulin-dependent diabetes mellitus, in order to determine whether this syndrome is caused by insulin 'deficiency, insulin resistance, or a combination of the two. Studies of insulin secretion have produced much controversy, owing in part to a failure to distinguish between patients having defects of different severity.

Thus, patients with impaired glucose intolerance, also referred to as having chemical diabetes (i.e. fasting glucose <140 mg/dl with abnormal oral glucose tolerance test) typically have normal or elevated plasma insulin levels after oral glucose administration, even when compared with control groups matched for weight (48). In contrast, patients with significant fasting hyperglycemia (i.e. overt diabetes) typically have insulin levels that are normal or high in the fasting state, but low after oral glucose administration (48). In the glucose intolerant, hyperinsulinemic group, insulin resistance seemed likely. In the overtly diabetic group, the state of insulin sensitivity was less clear. Insulin sensitivity was directly assessed in both groups with the euglycemic insulin clamp technique, and the findings were straightforward. Most patients with glucose intolerance displayed the predicted resistance to insulin (49, 50). Patients with fasting hyperglycemia displayed even greater degrees of insulin resistance (50).

As in obesity, the mechanism responsible for insulin resistance in Type II diabetes was probed by studying insulin receptors, and at the same time, assessing the shape of the in vivo dose response curve for insulin-mediated glucose disposal. Circulating monocytes and erythrocytes, as well as freshly isolated adipocytes, provide convenient tissues for the study of insulin receptors in these patients; and, in general, patients with impaired glucose tolerance and overt diabetes have fewer insulin receptors than controls on a per cell basis (50). Qualitative aspects of these receptors (kinetics of binding, etc) are not well studied, but are assumed to be normal. Despite the greater severity of insulin resistance in patients with overt fasting hyperglycemia vs those with impaired glucose tolerance, the severity of the binding defect is similar in the two groups (50). This was the first hint that defects apart from receptor binding might be important components of the insulin resistance of Type II diabetes. Further data on in vivo dose response curves for insulin-mediated glucose disposal support this notion. Thus, in patients with impaired glucose tolerance and mild insulin resistance, there is diminished insulin sensitivity that can be attributed solely to a decreased number of cellular insulin receptors (51). In patients with Type II diabetes and more severe insulin resistance, a receptor defect does account for reduced insulin sensitivity, but a postreceptor defect is also present and may be the dominant abnormality (51). Neither the biochemical nature of this apparent postreceptor defect nor the causal sequence leading to the abnormality are currently known. Although most patients with Type II diabetes are obese, the fact that obese and nonobese Type II diabetics have similar degrees of insulin resistance suggests that, whatever the additive effect of obesity, insulin resistance is a function of the diabetes itself. Hyperglycemia, elevated free fatty acid levels, or insulin deficiency could each be responsible for the increasingly severe postreceptor defect in Type II diabetes, as could a currently unknown factor. The fact that insulin binding and action are normal in fibroblasts cultured from these patients makes it more likely that the insulin resistance is caused by some aspect of the in vivo metabolic milieu (52, 53).

SYNDROMES OF EXTREME TISSUE RESISTANCE TO INSULIN   In contrast to obesity and diabetes, in which tissue resistance to insulin is typically modest, there is a group of syndromes in which tissue resistance to the actions of insulin is extreme (3). In addition to their clinical interest, these syndromes have led to important insights regarding the mechanism of action of insulin. Although clinically diverse in their manifestations, patients with these syndromes nearly all manifest the skin lesion acanthosis nigricans. This cutaneous disorder is characterized by symmetric, hyperpigmented, verrucous, hyperkeratotic thickening. It most often affects the nape of the neck, axillae, and groins, and it appears to be a cutaneous manifestation of severe target cell insulin resistance, regardless of the specific etiology. It is not known whether acanthosis occurring with malignancy has the same basis. The presence of acanthosis nigricans should raise suspicion of insulin resistance even in nondiabetic patients, since compensatory hyperinsulinemia may prevent the development of diabetes.

The Type B syndrome of insulin resistance with insulin receptor autoantibodies   Insulin receptor autoantibodies were first discovered during the evaluation of several patients with extreme insulin resistance in 1975, and since that time approximately 25 patients have been described (54, 55). Clinically, there is female preponderance, and the majority of patients have been Blacks, with several cases in Caucasians and Japanese. The mean age of onset is 43, with a range of 12 to 78 years of age.

The most common clinical presentation is symptomatic diabetes, with polyuria, polydipsia, and weight loss. Ketoacidosis is generally absent or mild. Resistance to exogenous insulin therapy is present from its initial use, and some patients fail to respond to over 100,000 units of insulin per day. A minority of patients have only mild glucose intolerance, or frank hypoglycemia in association with insulin resistance. These phenomena and the pathogenetic antibodies are discussed below.

Most of these patients had symptoms or laboratory tests suggestive of autoimmune disease including alopecia, vitiligo, arthralgias and arthritis, splenomegaly, Raynaud's phenomenon, enlarged salivary glands, elevated ESR, leukopenia, and hypergammaglobulinemia (55). One third of the cases could be classified as having a specific autoimmune syndrome such as Sjögren's syndrome or systemic lupus erythematosus.

Insulin receptors were studied on circulating monocytes and erythrocytes, as well as adipocytes of these patients, and insulin binding was
severely depressed (54). Unlike obesity and Type II diabetes, the receptor
defect appears to be that of reduced affinity for insulin (56).

The key to understanding this syndrome was the observation that sera
from affected patients could inhibit insulin binding to normal insulin receptors in vitro (57). It was subsequently proven that these sera contain antibodies, predominantly IgG, that bind to the insulin receptor molecule and
are capable of precipitating it from solution (58, 59). Titers vary over a wide
range, and tend to correlate with the clinical severity of the insulin resistance (55).

The ability of these antibodies to bind to the insulin receptor and inhibit
binding provided a convenient explanation for the observed insulin resistance. However, subsequent findings proved more complex. Exposure of
cells to these antibodies will elicit insulin-like effects acutely (4). This
finding raised a potential paradox between in vitro and in vivo observations.
The resolution came from in vitro studies in which the insulin-like effects
were seen to be transient, followed by insulin resistance due to a postreceptor desensitization (4). Persistent insulin-like action of these antibodies
could account for the hypoglycemia occurring during the course of some
of these patients.

Over several years of follow-up, patients with this syndrome have had a
variety of different outcomes (60). Remission of insulin resistance with
disappearance of receptor antibodies has been observed. Patients with refractory severe insulin resistance have been treated with a variety of regimens, including glucocorticoids, antimetabolites, and plasma exchange
(61). These have produced only limited success.

The Type A syndrome of insulin resistance   The initial description of
this syndrome described three young, thin, females with carbohydrate
intolerance (in one case manifested as overt diabetes), severe target cell
resistance to insulin, hyperandrogenism, and acanthosis nigricans (54).
The cellular basis for the insulin resistance has been investigated in
detail. Freshly obtained circulating monocytes displayed markedly decreased insulin binding, owing to a reduction in the number of available
binding sites (56).

Receptors on monocytes appeared to be qualitatively normal (56). Unlike obesity, insulin binding failed to increase after three days of fasting,
which suggests that insulin-induced down regulation might not account
for this condition (56). Further studies add support to the notion that
these patients might be suffering from a genetically determined disorder
of insulin receptors. First, two families were described with severe insulin

resistance and hyperandrogenism in multiple members (62, 63). In one family, a male was also insulin resistant, which demonstrated the nonessentiality of the hyperandrogenism in the genesis of the insulin resistance (62). Second, decreased insulin binding was seen in cells cultured from these patients and grown outside of the in vivo milieu (63, 64).

The mechanism by which insulin resistance due to a genetic defect at the level of insulin receptors causes ovarian hyperandrogenism is unknown, but the gonadal problem is often the most troubling clinical feature (65). Unlike patients with antireceptor antibodies, remissions have not been demonstrated. One patient with a similar clinical and biochemical profile had normal receptors on circulating monocytes, which suggested the presence of a postreceptor defect (66).

Another, presumably distinct, group of patients may be easily mistaken as having Type A syndrome. This is a fairly large group of obese, nondiabetic women with hyperandrogenism and acanthosis nigricans. Insulin resistance is at the severe end of that seen with obesity, but the resistance and the receptor defect are less marked than what is present in the classical Type A syndrome. Insulin binding increases with caloric restriction in these patients, and thus, they more closely resemble those patients with insulin resistance due to obesity (67).

Leprechaunism and lipoatrophic diabetes   Two other rare syndromes that involve extreme tissue resistance to insulin are leprechaunism and lipoatrophic diabetes. In addition to insulin resistance, the former syndrome affects infants with hirsutism, low birth weight, characteristic facial features, and failure to thrive (68, 69). Studies of insulin binding to circulating cells have been performed in only one case, and they were normal (70). Despite the syndromes' rarity, studies of fibroblasts from several patients yielded different results. In one study, insulin receptor binding was normal, and impaired insulin-stimulated glucose transport was ascribed to a postreceptor defect (70). In another study, insulin binding was reduced, and several qualitative abnormalities of insulin receptor binding were observed (71).

Lipoatrophic diabetes, although rare, probably represents a number of distinct clinical syndromes (72). Thus, the lipoatrophy can be congenital or acquired, complete or partial. This clinical heterogeneity may in part explain the discordant insulin-binding data, with binding to circulating monocytes or cultured skin fibroblasts reported to be normal, decreased, or even increased (72–74).

Literature Cited

1. Roth, J. 1973. *Metabolism* 22:1059–73
2. Roth, J., Kahn, C. R., Lesniak, M. A., Gorden, P., DeMeyts, P., Megyesi, K., Neville, D. M. Jr., Gavin, J. R. III, Soll, A. H., Freychet, P., Goldfine, I. D., Bar, R. S., Archer, J. A. 1975. *Rec. Prog. Horm. Res.* 31:95–139
3. Flier, J. S., Kahn, C. R., Roth, J. 1979. *N. Engl. J. Med.* 300:413–19
4. Kahn, C. R., Baird, K. L., Flier, J. S., Grunfeld, C., Harmon, J. T., Harrison, L. C., Karlsson, F. A., Kasuga, M., King, G. L., Lang, U. C., Podskalny, J. M., van Obberghen, E. 1981. *Rec. Prog. Horm. Res.* 37:477–538
5. Czech, M. P. 1981. *Am. J. Med.* 70:142–50
6. Zapf, J., Rinderknecht, E., Humbel, R. E., Froesch, E. R. 1978. *Metabolism* 27:1803–28
7. Rinderknecht, E., Humbel, R. E. 1978a. *J. Biol. Chem.* 253:2769–76
8. Rechler, M. M., Zapf, J., Nissley, S. P., Froesch, E. R., Moses, A. C., Podskalny, J. M., Schilling, E. E., Humbel, R. E. 1980. *Endocrinology* 107:1451–59
9. Muggeo, M., Ginsberg, B. H., Roth, J., Neville, D. M. Jr., DeMeyts, P., Kahn, C. R. 1979. *Endocrinology* 104:1393–1402
10. Jacobs, S., Hazum, E., Cuatracasas, P. 1980. *J. Biol. Chem.* 255:6937–40
11. Bar, R. S., Harrison, L. C., Muggeo, M. 1979. *Adv. Intern. Med.* 24:23–52
12. Gavin, J. R. III, Roth, J., Neville, D. M. Jr., DeMeyts, P., Buell, D. N. 1974. *Proc. Natl. Acad. Sci. USA* 71:84–88
13. Blackard, W. G., Guzelian, P. S., Small, M. E. 1978. *Endocrinology* 103:548–53
14. Kasuga, M., Kahn, C. R., Hedo, J. A., van Obberghen, E., Yarnada, K. M. 1981. *Proc. Natl. Acad. Sci. USA* 78:6917–21
15. Muggeo, M., Bar, R. S., Roth, J. 1977. *J. Clin. Endocrinol. Metab.* 44:1206–9
16. Thomopoulos, P., Kosmakos, F. C., Pastan, I., Lovelace, I. 1977. *Biochem. Biophys. Res. Commun.* 75:246–52
17. Merimee, T. J., Pulkkinen, A. J., Loften, S. 1976. *J. Clin. Endocrinol. Metab.* 43:1190
18. Jarett, L., Seals, J. R. 1979. *Science* 206:1407–8
19. Kasuga, M., Karlsson, F. A., Kahn, C. R. 1982. *Science* 215:185–87
20. Tager, H., Given, B., Baldwin, D., Mako, M., Markese, J., Rubenstein, A., Olefsky, J., Kobayashi, M., Kolterman, O., Poucher, R. 1979. *Nature* 281:122–25
21. Sherwin, R. S., Kramer, K. J., Tobin, J. D., Insel, P. A., Liljenquist, J. E., Berman, M., Andres, R. 1974. *J. Clin. Invest.* 53:1481–92
22. Kahn, C. R. 1978. *Metab. Clin. Exp.* 27:1893–1902
23. Roth, J., Grunfeld, C. 1981. *Textbook of Endocrinology,* ed. R. H. Williams pp. 15–72. Philadelphia: Saunders
24. Kahn, C. R., Rosenthal, A. 1979. *Diabetes Care* 2:283–95
25. Harrison, L., Flier, J. S. 1980. *Secondary Diabetes,* pp. 269–86. New York: Raven
26. Eigler, N., Sacca, L., Sherwin, R. S. 1979. *J. Clin. Invest.* 63:114–23
27. Kahn, C. R., Goldfine, I. D., Neville, D. M. Jr., DeMeyts, P. 1978. *Endocrinology* 103:1059–72
28. Olefsky, J. M., Johnson, J., Lin, F., Jen, P., Reaven, G. M. 1975. *Metabolism* 24:517–26
29. Olefsky, J. M. 1975. *J. Clin. Invest.* 56:1499–1508
30. Grunfeld, C., Baird, K., van Obberghen, E., Kahn, C. R. 1981. 109:1723–30
31. Beck Nielsen, H., DePirro, R., Pederson, O. 1980. *J. Clin. Endocrinol. Metab.* 50:1–4
32. Yasuda, K., Kitabchi, A. E. 1980. *Diabetes* 29:811–14
33. Fantas, I. G., Ryan, J., Hizaka, N., Gorden, P. 1981. *J. Clin. Endocrinol. Metab.* 52:953–60
34. Muggeo, M., Bar, R. S., Roth, J., Gorden, P. 1979. *J. Clin. Endocrinol. Metab.* 48:17–25
35. Maloff, B. L., Levine, J. H., Lockwood, D. H. 1980. *Endocrinology* 107:538–44
36. Karam, J. H., Grodsky, G. M., Forsham, P. H. 1963. *Diabetes* 12:196
37. Bagdade, J. D., Bierman, E. L., Porte, D. 1967. *J. Clin. Invest.* 46:1549
38. Rabinowitz, D., Zierler, K. L. 1962. *J. Clin. Invest.* 41:2173
39. Kahn, C. R. 1980. *Metabolism* 29:455–66
40. Kahn, C. R., Neville, D. M. Jr., Roth, J. 1973. *J. Biol. Chem.* 248:244
41. Bar, R. S., Gorden, P., Roth, J., Kahn, C. R., DeMeyts, P. 1976. *J. Clin. Invest.* 58:1123
42. Olefsky, J. M. 1976. *J. Clin. Invest.* 57:842–51
43. LeMarchand-Brustel, Y., Jeanrenaud, B., Freychet, P. 1978. *Am. J. Physiol.* 234:E348–58
44. Marshall, S., Olefsky, J. M. 1980. *J. Clin. Invest.* 66:763–72

45. Bar, R. S., Gorden, P., Roth, J., Kahn, C. R., DeMeyts, P. 1976. *J. Clin. Invest.* 58:1123–35
46. Olefsky, J. M. 1976. *J. Clin. Invest.* 57:1165–72
47. Kolterman, O. G., Insel, J., Saekow, M., Olefsky, J. M. 1980. *J. Clin. Invest.* 65:1273–84
48. Reaven, G. M., Bernstein, R., Davis, B., Olefsky, J. M. 1976. *Am. J. Med.* 60:80–88
49. Kalant, H., Csorba, T. R., Heller, N. 1963. *Metabolism* 12:1100
50. Olefsky, J. M., Reaven, G. M. 1977. *Diabetes* 26:680
51. Kolterman, O. G., Gray, R. S., Griffin, P., Burstein, J., Insel, J. A., Scarlett, J. A., Olefsky, J. M. 1981. *J. Clin. Invest.* 68:957–69
52. Howard, B. V., Hidaka, H., Ishibashi, F., Fields, R. M., Bennett, P. H. 1981. *Diabetes* 30:562–67
53. Prince, M. J., Tai, P., Olefsky, J. M. 1981. *Diabetes* 30:596–600
54. Kahn, C. R., Flier, J. S., Bar, R. S., Archer, J. A., Gorden, P., Martin, M. M., Roth, J. 1976. *N. Engl. J. Med.* 294:739–45
55. Flier, J. S. 1982. *Clin. Immunol. Rev.* 1:215–56
56. Bar, R. S., Muggeo, M., Kahn, C. R., Gorden, P., Roth, J. 1980. *Diabetologia* 18:209–16
57. Flier, J. S., Kahn, C. R., Roth, J., Bar, R. S. 1975. *Science* 190:63–65
58. Flier, J. S., Kahn, C. R., Jarrett, D. B., Roth, J. 1976. *J. Clin. Invest.* 58: 1442–49
59. Harrison, L. C., Flier, J. S., Kahn, C. R., Roth, J. 1979. *J. Clin. Endocrinol. Metab.* 48:59–65
60. Flier, J. S., Bar, R. S., Muggeo, M., Kahn, C. R., Roth, J., Gorden, P. 1978.

61. Muggeo, M., Flier, J. S., Abrams, R. A., Harrison, L. C., Deisseroth, A. B., Kahn, C. R. 1979. *N. Engl. J. Med.* 300:477–81
62. Flier, J. S., Young, J. B., Landsberg, L. 1980. *N. Engl. J. Med.* 300:970–73
63. Scarlett, J. A., Kolterman, O. G., Moore, P., Saelsow, M., Insel, J., Griffin, J., Mako, M., Rubenstein, A., Olefsky, J. 1982. *J. Clin. Endocrinol. Metab.* 55:123–30
64. Podskalny, J. M., Kahn, C. R. 1982. *J. Clin. Endocrinol. Metab.* 54:261–68
65. Flier, J. S. 1982. *N. Engl. J. Med.* 306:1537–44
66. Bar, R., Muggeo, M., Roth, J., Imerato-McGinley, J. 1978. *J. Clin. Endocrinol. Metab.* 47:620–25
67. Flier, J. S., Matteson, D. F., Eastman, R. C. 1982. *Diabetes* 31(2):3A (Abstr.)
68. Donohue, W., Uchida, I. 1954. *J. Pediatr.* 45:505
69. D'Ercole, A. J., Underwood, L., Groelke, J., Plet, A. 1979. *J. Clin. Endocrinol. Metab.* 48:495
70. Kobayashi, M., Olefsky, J. M., Elders, J., Mako, M. E., Givens, B. D., Schwedie, H. K., Fisler, R. H., Hintz, R. L., Horner, J. A., Rubenstein, A. H. 1978. *Proc. Natl. Acad. Sci. USA* 75:3469
71. Podskalny, J. M., Kahn, C. R. 1982. *J. Clin. Endocrinol. Metab.* 54:261–68
72. Wachslicht-Rodbard, H., Muggeo, M., Kahn, C. R., Savolakis, G. A., Harrison, L., Flier, J. S. 1981. *J. Clin. Endocrinol. Metab.* 52:416–25
73. Dorflier, H., Wieczorek, A., Wolfran, G., Zollner, N. 1977. *Res. Exp. Med.* 170:161
74. Rosenbloom, A . L., Goldstein, S., Yip, C. C. 1977. *J. Clin. Endocrinol. Metab.* 44:803

Ann. Rev. Med. 1983. 34:161–68

CONGESTIVE HEART FAILURE IN THE DIABETIC

Timothy J. Regan, M.D.

University of Medicine and Dentistry–New Jersey Medical School, 100 Bergen Street, Newark, New Jersey 07103

ABSTRACT

Heart failure seems to occur in adult-onset diabetics with a greater frequency than in the nondiabetic population, particularly in women. A number of such patients do not have significant occlusive disease of the major coronary arteries, or convincing small-vessel disease. A subclinical abnormality of myocardium in experimental diabetes and asymptomatic human diabetics supports the concept of a diabetic cardiomyopathy.

Introduction

Over the past two decades a variety of disciplines have contributed to an increased knowledge of the influence of diabetes on the heart. Clarification of the prevalence of other cardiovascular risk factors has been a key to delineating the types of heart disease involved. In a community-wide survey, elevated serum cholesterol levels were not found to occur more frequently in adult male diabetics than in normal individuals (1). A greater prevalence of hypercholesterolemia and obesity in female diabetics presumably contributes to the substantially higher mortality and morbidity than in age-matched control women. Controversy exists as to the incidence of hypertension in diabetics. Elevated blood pressure, particularly systolic levels presumed to be secondary to peripheral arterial atherosclerosis, may occur for the first time late in the course of the disease. It is of interest that the prevalence of hypertension among diabetic women was no greater than that among controls, whereas the prevalence in males was only moderately increased.

The incidence of cardiovascular disease appears, however, to be out of proportion to the prevalence of the other risk factors. Based on 20 years of surveillance of the Framingham population (2), the relative risk of conges-

161

0066-4219/83/0401-0161$02.00

tive heart failure for diabetics versus nondiabetics was approximately doubled for men and more than tripled for women after adjustment for other risk factors. This relative risk was somewhat higher than that for coronary heart disease as judged by clinical criteria.

Since ischemic cardiomyopathy is generally accepted as a diagnostic category, coronary disease must be considered in this discussion of congestive heart failure. The contribution of occlusive disease of the coronary arteries based on angiographic or pathologic criteria has been difficult to establish in the diabetic population. A review of ten autopsy studies performed between 1930 and 1962 (3) concluded that the risk ratio for coronary atherosclerosis in diabetics was approximately 2.1, without correction for other cardiac risk factors. More recent analyses reveal that insulin-requiring diabetics (juvenile-onset) have substantially more narrowing of extramural coronary vessels than do age-matched controls and the extent of coronary involvement is also greater (4). Hypertension, known to be frequently present in this small subset of diabetics, may have contributed to the arterial pathology. Several recent studies of adult-onset diabetics provide more equivocal results. In patients who succumbed after long-term follow-up in a diabetes clinic, autopsy revealed a similar narrowing of the major coronary arteries by atherosclerosis in diabetics with and without clinical evidence of coronary heart disease and nondiabetics with fatal coronary artery disease (5). However, the study did not include a control group of nondiabetics with mortality from causes other than coronary disease. Another study involved a retrospective review of medical records in which it was not entirely clear that diabetes was an established diagnosis in a number of patients (6). A European study revealed at most only a modest increase in the quantity of atherosclerotic disease in diabetics compared with age- and sex-matched controls (7).

It is noteworthy that in a recent large-scale cineangiographic study of patients suspected of having coronary artery disease, diabetes per se was not associated with significantly greater occlusive disease in men when corrected for the coexistence of other risk factors. However, coronary disease was significant in the subsets of women age 40–60 years (8). Finally, two studies of nonhuman male primates, in which atherosclerosis was produced over an 18-month period by feeding an atherogenic diet, indicated that at equivalent degrees of hypercholesterolemia the diabetic rhesus monkey manifested no greater degree of fatty streak lesions in coronary vessels than did nondiabetic animals (9). In examining the effects of alloxan diabetes upon the development of plaque lesions in the cynomolgus monkey, neither the degree nor the extent of atherosclerosis nor the physiologic response to coronary vasodilation were different in diabetic and nondiabetic animals (10).

Thus the potential for coronary artery disease to result in chronic heart failure as a consequence of a single large infarct or several infarctions may be more likely in the juvenile-onset diabetic. In the adult-onset diabetic female, diabetes per se may well entail a higher risk, but this is less evident for males.

Intramural Vessels

Obliterative disease of the small coronary arteries has been thought to be important in the pathogenesis of cardiac disease in diabetics. Thickened intramural arteries and occasional bridges of endothelial cells have been attributed to diabetes (11, 12). However, such lesions have also been observed in nondiabetics without evident effects on cardiac muscle (11). In another disease with small-vessel involvement, endomyocardial fibrosis (13), the process appears to be independent of tissue necrosis or fibrosis, presumably because the arterial disease is patchy and its progression sufficiently slow to permit collateral development. The failure to find demonstrable obstructive lesions of intramural vessels in the free wall of the left ventricle in recent autopsy studies of diabetics (4) suggests that small-vessel lesions in this disease state may have little or no relation to cardiac pathology.

In vivo myocardial biopsies were recently reported in 12 adult diabetics with cardiac symptoms. Structural changes in the microcirculation were not observed, a finding that was confirmed at autopsy in two of the patients (14) and was also observed in a recent small series of diabetics (15). Although a matter of continuing controversy, the majority of recent studies support the view that occlusive disease of the intramural arteries and arterioles is not usually sufficient to account for heart muscle pathology. It should be added that a preparation for fixing small vessels at postmortem revealed saccular microaneurysms of arteriolar and capillary vessels in three of six patients (16). No specific abnormalities were observed in the tissue around these vessels. Although fibrosis or myocardial degeneration was seen, these abnormalities also occurred in other areas of myocardium where no aneurysms were observed.

Subclinical Cardiomyopathy

To test the hypothesis that a portion of the diabetic population may have asymptomatic myocardial abnormalities, diabetic patients aged 20–56 years, who had no evidence of myocardial ischemia or other cardiovascular disease, underwent noninvasive measurement of the systolic time intervals for comparison with age-matched normals (17). Heart rate and arterial pressure were normal, but the diabetic subjects had a shorter left ventricular ejection time, a longer preejection period, and a higher ratio of preejection period to left ventricular ejection time, apparently unrelated to types of treatment. This ratio was not as elevated as in patients with overt heart failure. The abnormality was thought to be related to either increased wall stiffness or reduced contractility. It is relevant that patients with classic angina pectoris without cardiac decompensation usually have normal systolic time intervals at rest, so that myocardial ischemia appears to be improbable as a basis for the preclinical abnormality.

An additional report supports the hypothesis that some patients with diabetes mellitus have myocardial alterations without clinical manifestations; these may result in heart failure if the process develops fully (18). This study is of particular interest because the authors indicate that most normotensive persons with long-standing diabetes but without clinical evidence of heart disease may have a preclinical abnormality of the left ventricle without overt manifestations. A computerized echocardiographic technique showed that 60% had an abnormality during left ventricular diastole in which the normally close time interval between movements of the mitral valve and ventricular wall was absent. Since this alteration has been observed in patients with cardiomyopathy, it was concluded that a diffuse myopathic process was present. A more recent study of noncardiac middle-aged diabetic males demonstrated that fractional shortening of the left ventricle was significantly reduced (19). Exercise stress tests performed in some were uniformly negative.

Congestive Heart Failure

The noninvasive studies do not indicate the basis for the observed abnormalities and the relative role of impaired compliance or contractility. To explore the question of myopathy after the development of typical or atypical angina or dyspnea, left ventricular function was examined in uncomplicated adult diabetics with a familial history to determine whether symptoms depended on the presence of significant atherosclerosis (20). These patients were well controlled without ketosis on diet, insulin, or oral hypoglycemic agents and were without other cardiac risk factors.

There was no significant obstructive disease by coronary arteriography in 12 of 17 patients, and ventriculograms showed no evidence of regional contractile abnormalities or mitral valve lesions in the noncoronary group. The latter were also without hypertrophy but had a significant reduction of stroke volume and elevation of end-diastolic pressure at rest compared with control subjects of similar age. Since end-diastolic volume was significantly less than in controls, the reduced stroke volume appeared to be secondary to abnormal filling of the ventricle. Ejection fraction did not differ significantly from controls, but this may have been due to enhanced end-diastolic wall stiffness.

In diabetics with prior episodes of cardiac failure and normal coronary arteriograms, stroke volume was reduced more than in diabetic subjects without failure. This was not solely related to diminished diastolic filling of the ventricle; decreased pump function also contributed since ejection fraction was significantly reduced. Although the compliance abnormality was also more evident, the sequence of diminished diastolic compliance followed by impaired contractility may be important in pathogenesis.

Since myocardial ischemia on a microvascular basis could not be excluded in these patients, atrial pacing was induced to determine whether or not lactate production as evidence of inadequate coronary blood flow could be evoked. Lactate production was not encountered. Consequently, if abnormalities of small arteries or capillaries were present in these diabetic patients with altered ventricular function, they were apparently insufficient to restrict myocardial perfusion.

The change in cardiac function suggestive of enhanced wall stiffness may be related to altered muscle composition in the form of interstitial collagen accumulation observed in morphologic studies (20, 21). A diffuse distribution of this process throughout the left ventricle, as well as accumulation of triglyceride and cholesterol, supports the view that a cardiomyopathic process can exist in diabetes. The amount and distribution of glycoprotein in the interstitium may contribute to progression of the process. It is not yet known whether or not a primary effect on contractile protein or calcium transport occurs in diabetes to effect the onset of decompensation.

Pathogenesis

Abnormalities of the myocardium apparently independent of coronary atherosclerosis have been described in animals with spontaneous (22) or experimental diabetes (23, 24) as well as in human diabetes (20, 21). One of the features of the disease is the accumulation of collagen in the myocardial interstitium. This process can be affected by several variables. Chronic ketoacidosis in animals impairs cardiac protein synthesis (25) and may thus explain the absence of cardiac collagen increments in this circumstance (26). Counterregulatory hormones may have an influence. Growth hormone is considered to play an important role in the cardiovascular complications (27). In arterial myomedial cell cultures from normal rabbits, greater amounts of procollagen type I were produced in the presence of diabetic serum or normal serum with small increments of growth hormone (28). Glucose, insulin, lipids, and ketones were without effect. Although well-controlled diabetics appear to have normal serum growth hormone levels, when related to the level of hyperglycemia, the hormone level is significantly higher than in normals with equivalent hyperglycemia induced by glucose infusion (29).

Distinctly different cardiac abnormalities have been described in a rat model during severe chemically induced diabetes (26, 30). Depressed contractility, slowed relaxation, abnormal molecular properties of myosin, and impaired calcium transport have been observed. These are normalized after days of insulin replacement (30, 31), and may be at least partially dependent on correction of acidosis. The latter can impair developed tension and calcium exchange in nondiabetic heart muscle (32). It should be noted that the incidence of heart failure in human diabetics after prolonged untreated ketoacidosis is unknown.

Management

The influence of chronic treatment on the development and progression of the tissue complications of diabetes has been a matter of controversy. Long-term use of insulin in diabetic animals has apparently reduced the incidence of retinal microvascular disease (33), but the influence of this hormone on the myocardium is less clear. In the chronic canine model of mild diabetes (34), collagen accumulation and diminished myocardial compliance were unaffected by insulin control of postprandial hyperglycemia. Similarly the lipid abnormalities of diabetic nerve are reportedly not corrected by insulin therapy (35).

Treatment of the adult-onset diabetic is frequently approached by caloric restriction, perhaps combined with a modest exercise program that usually results in improved glucose tolerance. Although infrequent episodes of ketoacidosis or marked hyperglycemia may require intermittent use of insulin, a minority of adult-onset diabetics are believed to require long-term insulin therapy for metabolic control. In view of the uncertain status of tolbutamide, other oral hypoglycemic agents should be used if indicated. It is generally agreed that diabetics should not smoke cigarettes. Treatment for hypertension and hyperlipidemia is at least as important as in nondiabetics. Patients who develop heart failure requiring thiazide diuretics or those with angina requiring beta-blocking agents may run the risk of impaired insulin secretion. The latter problem is obviated by cardioselective agents with beta-1 action. Preload- and afterload-reducing agents for heart failure should be used cautiously in diabetics, since impaired arterial reflex responses due to autonomic dysfunction may be present. Digitalis is particularly useful in patients with atrial fibrillation and heart failure. An altered sensitivity of the myocardium to glycosides that is specific for diabetes has not been established.

Literature Cited

1. Garcia, M. J., McNamara, P. M., Gordon, T., Kannel, W. B. 1974. Morbidity and mortality in diabetics in the Framingham population. *Diabetes* 23: 105–11
2. Kannel, W. B., McGee, D. L. 1979. Diabetes and cardiovascular disease. The Framingham study. *J. Am. Med. Assoc.* 241:2035–38
3. Knowles, H. C. Jr. 1978. Coronary artery disease in diabetes: its development, course, and response to treatment. In *Diabetes and The Heart*, ed. S. Zoneraich, Ch. 8, pp. 113–22. Springfield, Ill: Thomas. 303 pp.
4. Crall, F. V. Jr., Roberts, W. C. 1978. The extramural and intramural coronary arteries in juvenile diabetes mellitus. Analysis of nine necropsy patients aged 19–38 years with onset of diabetes before age 15 years. *Am. J. Med.* 64:221–30
5. Waller, B. F., Palumbo, P. J., Lie, J. T., Roberts, W. C. 1980. Status of the coronary arteries at necropsy in diabetes mellitus with onset after age 30 years. Analysis of 229 diabetic patients with and without clinical evidence of coronary heart disease and comparison to 183 control subjects. *Am. J. Med.* 69:498–506
6. Vigorita, V. J., Moore, G. W., Hutchins, G. M. 1980. Absence of correlation between coronary arterial atherosclerosis and severity or duration of diabetes mellitus of adult onset. *Am. J. Cardiol.* 46:535–42
7. Vihert, A. M., Zhdanov, V. S., Matova, E. E. 1969. Atherosclerosis of the aorta and coronary vessels of the heart in cases of various disease. *J. Atheroscler. Res.* 9:179–92
8. Vlietstra, R. E., Frye, R. L. Kronmal, R. A., Sim, D. A., Phil, M., Tristani, F. E., Killip, T. III, and Participants in the Coronary Artery Surgery Study. 1980. Risk factors and angiographic coronary artery disease: a report from the coronary artery surgery study (CASS). *Circulation* 62:254–51
9. Haider, J., Yeh, C. K., Thomas, G., Oldewurtel, H. A., Lyons, M. M., Regan, T. J. 1981. Influence of diabetes on the myocardium and coronary arteries of rhesus monkey fed an atherogenic diet. *Circ. Res.* 41:1278–88
10. Haider, B., Lyons, M. M., Oldewurtel, H. A., Regan, T. J. 1982. Severity of obstructive atherosclerosis in the diabetic non-human primate. *Clin. Res.* 39(2):192A

11. Blumenthal, H. T., Alex, M., Goldenberg, S. 1960. Study of lesions of the intramural coronary artery branches in diabetes mellitus. *Arch. Pathol.* 70: 13–28
12. Hamby, I., Zoneraich, S., Sherman, L. 1974. Diabetic cardiomyopathy. *J. Am. Med. Assoc.* 229:1749–54
13. Farrer-Brown, G., Tarbit, M. H., Somers, K., Hutt, M. S. R. 1972. Microvascular study of hearts with endomyocardial fibrosis. *Br. Heart J.* 34:1250–62
14. Shirley, E. K., Proudfit, W. L., Hawk, W. A. 1980. Primary myocardial disease. Correlation with clinical findings, angiographic and biopsy diagnosis. Follow-up of 139 patients. *Am. Heart J.* 99:198–207
15. Baandrup, U., Oldsen, E. G. J. 1981. Critical analysis of endomyocardial biopsies from patients suspected of having cardiomyopathy. I: Morphological and morphometric aspects. *Br. Heart J.* 45:475–86
16. Factor, S. M., Okun, E. M., Minase, T. 1980. Capillary microaneurysms in the human diabetic heart. *N. Engl. J. Med.* 302:384–88
17. Ahmed, S. S., Regan, T. J., Jaferi, G. A., Narang, R. M. 1975. Preclinical abnormality of left ventricular function in diabetes mellitus. *Am. Heart J.* 89:153–58
18. Sanderson, J. E., Brown, D. J., Rivellese, A., Kohner, E. 1978. Diabetic cardiomyopathy? An echocardiographic study of young diabetics. *Br. Med. J.* 1:404–7
19. Abenavoli, T., Rubler, S., Fisher, V. J., Axelrod, H. I., Zuckerman, K. P. 1981. Exercise testing with myocardial scintigraphy in asymptomatic diabetic males. *Circulation* 63:54–63
20. Regan, T. J., Lyons, M. M., Ahmed, S. S., Levinson, G. E., Oldewurtel, H. A., Ahmad, M. R., Haider, B. 1977. Evidence for cardiomyopathy in familial diabetes mellitus. *J. Clin. Invest.* 60:885–99
21. Ledet, T. 1976. Diabetic cardiomyopathy: quantitative histological studies of the heart from young juvenile diabetics. *Acta Pathol. Microbiol. Scand. Sect. A* 84:421–28
22. Giacomelli, F., Wiener, J. 1979. Primary myocardial disease in diabetic mouse. An ultrastructural study. *Lab. Invest.* 40:460–73
23. Regan, T. J., Ettinger, P. O., Khan, M. I., Jesrani, M. U., Lyons, M. M., Ol-

dewurtel, H. A., Weber, M. 1974. Altered myocardial function and metabolism in chronic diabetes mellitus without ischemia in dogs. *Circ. Res.* 35:222–37

24. Baandrup, U., Ledet, T., Rasch, R. 1981. Experimental diabetic cardiopathy preventable by insulin treatment. *Lab. Invest.* 45:169–73

25. Pain, V. M., Garlick, P. J. 1974. Effects of streptozotocin diabetes and insulin treatment on the rate of protein synthesis in tissues of the rat in vivo. *J. Biol. Chem.* 249:4510–14

26. Fein, F. S., Kornstein, L. B., Strobeck, J. E., Capasso, J. M., Sonnenblick, F. H. 1980. Altered myocardial mechanics in diabetic rats. *Circ. Res.* 47:922–33

27. Merimee, T. J. 1978. A follow-up study of vascular disease in growth-hormone-deficient dwarfs with diabetes. *N. Engl. J. Med.* 298:1217–22

28. Ledet, T., Vuust, J. 1980. Arterial procollagen type I, type III, and fibronectin: effects of diabetic serum, glucose, insulin, ketone, and growth hormone studied on rabbit aortic myomedial cell cultures. *Diabetes* 29:964–68

29. Merimee, T. J., Fitzgerald, C. R., Gold, L. A., McCourt, J. P. 1979. Character-istics of growth hormone secretion in clinically stable diabetes. *Diabetes* 28:308–12

30. Dillmann, W. H. 1980. Diabetes mellitus induces changes in cardiac myosin of the rat. *Diabetes* 29:579–82

31. Fein, F. S., Strobeck, J. E., Malhotra, A., Scheuer, J., Sonnenblick, E. H. 1981. Reversibility of diabetic cardiomyopathy with insulin in rats. *Circ. Res.* 49:1251–61

32. Poole-Wilson, P. A., Langer, G. A. 1979. Effects of acidosis on mechanical function and Ca^{2+} exchange in rabbit myocardium. *Am. Physiol. Soc.* H525–33

33. Engerman, R., Bloodworth, J. M. B. Jr., Nelson, S. 1977. Relationship of microvascular disease in diabetes to metabolic control. *Diabetes* 26:760–69

34. Regan, T. J., Wu, C. F., Yeh, C. K., Oldewurtel, H. A., Haider, B. 1981. Myocardial composition and function in diabetes: the effects of chronic insulin use. *Circ. Res.* 41:1268–77

35. Clements, R. S. Jr., Stockard, C. R. 1980. Abnormal sciatic nerve myoinositol metabolism in the streptozotocin-diabetic rat. Effect of insulin treatment. *Diabetes* 27:227–35

Ann. Rev. Med. 1983. 34:169–77

DRUG SUPPRESSION OF THE ANGIOTENSIN SYSTEM IN CONGESTIVE HEART FAILURE

Jay M. Sullivan, M.D.

Division of Cardiovascular Diseases, The University of Tennessee Center for the Health Sciences, Memphis, Tennessee 38163

ABSTRACT

Congestive heart failure is frequently associated with elevated systemic vascular resistance. Lowering resistance can improve cardiac performance and alleviate symptoms. The angiotensin-converting enzyme inhibitors offer a new way to lower resistance and have certain advantages, including the inhibition of compensatory mechanisms. However, skillful use of these compounds demands a thorough understanding of their pharmacologic properties and of the pathophysiology of congestive heart failure.

INTRODUCTION

Sodium restriction, diuretics, and/or digitalis are still the initial choices in the treatment of congestive heart failure. Unfortunately, these measures are sometimes inadequate. When a surgical approach is not appropriate, other means must be found to improve the patient's condition. Over the past decade, vasodilator therapy has constituted a major therapeutic advance. Interruption of the renin-angiotensin system is a form of vasodilator therapy that may offer unique advantages as well as certain risks compared to other forms. To understand the use of the compounds involved, a brief review of circulatory regulation is in order.

169

0066-4219/83/0401-0169$02.00

REGULATION OF THE CARDIOVASCULAR AND RENIN-ANGIOTENSIN SYSTEMS

Blood pressure is the product of cardiac output and peripheral vascular resistance. The resistance component is subject to both intrinsic and extrinsic control (1). Intrinsic control includes the myogenic activity of vascular smooth-muscle cells in response to stretch and to vasoactive substances. Extrinsic control includes the activity of the autonomic nervous system and the effects of circulating hormones, e.g. catecholamines and angiotensin II.

Cardiac output is the product of heart rate and stroke volume. Heart rate is determined by the intrinsic rhythmicity of the sinoatrial node modulated by the interplay of the sympathetic and parasympathetic nervous systems. It is also influenced by circulating hormones such as epinephrine. Stroke volume is determined by the size of the left ventricle at the end of diastole and the amount of myocardial fiber shortening during systole (2). These, in turn, are determined by preload, contractility, and afterload. Preload, the amount of stretch on the resting myocardial fiber, is set by venous return, which in itself is a reflection of intravascular volume, venous tone, and several other factors. Within limits, a greater degree of stretch is followed by a greater contraction (the Frank-Starling mechanism). Contractility is determined by the amount of calcium reaching the active sites of the actin and myosin filaments during systole and by the response of the myocardium to norepinephrine. Afterload, overcome by the myocardium as it contracts, is determined by the size of the ventricle, or its radius, and by the intracavitary pressure generated therein, which is determined by the peripheral vascular resistance provided there is no outflow tract obstruction. The extent and velocity of myocardial contraction decreases as afterload is increased beyond a certain limit.

The renin-angiotensin-aldosterone system forms a feedback loop in the regulation of blood pressure (3). The liver synthesizes renin substrate, a glycoprotein, which is released into the circulation. Renin, a proteolytic enzyme, cleaves a decapeptide, angiotensin I, from the substrate molecule. During passage through the pulmonary circulation, angiotensin I is lysed by a converting enzyme, leaving the octapeptide angiotensin II, a potent vasopressor. The latter is inactivated by angiotensinases. Angiotensin II has several effects among which are vasoconstriction and aldosterone release. Aldosterone causes the distal tubules of the kidney to retain sodium.

The renin-angiotensin system works to maintain blood pressure in two major ways—by increasing effective blood volume and increasing peripheral vascular resistance. Further, angiotensin II acts directly on the juxtaglomerular cells to inhibit renin release, thus acting as a brake on that activity. Any manipulation that drops the blood pressure, blood volume, or serum sodium concentration tends to activate the feedback loop. Hemorrhage, hypotension, sodium depletion, gastrointestinal fluid loss, upright posture, and renal artery stenosis all stimulate renin release.

The release of renin is controlled by the interplay of a number of mechanisms by which the body adjusts to changing circumstances. The major ones involved are the vascular receptors in the afferent renal arterioles, the macula densa, the sympathetic nervous system, and certain blood-borne substances. The vascular receptor comprises the juxtaglomerular cells and portions of the afferent glomerular arteriole that respond to altered wall tension caused by changes in perfusion pressure, sympathetic nerve activity, and intrinsic modifications in vascular smooth-muscle during renal autoregulation. The macula densa responds to changes in the rate of sodium delivery, but the relative importance of this mechanism in the control of renin release is not clear. The circulating agents known to affect renin release include sodium, potassium, angiotensin II, catecholamines, estrogens, adrenal steroids, and antidiuretic hormone (ADH).

Although the renal sympathetic nerves are important modulators of renin release, they are not essential for it. Increased renin secretion in response to sodium depletion has been demonstrated in dogs with bilateral renal denervation.

Aldosterone and angiotensin II are the two effector compounds in this system that act directly on tissues. Potassium and ACTH stimulate aldosterone secretion as does angiotensin II, whereas large increases in plasma sodium concentration inhibit aldosterone release.

If plasma renin activity (PRA) is measured in a group of normal subjects of comparable age under standard conditions of posture, activity, diet, and time of day, values will be found to fall within a relatively narrow range. In about 30% of hypertensive patients PRA is below this range, in about 10% it is above. A greater fall in blood pressure and vascular resistance can be expected with converting enzyme inhibition in patients with higher levels of renin activity (4).

PATHOPHYSIOLOGY AND TREATMENT OF CONGESTIVE HEART FAILURE

The usual form of congestive heart failure is characterized by a decrease in myocardial contractility (2). Thus, to maintain a cardiac output sufficient to meet the metabolic demands of the body, a higher ventricular filling pressure is needed. However, as pressure rises to levels exceeding the oncotic pressure of plasma, fluid leaves the capillaries, enters the interstitial space, and causes congestive symptoms such as dyspnea, orthopnea, and dependent edema. As cardiac output falls, the symptoms of fatigue appear.

In an attempt to maintain blood pressure in the face of a falling cardiac output, the baroreceptor reflex is activated; this increases the activity of the sympathetic nervous system. In turn, increased release of catecholamines is followed by increases in heart rate, contractility (when possible) with greater ventricular emptying, venoconstriction, increased peripheral vascular resistance, renal renin release, and adrenal epinephrine release. These events serve to maintain cardiac output, thus maintaining arterial pressure in the usual range.

However, a price is paid for maintaining the integrity of the circulation through these mechanisms. Ventricular filling pressure is high, because stroke volume is maintained by the Frank-Starling mechanism plus increased venous return as sympathetic activation increases venous tone. Therefore, ventricular size is increased. Additionally, sympathetic activation results in increased peripheral vascular resistance. This effect is amplified by renin release, which allows formation of angiotensin II, with additional vasoconstriction, and stimulation of aldosterone release with consequent retention of water and sodium, expansion of intravascular volume, and further increase in venous return, ventricular filling pressure, and ventricular dimension.

The Law of Laplace states that tension in the wall of a sphere is directly related to the radius of the sphere and the pressure contained in the sphere. In the case of the left ventricle, this tension must be generated to allow ejection to occur; the greater the size of the ventricle and height of the pressure, the more the work. However, the normal ventricle is capable of meeting this work load, even though hypertrophy might be necessary. In a diseased left ventricle, increase in size or pressure results in a fall in ejection. The greater the disease, the greater is the degree of fall for a given increase in size or pressure. Similarly, the greater is the increase in ventricular performance as size or pressure is decreased. However, because of the importance of the Starling mechanism in maintaining ejection, an isolated decrease in size alone (i.e. after a diuretic) can be followed by a decrease in output, thus increasing symptoms of forward failure.

The agents available for increasing contractility—digitalis, catecholamines, and amrinone—all have therapeutic ceilings that may not be adequate for the degree of myocardial impairment. Thus, reduction of impedance to left ventricular ejection, by reducing arterial pressure, or even by slightly decreasing total peripheral resistance, can result in improved ventricular performance (5). The first attempt to use this approach was made by Burch (6), who used the ganglion-blocking agent trimethaphan to treat congestive heart failure.

Several vasodilating agents, e.g. hydralazine, prazosin, trimazosin, nitroprusside, nitrates, minoxidil, and nifedipine, have been used to reduce afterload in the treatment of congestive heart failure, at times very successfully (4). The long-term effect of vasodilation on mortality and morbidity in such patients is currently under scrutiny in a multicenter study. Of the factors limiting the efficacy of directly acting vasodilators in congestive heart failure, three are of particular importance: (*a*) progression of underlying disease, (*b*) tachyphylaxis, and (*c*) compensatory mechanisms. When a vasodilator is given, resistance falls, the baroreceptor reflex is activated, angiotensin II and aldosterone levels rise, sodium and water retention are stimulated, and expansion of intravascular volume and vasoconstriction blunt the initial favorable response to vasodilator therapy.

One way around this dilemma is to use an agent that lowers afterload through an effect on total peripheral resistance, blocks the renin-angiotensin-aldosterone system, and inhibits, at least partially, compensatory mechanisms.

PHARMACOLOGIC SUPPRESSION OF THE ANGIOTENSIN SYSTEM

The negative feedback loop controlling effective blood volume can be interrupted in a number of ways. Agents that inhibit sympathetic transmission decrease the release of renin. Agents that block beta-1-adrenergic receptors inhibit renin release, especially if the system has been stimulated previously (7). Antibodies have been made that inhibit renin after its release from the juxtaglomerular cells. Compounds that inhibit the enzyme kininase II prevent the conversion of the inactive decapeptide to the active octapeptide, angiotensin II (8). Saralasin and other compounds under development block angiotensin II receptors and thus prevent its physiologic effects (9). Finally, the properties of effector compounds such as aldosterone can be blocked by spironolactone.

Saralasin

The parenteral compound saralasin is a specific competitive antagonist of angiotension with partial agonist properties (9). Infusion into a hypertensive patient with high plasma renin activity results in a fall in blood pressure; infusion into a volume-expanded patient with low plasma renin activity results in a brief hypertensive response. Saralasin was used by Gavras et al (10) to control congestive heart failure preoperatively in a patient with ischemic heart disease and severe renovascular hypertension; the patient experienced a two-fold increase in cardiac output, a 50% fall in vascular resistance, and a decrease in left ventricular end-diastolic pressure from 26 to 5 mmHg. However, the usefulness of this compound is limited by its parenteral requirement, short duration of action, and partial agonist properties.

The Angiotensin-Converting Enzyme Inhibitors

A number of compounds that inhibit kininase II, an enzyme that converts angiotensin I to angiotensin II and also lyses bradykinin (11), are under development or undergoing various phases of clinical testing. Published reports have reached the medical literature concerning the use of two of these compounds in the treatment of congestive heart failure—teprotide and captopril.

TEPROTIDE   This nonapeptide was originally isolated from the venom of the Brazilian pit viper *Bothrops jararaca* (12). It was widely used in studies to determine the role of the renin-angiotensin system in various experimental and clinical forms of hypertension. The short-term hemodynamic effects of this compound are due to a fall in plasma angiotensin II levels rather than an increase in levels of bradykinin, an arteriolar vasodilator. In 1978, Curtiss et al (13) and Gavras et al (14) simultaneously published reports describing the acute effects of teprotide infusions in patients with congestive heart failure. Curtiss and his co-workers (13) treated 15 normotensive patients with severe chronic left ventricular failure due to ischemic heart disease or cardiomyopathy. Twenty minutes after the last gradual dose of teprotide, arterial pressure fell 11%, pulmonary capillary wedge pressure fell 23%, and cardiac output rose 21%. The response was greatest in those with high plasma renin activity. Gavras and his colleagues (14) made similar observations in four normotensive and four hypertensive patients, thus supporting the concept that the renin-angiotensin system plays an important role in maintaining elevated systemic vascular resistance in congestive heart failure. Faxon et al (15) studied 10 patients with severe refractory congestive heart failure again with similar results and in addition found no change in calf venous capacitance, which suggests that teprotide does not reduce wedge pressure by venodilatation.

CAPTOPRIL   Studies of the structure of the active portions of teprotide combined with insight gained in the synthesis of inhibitors of carboxypeptidase A, an enzyme similar to kininase II, led to the development of captopril by Ondetti, Rubin & Cushman in 1977 (8). As captopril is orally active, its potential for the long-term treatment of congestive heart failure is greater than saralasin or teprotide. In studies of hypertensive subjects, captopril was found to lower total peripheral resistance (16, 17) with little effect on cardiac output. Subsequently, Sullivan and co-workers (18) observed a fall in venous compliance during long-term captopril therapy. Although the mechanism of the acute fall in resistance appears to involve reduction in circulating angiotensin II levels, whether this effect is sufficient alone to explain the long-term effect is an unresolved matter. Other possibilities include effects on bradykinin, on prostaglandin metabolism in the kidney or in blood vessels, or on the central and sympathetic nervous system.

A number of groups have studied the acute and chronic hemodynamic effect of captopril in the treatment of refractory congestive heart failure. The degree of interest in this agent is evidenced by the publication of 19 abstracts and 5 papers describing the use of captopril for the treatment of congestive heart failure in 1979 alone. These publications all showed that captopril's hemodynamic effects were similar to those of teprotide (19–22). Subsequent studies have demonstrated a long-term beneficial effect of captopril. For example, Dzau et al (23) found in patients who had had six months of therapy a significant increase in ejection fraction from 12 ± 3 to $26\pm7\%$, and a sustained reduction in New York Heart Association functional class from IV to II. Sharpe et al (24) treated 18 patients with captopril, noting maximal hemodynamic improvement six to seven hours after doses of 6.25 to 12.5 mg. Ten patients, followed for three months, showed a sustained improvement in New York Heart Association functional class. Moreover, treadmill exercise duration increased significantly from 6.4 ± 6.5 min to 13.2 ± 8.4 min at three months. At the same time, echocardiographic studies showed a reduction in left ventricular dimension and an increase in fractional shortening. Levine et al (25) also noted improved exercise tolerance with long-term treatment.

Creager et al (26) studied the renal and regional hemodynamic effects of captopril in congestive heart failure. Previously, Hollenberg et al (27) had demonstrated that teprotide increased glomerular filtration rate. In congestive states, Creager and his co-workers (26) showed that captopril caused a 60% increase in renal blood flow, no change in glomerular filtration rate, and a 19% fall in filtration fraction. In this group of patients, plasma aldosterone fell by 63% and urine sodium excretion doubled. Plasma norepinephrine levels also decreased significantly. Since administration of a direct-acting vasodilator reflexively activates the sympathetic nervous system and sodium retention, captopril appears to offer theoretical advantages in the treatment of congestive heart failure. However, reports of neutropenia, agranulocytosis, and proteinuria during captopril treatment sound a note of caution.

MK-421 (ENALAPRIL)   MK-421 (Enalapril) has received extensive clinical testing in the treatment of hypertension. This compound appears to be equivalent to captopril in potency but has a longer duration of action. Reports of its use in congestive heart failure have not yet been published.

CONCLUSIONS

Agents that interrupt the renin-angiotensin system offer a promising new approach to the treatment of congestive heart failure. Comparative studies are needed to assess the advantages of this approach relative to other vasodilators and to determine whether the therapeutic efficacy is long lasting.

Literature Cited

1. Folkow, B., Neil, E. 1971. Principles of vascular control. In *Circulation*, pp. 285–306. New York: Oxford Univ. Press. 593 pp.
2. Braunwald, E., Ross, J. Jr., Sonnenblick, E. H. 1976. *Mechanisms of Contraction of the Normal and Failing Heart*, pp. 269–92. Boston: Little, Brown. 417 pp. 2nd ed.
3. Davis, J. O. 1971. What signals the kidney to release renin? *Circ. Res.* 28:301–6
4. Laragh, J. H., Baer, L., Brunner, H. R., Buhler, F. R., Sealey, J. E., Vaughan, E. D. Jr. 1972. Renin, angiotensin, and aldosterone systems in pathogenesis and management of hypertensive vascular disease. *Am. J. Med.* 52:633–52
5. Cohn, J. N., Franciosa, J. A. 1977. Vasodilator therapy of cardiac failure. *N. Engl. J. Med.* 297:27–31, 254–58
6. Burch, G. E. 1956. Evidence for increased venous tone in chronic congestive heart failure. *Arch. Intern. Med.* 98:750–66
7. Sullivan, J. M., Adams, D. F., Hollenberg, N. K. 1976. Beta blockade in essential hypertension. Reduced renin release despite renal vasoconstriction. *Circ. Res.* 39:532–36
8. Ondetti, M. A., Rubin, B., Cushman, D. W. 1977. Design of specific inhibition of angiotensin converting enzyme: new class of orally active antihypertensive agents. *Science* 196:441–44
9. Streeten, D. H. P., Anderson, G. H., Freiberg, J. M., Dalakos, T. G. 1975. Use of angiotensin II antagonist (Saralasin) in the recognition of "angiotensinogenic" hypertension. *N. Engl. J. Med.* 292:657–65
10. Gavras, H., Flessas, A., Ryan, T. J., Brunner, H. R., Faxon, D. P., Gavras, I. 1977. Angiotension II inhibition. Treatment of congestive cardiac failure in high-renin hypertension. *J. Am. Med. Assoc.* 238:880–82
11. Erdös, E. E. 1975. Angiotensin I converting enzyme. *Cir. Res.* 36:247–55
12. Ondetti, M. A., Williams, N. J., Sabo, E. F., Pluscec, J., Weaver, E. R., Kocy, O. 1971. Angiotensin-converting enzyme inhibitors from the venom of *Bothrops jararaca:* isolation, elucidation of structure and synthesis. *Biochemistry.* 10:4033–39
13. Curtiss, C., Cohn, J. N., Vrobel, T., Franciosa, J. A. 1978. Role of the renin-angiotensin system in the systemic vasoconstriction of chronic congestive heart failure. *Circulation* 58:763–69
14. Gavras, H., Faxon, D. P., Berkoben, J., Brunner, H. R., Ryan, T. J. 1978. Angiotensin converting enzyme inhibition in patients with congestive heart failure. *Circulation* 58:770–76
15. Faxon, D. P., Creager, M. A., Halperin, J. L., Gavras, H., Coffman, J. D., Ryan, T. J. 1980. Central and peripheral hemodynamic effects of angiotensin inhibition in patients with refractory congestive heart failure. *Circulation* 61: 925–30
16. Cody, R. J. Jr., Tarazi, R. C., Bravo, E. L., Fouad, F. M. 1978. Haemodynamics of orally-active converting enzyme inhibitor (SQ 14,225) in hypertensive patients. *Clin. Sci. Mol. Med.* 55: 453–59
17. Sullivan, J. M., Ginsburg, B. A., Ratts, T. E., Johnson, J. G., Barton, B. R., Kraus, D.H., McKinstry, D. N., Muirhead, E. E. 1979. Hemodynamic and antihypertensive effects of captopril, an orally active angiotensin converting enzyme inhibitor. *Hypertension* 1: 397–401
18. Sullivan, J. M., Taylor, J. C., Patrick, D. R., Johnson, J. G., Ratts, T. E., Muirhead, E. E. 1982. Long-term captopril therapy: evolving hemodynamic effects. *J. Clin. Pharmacol.* 22:976–84
19. Atkinson, A. B., Robertson, J. I. S. 1979. Captopril in the treatment of clinical hypertension and cardiac failure. *Lancet* 2:836–39
20. Davis, R., Ribner, H. S., Keung, E. L., Sonnenblick, E. H., LeJemtel, T. H.

1979. Treatment of chronic congestive heart failure with captopril, an oral inhibitor of angiotensin-converting enzyme. *N. Engl. J. Med.* 301:117–21

21. Tarazi, R. C., Fouad, F. M., Ceimo, J. K., Bravo, E. L. 1979. Renin, aldosterone and cardiac decompensation: studies with an oral converting-enzyme inhibitor in heart failure. *Am. J. Cardiol.* 44:1013–18

22. Turini, G. A., Gribic, M., Brunner, H. R., Waeber, B., Gavras, H. 1979. Improvement of chronic congestive heart failure by oral captopril. *Lancet* 1:1213–15

23. Dzau, V. J., Colucci, W. S., Williams, G. H., Curfman, G., Meggs, L., Hollenberg, N. K. 1980. Sustained effectiveness of converting-enzyme inhibition in patients with severe congestive heart failure. *N. Engl. J. Med.* 302:1373–79

24. Sharpe, D. N., Coxon, R. J., Douglas, J. E., Long, B. 1980. Low dose captopril in chronic heart failure: acute haemodynamic effects of long-term treatment. *Lancet* 2:1154–57

25. Levine, T. B., Franciosa, J. A., Cohn, J. N. 1980. Acute and long-term response to an oral converting-enzyme inhibitor, captopril, in congestive heart failure. *Circulation* 62:35–41

26. Creager, M. A., Halperin, J. L., Bernard, D. B., Faxon, D. P., Melidossian, C. D., Gavras, H., Ryan, T. J. 1981. Acute regional circulatory and renal hemodynamic effects of converting-enzyme inhibition in patients with congestive heart failure. *Circulation* 64:483–89

27. Hollenberg, N. K., Swartz, S. L., Passan, D. R., Williams, G. H. 1979. Increased glomerular filtration rate after converting-enzyme inhibition in essential hypertension. *N. Engl. J. Med.* 301:9–12

Ann. Rev. Med. 1983. 34:179–94

THE ROLE OF DIET IN THE ETIOLOGY AND TREATMENT OF ATHEROSCLEROSIS

Paul Samuel, M.D., Donald J. McNamara, Ph.D., Joseph Shapiro, M.D.

The Rockefeller University, New York, New York 10021; The Long Island Jewish-Hillside Medical Center, New Hyde Park, New York 11042; and the Albert Einstein College of Medicine, Bronx, New York 10461

ABSTRACT

The role of various dietary constituents in the etiology of hyperlipidemia and cardiovascular disease is examined in light of currently available data from epidemiological and clinical studies. Recommendations regarding the dietary management of the hyperlipidemic patient at risk are presented and the advisability of generalized dietary guidelines for the public examined. The certainties, which are few, and the uncertainties, which are numerous, regarding the cause and effect relationship between diet, hyperlipidemia, and cardiovascular disease suggest that dietary intervention to treat the hyperlipidemic patient is a rational first step but that the generalization of this approach for the public may be premature.

INTRODUCTION

In the course of the past three decades few issues have generated more discussion, argument, and controversy in the field of medicine or public health than the effect of diet on heart disease. Can diet prevent or even reverse arteriosclerosis, a disease affecting practically all of us in this society, an epidemic of unprecedented proportion in the history of the species? The confusion of the public is apparent, the opinion of the medical profession is divided, and the public policymaker is inundated with almost daily conflicting advice and information. What gave rise to this chaos? Where are we, how did we get there, and where do we go from here?

179

0066-4219/83/0401-0179$02.00

For thousands of years mankind struggled for food. During the past two hundred years, however, the advent of modern agriculture and industry has changed the life of Western man. A hundred years ago overnutrition (i.e. obesity) was a status symbol; the caricature of the rich, fat banker with a top hat and a big cigar, is familiar to all. Even today, there are still many countries on the globe where obesity is an exterior sign of success. It is alleged that in the Western world we are now paying the price for our opulence: arteriosclerosis, diabetes, hypertension, and perhaps some forms of cancer, to mention just a few. Can this idea withstand critical examination?

The average American diet contains about 40–45% of the total calories as fat, with a polyunsaturated-to-saturated (P/S) fat ratio of 0.4, 15–20% of total calories as protein, and the rest as carbohydrates. The daily cholesterol content of this diet is around 400–800 mg, and the fiber content is no more than 2–5 grams. In the 1950s and 1960s, facing an increasing rate of coronary heart disease, the horrified public was offered a number of modifications to this diet, especially those patients whose plasma lipids (and thus the risk of coronary disease) were excessively elevated. The thoughtful American Heart Association (1) and a number of other centers advanced the concept of the "prudent diet": decrease the fat content to 35% (with a P/S fat ratio of 1.5 or higher), decrease the daily intake of cholesterol to 250 mg or less (a single egg contains that much) with 15% as protein and the rest as carbohydrates. On the other hand, the Food and Nutrition Board of the National Academy of Sciences, after careful examination of the available data, could not find sufficient supporting evidence to recommend any dietary modifications for the general public, and especially to those who are enjoying good health (2). On the other side of the debate, public policymakers held Senate hearings and recommended a diet containing only 10–20% of the total calories as fat. Under these circumstances, how can the practicing physician answer when a patient asks for dietary instructions?

Arteriosclerosis is a multifactorial disease: heredity, diet, hypertension, diabetes, possible viral injury to the arterial wall, cigarette smoking, stress and strain, and perhaps many other factors may all play a role in the etiology and development of the disease. In the present article we consider the possible role of diet and its influences on plasma lipid levels and heart disease risk. The "lipid hypothesis" stipulates that increased levels of plasma lipids (more specifically cholesterol or LDL-cholesterol) will increase the degree of development of arteriosclerosis (and vice versa). We will not defend the lipid hypothesis, but we assume that it is valid. We may be right or wrong. Nonetheless, the following discussion and arguments are based on the validity of this probable, but as-yet unproven, theory.

EPIDEMIOLOGICAL EVIDENCE

The epidemiological data relating diet, plasma lipid levels, and coronary heart disease (CHD) come from four primary sources: (a) analysis of dietary patterns and disease incidences among nations; (b) analysis of autopsy data from different countries; (c) studies of populations in various nations; and (d) analysis of the effects of migration on dietary patterns and CHD incidence (3). Statistical analyses of the data suggest that certain nutrients may be involved in the development of hyperlipidemia and its associated risk of atherosclerosis and CHD incidence. In general these epidemiological studies demonstrate increased CHD in societies that have high intakes of total calories, total fat, saturated fat, animal protein, cholesterol, and sugar. Obviously a number of these dietary constituents are related (saturated fat–animal protein–cholesterol), and it is often difficult to separate out specific effects of a given nutrient on CHD incidence.

It should be noted that epidemiological studies compare populations differing in many respects other than dietary intakes. Thus comparing dietary patterns of an undernourished, lean, manual-laboring society to an overweight, sedentary population may be investigating more than simply dietary influences. Nevertheless, the epidemiological studies of the relationships between what a population eats and its incidence of specific diseases provide valuable data to guide the intrapopulation studies of nutrient intake and disease incidence.

With these considerations in mind, the following section addresses the findings from population studies relating dietary fat quality and quantity, cholesterol quantity, carbohydrate intake, and dietary protein intake to the risk of CHD.

Dietary Fat: Quantity and Quality

The Seven-Country Study of Keys and co-workers (4) is one of the most comprehensive investigations of the relationship between dietary intake patterns and CHD incidence in broad-based populations. This prospective study of 12,000 men age 40–59 years in 18 cohorts has been carried out for over ten years (5) and has demonstrated a positive correlation between the saturated fat intake, as a percentage of total calories, and the five-year CHD incidence. For these groups saturated fat intake was positively correlated with serum cholesterol, which was positively correlated with CHD.

The Seven-Country Study also demonstrates that the total calories derived from dietary fat is positively correlated to disease incidence. Similar data were reported by the International Atherosclerosis Project (6), which demonstrated a positive relationship between the saturation of dietary fat, serum cholesterol levels, and CHD.

The Ni Hon-San Study (7) of CHD mortality in Japanese men living in Japan, Hawaii, and San Francisco showed that, as the populations moved east, total fat intake in the diet, saturated fat intake, mean body weight, and serum cholesterol levels all increased, as did the incidence of CHD deaths. Undoubtedly other life-style factors also changed as these populations moved and, while it may not be possible to demonstrate a clear cause and effect relationship, the data are consistent with other epidemiological findings.

The data of these cross-cultural studies would be strengthened if they could be verified within a population. Unfortunately, this has not been accomplished though tested in a variety of studies (8, 9) attempting to relate plasma cholesterol levels and dietary patterns within groups. Many reasons for this failure have been suggested, including the homogeneity of the dietary pattern, the large degree of genetic and metabolic heterogeneity within a population, the methods used for measuring nutrient intakes, and/or various confounding variables such as other risk factors. Irrespective of the possible causes, the failure to verify the international findings by intranational data suggests to some that the statistical relationships between dietary fat intake, elevated serum cholesterol levels, and CHD incidence may not be as straightforward as originally perceived.

Dietary Cholesterol

For the epidemiologist it has been difficult to demonstrate direct causal relationship between dietary cholesterol intake, hypercholesterolemia, and CHD mortality simply because most cholesterol-rich foods also contain large amounts of saturated fat. Thus, demonstrating independence of effect has been virtually impossible. When the associated variables are factored out of the statistical analysis, dietary cholesterol alone appears to have little influence on CHD incidence (population studies) or on plasma cholesterol levels (cross-sectional studies).

Dietary Carbohydrate and Protein

The relationship between dietary carbohydrate intake, hypercholesterolemia, and CHD mortality is usually seen as a negative correlation in population studies. This observation is probably due to the fact that societies with a high carbohydrate intake also have a low fat intake and a low incidence of CHD. The available evidence would suggest that the negative correlation between dietary carbohydrate intake and CHD is more a function of the decreased dietary fat content than of an increased carbohydrate intake. Some studies suggest that a positive correlation exists between sucrose intake and CHD; yet sucrose intake is correlated with saturated fat intake. Once this variable is controlled for, the statistically significant relationship between sucrose and CHD is lost (3). Thus, the epidemiological data do not suggest a link between dietary carbohydrate intake, either simple or complex, and CHD risk.

A more complex problem is encountered in attempting to judge the effects of dietary protein, animal versus vegetable, on plasma lipids and CHD incidence since intake of animal protein usually involves intake of saturated animal fat and cholesterol. For these reasons one cannot state whether the sources of dietary protein in any way affect serum lipid levels or CHD incidence from the available epidemiological data.

Clinical Trials

There have been eight major clinical trials testing the "lipid hypothesis" by dietary interventions (reviewed in References 10 and 11). These studies were carried out as primary or secondary intervention trials and, with the exception of the Oslo Heart Study, the patients did not necessarily have hyperlipidemia. In the seven trials with an average plasma cholesterol level of 260 mg/dl, the decrease in plasma cholesterol achieved by dietary management ranged from 7 to 16% (mean 11%) and the data suggested, but could not demonstrate, a benefit in terms of new events of CHD. The Oslo Heart Study (average plasma cholesterol 323 mg/dl) clearly demonstrated that in healthy middle-aged men at high risk for CHD the dietary reduction of plasma cholesterol levels (13% reduction) and decreased smoking significantly reduced the incidence of the first event of myocardial infarction and sudden death. This study supports the use of aggressive intervention on multiple risk factors in high-risk individuals to decrease CHD incidence; whether such benefits could be achieved in the general population has yet to be demonstrated.

One unexpected finding from the epidemiological studies is that, within various populations, CHD incidence is only increased in those individuals having plasma cholesterol levels in the upper two quintiles of the population (12). For subjects having plasma cholesterol levels in the first three quintiles of the distribution there is little difference in CHD mortality; the third quintile is the population mean. This has led to the questioning of the rationale of generalized dietary guidelines for the general population since there may be little value in lowering plasma cholesterol levels except in those individuals with cholesterol concentrations in the top two quintiles (13).

EXPERIMENTAL STUDIES

Dietary Cholesterol

One of the major controversies in the field of nutrition is the effect of dietary cholesterol on plasma cholesterol levels and its impact on health and disease. According to some reports, plasma cholesterol levels will increase with increased dietary cholesterol intake (14) largely consisting of a marked elevation of LDL- and a moderate rise in HDL-cholesterol. (15). However, other authorities suggest that decreasing cholesterol intake makes no sense, since increased dietary cholesterol has no major effect on blood lipids (16, 17) primarily owing to feedback inhibition of endogenous cholesterol synthesis. Should dietary cholesterol intake decrease, the same feedback mechanism would be released resulting in an *increased* cholesterol synthesis in body tissues, thereby maintaining the same daily total input and an unchanged plasma cholesterol level. In fact, in carefully controlled metabolic ward studies, increased dietary cholesterol intake resulted in plasma cholesterol levels that rose in some and fell or remained unchanged in others (18, 19). It was completely impossible to define or to predict the individual patient's response to this "cholesterol challenge."

Can we explain these discrepancies, and how can we attempt to define the operative mechanisms? Figure 1 shows the "balance" of cholesterol in the plasma-pool of the body; in the adult human the mass of this pool is about 6 gm. Input occurs through the two top faucets: diet (~300 mg/day, 50% absorbed of 600 mg) and synthesis (~800 mg/day). In order to maintain the steady state (and plasma cholesterol levels are remarkably constant), the exact amount entering the pool must leave it day after day. The only excretion of cholesterol or its end products from the body is in the feces (we have no enzymes to decompose the cholesterol ring system). Indeed, about 800 mg of neutral sterols (unabsorbed cholesterol and its bacterial conversion products) appear daily in the stools, and about 250 mg of bile acids (converted from cholesterol by the liver) are excreted. (See two bottom faucets in Figure 1). The remaining 50 mg are used for steroid hormone production and/or are excreted through the skin. However, a third faucet on the bottom of Figure 1 communicates with the tissues. We know that tissue cholesterol is constantly exchanged with the plasma, and tracer ex-

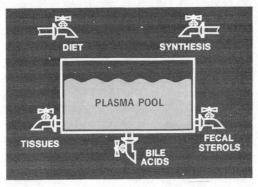

Figure 1   Cholesterol balance in the plasma pool (see text for explanation).

periments show that it takes about a year for most "tissue pools" to become equilibrated with the plasma pool (20, 21).

A careful inspection of Figure 1 indicates that reduction of plasma cholesterol levels by *whatever* means (diet, drug therapy, etc) can only be achieved by one of the following mechanisms:

1. Reduction of dietary cholesterol or its absorption;
2. Reduction of cholesterol synthesis;
3. Increase of the fecal excretion of cholesterol end products (neutral sterols and/or bile acids);
4. Transfer of cholesterol from the plasma pool to the tissues.

There is evidence that a feedback control mechanism may be operative between these four functions. However, the degree and effectiveness of the feedback control varies from individual to individual; in some it is extremely effective, in others it is practically absent. With presently available technology the effectiveness of this mechanism can be tested. The method consists of measuring cholesterol absorption, synthesis, and excretion during the feeding of a low-cholesterol diet and comparing the results to those of a regimen of markedly increased dietary cholesterol. What will be the reaction of the individual to this cholesterol load, and which of the four functions, if any, will be activated?

The exact mechanism of the absorption of cholesterol through the brush border of the gut wall is not completely understood, in spite of the enlightened efforts of many excellent laboratories over the past decades. Only about 50% of the intraluminal cholesterol is absorbed from the gut, contrary to many other dietary components such as neutral fats or carbohydrates, which have a nearly complete (>90%) single-passage absorption. The rate of cholesterol absorption remains around 50% from an intake of a few milligrams up to about 2000 mg per day (18). Above this level the rate of *percentage* absorption begins to fall and settles around 25% (at levels of 2000–3000 mg of daily dietary cholesterol) (18). It is peculiar that within the physiologic range of dietary intake of this compound the rate of absorption remains constant, and even at relatively low levels it is incomplete. We measured the rate of cholesterol absorption in a group of 41 outpatients on a low cholesterol diet (~240 mg daily). The mean absorption was ~145 mg/day (60%). When the daily cholesterol intake was increased to ~830 mg, the rate of absorption showed no change: about the same percentage, ~435 mg/day (53%), was absorbed (22). Therefore, when daily dietary cholesterol intake is increased, let us say, from 300 to 1000 mg, we are loading the system, increasing the daily input from the diet from ~150 to

~500 mg. What happens to cholesterol synthesis, excretion, and tissue transfer?

It should be emphasized that to answer this question the study of each individual patient necessitates several months of hospitalization on the metabolic ward, controlled feeding by a diet of exactly known constituents, the attainment of the metabolic steady state, and the precise monitoring and analysis of the daily fecal neutral sterol and bile acid excretion. Consequently, the total number of patients studied and the data published in the world literature are extremely limited: 15 patients, from three laboratories. (18, 19, 23). In these 15 subjects the response to an increased dietary cholesterol load was as follows: In 5 patients cholesterol synthesis was suppressed or markedly reduced; in 6 patients the fecal excretion of cholesterol end products (neutral sterols and bile acids) was increased; and in 4 patients the ingested cholesterol was stored in the tissues.

What characterizes the 4 patients unable to compensate? Can we define their clinical or biochemical characteristics and eventually predict who can eat cholesterol and who should not? On the basis of the available information we cannot define this segment of our population. Undoubtedly, many more studies will be necessary to obtain this very important information.

Thus, both sides of the dietary cholesterol debate are right. Some of us can neutralize increased dietary cholesterol intake by precise compensating mechanisms, namely reduced cholesterol synthesis and/or increased fecal excretion of cholesterol end products. However, in some others these mechanisms are apparently lacking. It seems to us, that one of the most important areas for future research in this field is to work out fast, precise, inexpensive, and reliable methods to define these variables and their importance in health and disease.

Dietary Fat and Carbohydrate

The argument concerning the fat content of the diet involves two major issues: quantity and quality. Will a low-fat diet reduce plasma lipids? It is almost impossible to answer this question directly, inasmuch as in most available experimental studies reduced fat content coincided with markedly decreased dietary cholesterol intake. When both dietary fat and cholesterol are reduced, serum cholesterol levels tend to decrease (24, 25). In one study, switching from an approximate fat content of 40–45% of the total calories (with a P/S fat ratio of 0.5, thus mostly saturated) to a practically fat-free diet (rice diet) reduced serum cholesterol levels by an average of 22%, and in some patients by as much as 30% (25). Some investigators ascribed this effect to the reduced fat content (24), whereas others thought it was due purely to reduced cholesterol intake (23). It is interesting that as early as 1955 Hatch and associates (24) noted that the isocaloric exchange of dietary fats for carbohydrates induced hypertriglyceridemia in about one fifth of the patients studied.

The effect of dietary exchange of carbohydrates for fats was investigated by Schreibman et al (26) under strictly controlled metabolic ward conditions in hyperlipidemic patients fed liquid-formula diets. The daily dietary cholesterol content was kept very low (<45 mg/day), and was identical during the low- and high-fat regimens. Dextrose was exchanged isocalorically for polyunsaturated fats, and the fat content of the diet ranged from 70% of the total calories to 45%, 40%, 20%, and fat free. Carbohydrates caused an increase of plasma triglycerides in each patient, and a rise in plasma cholesterol in 7 of 10 subjects; plasma cholesterol decreased only in one patient and remained unchanged in two. In these last 3 patients, fecal steroid excretion increased; in the others it remained unchanged or even decreased. During the administration of high-carbohydrate diets LDL-cholesterol increased and HDL-cholesterol decreased (26).

It seems to us that the exchange of dietary saturated fats (together with cholesterol) for carbohydrates may be beneficial; however, exchanging carbohydrates for polyunsatured fats isocalorically may cause a shift toward a more atherogenic lipid profile. Some authors disagree with this concept (15), and argue that the hypertriglyceridemic effect of high dietary carbohydrate is only transitory. They report a return to baseline triglycerides after 4 weeks, following a short period of elevated levels (15). However, in Schreibman's experiments the high-carbohydrate feeding was maintained for 40–70 days and triglyceride levels remained high throughout the study (26). It is, nonetheless, a fact that populations consuming a high-carbohydrate, low-fat, low-cholesterol diet over a lifetime have no elevated plasma triglyceride levels. Whether the determining factor in these populations is the diet or some other component of a markedly different life-style is not known at present.

The second question is the qualitative difference between fats, more specifically the well-known effect of saturated (animal) vs polyunsaturated (vegetable) fats on plasma cholesterol levels. In 1956 Sinclair (27) proposed that the degree of saturation or unsaturation of dietary fatty acids had a considerable influence in health and disease in general, and on plasma lipid levels in particular. Since then, as is well known, a massive array of literature has appeared on this subject.

The point that fats high in polyunsaturated fatty acids reduce plasma lipid levels was conclusively proved by Ahrens and co-workers in 1957 (28). However, the mechanism of action in reducing plasma cholesterol levels is still disputed. Connor et al (29) and Nestel et al (30) claim that polyunsaturated fats increase excretion of fecal steroids, but other workers have not been able to demonstrate this effect (31). Thus, the mechanism of plasma cholesterol reduction was explained in these studies by a shifting of cholesterol from the plasma pool into the tissues (31). It was assumed that the shift occurs into "bulk tissue," namely to muscle, adipose, or connective tissues. The calculated mass of cholesterol thus shifted from the plasma pool varies from 200 to 4000 mg. The estimated size of the mass of cholesterol in bulk tissue is about 50 g, thus the shift produces only an insignificant increase (31). Nevertheless, it has not been shown that this "shifted cholesterol" does not go to the intima of the arterial wall. There is general agreement that dietary polyunsaturated fatty acids reduce LDL-cholesterol; HDL-cholesterol may go up or down or may remain unchanged (32).

Recently, a series of papers appeared expressing some reservation on the use of fats high in polyunsaturated fatty acids. In most instances the authors expressed their fears that these substances may be carcinogenic or have cancer-potentiating effects (33). In our opinion, the evidence at hand connecting polyunsaturated fats to carcinogenesis is weak and insufficient to warrant discontinuation of the present trend. However, this concept has had its impact in that current dietary recommendations suggest a dietary fat intake of 30% of the calories; 10% of each type of fat, saturated, monounsaturated, and polyunsaturated. Until further data are obtained, a definitive statement cannot be made.

A word about refined carbohydrates is in order. In the early 1960s several groups reported that the exchange of starch for sucrose in the diet resulted in increased serum lipids (34). However, in later investigations this finding was not always reproduced. Again, only further studies will answer the question.

Dietary Protein

The exchange of mixed dietary protein, mainly of animal origin, for soybean protein was reported to reduce serum cholesterol levels moderately but significantly (35). LDL-cholesterol decreased, HDL-cholesterol remained unchanged or slightly diminished. The fat, carbohydrate, and sterol content of the diet remained unchanged in these experiments. Although in one report no difference was found in serum lipids when animal proteins were exchanged for soybean protein (36), in the majority of these studies the experimental data again seem to suggest the detrimental effects of carnivoricity.

Dietary Fiber

In 1954 Walker & Arvidsson (37) proposed that one of the important factors responsible for low plasma lipid levels in some indigenous African populations was the fiber content of their diet. In a later article Burkitt et al (38) generalized this theory, and proposed that high dietary fiber can prevent a number of diseases, particularly of the large bowel, and some other ailments like atherosclerosis that have become prevalent in Western society. Indeed, the average daily fiber content of the Western diet is estimated to be 2–5 g, whereas an 18–35-g/day intake is reported in more primitive cultures (38).

On the basis of the available experimental evidence it is difficult to assign a central role to dietary fiber alone in keeping plasma lipid levels at a very low plateau. Reports from a number of laboratories failed to show any effect of dietary bran, pectin, cellulose, wheat fiber, mixed cereals, or bagasse (39). On the other hand, a number of authors reported significant reductions of serum cholesterol and triglyceride levels with the use of bran, pectin, and, particularly, guar gum (40, 41). This coincided with decreased levels of LDL- and no change in HDL-cholesterol concentrations. Increased intestinal transit times with larger stool weights and decreased bacterial transformation of intraluminal bile acids were reported (38).

In our hands, the daily administration of 30 gm of guar gum in strictly controlled metabolic ward studies decreased plasma cholesterol levels by 14%, plasma triglycerides by 19%, cholesterol absorption from 66 to 49%, and significantly increased fecal neutral and acidic steroid excretions (P. Samuel, unpublished data). However, guar gum mix is a bad-tasting glue-like mixture, with a very poor patient acceptance. Perhaps in the form of "crispbread" as proposed by Jenkins (41) it could become more acceptable for ingestion.

Alcohol Consumption

During the past decade a considerable number of epidemiologic studies almost uniformly demonstrated that the consumption of moderate amounts of alcohol increased the level of HDL-cholesterol and decreased the risk of coronary artery disease (42). However, experimental data on the effect of ethanol intake are rather scarce and controversial. There is general agreement that alcohol further increases plasma triglyceride levels in patients with hypertriglyceridemia, concomitant with increased VLDL concentrations, with no change in other lipid parameters (43). Belfrage et al (44) in healthy volunteers supplemented a mixed diet with 75 g of ethanol daily. This resulted in a significant increase of HDL-cholesterol, which appeared 3 weeks after alcohol was added to the regimen. Conversely, in the study of Glueck et al, the isocaloric substitution of ethanol for carbohydrate failed to alter any of the lipid parameters in healthy young males (45). This was, however, a short-term study (2 weeks), and it seems possible that the alleged "beneficial" effects of moderate alcohol consumption are the results of long-term perseverance.

DISCUSSION, PRACTICAL APPROACH, AND RECOMMENDATIONS

The State of the Art

More than half of the American population dies of cardiovascular diseases, the majority of which are the result of the underlying process of arteriosclerosis. Simply put, the disease consists of the deposition of cholesterol in the intimal wall, which in turn decreases or obstructs blood flow through the lumen of the blood vessel. We are not born with atherosclerosis, so somehow this cholesterol has to get there. During the past decade a series of elegant experiments (46) in the laboratory of Goldstein and Brown demonstrated the possible mechanisms of the development of this disease in patients with familial hypercholesterolemia. Cellular cholesterol synthesis, and ultimately tissue deposition of cholesterol, was found to be a function of feedback mechanisms, dependent on the binding of circulating LDL-cholesterol by decreased or absent cell-surface receptors in these patients. Although the theory and the model were generalized, it must be pointed out that familial hypercholesterolemia is a relatively rare disease, certainly affecting less than 5% of the population, compared to the numbers affected by arteriosclerosis, namely all of us. What happens to the remaining more than 95% of the general public?

It must be clearly stated that arteriosclerosis is *not* a genetic but an *environmental disease.* Regardless of its primary cause or causes, it does not develop, or develops to a much lesser extent, in populations having low cholesterol concentrations, whereas its prevalence is overwhelming in those whose cholesterol concentrations are at Western levels (see the section on epidemiology). One could conclude that we are all environmentally hypercholesterolemic, and what we call "normal" in our population should rather be termed "average," undoubtedly an abnormally high level for the human species.

What causes this environmental catastrophe? Obviously, we do not have all the answers. Diet is perhaps one of the most important components of the environment. However, as shown in the foregoing paragraphs, the evidence is meager to incriminate diet as the sole factor. Many components and variables are unknown, and the little we know remains largely obscure when it comes to explaining by what mechanisms diet and the environment in general can affect plasma lipid levels and the development of the disease.

It seems to us, that the bottom line concerns the whole-body metabolism of cholesterol; namely dietary intake (or absorption), body synthesis, transport in the plasma (which lipoproteins carry cholesterol), fecal excretion of cholesterol and its end products, and possible shifts to or from the tissues

(See Figure 1). The final balance and outcome may well depend on these, or on the prevalence of one of these factors in each individual.

Diet and the Patient with Hyperlipidemia or Proven Vascular Disease

The primary treatment of hyperlipidemia is diet. In our institution, in 1400 proven hyperlipidemic male outpatients, a carefully regulated low-fat (35%) (high in polyunsaturated fatty acids), low-cholesterol (<250 mg/day) diet (reduced in calories when necessary) decreased plasma lipid levels over a 6-month period in 20% of the participants to "normal" levels (to or below the 95th percentile) (R. Palmer, personal communication). It is indeed the general rule that in patients with hyperlipidemia or vascular disease, before instituting drug therapy, a 3–6-month dietary trial is in order, possibly under the supervision of an experienced nutritionist.

But the question is: can diet induce the regression of atherosclerosis? Again the honest answer is: we don't know. The data on the epidemiologic trials are at best inconclusive in our view. Blankenhorn et al (47) demonstrated regression of atherosclerotic lesions measured by sophisticated computerized angiographic methods, following combined dietary and drug treatment.

Thus, the scarce data seem to indicate that atherosclerosis can regress, perhaps by the combination of vigorous dietary and drug therapy, perhaps even by diet alone. It is, therefore, our opinion that strictly enforced dietary measures are indicated in patients with hyperlipidemia or evidence of vascular disease due to atherosclerosis, in individuals with a heavy family history of the disease, or in subjects with other major risk factors (hypertension, diabetes, etc). The degree of success of the dietary treatment in these patients is difficult to measure. However, decreasing the levels of plasma lipids by dietary changes should undoubtedly be a first step.

Diet and the Healthy General Population

The plethora of popular literature and material in the public media has significantly changed the diet of the American population during the past two decades (48). Concomitantly, between 1969 and 1977 mortality from coronary heart disease has declined by 23% (48). On careful analysis one cannot ascribe this improvement to dietary changes alone. Many other factors enter the equation: improved coronary care units, new drugs, better surgical and diagnostic techniques, control of hypertension, decreased cigarette smoking, etc.

Should we, under these circumstances, recommend a change of diet to the American public at large? Such recommendation would assume that dietary changes can prevent atherosclerosis. We showed in the foregoing that such proof is not yet available. Should the public policymaker decide to recommend major dietary changes, who would pay for the multibillion-dollar expenditure that this may entail? The food industry? The public? Probably the public. In our view at present it is not justified to make such broad-scale recommendations.

SUMMARY

Our knowledge of the role of diet in the prevention and treatment of arteriosclerosis is at a crossroad. The available evidence is at best ambiguous. We do not know if arteriosclerosis can be cured or prevented by diet alone. Indeed, we have yet to demonstrate that reduction of plasma lipid levels by any intervention can decrease cardiovascular disease mortality. The complexity of the problem originates from the multifactorial etiology of the disease, the indecisiveness of epidemiological studies, and the incompleteness of experimental data available to date. To overcome these gaps we need to perfect experimental methods, carry out large and carefully organized controlled trials, and foremost we need new ideas and approaches concerning the mechanisms by which environmental factors, such as diet, influence plasma lipids and the development of the disease.

Based on a careful review of what we know and what we don't know, we recommend that patients with hyperlipidemia, evidence of atherosclerotic vascular disease, heavy family history of vascular disease, and/or the presence of other major risk factors be vigorously treated with diet. However, we feel that the evidence available is insufficient to recommend a radical (and expensive) change in the dietary habits of the general population at this time.

Prior to recommending any specific dietary guidelines to the general public it should be demonstrated that (a) the diet will significantly reduce plasma cholesterol levels in a majority of the population; (b) the risk of cardiovascular disease can be reduced by reducing plasma cholesterol levels; and (c) the proposed diet is free of any potential long-term side effects. At this time none of these points has been answered for any of the recommended diets. Under these circumstances it seems to us that the physician should use his or her judgment in the case of each individual or family in weighing the possible benefits of a strictly enforced prudent diet against the inconvenience of a moderate degree of long-term discipline, and the regimentation and occasional frustration such a diet may entail.

Literature Cited

1. Atherosclerosis Study Group. 1970. Primary prevention of the atherosclerotic disease. *Circulation* 42: Suppl. I, pp. 55–95
2. Food and Nutrition Board, National Research Council. 1980. *Guidelines Toward Healthful Diets.* Washington, DC: Natl. Acad. Sci.
3. Stamler, J. 1979. Population studies. In *Nutrition, Lipids, and Coronary Heart Disease,* ed. R. Levy, B. Rifkind, B. Dennis, N. Ernst, pp. 25–88. New York: Raven
4. Keys, A., ed. 1970. Coronary heart disease in seven countries. *Circulation* 41: Suppl. I
5. Keys, A. 1980. *Seven Countries: A Multivariate Analysis of Death and Coronary Heart Disease.* Cambridge, Mass: Harvard Univ. Press
6. McGill, H. C., ed. 1968. *The Geographic Pathology of Atherosclerosis.* Baltimore, Md: Williams & Wilkins
7. Marmot, M. G., Syme, S. L., Kagan, H., Kato, H., Cohen, J. B., Belsky, J. 1975. Epidemiologic studies of coronary heart disease and stroke in Japanese men living in Japan, Hawaii, and California: prevalence of coronary and hypertensive heart disease and associated risk factors. *Am. J. Epidemiol.* 102:514–28
8. Nichols, A. B., Ravenscroft, C., Lamphier, D. E., Ostrander, L. D. 1977. Daily nutritional intake and serum lipid levels, the Tecumseh study. *Am. J. Clin. Nutr.* 29:1384–92
9. Herschcopf, R. J., Elahi, D., Andres, R., Baldwin, H. L., Raizes, G. S., Schocken, D. D., Tobin, J. D. 1982. Longitudinal changes in serum cholesterol in man: an epidemiologic search for an etiology. *J. Chron. Dis.* 35: 101–14
10. Ahrens, E. H. Jr. 1976. The management of hyperlipidemia: whether rather than how. *Ann. Intern. Med.* 85:87–93
11. Hjermann, I., Velve Byre, K., Holme, I., Leren, P. 1981. Effect of diet and smoking intervention on the incidence of coronary heart disease. *Lancet* 2:1303–10
12. Carlson, L. A. 1982. Serum lipids and atherosclerosis disease. In *Metabolic Risk Factors in Ischemic Cardiovascular Disease,* ed. L. A. Carlson, B. Pernow, pp. 1–16. New York: Raven
13. McNamara, D. J. 1982. Diet and hyperlipidemia: a justifiable debate. *Arch. Intern. Med.* 142:1121–24
14. Mattson, F. H., Erickson, B. A., Kligman, A. M. 1972. Effect of dietary cholesterol in man. *Am. J. Clin. Nutr.* 25:589–94
15. Connor, W. E., Connor, S. L. 1977. Dietary treatment of hyperlipidemia. In *Hyperlipidemia, Diagnosis and Therapy,* ed. B. M. Rifkind, R. I. Levy, pp. 283–84. New York, San Francisco, London: Grune & Stratton
16. Mann, G. V. 1977. Diet-heart: end of an era. *N. Engl. J. Med.* 297:644–50
17. Samuel, P., McNamara, J. J., Ahrens, E. H. Jr., Crouse, J. R., Parker, T. 1982. Further validation of the plasma isotope ratio method for measurement of cholesterol absorption in man. *J. Lipid Res.* 23:480–89
18. Qintao, E., Grundy, S. M., Ahrens, E. H. Jr. 1971. Effects of dietary cholesterol on the regulation of total body cholesterol in man. *J. Lipid Res.* 12:233–47
19. Nestel, P. J., Poyser, A. 1976. Changes in cholesterol synthesis and excretion when cholesterol intake is increased. *Metabolism* 25:1591–99
20. Samuel, P., Perl, W. 1970. Long-term decay of serum cholesterol radioactivity: body cholesterol metabolism in normals and in patients with hyperlipoproteinemia and atherosclerosis. *J. Clin. Invest.* 49:346–57
21. Samuel, P., Lieberman, S. 1973. Improved estimation of body masses and turnover of cholesterol by computerized input-output analysis. *J. Lipid Res.* 14:189–96
22. McNamara, D. J., Kolb, R., Parker, T., Batwin, H., Brown, C., Samuel, P., Ahrens, E. H. Jr. 1981. Diet and cholesterol homeostasis in man. *Arteriosclerosis* 1:369a
23. Lin, D. S., Connor, W. E. 1980. The long-term effects of dietary cholesterol upon the plasma lipids, lipoproteins, cholesterol absorption, and the sterol balance in man. The demonstration of feedback inhibition of cholesterol biosynthesis and increased bile acid excretion. *J. Lipid Res.* 21:1042–52
24. Hatch, F. T., Abell, L. L., Kendall, F. E. 1955. Effects of restriction of dietary fat and cholesterol upon serum lipids and lipoproteins in patients with hypertension. *Am. J. Med.* 19:48–60
25. Samuel, P., Meilman, E. 1967. Dietary lipids and reduction of serum cholesterol levels by neomycin in man. *J. Lab. Clin. Med.* 70:471–79

26. Schreibman, P. H., Ahrens, E. H. Jr. 1976. Sterol balance in hyperlipidemic patients after dietary exchange of carbohydrate to fat. *J. Lipid Res.* 17:97–105

27. Sinclair, H. M. 1956. Deficiency of essential fatty acids and atherosclerosis, et cetera. *Lancet* 1:381–83

28. Ahrens, E. H. Jr., Hirsch, J., Insull, W. Jr., Tsaltas, T. T., Blomstrand, R., Peterson, M. L. 1957. The influence of dietary fats on serum-lipid levels in man. *Lancet* 1:943–53

29. Connor, W. E., Witiak, D. T., Stone, D. B., Armstrong, M. L. 1969. Cholesterol balance and fecal neutral steroid and bile acid excretion in normal man fed dietary fats of different fatty acid composition. *J. Clin. Invest.* 48:1363–75

30. Nestel, P. J., Havenstein, N., Homma, Y., Scott, T. W., Cook, L. J. 1975. Increased sterol excretion with polyunsaturated-fat high cholesterol diets. *Metabolism* 24:189–98

31. Grundy, S. M., Ahrens, E. H. Jr. 1970. The effects of unsaturated dietary fats on absorption, excretion, synthesis, and distribution of cholesterol in man. *J. Clin. Invest.* 49:1135–52

32. Eder, H. A., Gidez, L. I. 1982. The clinical significance of the plasma high density lipoproteins. *Med. Clin. North Am.* 66:431–40

33. Jones, R. J. 1981. Cholesterol, coronary disease, and cancer. *J. Am. Med. Assoc.* 245:2060

34. Keys, A., Anderson, J. T., Grande, F. 1960. Diet-type (fat constant) and blood lipids in man. *J. Nutr.* 70:257–66

35. Shorey, R. L., Bazan, B., Lo, G. S., Steinke, F. H. 1981. Determinants of hypocholesterolemic response to soy and animal protein-based diets. *Am. J. Clin. Nutr.* 34:1769–78

36. Van Raaij, J. M. A., Katan, M. B., Hautvast, J. G. A. 1979. Casein, soya protein, serum cholesterol. *Lancet* 2:958

37. Walker, A. R. P., Arvidsson, U. B. 1954. Fat intake, serum cholesterol concentration, and atherosclerosis in the South African Bantu. *J. Clin. Invest.* 33:1358–65

38. Burkitt, D. P., Walker, A. R. P., Painter, N. S. 1972. Effect of dietary fiber on stools and transit-times, and its role in the causation of disease. *Lancet* 2:1408–12

39. Raymond, T. L., Connor, W. E., Lin, D. S., Warner, S., Fry, M. M., Connor, S. L. 1977. The interaction of dietary fibers and cholesterol upon the plasma lipids and lipoproteins, sterol balance and bowel function in human subjects. *J. Clin. Invest.* 60:1429–37

40. Fahrenbach, M. J., Riccardi, B. A., Saunders, J. C., Lourie, I., Heider, J. G. 1965. Comparative effects of guar gum and pectin on human serum cholesterol levels. *Circulation* 31:II–11–12 (Abstr.)

41. Jenkins, D. J. A., Reynolds, D., Slavin, B., Leeds, A. R., Jenkins, A. L., Jepson, E. M. 1980. Dietary fiber and blood lipids: treatment of hypercholesterolemia with guar crispbread. *Am. J. Clin. Nutr.* 33:575–81

42. Ernst, N., Fisher, M., Smith, W., Gordon, T., Rifkind, B. M., Little, J. A., Mishkel, M. A., Williams, O. D. 1980. The association of plasma high density lipoprotein cholesterol with dietary intake and alcohol consumption. *Circulation* 62:(Suppl.) IV–41–52

43. Kudzma, D. J., Shonfeld, G. 1971. Alcoholic hyperlipidemia: induction by alcohol but not by carbohydrate. *J. Lab. Clin. Med.* 77:384–95

44. Belfrage, P., Berg, B., Hagerstrand, I., Nilson-Ehle, P., Tornzvist, H., Wiebe, T. 1977. Alterations of lipid metabolism in healthy volunteers during long-term ethanol intake. *Eur. J. Clin. Invest.* 7:127–31

45. Glueck, C. J., Hogg, E., Allen, C., Gartside, P. S. 1980. Effects of alcohol ingestion on lipids and lipoproteins in normal man: isocaloric metabolic studies. *Am. J. Clin. Nutr.* 33:2287–93

46. Fredrickson, D. S., Goldstein, J. L., Brown, M. S. 1978. The familial hyperlipoproteinemias. In *The Metabolic Basis of Inherited Disease,* ed. J. B. Stanbury, J. B. Wyngaarden, D. S. Fredrickson, pp. 604–55. New York: McGraw-Hill

47. Blankenhorn, D. H., Brooks, S. H., Selzer, R. H. 1978. The rate of atherosclerosis change during treatment of hyperlipidemia. *Circulation* 57:355–61

48. Levy, R. 1981. Declining mortality in coronary heart disease. *Arteriosclerosis* 1:312–25

Ann. Rev. Med. 1983. 34:195–204

IMMUNOREGULATORY MECHANISMS IN NONSPECIFIC INFLAMMATORY BOWEL DISEASE

R. G. Strickland, M.D.

Department of Medicine, University of New Mexico School of Medicine, Albuquerque, New Mexico, USA 87131

D. P. Jewell, D.Phil.

Gastroenterology Unit, The Radcliffe Infirmary, Oxford OX2 6HE, England

ABSTRACT

Little is known of either the etiology or the pathogenesis of nonspecific inflammatory bowel disease (IBD). One hypothesis proposes the presence of a disorder of immune regulation as an initiating or perpetuating mechanism of continued bowel wall inflammation in these diseases. This chapter examines the basis for this proposal and reviews recent studies directed toward the demonstration of defective immunoregulatory mechanisms in IBD.

INTRODUCTION

Recent studies have established that normal immune responses depend on a complex balance between effector and regulator cells. Particularly well defined are those regulatory systems concerned with the modulation of T-cell or B-cell effector function by inducer (helper) or suppressor influences (1). Less well defined, yet of increasing interest as components of the immunoregulatory network, are the NK-K cell system of natural and antibody-dependent cytotoxicity (2) and the monocyte-macrophage system (3). Functional assays of these immunoregulatory mechanisms together with measurements of regulator-cell subpopulations by the use of monoclonal antibodies (4) are being extensively applied to the study of normal immune

195

responses and of human diseases that may have an immune pathogenesis. Indeed it is already apparent that some autoimmune diseases are associated with a lack of T-suppressor function (5) and conversely that some immunodeficiency disorders may result from excess T-suppressor function (6).

This chapter reviews current investigations of immune regulation in a group of disorders less certainly related to autoimmunity or immunodeficiency—namely the nonspecific inflammatory bowel diseases (IBD), which include ulcerative colitis and proctitis (UC) and Crohn's disease of the gastrointestinal tract (CD).

ETIOLOGY AND PATHOGENESIS OF IBD

Designation of these disorders as nonspecific reflects the continuing lack of understanding of their etiology. Indirect evidence supports an interaction between genetic, immunologic, and environmental (possibly microbial) factors in their pathogenesis. Moreover, studies of these potentially pathogenic factors in UC and CD suggest that the two disorders are related in spite of differences in the intestinal pathology evident between them.

IMMUNOLOGIC OBSERVATIONS IN IBD

Interest in the possible participation of immunologic reactions in IBD (see 7 for detailed review) derives from the recognition that the gut-associated lymphoid tissue (GALT) is a major component of the body's immune system and is clearly expanded in UC and CD. Quantitative increases in plasma cells, T and B cells, and macrophages are consistent components of the chronic mucosal inflammation in these conditions. In addition, IBD may be associated with other more clearly immune-related disorders, and both UC and CD show therapeutic responsiveness to immunosuppressive drugs.

Immune responses to gut-associated antigens have been widely reported in both UC and CD. These include the presence of circulating antibodies to colonic bacteria, dietary antigens, and colonic epithelial cells. Cell-mediated immunity to crude colonic antigens and the enterobacterial antigen of Kunin is also demonstrable. Earlier work showing that peripheral blood lymphocytes from patients with either UC or CD are cytotoxic to colon epithelial cells in vitro has been recently confirmed.

A major question posed by these observations of enhanced systemic and mucosal immunologic activity in UC and CD concerns the mechanism(s) by which they arise. One explanation is that an increased permeability of the intestine in IBD results in increased antigen absorption and enhanced exposure of GALT to gut-associated antigens. Alternatively, increased responses to these antigens may be the result of a fundamental defect in immunoregulation in UC and CD. An immunoregulatory defect, if present, might explain the well-established increased risk of colonic malignancy in both UC and CD.

IMMUNE REGULATION IN IBD—INDIRECT OBSERVATIONS

Humoral Immunity

Initial studies provided no evidence for the presence of a general disturbance of humoral immunity in either UC or CD (reviewed in 7). Thus, serum concentrations of immunoglobulins and complement components are either normal or variably raised during disease relapses, and antibody responses to extrinsic antigens administered parenterally are normal. Total circulating B cells are either normal or slightly increased and no consistent abnormality in numbers of B-cell subclasses has been observed. However, recent work has renewed interest in abnormalities of humoral immunity in IBD. MacDermott et al (8) reported increased spontaneous synthesis and secretion of IgG, IgM, and particularly IgA by peripheral blood mononuclear cells from patients with UC or CD when cultured in vitro for 12 days. Ginsburg et al (9) demonstrated the presence of circulating B cells with a homogenous amount of light chain of only one type on their surface in patients with UC or CD. It is possible that these observations (if confirmed) may reflect defective regulation of B-cell function in these disorders.

Antilymphocyte Antibodies

The occurrence of circulating IgM cold-reactive antilymphocyte antibodies in UC and CD is not surprising since such antibodies are present in a wide range of diseases associated with heightened immunity. Of greater interest is the observation (10) now confirmed (11) that a significant proportion of unaffected relatives of patients with IBD also have circulating antilymphocyte antibodies. It has been suggested that these findings may indicate common exposure to environmental (infectious) agent(s) in IBD families (10). Alternatively, since circulating antibodies to Escherichia coli and to colon epithelium are also observed in a proportion of unaffected IBD relatives (12), the findings may reflect an underlying genetically determined abnormality in immune regulation in IBD.

Cell-Mediated Immunity

The results of studies of cellular immunity in UC and CD have been highly variable (reviewed in 7). Reports of anergy, depressed in vitro lymphocyte proliferative responses to nonspecific mitogens, and decreased circulating

T-cell numbers (particularly prominent in CD) have been matched by other studies showing no substantial alteration in these measurements. It is likely that any observed alterations are a secondary consequence of IBD or its nutritional sequelae rather than of primary (etiologic) significance. On the other hand, studies of peripheral blood lymphocyte responses to allogeneic stimulation in one-way mixed lymphocyte cultures (MLR) in IBD have consistently shown reduced MLR in a significant proportion of such patients (13–15). Among the possible mechanisms for this abnormality is a disturbance in immunoregulatory function.

IMMUNE REGULATION IN IBD—DIRECT OBSERVATIONS

There are a number of recent studies that more directly examine immunoregulatory mechanisms in patients with UC or CD. They include observations of mononuclear-cell (MNC) function and the phenotypes of immunoregulatory-cell subpopulations in both the peripheral blood and intestinal mucosa.

Peripheral Blood Studies

SUPPRESSOR CELL FUNCTION   A number of studies indicate that suppressor-cell activity of peripheral blood MNC from patients with IBD may be normal, reduced, or increased. There is growing evidence that suppressor mechanisms are heterogeneous in nature (16) and the apparent disparity between these studies may therefore reflect the fact that the different assay systems measure distinct suppressor-cell functions. Thus Conconavalin-A-inducible suppressor activity is consistently reduced in active but not inactive IBD (17–19). Spontaneous suppressor activity (20) and autologous MLC-induced T suppression (21) are reduced independently of disease activity. A study of T-cell suppression of antibody synthesis revealed the presence of covert suppressor cells that cause profound reductions in B-cell IgM synthesis in 50% of patients with CD (22). Increased suppressor activity in a further study (23) may reflect enhanced function of a prostaglandin-sensitive monocyte subpopulation in some patients with IBD.

NK-K CELL FUNCTION   Interest in alterations of natural killer (NK) and antibody-dependent K-cell activity in IBD derives from both general considerations (such as their putative role in immune surveillance against neoplasia) and the possible role of these cells in producing the in vitro cytotoxicity of IBD lymphocytes against colon epithelial cells. The effector cell in this system is an Fc receptor-bearing lymphocyte and the reaction is consistent with an NK or K-cell-mediated effect. Studies of peripheral blood NK- or K-cell function against nonspecific target cells in IBD reveal either normal (24) or reduced (25, 26) NK, and normal (27) or enhanced (29) K-cell activities. These variable results are at present unexplained. However, it is increasingly evident that NK and K cells are themselves subject to a number of regulatory influences (2, 29) that may be altered in IBD. These include interferon (30), prostaglandins (31), and plasminogen activator (32, 33).

MONOCYTE FUNCTION   Patients with UC or CD frequently show an absolute monocytosis during disease relapses. The turnover of monocytes is also increased. The monocytes appear to be "activated" in so far as they show enhanced phagocytosis and intracellular killing, increased concentrations of lysosomal enzymes, and increased cell movement. These markers of activation are all related to disease activity and are therefore probably secondary to the inflammatory response (34). Nevertheless, it is also possible that increased monocyte activity may influence other immune effector functions in IBD. Thus increased prostaglandin-sensitive suppressor function and altered NK activity in IBD may actually result from cellular interactions with monocytes or from mediators such as prostaglandins, plasminogen activator, or reactive metabolites of oxygen (35) released by these cells.

CIRCULATING IMMUNOREGULATORY CELL SUBSETS   Initially, circulating T-cell subsets in patients with IBD were studied using the $T\mu/T\gamma$ system to define inducer and suppressor cells respectively (19, 36, 37). These immunoglobulin markers no longer provide a satisfactory way of defining T-cell subsets and have been superseded by the use of specific monoclonal antibodies. The results published so far are conflicting (24, 38–41); however, the reported differences are small and, in general, there appears to be no major change in either the absolute numbers or the proportions of these subsets, or in the ratio of inducer- to suppressor-cytotoxic cells in these patients. So far, there is no study reported that correlates phenotype with function of either inducer- or suppressor-cytotoxic cells in patients with IBD.

Monoclonal antibodies to identify monocytes (OKM-1) and NK-K cells (HNK-1) are currently being investigated in IBD.

Studies of Intestinal Mucosal Mononuclear Cells

The current emphasis on the study of intestinal mucosal MNC in IBD is appropriate since a fundamental defect in immune regulation may be present in cells derived from the target organ itself, a defect not reflected in similar cells present in more remote sites such as the systemic circulation. Two experimental approaches are currently being undertaken. One involves the evaluation of MNC isolated in suspension from surgically resected bowel mucosa by either enzymatic (42, 43) or mechanical (44, 45) separation techniques. The other approach involves an enumeration of MNC subsets *in situ* on mucosal tissue sections using cell-labelling techniques with a variety of monoclonal antibodies directed toward regulator-cell subpopulations (46, 47).

NORMAL INTESTINAL MNC   Isolated *normal* intestinal MNC display significant functional differences from autologous peripheral blood MNC. Thus intestinal MNC show enhanced spontaneous antibody secretion, particularly of IgA (8), enhanced spontaneous and enterobacterial-stimulated lymphocyte proliferation (48), variable differences in proliferative (44, 49–51) and cytotoxic (51–54) responses to nonspecific mitogens, and striking reductions or even absence of NK and K-cell cytotoxicity (49, 51–58), particularly when cell lines are used as targets. Intestinal MNC are also responsive in an allogeneic mixed lymphocyte reaction, albeit less vigorously than autologous peripheral blood MNC (PBL). However, in contrast to PBL, they do not subsequently function as effector cells in cell-mediated lympholysis (50). Normal intestinal MNC are more closely associated with macrophages than are peripheral blood MNC, and intestinal macrophages themselves are larger, spread more actively, and show greater phagocyte capacity than peripheral blood monocytes (47). Suppressor-cell function of isolated intestinal MNC appears to be equivalent to that observed in peripheral blood MNC (49).

The distributions of regulator-cell subpopulations *in situ* in normal intestinal mucosa were recently examined (46, 47). The intra-epithelial lymphocytes are predominantly T cells (>90%), and the majority of them (>80%) express the phenotype of the suppressor-cytotoxic T-cell subpopulation. The lamina propria T cells are more heterogeneous, with only 40% displaying the suppressor-cytotoxic marker; the remainder appear to be inducer (helper) T cells. Large numbers of macrophages bearing Ia antigen are also present in this site (47). Moreover, morphologic and histochemical differences between lamina propria macrophages in small and large intestine are apparent (59), which may reflect functional differences such as the type of antigen presentation at these two sites.

INTESTINAL MNC IN IBD   Much of the work relating to intestinal MNC in IBD is preliminary and not confirmed by independent laboratories. In addition there continues to be some concern regarding the methods of intestinal MNC isolation and the effect that these procedures themselves may have on a number of the functional assays (53, 56).

With these reservations, some functional differences have been observed between IBD and normal intestinal MNC. First, IBD intestinal MNC (particularly from CD) contain many "activated" T cells and show greater responsiveness to bacterial antigens (48). Second, MNC from either CD or UC intestine have been reported to show *decreased* spontaneous antibody secretion, particularly of IgA (8). Third, using a co-culture assay with autologous mitomycin-treated peripheral blood lymphocytes, Goodacre & Bienenstock (60) found *decreased* suppressor-cell activity in MNC isolated by mechanical separation from CD intestine. This effect was associated with an *enhanced* proliferative response of the intestinal MNC to phytohemagglutinin-P. An earlier report (49) describing normal suppressor-cell function in IBD intestinal MNC utilized an enzymatic isolation technique and a different suppressor-cell assay (Conconavalin-A-inducible suppression). Despite these functional differences, preliminary studies of inducer- and suppressor-cytotoxic subpopulations in IBD mucosal sections or isolated intestinal MNC preparations have not shown any substantial qualitative changes from those present in noninflamed intestine (61).

NK and K cytotoxic functions of MNC isolated from IBD intestine have not differed significantly from those of normal intestinal MNC (44, 49, 51–55, 57–58). The presence of K cells in mesenteric lymph nodes of patients with Crohn's disease but not in control mesenteric nodes (27), although intriguing, requires confirmation. In addition studies have thus far utilized nonspecific target cells, and cytotoxicity of intestinal MNC toward colonic epithelial targets has not yet been reported. With regard to intestinal macrophage function, no studies have yet examined the properties of these cells in IBD. However, histochemical studies on IBD tissue sections showed that morphologic changes are present (59). Whether these changes represent macrophage alteration within the mucosa is not known.

CONCLUSIONS

The precise role of immunologic processes in UC or CD is not yet established. Although their participation as effector mechanisms in the intestinal damage seems probable, it remains uncertain whether such mechanisms initiate inflammation or merely perpetuate it. With these uncertainties it is not surprising that studies of immunoregulatory dysfunction as a possible basis for immunologic intestinal damage in IBD are at present inconclusive. There is as yet no evidence for the existence of a uniform abnormality of systemic or mucosal immunoregulation in these disorders. However, the data reviewed here strongly indicate the need for continued investigation of such a possibility. Future research efforts should continue to focus on intestinal MNC and be directed toward extensive correlative and parallel studies of both function and cell phenotypic expression.

ACKNOWLEDGMENT

R. G. Strickland gratefully acknowledges support from the US Public Health Service Grant AM27354.

Literature Cited

1. Cantor, H., Boyse, E. A. 1977. Regulation of the immune response by T cell subclasses. In *Contemporary Topics in Immunobiology,* ed. D. Stutman, 7:47–67. New York: Plenum
2. Herberman, R. B., Djeu, J. Y., Kay, H. D., Ortaldo, J. R., Riccardi, C., Bonnard, G. D., Holden, H. T., Fagnani, R., Santoni, A., Pucetti, P. 1979. Natural killer cells: Characteristics and regulation of activity. *Immunol. Rev.* 44:43–70
3. Nelson, D. S. 1981. Macrophages: progress and problems. *Clin. Exp. Immunol.* 45:225, 233
4. Reinherz, E. L., Schlossman, S. F. 1980. Regulation of the immune response—inducer and suppressor T-lymphocyte subsets in human beings. *N. Engl. J. Med.* 303:370–73
5. Strelkauskas, A. J., Callery, R. T., McDowell, J., Borel, Y., Schlossman, S. T. 1978. Direct evidence for loss of human suppressor cells during active autoimmune disease. *Proc. Natl. Acad. Sci. USA* 75:5150–54
6. Waldmann, T. A., Durm, V., Broder, S., Blackmann, M., Blaese, R. H., Strober, W. 1974. Role of suppressor T cells in pathogenesis of common variable hypogammaglobulinaemia. *Lancet* 2: 609–13
7. Kirsner, J. B., Shorter, R. G. 1982. Recent developments in "non-specific" inflammatory bowel disease. *N. Engl. J. Med.* 306:837–48
8. MacDermott, R. P., Nash, G. S., Bertovich, M. J., Seiden, M. V., Bragdon, M. J., Beale, M. G. 1981. Alterations of IgM, IgG, and IgA synthesis and secretion by peripheral blood and intestinal mononuclear cells from patients with ulcerative colitis and Crohn's disease. *Gastroenterology* 81:844–52
9. Ginsburg, C. H., Ault, K. A., Falchuk, Z. M. 1981. Monoclonal B lymphocytes in the peripheral blood of patients with inflammatory bowel disease. *Gastroenterology* 81:1111–14
10. Korsmeyer, S. J., Williams, R. C. Jr., Wilson, I. D., Strickland, R. G. 1975. Lymphocytotoxic antibody in inflammatory bowel disease—a family study. *N. Engl. J. Med.* 293:1117–20

11. Kuiper, J., Weterman, I. T., Biemond, I., Castelli, R. C., Van Rood, J. J., Pena, A. S. 1981. Lymphocytotoxic antibodies in patients with Crohn's disease and family members. In *Developments in Gastroenterology—Recent Advances in Crohn's Disease,* ed. A. S. Pena, I. T. Weterman, C. C. Booth, W. Strober, 1:341–47. The Hague: Martinus Nijhoff. 549 pp.
12. Lagercrantz, R., Perlmann, P., Hammarstrom, S. 1971. Immunological studies in ulcerative colitis v. family studies. *Gastroenterology* 60:381–89
13. Richens, E. R., Williams, M. J., Gough, K. R., Ancill, R. J. 1974. Mixed-lymphocyte reaction as a measure of immunologic competence of lymphocytes from patients with Crohn's Disease. *Gut* 15:24–28
14. Auer, I. O., Buschmann, C. H., Ziemer, E. 1978. Immune status in Crohn's Disease. 2. Originally unimpaired primary cell-mediated immunity *in vitro. Gut* 19:618–26
15. Fiske, S. C., Falchuk, Z. M. 1980. Impaired mixed-lymphocyte culture reactions in patients with inflammatory bowel disease. *Gastroenterology* 79:682–86
16. Lobo, P. I., Spencer, C. E. 1979. Inhibition of humoral and cell-mediated immune responses in man by distinct suppressor cell systems. *J. Clin. Invest.* 63:1157–63
17. Hodgson, H. J. F., Wands, J. R., Isselbacher, K. J. 1978. Decreased suppressor cell activity in inflammatory bowel disease. *Clin. Exp. Immunol.* 32: 451–58
18. Knapp, W., Smolen, J. S., Gangl, A., Menzel, E. J., Wolf, C. H. 1981. Con A-induced suppressor cell activity in IBD and other inflammatory diseases. See Ref. 11, 1:380–85
19. Shorter, R. G., ReMine, S. G., Bartnik, W. 1981. T cells and Conconavalin-A-induced suppressor cell activity *in vitro* in colonic inflammatory bowel disease and colo-rectal cancer. See Ref. 11, 1:448–55
20. Victorino, R. M. M., Hodgson, H. J. F. 1981. Spontaneous suppressor cell func-

tion in inflammatory bowel disease. *Dig. Dis. Sci.* 26:801–6
21. Ginsburg, C. H., Falchuk, Z. M. 1980. Defective autologous mixed-lymphocyte culture reactions and suppressor T cell generation in patients with inflammatory bowel disease. *Gastroenterology* 78:1173 (Abstr.)
22. Elson, C. O., Graeff, A. S., James, S. P., Strober, W. 1981. Covert suppressor T cells in Crohn's Disease. *Gastroenterology* 80:1513–21
23. Holdstock, G., Chastenay, B. F., Krawitt, E. L. 1981. Increased suppressor cell activity in inflammatory bowel disease. *Gut* 22:1025–30
24. Brown, T. E., Bankhurst, A. D., Strickland, R. G. 1982. Natural killer (NK) function and lymphocyte subpopulation profiles in inflammatory bowel disease. *Gastroenterology* 82:1026 (Abstr.)
25. Auer, I. O., Zimer, E., Sommer, H. 1980. Immune status in Crohn's Disease v. decreased *in vitro* natural killer cell activity in peripheral blood. *Clin. Exp.* 42:41–49 *Immunol.*
26. Ginsburg, C. H., Ault, K. A., Falchuk, Z. M. 1981. Defective natural killer cell activity in patients with inflammatory bowel disease: evidence for a primary effect. *Gastroenterology* 80:1156 (Abstr.)
27. Britton, S., Eklund, A. E., Bird, A. G. 1978. Appearance of killer (K) cells in the mesenteric lymph nodes in Crohn's Disease. *Gastroenterology* 75:218–20
28. Eckhardt, R., Kloos, P., Dierich, M. P., Meyer Zum Büschenfelde, K. H. 1977. K-lymphocytes (killer cells) in Crohn's Disease and acute virus B-hepatitis. *Gut* 18:1010–16
29. Nair, M. P. N., Schwartz, S. A. 1981. Suppression of natural killer activity and antibody-dependent cellular cytotoxicity by cultured human lymphocytes. *J. Immunol.* 126:2221–29
30. Ginsburg, C. H., Dambrauskas, J. T., Levin, M., Ault, K. A., Falchuk, Z. M. 1982. Interferon in inflammatory bowel disease: production and effect on the natural killer cell. *Gastroenterology* 82:1067 (Abstr.)
31. Droller, M. J., Schneider, M. U., Perlman, P. 1978. A possible role of prostaglandins in the inhibition of natural and antibody-dependent cell-mediated cytotoxicity against tumour cells. *Cell. Immunol.* 39:165–77
32. Wainberg, M. A., Israel, E., Margolese, R. G. 1982. Further studies on the mitogenic and immune-modulating effects of

plasminogen activator. *Immunology* 45:715–20
33. Doe, W. F., Dorsman, B. 1982. Chronic inflammatory bowel disease—increased plasminogen-activator secretion by mononuclear phagocytes. *Clin. Exp. Immunol.* 48:256–60
34. Mee, A. S., Jewell, D. P. 1980. Monocytes in inflammatory bowel disease: monocyte and serum lysosomal enzyme activity. *Clin. Sci.* 58:295–300
35. Seaman, W. E., Gindhart, T. D., Blackman, M. A., Dalal, B., Talal, N., Werb, Z. 1982. Suppression of natural killing *in vitro* by monocytes and polymorphonuclear leukocytes. Requirement for reactive metabolites of oxygen. *J. Clin. Invest.* 69:876–88
36. Victorino, R. M. M., Hodgson, H. J. F. 1980. Alteration in T lymphocyte subpopulations in inflammatory bowel disease. *Clin. Exp. Immunol.* 41:156–65
37. Pena, A. S., Cnossen, J., Damsteeg, M. G., Weterman, I. T., Meijer, C. J. L. M. 1981. T-cell subpopulations in Crohn's Disease. See Ref. 11, 1:403–6
38. Godin, N. J., Winchester, R., Sachar, D. B., Janowitz, H. D. 1982. Activity in inflammatory bowel disease is associated with a significant increase in ratio of helper to suppressor T cells. *Gastroenterology* 82:1069 (Abstr.)
39. Hanauer, S. B., Kluskens, L. F., Yuan, S.-Z., Kraft, S. C. 1982. Monoclonal antibody studies of circulating lymphocytes in Crohn's Disease. *Gastroenterology* 82:1079 (Abstr.)
40. James, S. P., Graeff, A. S., Cossman, J., Neckers, L. M., Strober, W. 1982. Deficiency of helper/inducer T cell subset in patients with mild Crohn's Disease. *Gastroenterology* 82:1092 (Abstr.)
41. Selby, W. S., Jewell, D. P. 1982. T lymphocyte subsets in inflammatory bowel disease: peripheral blood. *Gut.* In press
42. Bull, D. M., Bookman, M. A., 1977. Isolation and functional characterization of human intestinal mucosal lymphoid cells. *J. Clin. Invest.* 59:966–74
43. Bartnik, W., ReMine, S. G., Chiba, M., Thayer, W. R., Shorter, R. G. 1980. Isolation and characterization of colonic intraepithelial and lamina proprial lymphocytes. *Gastroenterology* 78:976–85
44. Clancy, R. 1976. Isolation and kinetic characteristics of mucosal lymphocytes in Crohn's Disease. *Gastroenterology* 70:177–80
45. Goodacre, R., Davidson, R., Singal, D., Bienenstock, J. 1979. Morphologic and functional characteristics of human intestinal lymphoid cells isolated by a me-

chanical technique. *Gastroenterology* 76:300–8

46. Selby, W. S., Janossy, G., Jewell, D. P. 1981. Immunohistological characterization of intraepithelial lymphocytes of the human gastrointestinal tract. *Gut* 22:169–76

47. Selby, W. S., Janossy, G., Goldstein, G., Jewell, D. P. 1981. T lymphocyte subsets in human intestinal mucosa: the distribution and relationship to MHC-derived antigens. *Clin. Exp. Immunol.* 44:453–58

48. Fiocchi, C., Battisto, J. R., Farmer, R. G. 1981. Studies on isolated gut mucosal lymphocytes in inflammatory bowel disease. Detection of activated T cells and enhanced proliferation to *staphylococcus aureus* and lipopolysaccharides. *Dig. Dis. Sci.* 36:728–36

49. Fiocchi, C., Battisto, J. R., Farmer, R. G. 1979. Gut mucosal lymphocytes in inflammatory bowel disease. Isolation and preliminary functional characterization. *Dig. Dis. Sci.* 24:705–17

50. MacDermott, R. P., Bragdon, M. J., Jenkins, K. M., Franklin, G. O., Shedlofsky, S., Kodner, I. J. 1981. Human intestinal mononuclear cells II. Demonstration of a naturally occurring subclass of T cells which respond in the allogeneic mixed-leukocyte reaction but do not effect cell-mediated lympholysis. *Gastroenterology* 80:748–57

51. Bland, P. W., Britton, D. C., Richens, E. R., Pledger, J. V. 1981. Peripheral, mucosal and tumour-infiltrating components of cellular immunity in cancer of the large bowel. *Gut* 22:744–51

52. MacDermott, R. P., Franklin, G. O., Jenkins, K. M., Kodner, I. S., Nash, G. S., Weinrieb, I. J. 1980. Human intestinal mononuclear cells. I. Investigation of antibody-dependent, lectin-induced, and spontaneous cell-mediated cyto-

toxic capabilities. *Gastroenterology* 78:47–56

53. Chiba, M., Bartnik, W., ReMine, S. G., Thayer, W. R., Shorter, R. G. 1981. Human colonic intra-epithelial and lamina proprial lymphocytes: cytotoxicity *in vitro* and the potential effects of the isolation method on their functional properties. *Gut* 22:177–86

54. Falchuk, Z. M., Barnard, E., Machado, I. 1981. Human colonic mononuclear cells: studies of cytotoxic function. *Gut* 22:290–94

55. Clancy, R., Pucci, A. 1978. Absence of K cells in human gut mucosa. *Gut* 19:273–76

56. Bland, P. W., Richens, E. R., Britton, D. C., Lloyd, J. V. 1979. Isolation and purification of human large bowel mucosal lymphoid cells: effect of separation technique on functional characteristics. *Gut* 20:1937–46

57. Bookman, M. D., Bull, D. M. 1979. Characteristics of isolated intestinal mucosal lymphoid cells in inflammatory bowel disease. *Gastroenterology* 77:503–10

58. Chiba, M., Shorter, R. G., Thayer, W. R., Bartnik, W., ReMine, S. 1979. K-cell activity in lamina proprial lymphocytes from the human colon. *Dig. Dis. Sci.* 24:817–22

59. Selby, W. S., Poulter, I., Hobbs, S., Janossy, G., Jewell, D. P. 1982. Heterogeneity of HLA-DR-positive human intestinal lamina propria histocytes. *Gut* 23:A460 (Abstr.)

60. Goodacre, R. L., Bienenstock, J. 1982. Reduced suppressor cell activity in intestinal lymphocytes from patients with Crohn's Disease. *Gastroenterology* 82:653–58

61. Selby, W. S., Janossy, G., Bofill, M., Goldstein, G., Jewell, D. P. 1982. Mucosal lymphocyte subpopulations in inflammatory bowel disease. *Gut.* In press

Ann. Rev. Med. 1983. 34:205–17
Copyright © 1983 by Annual Reviews Inc. All rights reserved

DERMATOLOGIC MANIFESTATIONS OF INFECTION IN THE COMPROMISED HOST

John S. Wolfson, M.D., Arthur J. Sober, M.D., and Robert H. Rubin, M.D., F.A.C.P.

The Infectious Disease Unit of the Medical Service and the Dermatology Service of the Massachusetts General Hospital and the Departments of Medicine and Dermatology of the Harvard Medical School, Boston, Massachusetts 02114

ABSTRACT

The skin occupies an important position in the prevention and evaluation of infection in patients who are immunocompromised. The skin can provide a portal of entry for both locally invasive and disseminated infection; and, not infrequently, skin lesions may be the first sign of disseminated infection from other primary sites. The first clinical principle in approaching this problem is that the skin must be protected from trauma, maceration, or alteration in its normal microbial flora. The second principle is that any lesion, no matter how innocuous, should be carefully evaluated in this patient population. Since the gross morphology of the lesion is so frequently modified by the altered inflammatory response of the immunocompromised patient, an aggressive biopsy approach is essential for diagnosis and therapy.

INTRODUCTION

Perhaps in no other area of infectious disease is the challenge of patient management so compelling as in the care of the patient with major abnormalities of host defense—the compromised host. Several factors contribute to this: the array of potential pathogens is most imposing; the clinical presentation, course, and impact of even the most common infectious process may be greatly modified or obscured by the underlying immunocom-

205

promising illness and its treatment; multiple organ systems may be simultaneously involved; and meaningful survival is dependent on rapid diagnosis and initiation of effective therapy.

The skin occupies a central position in any consideration of infection in the compromised host. First, it and the mucosal surfaces of the body are the primary host barriers against infection. One would predict that these primary barriers would assume an even greater importance in patients whose secondary defenses—phagocytosis, cell-mediated immunity, antibody production, etc—are impaired. Second, the unusually rich blood supply of the skin provides an opportunity for metastatic spread of infection both *from* the skin as the initial portal of entry and *to* the skin from other sources (Figure 1). Third, skin infections are common, accounting for 22–33% of infections in different immunocompromised patient populations. Finally, the availability of the skin for examination and biopsy provides an "early warning system" to the clinician that serious infection may be present (1, 2). It is the purpose of this review to develop a logical approach to the dermatologic manifestations of infection in the compro-

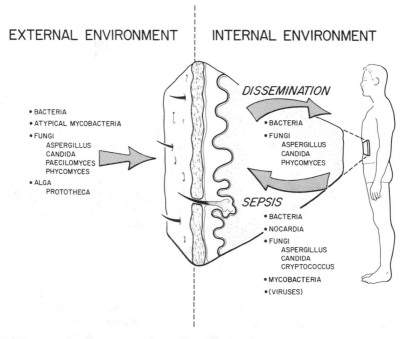

Figure 1   Schematic representation of skin's important role in the occurrence of both localized and disseminated infection in the compromised host. Not only can the skin be the primary portal of entry, it can also be an important manifestation of disseminated infection originating from other bodily sites.

mised host so that this primary barrier may be best protected and this early warning system be best utilized.

THE SKIN AS A BARRIER TO INFECTION

Ordinarily, the skin is quite resistant to microbial invasion. Although such specific components of the host defense system as cell-mediated immunity and antibody production clearly play a role in protecting the skin against infection, the mechanisms by which this is accomplished are poorly understood. At present, the most important elements of microbial resistance that have been defined are nonspecific. The intact keratinized layers of the epidermis prevent penetration by microorganisms, the relative dryness of the skin limits the growth of such moisture-requiring organisms as the aerobic gram-negative bacilli and *Candida* species, and the suppressant effect of the normal skin flora significantly retards pathogen colonization (so-called bacterial interference) (3, 4). Thus, one would predict that the skin would become a portal of entry for potentially serious infection under the following circumstances: when the surface layer of keratin is destroyed or bypassed by trauma or the introduction of such foreign materials as intravenous catheters; when the skin is kept moist and becomes macerated, as under occlusive dressings; and when broad spectrum antimicrobial therapy has been administered, thus altering the normal flora and abrogating its beneficial bacterial interference effect. Perhaps the outstanding clinical example of this phenomenon has been the occurrence of invasive fungal infection in immunocompromised patients whose skin has been macerated by occlusive dressings or tape. As delineated in Figures 2*a*, *b*, and *c*, the implications for the practicing physician are clear—great care must be taken in these compromised hosts in protecting the nonspecific defenses of the skin.

The importance of guarding the integrity of the skin in this patient population is further underlined by a careful analysis of the occurrence of wound infection in immunocompromised patients undergoing surgery. Perhaps the best data in this area come from the renal transplant experience, where the incidence of post-transplant wound infection is as high as 56%. The effects of such infections can be quite great, particularly when they extend to the perinephric space, with 75% of deep perinephric infections resulting in the need for transplant nephrectomy, and with many lives lost due to systemic sepsis originating from this site or from the development of a mycotic aneurysm in the area of the vascular anastomoses. That wound infection should be common in the renal transplant recipient is not surprising, given the combined diverse effects of chronic uremia, possible protein malnutrition, immunosuppressive therapy, and the like on wound healing

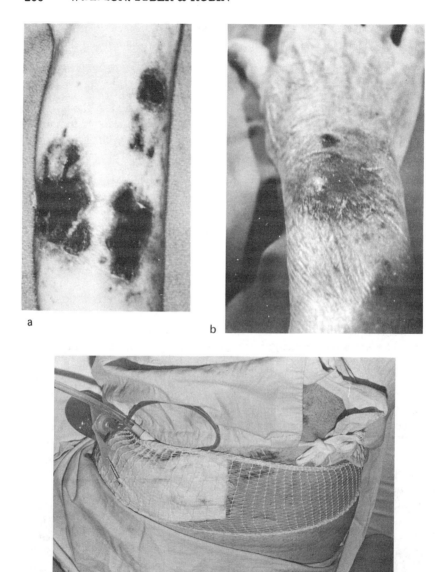

Figure 2a   Invasive Aspergillus infection in a patient with systemic lupus erythematosis who was receiving high-dose corticosteroid therapy. The Aspergillus infection began at a site where intravenous equipment was kept in place by a board and adhesive tape.

Figure 2b   Disseminated candidal infection originating at a site of intravenous therapy extravasation in a patient with aplastic anemia.

Figure 2c   Surgical dressings being held in place atraumatically in a renal transplant patient by a "girdle" of Surgiflex® netting.

and resistance to infection (1). However, data generated by the University of Minnesota transplant group show that the most important factors in the occurrence of wound infection are technical complications. In 439 kidney transplant recipients, the incidence of wound infection was 6.1% (comparable to that seen in nonimmunosuppressed patients), with all of these being clinically trivial, superficial infections (5). The unavoidable conclusion is that the most important factor in the prevention of wound sepsis in the transplant recipient, and presumably other immunocompromised patients, is the technical quality of the surgery performed and the amount of compromise made to the integrity of the skin (1, 5).

CLASSIFICATION OF SKIN INFECTION

Microbial invasion of the skin and subcutaneous tissue as it occurs in immunocompromised patients can be conveniently grouped into four categories: (a) primary skin infection typical of that occurring in nonimmunocompromised patients, albeit with the potential for more serious consequences; (b) widespread cutaneous involvement with infectious agents commonly producing localized and/or trivial infection in the normal host; (c) disseminated systemic infection metastatic to the skin from a noncutaneous portal of entry; and (d) primary skin infection due to opportunistic agents that rarely produce significant disease in the nonimmunosuppressed population but that can produce localized or disseminated disease in compromised patients (1, 2).

Typical Primary Skin Infection

Both the incidence and severity of such conventional forms of cutaneous infection as cellulitis are increased in immunocompromised patients. As in normal hosts, such infections are commonly due to such gram-positive organisms as Group A Streptococci and *Staphylococcus aureus.* However, the possibility of more unusual causes of infection must be kept in mind. Thus, in granulocytopenic patients, cellulitis (particularly due to Enterobacteriaceae, Pseudomonas, or anaerobes) is not uncommon; in patients with leukemia or disorders of cell-mediated immunity, cellulitis due to such fungal agents as *Cryptococcus neoformans* or *Candida* species (see below) can occur. Therefore, for the clinician dealing with cellulitis, carbuncles, etc—routine-appearing skin infections—it must be emphasized that the possibility of more exotic (and antimicrobial-resistant) infection is always present, and an aggressive policy of biopsying skin lesions for gram stain, culture, and pathologic analysis must be pursued (2). The preferred technique for biopsy is a generous wedge excision, half of which is sent to the pathology laboratory for routine processing and special stains (for fungi, mycobacteria, and conventional bacteria) and half to the microbiology laboratory for culture.

One group of patients at particular risk for recurrent cellulitis is comprised of those individuals receiving chronic corticosteroid therapy. Steroids depress proliferation of fibroblasts and inhibit deposition of collagen and synthesis of mucopolysaccharides; the end result is skin that becomes thin and atrophic, with poor wound healing and scar formation. Thus, minor injuries tend to persist and provide a portal of entry for potential pathogens. In renal transplant patients, and presumably among other patients receiving comparable doses of corticosteroids, we have observed a particular example of this phenomenon, which we have euphemistically termed "transplant elbow"—recurrent staphylococcal cellulitis about the elbow, frequently associated with spread to the olecranon bursa. These patients all had two adverse effects of corticosteroid therapy—the previously noted attenuation of skin tensile strength and susceptibility to trauma, plus a steroid-induced proximal myopathy of their legs so that they could not rise from a sitting position without pushing off with their elbows and thus traumatizing them. Recurrent bouts of cellulitis occurred until adequate protection could be provided for the elbows and the steroid-induced myopathy was lessened by decreasing the steroid dose (2).

Unusually Widespread Cutaneous Infection

Included in this category of infection are those caused by viruses and skin dermatophytes. Although each of these infections occurs not uncommonly in normal individuals, in immunosuppressed patients they are more common, more extensive, and may be associated with serious systemic consequences.

VIRAL INFECTION OF THE SKIN   Human warts are caused by a DNA papillomavirus. Although single verrucous lesions are common in normal individuals, in patients receiving chronic immunosuppressive therapy warts may be so numerous as to be disfiguring. The best documented example of this phenomenon is that seen in renal transplant patients. Approximately 40% of renal transplant patients will develop warts, with 1–5% having extensive disease. Immunosuppressive therapy apparently reactivates latent papillomavirus in most instances of wart disease, so it is not surprising that the incidence of such lesions is directly related to the duration of immunosuppression. Of importance, malignant transformation has been documented in such warts, particularly in sun-exposed areas (2, 6, 7). Recently, Ostrow et al (8) demonstrated human papillomavirus DNA in cutaneous primary and metastasized squamous cell carcinomas from patients with chronic wart disease. Clinical management of warts in immunosuppressed patients is centered on avoiding sun exposure and the use of the usual local methods that are employed in the normal host. Often these methods do not work particularly well, and prevention and management of malignant degeneration is all that can be accomplished.

Herpes simplex virus (HSV) is a common cause of mucocutaneous infection in both normal and immunocompromised patients. Although recurrent, localized, nasolabial and anogenital infection is the most common clinical manifestation of HSV infection in both groups of patients, more severe consequences may be seen in certain patients with altered immunity (9):

1. Chronic, large, ulcerated lesions persisting for weeks to months (so-called herpes phagenda) may be observed in transplant patients, patients with hematological malignancies, and patients with the newly described acquired immunodeficiency syndrome (AID syndrome). Particularly when occurring in the anogenital area, such lesions may provide a portal of entry for bacteria that will cause severe local superinfection or septicemia.
2. Dissemination from cutaneous sites is uncommon, but has been noted in transplant patients, neonates, patients with hematologic malignancy, and men with the AID syndrome.
3. Patients with orolabial HSV infection may develop associated esophageal and respiratory tract infection. Usually these occur in patients with HSV infection where mucosa has been traumatized by a nasogastric or endotracheal tube, and such manipulations should be avoided in immunocompromised patients with orolabial HSV.

Until recently, therapy of HSV infection in immunocompromised patients was difficult at best, chiefly consisting of decreasing immunosuppressive therapy. Recent trials of intravenous acyclovir in immunocompromised patients have been promising, with localized disease responding quite nicely (10, 11). However, if the immunocompromised state that led to severe herpetic infection cannot be corrected, then the HSV infection may recur as soon as the acyclovir is discontinued. This has been our experience with both renal transplant patients continued on high-dose immunosuppressive therapy (particularly antithymocyte globulin), and patients with the AID syndrome and severe anogenital HSV infection.

Primary varicella-zoster virus (VZV) infection can have catastrophic consequences in such immunocompromised patients as transplant patients, those with hematologic malignancy, and some individuals with congenital or acquired immunodeficiency diseases (particularly those with major defects in cell-mediated immunity). Thus, any such individual without prior history of chickenpox, particularly when this is confirmed by a negative antibody test, should receive zoster immune globulin within 72 hours of a significant exposure (9).

Reactivated VZV infection is common in immunocompromised patients; thus, 13–15% of Hodgkin's disease patients, 7–9% of non-Hodgkin's lymphoma and renal transplant patients, and 1–3% of patients with solid tumors develop clinical zoster. Although disseminated disease with visceral involvement is quite uncommon in such moderately immunocompromised patients as renal transplant recipients, 15–30% of Hodgkin's disease patients with zoster will disseminate. The problem is even greater in bone marrow transplant patients: approximately half will develop VZV infection; of these one third will disseminate and another 15–20% will develop an atypical generalized zoster that may be thought of as "recurrent chickenpox." Because the consequences of such disseminated VZV infections can be so great, much effort has been devoted to developing effective therapy. Adenine arabinoside, human leukocyte interferon, and acyclovir all appear to be quite promising for this purpose (9).

DERMATOPHYTE INFECTION Immunosuppressed patients, particularly those receiving corticosteroid therapy, have both an increased incidence and severity of dermatophyte infection. Although systemic dissemination of these organisms is rare, local disease, particularly on the extremities, can be extensive—causing disfigurement and providing a portal of entry for bacteria, which then may cause serious superinfection (2). Carefully performed studies of apparently normal skin in renal transplant patients and patients with cancer have shown both an increased rate of colonization with dermatophytes when compared with normal individuals, and also colonization at sites such as the back, chest, and abdomen, which are normally free of such colonization (6, 12). Presumably, small breaks in the integrity of the skin then permit these colonizers to establish infection, and the impaired cell-mediated immunity of these patients fails to eradicate it. Topical therapy and treatment with griseofulvin in these patients, particularly those with extensive disease, usually fails. Recently we treated four renal transplant patients with extensive dermatophyte infection with ketoconazole at a dose of 400 mg per day, with striking success for as long as the drug was administered. However, cessation of the drug after periods of two to three months is frequently associated with relapse (2).

Disseminated Infection Metastatic to the Skin

Hematogenous dissemination of infection to the skin from a distant primary site occurs not uncommonly in patients with impaired host defenses. Three groups of organisms are responsible for this category of cutaneous infection in the compromised host: *Pseudomonas aeruginosa* and, to a much lesser extent, other gram-negative bacilli; the endemic systemic mycoses (*Histoplasma capsulatum, Coccidioides immitis,* and *Blastomyces dermatitidis*); and the opportunistic fungi (*Aspergillus* species, *Cryptococcus neoformans, Candida* species, and the *Mucoraceae*) and *Nocardia* species.

PSEUDOMONAS AERUGINOSA INFECTION   The basic pathology of Pseudomonas infection is a necrotizing vasculitis, which in the skin results in several types of skin lesions, the most important of which are vesicles and bullae, which may become hemorrhagic; a gangrenous cellulitis, which is a sharply demarcated, superficial, necrotic lesion not too dissimilar from a decubitus ulcer but which occurs on nonpressure areas; a nodular cellulitis, which is red, warm, and often fluctuant; macular or papular/nodular lesions; and ecthyma gangrenosum. This last is the lesion classically associated with Pseudomonas sepsis and is characterized by a round, indurated, ulcerated lesion with a central area of black necrosis surrounded by erythema. This lesion may evolve from an earlier vesicle, and is most commonly found in the perineal or axillary regions. Material aspirated from each of these lesions will usually yield the organism both on gram stain and culture. On occasion, other gram-negative organisms can cause similar cutaneous manifestations (13, 14).

The clinical setting in which such life-threatening Pseudomonas infection occurs is usually the patient with leukemia and profound granulocytopenia, with the portal of entry being the gastrointestinal tract. Any such patient who develops these skin lesions should undergo prompt aspirational biopsy, blood culturing, and then initiation of therapy with an antipseudomonal penicillin and an aminoglycoside. These dermatologic findings clearly are a mark of life-threatening septicemia.

SYSTEMIC MYCOTIC INFECTION   In the United States there are three major endemic fungal infections—blastomycosis, coccidiodomycosis, and histoplasmosis—that share a number of characteristics. These infections occur in circumscribed geographic areas where the infecting agents are found in the soil, are aerosolized, and infect via the respiratory tract a large segment of the population. As with tuberculosis, asymptomatic or minimally symptomatic primary pulmonary infection is the most common result, but disseminated infection can occur, especially in individuals with impaired cell-mediated immunity. Although progressive primary infection with each of these three agents may occur in immunocompromised patients, endogenous reactivation appears to be more common. Because of this, a detailed epidemiologic history is essential, as individuals who acquired their dormant mycotic infection many years previously while resident in an endemic area may reactivate while living in a nonendemic area following renal transplantation or the development of other immunosuppressing illness (1).

Disseminated fungal infection involving the skin has been reported for all three agents but appears to be most common with *Histoplasma capsulatum* infection. Thus, 47% of renal transplant patients with disseminated histoplasmosis have skin lesions relatively early in their clinical course, often as the presenting manifestation. The range of skin abnormalities observed may be very great: cellulitis mimicking bacterial cellulitis is the most common finding, but papules, ulcers, and a diffuse, exfoliative erythroderma have all been reported (15, 16). Similar manifestations may be noted with disseminated mycobacterial infection on occasion, with cutaneous *M. kansasii, M. avium-intracellulare,* and *M. tuberculosis* infections all having been reported in immunocompromised patients (17, 18). The message for the clinician is clear: skin lesions may be an early warning of disseminated infection, but no morphologic appearance is pathognomonic, and early biopsy is mandatory.

OPPORTUNISTIC FUNGAL AND NOCARDIAL INFECTION   Infections due to *Aspergillus* species, *Cryptococcus neoformans, Mucoraceae,* and *Nocardia* species share several characteristics. Invasive infection with these relatively ubiquitous organisms is primarily observed in immunocompromised patients. The primary site of infection is the respiratory tract, but blood vessel invasion and hematogenous dissemination occur relatively early in the course of the illness. Not uncommonly, the site of metastasis may be the initial clinically recognized event. When such a site is the skin, early diagnosis can be life-saving. In recent years, we observed two patients with cryptococcal infection, one with Aspergillus, one with Nocardia, and one with Mucor infection of the skin, in whom the cutaneous manifestations were the first signs of disseminated opportunistic infection—the primary pulmonary site of infection having gone unrecognized. Again, the range of cutaneous presentation may be very great, from an unimpressive papule to an extensive cellulitis, with nodules, pustules, and ulcerations being well described (2).

The importance of early biopsy in the management of such patients is illustrated by two contrasting cases. The first was a renal transplant patient who eventually died with cryptococcal meningitis despite intensive therapy with amphotericin B and 5-fluorocytosine. When he presented with his meningitis, an insignificant-appearing papule was noted on the dorsum of his foot. Biopsy of this papule revealed cryptococcal infection. In retrospect, this early warning had been present for more than two months prior to the onset of the neurologic disease, and had been ignored. The second patient, also a renal transplant patient, presented with an asymptomatic nodule on his scalp. Excisional biopsy revealed cryptococcal infection; evaluation for central nervous system infection was negative, and he was treated effectively with a total of one gram of amphotericin B for this early harbinger of disseminated infection (1, 2).

The same concerns apply to candidal infection. The only difference from the other disseminated opportunistic infections is that the portal of entry is rarely the lung, but more commonly the gastrointestinal tract or an infected intravascular catheter. This most common of all disseminated opportunistic fungal infections will manifest skin lesions in approximately 15% of cases. In leukemic or severely neutropenic patients, a particular clinical syndrome that has been emphasized is the association of multiple erythematous, maculopapular skin lesions, myalgias (due to candidal myositis), and fever with positive blood cultures for *Candida* species. Occasionally, candidal chorioretinitis may also be present. *C. tropicalis* appears to be the candidal species most likely to produce this syndrome (19–22).

It is important to emphasize that the biopsy findings in disseminated candidiasis are very different from those observed with the more benign superficial candidal colonization syndromes that typically occur in moist, intertriginous areas of the skin. With superficial candidiasis, the organism is localized to the epidermis in subcorneal neutrophilic pustules. In disseminated disease the epidermis is intact, but pseudohyphal elements and blastospores are localized in the dermis, particularly in association with vascular structures. Variable degrees of inflammatory response may be present, as well as leukocytoclastic angiitis. Again, early diagnosis by biopsy is the key to life-saving therapy, as blood cultures and other diagnostic studies (such as antibody tests) are frequently negative despite disseminated disease (19).

Opportunistic Primary Skin Infections

The final category of cutaneous infection to be considered in immunocompromised patients is that caused by opportunistic pathogens that rarely cause such infection in the normal host but that can invade the skin in this population. In all instances of this category some form of injury to the skin has provided the opportunity for these relatively nonvirulent microbes to invade, and, because the secondary host defenses are impaired, significant local or disseminated disease may result.

Important causes of localized disease include the following: the fungi *Paecilomyces, Penicillium, Alternaria, Fusarium,* and *Trichosporon;* the atypical mycobacterium *M. marinum;* and the alga *Prototheca wickerhamii* (1, 2). In the case of the fungi, physical trauma to the skin is an invariable first step prior to the development of infection. We find that the shins are a particularly common site for this form of infection to occur. In the case of *M. marinum* (23) and *Prototheca wickerhamii* (24, 25) infection, water-immersion injury to the skin is the usual prerequisite. Thus, we have seen extensive *M. marinum* infection on the fingers and arm (spreading in sporo-trichoid fashion) invading underlying bones and joints in a renal transplant patient who was working with an aquarium. A similar clinical presentation was noted in another renal transplant patient whose work required immersion of his hands in water (2).

Far more pernicious is primary cutaneous infection observed with *Aspergillus, Candida,* and *Rhizopus* species (a member of the Mucoraceae). Both invasive aspergillosis and disseminated candidiasis with the skin as the primary site of infection have been observed in patients whose skin has been injured by intravenous therapy—usually due to trauma induced by adhesive tape on the boards used to secure intravenous equipment or due to intravenous infiltration and hematoma formation (Figures 2*a* and 2*b*) (26, 27). In the case of *Rhizopus,* fungal spores contaminating Elastoplast® tape used for occlusive dressings resulted in both locally invasive and disseminated infection requiring extensive local debridement and extended courses of amphotericin B therapy. Here the pathogenesis is clear: maceration and trauma in the skin followed by direct inoculation of the fungus in the face of compromised host defense (28, 29). Because of these occurrences, we do not use Elastoplast® occlusive dressings in immunocompromised patients and we inspect daily all areas of the skin to which dressings are applied. Paper tape is preferred over adhesive tape, and new techniques of securing surgical dressings that employ "girdles" of elasticized netting such as Surgiflex® rather than tape are utilized whenever possible (Figure 2*c*).

Literature Cited

1. Rubin, R. H. 1981. Infection in the renal transplant patient. In *Clinical Approach to Infection in the Compromised Host,* ed. R. H. Rubin, L. S. Young, pp. 553–606. New York: Plenum Med.
2. Wolfson, J. S., Sober, A. J., Harrist, T. J., Rubin, R. H. 1983. Dermatologic and dermatopathologic manifestations of infection in immunocompromised patients. Submitted for publication
3. Weinberg, A. N., Swartz, M. N. 1979. General considerations of bacterial diseases. In *Dermatology in General Medicine,* ed. T. B. Fitzpatrick, A. Z. Eisen, K. Wolff, I. W. Freedberg, K. F. Austen, pp. 1415–26. New York: McGraw-Hill
4. Kligman, A. M., Leyden, J. J., McGinley, K. J. 1976. Bacteriology. *J. Invest. Dermatol.* 67:160–68
5. Kyriakides, G. K., Simmons, R. L., Najarian, J. S. 1975. Wound infections in renal transplant wounds: pathogenetic and prognostic factors. *Ann. Surg.* 186:770–75
6. Koranda, F. C., Dehmel, E. M., Kahn, G., Penn, I. 1974. Cutaneous complications in immunosuppressed renal homograft recipients. *J. Am. Med. Assoc.* 229:419–24
7. Mullen, D. L., Silverberg, S. G., Penn, I., Hammond, W. S. 1976. Squamous cell carcinoma of the skin and lip in renal homograft recipients. *Cancer* 37:729–34
8. Ostrow, R. S., Bender, M., Niimura, M., Seki, T., Kawashima, M., Pass, F., Faras, A. J. 1982. Human papillomavirus DNA in cutaneous primary and metastasized squamous cell car-

cinomas from patients with epidermodysplasia verruciformis. *Proc. Natl. Acad. Sci. USA* 79:1634–38

9. Hirsch, M. S. 1981. Herpes group virus infections in the compromised host. See Ref. 1, pp. 389–415

10. Mitchell, C. D., Bean, B., Gentry, S. R., Groth, K. E., Boen, J. R., Balfour, H. H. Jr. 1981. Acyclovir therapy for mucocutaneous herpes simplex infections in immunocompromised patients. *Lancet* 1:1389–92

11. Chou, S., Gallagher, J. G., Merigan, T. C. 1981. Controlled clinical trial of intravenous acyclovir in heart-transplant patients with mucocutaneous herpes simplex infection. *Lancet* 1:1392–94

12. Alteras, I., Aryeli, G., Feuerman, E. J. 1980. The prevalence of pathogenic and potentially pathogenic fungi on the apparently healthy skin of patients with neoplastic diseases. *Mycopathologia* 71: 85–87

13. Weinberg, A. N., Swartz, M. N. 1979. Gram-negative coccal and bacillary infections. See Ref. 3, pp. 1445–59

14. Forkner, C. E., Jr., Frei, E. III, Edgecomb, J. H., Utz, J. P. 1958. Pseudomonas septicemia: observations on twenty-three cases. *Am. J. Med.* 25:877–89

15. Davies, S. F., Sarosi, G. A., Peterson, P. K., Khan, M., Howard, R. J., Simmons, R. L., Najarian, J. S. 1979. Disseminated histoplasmosis in renal transplant recipients. *Am. J. Surg.* 137: 686–91

16. Farr, B., Beacham, B. E., Atuk, N. O. 1981. Cutaneous histoplasmosis after renal transplantation. *South. Med. J.* 74:635–37

17. Lloveras, J., Peterson, P. K., Simmons, R. L., Najarian, J. S. 1982. Mycobacterial infections in renal transplant recipients: seven cases and a review of the literature. *Arch. Intern. Med.* 142: 888–92

18. Sanderson, T. L., Moskowitz, L., Hensley, G. T., Cleary, T. J., Penneys, N. 1982. Disseminated *Mycobacterium avium-intracellulare* infection appearing as a panniculitis. *Arch. Pathol. Lab. Med.* 106:112–14

19. Ray, T. L. 1980. Fungal infections in the immunocompromised host. *Med. Clin. North Am.* 64:955–68

20. Wingard, J. R., Merz, W. G., Saral, R. 1979. *Candida tropicalis:* a major pathogen in immunocompromised patients. *Ann. Intern. Med.* 91:539–43

21. Bodey, G. P., Luna, M. 1974. Skin lesions associated with disseminated candidiasis. *J. Am. Med. Assoc.* 229 :1466–68

22. Balandran, L., Rothschild, H., Pugh, N., Seabury, J. 1973. A cutaneous manifestation of systemic candidiasis. *Ann. Intern. Med.* 78:400–3

23. Gombert, M. E., Goldstein, E. J. C., Corredo, M. L., Stein, A. J., Butt, K. M. H. 1981. Disseiminated *Mycobacterium marinum* infection after renal transplantation. *Ann. Intern. Med.* 94: 486–87

24. Wolfe, I. D., Sacks, H. G., Samorodin, C. S., Robinson, H. M. 1976. Cutaneous protothecosis in a patient receiving immunosuppressive therapy. *Arch. Dermatol.* 112:829–32

25. Venezio, F. R., Lavoo, E., Williams, J. E., Zeiss, C. R., Caro, W. A., Mangkornkanok-Mark, M. , Phair, J. P. 1982. Progressive cutaneous protothecosis. *Am. J. Clin. Pathol.* 77:485–93

26. Prystowsky, S. D., Vogelstein, B., Ettinger, D. S., Merz, W. G., Kaizer, H., Sulica, V. I., Zinkham, W. H. 1976. Invasive aspergillosis. *N. Engl. J. Med.* 295:655–58

27. Granstein, R. D., First, L. R., Sober, A. J. 1980. Primary cutaneous aspergillosis in a premature neonate. *Br. J. Dermatol.* 103:681–84

28. Gartenberg, G., Bottone, E. J., Keusch, G. T., Weitzman, I. 1978. Hospital-acquired mucormycosis (*Rhizopus rhizopodiformis*) of skin and subcutaneous tissue. *N. Engl. J. Med.* 299: 1115–18

29. Dennis, J. E., Rhodes, K. H., Cooney, D. R., Roberts, G. D. 1980. Nosocomial *Rhizopus* infection (zygomycosis) in children. *J. Pediatr.* 96:824–28

Ann. Rev. Med. 1983. 34:219–29

MECHANISMS AND DISORDERS OF GASTRIC EMPTYING

J. N. Hunt, M.D., Ph.D.

Department of Physiology, Baylor College of Medicine, Houston, Texas 77030

ABSTRACT

The stomach converts food into fragments and then liquifies it before emptying it into the duodenum. Gastric emptying of liquid foodstuffs is so controlled that about 200 kcal/hr are delivered to the duodenum. The volume of the meal, its energy density (kcal/ml), and the proportions of fat, carbohydrate, and protein in the meal have minor effects on the rate of gastric emptying of energy. Regulation is achieved through the osmotic effect and calcium binding of the products of digestion in the duodenum. There are no receptors that respond to energy.

INTRODUCTION

The aim of this review is to blend some new ideas with old ones to give a framework for discussion of gastric emptying in a clinical setting. Most of the work cited here was performed in man. Preference has been given to the most recent work.

THE ROLE OF THE STOMACH IN METABOLISM

Our rate of intake of energy as food has peaks and valleys. Storage in the stomach and regulated gastric emptying smooth out the flow of energy into the small intestine and thence into the portal blood (1). The rate of intestinal absorption usually is limited by the rate at which the stomach transfers material to the duodenum (2). If food enters the intestine unduly rapidly, the osmotic effects of the products of digestion may cause water to accumulate in the lumen with resultant discomfort, or diarrhea, that may be mediated partly through the release of vasoactive intestinal peptide (3). A high rate of entry of glucose into the portal blood, and its storage as glycogen,

219

may cause symptoms because of a sudden redistribution of the potassium that enters the cells with glucose. Later there may be hypoglycemia because the secretion of insulin is overstimulated by the high concentration of glucose in the plasma. When the stomach has emptied and absorption of glucose stops, the high concentration of insulin in the plasma causes a rapid fall in blood sugar (4). Surgical operations that are designed to reduce gastric secretion of acid may cause symptoms that are attributed, sometimes wrongly (5), to unduly rapid initial emptying or to unduly slow later emptying. After vagotomy both may occur sequentially with the same meal (6). It seems likely that the long-term regulation of food intake is mediated partly through short-term effects of gastric distension (7, 8).

THE RECEPTIVE FUNDUS AND THE GRINDING ANTRUM

Here follow some impressions of gastric functions that are currently held, mainly on the basis of studies in dogs by Cannon (9), Code & Carlson (10), Kelly (11), and Werle et al (12). The stomach receives the first mouthfuls of a meal, and soon transfers some to the duodenum. The constituents of the meal, in proportion to the concentration of their products of digestion in the *duodenum*, stimulate receptors that slow gastric emptying. The fundus and proximal corpus [the proximal stomach (11)] are made to relax by impulses in the vagus. The proximal stomach accepts the main bulk of the meal. The surface of the mass of food in the corpus is in contact with the region of the epithelium with the highest density of cells that secrete pepsinogen, acid, and intrinsic factor.

The fuller the stomach, the more distal is the site at which gastric peristaltic waves appear (9). After a meal, the food in the proximal stomach is left relatively undisturbed while peristalsis drives food and secretions from the distal corpus into the antrum three times per minute. The antral content is vigorously retropulsed into the corpus by a contraction of the whole antrum while the pylorus is closed. About twice per minute, 1 to 5 ml of antral contents escape into the duodenum and decrease duodenal pH (13).

THE STOMACH AS AN ELECTROMECHANICAL PUMP

The stomach and duodenum will pump gastric contents in vitro without any connection to the central nervous system (14). The control system of gastric peristalsis is built into the stomach (15). As in the heart, changes in membrane potential occur spontaneously in one region of the stomach, the mid corpus, and act as a pacemaker for the distal corpus and the antrum. The pacesetter potential, a decrease in transmembrane potential, sweeps slowly from the corpus to the antrum and sets peristaltic contractions at three per minute. Any fall in transmembrane potential increases the inward flux of calcium into the smooth muscle. The inward flux of calcium sets free more bound calcium held within the muscle cell. The increase in the concentration of ionic calcium at the activation sites of the muscle fibers causes contraction.

The Transmembrane Potential and the Tension of Gastric Circular Muscle

The inside of smooth muscle cells, indeed of all cells, is electronegative to the fluid between the cells. The less this potential difference between inside and outside, the more contracted the muscle. This is true for the standing potential, for the plateau potentials that follow the pacesetter potentials, and for the spike potentials that occur during some plateau potentials. These three types of fluctuation all occur before and during contraction and appear to cause the contraction by regulating the intracellular concentration of calcium ion.

The transmembrane potential of gastric circular smooth muscle is –48 mV in the fundus, increasing steadily to –71 mV in the terminal antrum. The threshold for the relation between decrease in negativity of potential and increase in mechanical tension is about –50 mV in the fundus. At –48 mV the calcium channel is held slightly open. As a result there is continuous active tone in the fundus. The proximal stomach does not show 3/min contractions, but it acts as a hopper with variable capacity. Nerve impulses in the vagus can cause the muscle to relax as the stomach fills with food. The transmitter is not known, but it is neither acetylcholine nor epinephrine. After vagal denervation of the fundus, the muscle is less compliant. As a result, fundal pressure rises when the stomach fills (16) and the initial gastric emptying of liquids is more rapid (6). In patients who have Chagas' disease, the intramural plexus is damaged. They have a noncompliant fundus and show rapid gastric emptying of saline (17). The converse, slow gastric emptying, is seen in some but not in all diabetics with peripheral neuropathy (18). Metoclopramide is a specific remedy (19). Increased frequency of pacesetting potentials, up to 8/min is associated sometimes, but not always, with slow gastric emptying (20).

THE MECHANICAL EVENTS OF REGULATED GASTRIC EMPTYING

It is not clear how the mechanical activation of the fundus, corpus, antrum, and duodenum changes as the rate of gastric emptying of food moves from fast to slow. Each episode of gastric emptying lasts one or two seconds, and may involve the passage of only a few milliliters of contents through a tube as wide as the aorta. It is not surprising that the pressure gradient, the driving force to such movements, is too small to measure (13). Large pressure gradients between the antrum and the duodenal bulb are likely to signify that the pylorus is closing, or closed, or that the gastric content contains solid material (21).

Is Gastric Emptying Controlled through the Proximal Stomach?

A slow rate of emptying of a meal might be explained by the proximal stomach relaxing and thus not loading the gastric contents into the antrum (11). A meal given down a tube, which presumably does not cause receptive relaxation, empties faster than does a swallowed meal (22). Moreover, a suspension of fat, which normally empties very slowly, produced long-lasting relaxation of the proximal stomach. The short (10 sec) latency almost demands the interpretation that these effects are initiated through nerves, presumably the vagi (23). In dogs, and presumably in man, even the rapid gastric emptying of saline coincides with antral peristalsis (24).

If fundal pressure were the main determinant of gastric emptying under some conditions, it ought to be possible to show that venting the fundus to the atmosphere slows the rate of gastric emptying. Attempts to do so have not succeeded. Moreover, the fractional rate of emptying of 25-ml instillations (25), which can hardly distend the proximal stomach of man, is much the same as that for larger meals that could fill it. On the other hand, a presumed increase in filling of the antrum when the subject turns from the left to the right side increases the rate of emptying of saline (26).

Do the Antrum and Pylorus Control Gastric Emptying?

Chyme can enter the duodenal bulb, as judged from a fall in pH, without any passage of radio-opaque contents being observable by X rays, and without any measured gradient of pressure (13). The rate of emptying of barium is the same as that of water (27). By putting a light in the duodenum and a photocell in the antrum, Berger (23) was able to show that the pylorus closed momentarily three times per minute when the stomach was emptying air. Intraduodenal injection of saline stopped the 3/min closure of the pylorus for some seconds, whereas a 10% solution of glucose, which slows gastric emptying, *stopped* pyloric closure for four minutes. Apparently slowing of gastric emptying is not mediated by long-lasting closure of the pylorus, although the early onset of pyloric closure during antral systole could limit the amount ejected into the duodenum. However, for at least half of the 20 seconds of each gastric cycle there is a free passage to the duodenal bulb from the proximal stomach (23). In dog and in man, with slowly emptying test solutions there is to-and-fro movement of gastric contents across the pylorus (28). If these statements are correct, it follows that the moment-to-moment resistance to flow through the pylorus must be provided by structures distal to the pylorus (29).

Do Changes in Duodenal Receptivity Control Gastric Emptying?

Increased intestinal activity usually corresponds to a reduced rate of distal flow of luminal contents (30). Studies in dogs show that an instillation of sodium oleate, which emptied from the stomach slowly, halved antral propulsive activity but increased duodenal contractile activity fifteen-fold (31). This implies that increased duodenal resistance has a major effect on slowing gastric emptying. The finding that myotomy of the first and second part of the duodenum in dogs reduces duodenal contractile activity and increases the rate of gastric emptying of food (32) supports the notion that duodenal resistance slows gastric emptying.

If decreased duodenal compliance were responsible for slowing gastric emptying, it might be expected that there would be increased frequency of duodeno-gastric reflux with solutions that empty from the stomach slowly. This result has been reported for meals containing fat (28).

Records of falls in pH in the duodenal bulb (13) indicate the minimal frequency of antral ejection. After a meal of meat and two vegetables, the frequency of falls in bulbar pH reached 3/min in the first hour but decreased to about 2/min for the next 3 hours. However, one of the records shows large falls in pH occurring 7 times in 10 min with minor falls between. One interpretation might be that chyme accumulates in the duodenal bulb and causes a gradual inhibition of antral propulsion or relaxation of the proximal stomach.

It seems that the stomach does not expel a new bolus into the duodenum until the earlier bolus is cleared (33). The clearance is rapid in patients with duodenal ulcer, who have rapid gastric emptying (34). From this it might be inferred that the rate of gastric emptying is limited by the rate of duodenal clearance. It may be that the whole duodenum acts as a mixing and digesting chamber whose rate of clearance is related to the concentration of the digestion products stimulating receptors in its walls. This changes the question from "How is the emptying of the stomach controlled?" to "How is the emptying of the duodenum controlled?"

This proposal would explain the recent findings in a patient who had normal rapid gastric emptying of saline but failed to clear his stomach of a liquid diet. At operation he was found to have a carcinoma of the head of the pancreas that could have kept partly digested food in the duodenum and thus maintained resistance to further gastric emptying. Saline in the duodenum is a minimal stimulus to receptors, so that duodenal resistance would be low with saline (22).

THE FRAGMENTATION OF FOOD BY THE STOMACH

The antrum has remarkable ability to fragment foods and to pass into the duodenum only those particles less than 1 mm in size (35). This breaking up of food is more a mechanical process than enzymatic digestion. The breaking up of liver chunks and the separation of the particles larger than 1 mm is less effective after vagotomy and pyloroplasty. It may appear that the stomach empties different solids at different rates, but for the most part this distinction can be explained by different rates of fragmentation in the stomach before emptying occurs. The stomach probably routinely empties the liquid, and liquified, parts of a meal before all of the solids have been broken down (11). Some of this new quantitative information about the rates of gastric emptying of liquified solids should be interpreted wth caution, as it is based on studies with radionuclide markers that have technical uncertainties (36).

GASTRIC EMPTYING OF ENERGY

To summarize what follows, the control of the gastric emptying of food results in the transfer of energy to the duodenum at a rate independent of the proportions of fat, carbohydrate, and protein yielding the energy. The greater the energy density (kcal/ml) of a meal, the less is the volume emptied per minute. However, doubling the energy density of a meal does not reduce the volume rate of emptying by half. The result is that the rate of gastroduodenal transfer of energy (volume transferred X energy density) increases somewhat with increase in energy density of meals (37). The rate of emptying of meals increases only moderately as their volume is increased, say from 300 to 600 ml, when the energy density is constant. The usual rate of gastroduodenal transfer of energy with liquid meals, about 200 kcal/hr in lean males (personal observation), is twice a person's overall metabolic rate, so that in principle the stomach could transfer a day's food to the duodenum in about 12 hours. The same relation between metabolism and rate of gastric emptying may be computed for infants (38). The elderly have slow gastric emptying (39).

DUODENAL RECEPTORS THAT SLOW GASTRIC EMPTYING

Fat, carbohydrate, protein, and acids all slow gastric emptying as compared with saline (40). It is proposed that the spaces between the duodenal enterocytes (41) can act as the single transducer for all four stimuli. Also, the sensitivity of the duodenal receptor mechanism is such that gastric contents with equal concentrations of fat, carbohydrate, and protein, expressed as kcal of metabolically available energy per milliliter, slow gastric emptying equally (37). Duodenal receptors are stimulated by the osmotic effects and affinity for calcium (42) of the digestion products formed in the duodenal lumen and in the absorbing cells. The association of energy and stimulation is not essential, since noncalorigenic materials such as potassium chloride (43) stimulate the same receptor and slow gastric emptying (44).

Isocaloric Slowing by Starch and Sugars

In man, as distinct from dog (45), there are osmoreceptors in the duodenal but not in the gastric or jejunal epithelium (46). After the digestion of starch to glucose in the lumen of the duodenum by pancreatic amylase, and by maltase at the surface of the duodenal epithelial cells (47), isocaloric solutions of starch or glucose give equal concentrations of glucose and equal osmotic effects. This explains how they slow gastric emptying equally (48). It is also consistent with the finding that in patients who do not digest starch normally, because they are deficient in pancreatic amylase, starch solutions emptied as fast as water. Glucose slowed gastric emptying in the usual way, which demonstrated that the receptors were normally responsive (49).

The Lateral Intercellular Space as the Transducer of Duodenal Stimuli

The disaccharide maltose is hydrolyzed to glucose by maltase, which is fixed in the surface of the duodenal epithelium. The osmoreceptive transducer must be functionally deep to the maltase, since maltose slows gastric emptying as though it were having an osmotic effect after being split to glucose (47). Diglycine slows gastric emptying as though it had been completely split into two molecules of glycine (41). This split occurs within the enterocyte and should *increase* the net osmotic flux of water into the cell. Yet mannitol, an osmotically active substance confined to the duodenal lumen (50), slows gastric emptying even though it *reduces* the flux of water into the enterocyte. However, mannitol does shrink the lateral spaces around the enterocytes (51). It would be expected also that the formation of glycine from diglycine inside the enterocyte would shrink the lateral spaces by reducing the flux of water from cell to space. Thus it is proposed that the shrinking of the lateral intercellular spaces initiates a signal that slows gastric emptying (41).

Slowing by Protein

Casein and glucose slow gastric emptying equally on a gram-for-gram basis, but undenatured egg albumin has little effect. This implies that only readily digested proteins can slow gastric emptying as effectively as glucose (52).

Denaturing egg albumin by boiling increases the rate of its digestion and increases the slowing of gastric emptying that it causes. Most amino acids slow gastric emptying by acting as weak acids (53, 54).

Slowing by Triglycerides

Dietary fats slow gastric emptying only if they are digested in the duodenum to anions of fatty acids (55, 56). The long-chain fatty acids are much more effective than the short-chain ones (57). They probably slow gastric emptying by binding to calcium on the tight junctions, opening them, and shrinking the lateral intercellular spaces by causing them to drain into the duodenal lumen (42, 57a).

GASTRIC PROPULSIVE POWER AND THE DUODENAL BRAKE

The stomach can empty saline about ten times faster than it usually empties food. When the stomach is emptying food, gastric propulsive activity is held in check by a duodenal brake. Gastric propulsive power can be assessed from the rate of emptying of saline. Saline (120 mM) is a minimal stimulus to the duodenal receptors that slow gastric emptying. Thus the rate of gastric emptying of 750 ml of saline gives an index of the stomach's inherent rate of emptying. The reactivity and power of the system of duodenal receptors, the duodenal brake that slows gastric emptying in response to the products of digestion of food, can be assessed from the slowing of gastric emptying caused by a range of concentrations of glucose. Since the usual rate of emptying of food, 3 to 6 ml/min, is less than a tenth of the maximal rate of emptying with saline, the duodenal brake appears to control the emptying of food. It is defective in patients who have duodenal ulcer (34). The clearance rate of the duodenal bulb seems proportional to the ratio of antegrade to retrograde duodenal peristalsis, which is 1.3 in normals but 2.8 in patients with duodenal ulcer. This may account for the low pH in the duodenal bulb (58). The signal is relayed from the duodenal epithelium by vagal afferents and/or hormones (59–61). The effect is that the frequency, and possibly the volume, of each ejection of food into the duodenum becomes less.

ACKNOWLEDGMENTS

This work was supported in part by grant AM 26665 from the National Institutes of Health and the General Medical Research Trust, London. The author is grateful to Miss Ann Thompson for assistance in preparing the manuscript.

Literature Cited

1. Lagerlof, H. O., Johansson, C., Ekelund, K. 1976. Human gastric and intestinal response to meals studied by a multiple indicator dilution method. *Mt. Sinai J. Med.* 43(part II):1–98
2. Evensen, O. K. 1942. Alimentary hypoglycemia after stomach operations and influence of gastric emptying on glucose tolerance curve. *Acta Med. Scand. Suppl.* 126:1–388
3. Sagor, G. R., Bryant, M. G., Ghatei, M. A., Kirk, R. M., Bloom, S. R. 1981. Release of vasoactive intestinal peptide in the dumping syndrome. *Br. Med. J.* 282:507–10
4. Smith, W. H., Fraser, R., Staynes, K., Willcox, J. M. 1953. The causes of postprandial attacks of palpitation and weakness after gastric operation. *Q. J. Med.* 22:381–404
5. Gulsrud, P. O., Taylor, I. L., Watts, H. D., Cohen, M. B., Elashoff, J., Meyer, J. H. 1980. How gastric emptying of carbohydrate affects glucose tolerance and symptoms after truncal vagotomy with pyloroplasty. *Gastroenterology* 78:1463–71
6. Donovan, I. A. 1976. The different components of gastric emptying after gastric surgery. *Ann. R. Coll. Surg. Engl.* 58:368–73
7. Hunt, J. N. 1980. A possible relation between the regulation of gastric emptying and food intake. *Am. J. Physiol.* 239:G1-G4
8. Moran, T. H., McHugh, P. R. 1982. Cholecystokinin suppresses food intake by inhibiting gastric emptying. *Am. J. Physiol.* 242:R491 97
9. Cannon, W. B. 1911. The nature of gastric peristalsis. *Am. J. Physiol.* 29:250–66
10. Code, C. F., Carlson, H. C. 1968. Motor activity of the stomach. In *Handbook of Physiology,* Sect. 6: Alimentary Canal, ed. C. F. Code, 4:1903–16. Washington, DC: Am. Physiol. Soc. 770 pp.
11. Kelly, K. A. 1981. Motility of the stomach and gastroduodenal junction. In *Physiology of the Gastrointestinal Tract,* ed. L. R. Johnson, 1:393–410. New York: Raven. 772 pp.
12. Werle, J. M., Brody, D. A., Ligon, E. W. Jr., Read, M. R., Quigley, J. P. 1941. The mechanics of gastric evacuation. *Am. J. Physiol.* 131:606–14
13. Rhodes, J., Goodall, P., Apsimon, H. T. 1966. Mechanics of gastroduodenal emptying. A study of gastric and duodenal emptying with miniature balloons and intestinal glass electrodes. *Gut* 7:515–20
14. Armitage, A. K., Dean, A. C. B. 1963. Function of the pylorus and pyloric antrum in gastric emptying. *Gut* 4:174–78
15. Szurszewski, J. H. 1981. Electrical basis for gastrointestinal motility. See Ref. 11, 2:1435–66
16. Jahnberg, T., Martinson, J., Hultén, L., Fasth, S. 1975. Dynamic gastric response to expansion before and after vagotomy. *Scand. J. Gastroenterol.* 10:593–98
17. Oliveira, R. B., Troncon, L. E. A., Meneghelli, U. G., Padovan, W., Dantas, R. O., de Godoy, R. A. 1980. Impaired gastric accommodation to distension and rapid gastric emptying in patients with Chagas' disease. *Dig. Dis. Sci.* 25:790–94
18. Scarpello, J. H. B., Barber, D. C., Hague, R. V., Cullen, D. R., Sladen, G. E. 1976. Gastric emptying of solid meals in diabetics. *Br. Med. J.* 2:671–73
19. Snape, W. J. Jr., Battle, W. M., Schwartz, S. S., Braunstein, S. N., Goldstein, H. A., Alavi, A. 1982. Metoclopramide to treat gastroparesis due to diabetes mellitus. A double blind, controlled trial. *Ann. Intern. Med.* 96:444–46
20. Stoddard, C. J., Smallwood, R. H., Duthie, H. L. 1981. Electrical arrhythmias in the human stomach. *Gut* 22:705–12
21. Rees, W. D. W., Go, V. L. W., Malagelada, J.-R. 1979. Antroduodenal motor response to solid-liquid and homogenized meals. *Gastroenterology* 76:1438–42
22. Hunt, J. N. 1956. Some properties of an alimentary osmoreceptor mechanism. *J. Physiol. London* 132:267–88
23. Berger, T. 1969. Studies on the gastric emptying mechanism in healthy persons and patients after partial gastrectomy. *Acta Chir. Scand. Suppl.* 404:5–51
24. Prove, J., Ehrlein, H.-J. 1982. Motor function of gastric antrum and pylorus for evacuation of low and high viscosity meals in dogs. *Gut* 23:150–56
25. Erskine, L., Hunt, J. N. 1981. The gastric emptying of small volumes given in quick succession. *J. Physiol. London* 313:335–41
26. Burn-Murdoch, R., Fisher, M. A., Hunt, J. N. 1980. Does lying on the right side increase the rate of gastric emptying? *J. Physiol. London* 302:395–98

27. Ramsbottom, N., Knox, M. T., Hunt, J. N. 1977. Gastric emptying of barium sulphate suspension compared with that of water. *Gut* 18:541–42

28. Sonnenberg, A., Muller-Lissner, S. A., Weiser, H. F., Muller-Duysing, W., Heinzel, F., Blum, A. L. 1982. Effect of liquid meals on duodenogastric reflux in humans *Am. J. Physiol.* 243:G42–G47

29. Miller, J., Kauffman, G., Elashoff, J., Ohashi, H., Carter, D., Meyer, J. H. 1981. Search for resistances controlling canine gastric emptying of liquid meals. *Am. J. Physiol.* 241:G403–15

30. Gregory, R. A. 1950. Some factors influencing the passage of fluid through intestinal loops in dogs. *J. Physiol. London* 111:119–37

31. Weisbrodt, N. W., Wiley, J. N., Overholt, B. F., Bass, P. 1969. A relation between gastroduodenal muscle contractions and gastric emptying. *Gut* 10:543–48

32. Bortolotti, M., Pandolfo, N., Nebiacolombo, C., Labò, G., Mattioli, F. 1981. Modifications in gastroduodenal motility induced by the extramucosal section of circular duodenal musculature in dogs. *Gastroenterology* 81:910–14

33. Borgstrom, S., Arborelius, M. Jr. 1975. Influence of a fatty acid on duodenal motility. *Scand. J. Gastroenterol.* 10:599–601

34. Stubbs, D. F., Hunt, J. N. 1975. A relation between the energy of food and gastric emptying in men with duodenal ulcer. *Gut* 16:693–94

35. Meyer, J. H., Ohashi, H., Jehn, D., Thomson, J. B. 1981. Size of liver particles emptied from the human stomach. *Gastroenterology* 80:1489–96

36. Christian, P. E., Moore, J. G., Sorenson, J. A., Coleman, R. E., Welch, D. M. 1980. Effects of meal size and correction technique on gastric emptying time: Studies with two tracers and opposed detectors. *J. Nucl. Med.* 21:883–85

37. Hunt, J. N., Stubbs, D. F. 1975. The volume and energy content of meals as determinants of gastric emptying. *J. Physiol. London* 245:209–25

38. Husband, J., Husband, P., Mallinson, C. N. 1970. Gastric emptying of starch meals in the newborn. *Lancet* 2:290–92

39. Evans, M. A., Triggs, E. J., Cheung, M., Broe, G. A., Creasey, H. 1981. Gastric emptying rate in the elderly: Implications for drug therapy. *J. Am. Geriatr. Soc.* 29:201–5

40. Hunt, J. N., Knox, M. T. 1968. Regulation of gastric emptying. See Ref. 10, pp. 1917–35

41. Barker, G. R., Cochrane, G. M., Corbett, G. A., Dufton, J. F., Hunt, J. N., Roberts, S. K. 1978. Glucose, glycine and diglycine in test meals as stimuli to a duodenal osmoreceptor slowing gastric emptying. *J. Physiol. London* 283:341–46

42. Hunt, J. N., McHugh, P. R. 1982. Does calcium mediate the slowing of gastric emptying in primates? *Am. J. Physiol.* 243:G200–3

43. Barker, G. R., Cochrane, G. M., Corbett, G. A., Hunt, J. N., Roberts, S. K. 1974. Actions of glucose and potassium chloride on osmoreceptors slowing gastric emptying. *J. Physiol. London* 237:183–86

44. Bell, F. R., Webber, D. E. 1979. A comparison of duodenal osmolality and energy content as controlling factors of gastric emptying in the calf. *J. Physiol. London* 297:379–85

45. Cooke, A. R. 1977. Localization of receptors inhibiting gastric emptying in the gut. *Gastroenterology* 72:875–80

46. Meeroff, J. C., Go, V. L. W., Phillips, S. F. 1975. Control of gastric emptying by osmolality of duodenal contents in man. *Gastroenterology* 68:1144–51

47. Elias, E., Gibson, G. J., Greenwood, L. F., Hunt, J. N., Tripp, J. H. 1968. The slowing of gastric emptying by monosaccharides and disaccharides in test meals. *J. Physiol. London* 194:317–26

48. Hunt, J. N. 1960. The site of receptors slowing gastric emptying in response to starch in test meals. *J. Physiol. London* 154:270–76

49. Mallinson, C. N. 1968. Effect of pancreatic insufficiency and intestinal lactase deficiency on the gastric emptying of starch and lactose. *Gut* 9:737 (Abstr.)

50. Saunders, D. R., Wiggins, H. S. 1981. Conservation of mannitol, lactulose, and raffinose by the human colon. *Am. J. Physiol.* 241:G397–G402

51. McElligott, T. F., Beck, I. T., Dinda, P. K., Thompson, S. 1975. Correlation of structural changes at different levels of the jejunal villus with positive and negative net water transport *in vivo* and *in vitro*. *Can. J. Physiol. Pharmacol.* 53:439–50

52. Burn-Murdoch, R. A., Fisher, M. A., Hunt, J. N. 1978. The slowing of gastric emptying by proteins in test meals. *J. Physiol. London* 274:477–85

53. Fisher, M., Hunt, J. N. 1977. Effects of hydrochlorides of amino acids in test meals on gastric emptying. *Digestion* 16:18–22

54. Hunt, J. N., Knox, M. T. 1972. The slowing of gastric emptying by four strong acids and three weak acids. *J. Physiol. London* 222:187–208

55. Knox, M. T., Mallinson, C. N. 1971. Gastric emptying of fat in patients with pancreatitis. *Rend. Rom. Gastroenterol.* 3:115–16

56. Morgan, R. G. H., Simmonds, W. J. 1962. The relative effects of diversion of bile to the ileum or to the urinary bladder on fat absorption and gastrointestinal motility in the rat. *Q. J. Exp. Physiol.* 47:352–59

57. Hunt, J. N., Knox, M. T. 1968. A relation between the chain length of fatty acids and the slowing of gastric emptying. *J. Physiol. London* 194:327–36

57a. Hunt, J. N. 1983. Does calcium mediate slowing of gastric emptying by fat in humans? *Am. J. Physiol.* In press

58. Borgstrom, S., Arborelius, M. Jr. 1978. Duodenal motility pattern in duodenal ulcer disease. *Scand. J. Gastroenterol.* 13:349–52

59. Leek, B. F. 1977. Abdominal and pelvic visceral receptors. *Br. Med. Bull.* 33:163–68

60. Strunz, U. 1979. Hormonal control of gastric emptying. *Acta Hepatogastroenterol.* 26:334–41

61. Valenzuela, J. E., Defilippi, C. 1981. Inhibition of gastric emptying in humans by secretin, the octapeptide of cholecystokinin, and intraduodenal fat. *Gastroenterology* 81:898–902

Ann. Rev. Med. 1983. 34:231–45

THE DIAGNOSIS AND TREATMENT OF MAJOR DEPRESSIVE DISORDER IN CHILDHOOD

Joaquim Puig-Antich, M.D., and Burt Weston, M.D.

Department of Psychiatry, Columbia University College of Physicians and Surgeons, and the New York State Psychiatric Institute, New York, New York 10032

ABSTRACT

The authors review the evidence supporting the hypothesis of similarity or identity of prepubertal and adult major depressive disorders and give a state-of-the-art account of current assessment techniques, diagnosis, and treatment methods of prepubertal major depression. This is an area of child psychiatry where recent psychobiological research advances are fueling profound changes in traditional nosology and therapeutics. In addition, further understanding of early onset major depression is likely to throw considerable light on the nature and pathophysiology of depressive illness across ages.

DIAGNOSTIC CRITERIA AND ASSESSMENT METHODS

The existence of the clinical diagnosis of depressive disorder was not mentioned in any standard child psychiatry textbook until 1976 (1). Although a large segment of child psychiatrists held that severe depression did not exist in children (2), this position, while quite prevalent, was based on data-free, *a priori* theoretical assumptions.

The 1970s witnessed repeated challenges to this early notion. The first challenge came from the concept of "masked" depression (3, 4). This provi-

231

sional diagnosis assumed that, for developmental reasons, a child's depressive symptomatology was almost always "masked" behind a variety of nondepressive symptoms ("depressive equivalents") and simply had to be inferred. This was a "diagnosis" without operational criteria. There was no way of distinguishing the child whose "equivalent" symptoms were secondary to "masked" depression from the child in whom the same symptoms were primary. The symptoms more frequently mentioned as possible "depressive equivalents" were hyperactivity, enuresis, conduct disorder, phobias, etc. This concept did not survive the passage of time. Pearce (5) found no association between depressive mood and so-called depressive equivalents. Kovacs & Beck (6) reviewed the pertinent literature and concluded that such depressive equivalents were no more than presenting complaints. Other developments, which are summarized in this chapter, led the proponents of "masked" depression to formally abandon the concept in favor of the systematic use of operationalized diagnostic criteria (7).

The second challenge came from the progress in assessment of child psychiatric symptoms, and from the demonstrated feasibility of using unmodified diagnostic criteria for adult major depression to identify the same disorder in children (8) and adolescents (9–11).

Ling et al (12) modified research diagnostic criteria for adult major depression (13) to identify depressive children among consecutive cases presenting with headache as the main complaint. Since then many investigators (14–18) have used different modifications of adult criteria to obtain interview data from a variety of sources (parent, child, teacher). They identified depressed children using different samples (inpatients, outpatients, learning disabled, pediatric patients, and offspring of parents with affective disorders). Puig-Antich et al (8) and Strober et al (10) were the first to use unmodified research diagnostic criteria (RDC) (19) in child and adolescent psychiatric samples. From all such studies, the consensus is that this strategy is feasible and practical. This is reflected in the official American Psychiatric Association (APA) classification of mental disorders (DSM-III) where the same diagnostic criteria for major depression are used for all age groups (20).

Two main criticisms have been made of this approach:

1. Fitting a particular set of diagnostic criteria to a patient's symptoms is not sufficient description of that patient. There is no question that within any diagnostic group no two patients are identical. There is variability in symptom combinations within a syndrome and in associated symptoms, as well as in other parameters such as patterns of relationships, life events, antecedents, etc. This criticism falsely attributes the aim of fully characterizing all patients to the strategy of using diagnostic criteria, an aim that their original proponents (13, 19) never claimed they had. The aim was to reduce heterogeneity within diagnostic groups. This criticism is, therefore, invalid.

2. The second criticism, formulated mainly by Kovacs, claims that, although adult criteria for major depression clearly identify the most severe group of childhood depressives, we have no evidence that the lower diagnostic limit for major depression in adults is also correct for prepubertal children. Kovacs hypothesized that children with depressive mood, but with only two or three symptoms in the depressive syndrome (dysthymic disorder, minor depression), may be identical to major depressive children. This hypothesis is consistent with Kovacs' recent follow-up data (21), which indicate that the rates of recurrent major depressive episodes in nonpharmacologically treated prepubertal minor and major depressives are quite similar. Thus, the use of adult diagnostic criteria for the diagnosis of major depression in children and adolescents is well established at present, although evidence is emerging that the lower limit of the diagnosis of major depression may have to be lowered further in prepuberty.

The use of strictly defined diagnostic criteria reduces only one of the two main sources of unreliability: criterion variance. Diagnostic criteria are not very helpful if the decision about their presence or absence in a particular patient is left to each clinician's preferences, habits, biases, or inferences. Thus, as it became clear that diagnostic criteria for major depression were useful in children, several investigators proceeded to reduce assessment variance by developing semistructured interview methods all based, to a certain degree, on existing methods in adult psychiatric research (22). The most widely used at present are the Interview Schedule for Children (ISC) by Kovacs, the Child Depression Rating Scale (CDRS) by Poznanski, and the Schedule for Affective Disorders and Schizophrenia (K-SADS-P) for School Age Children by Puig-Antich and Chambers. The latter also has a companion interview for past episodes of child or adolescent psychiatric disorder (K-SADS-E) (23).

The use of symptom-oriented semistructured interviews is not new in child psychiatry. At least two different groups (24, 25) had already demonstrated that this assessment technique was feasible and reliable in children; nevertheless it had little impact on child psychiatric practice, where play interviews remained the cornerstone of assessment. The awareness that nonaphasic, normally intelligent children 6 years or older are as a group reliable informants (26) gives the clinician a choice of what assessment technique to use. Play interviews are excellent methods to assess worries, preoccupations, "deep" psychological conflicts, and symbolic meanings, but by and large they do not assess symptoms. For symptomatic assessment, in order to achieve a diagnosis of affective disorder, the use of structured interviews is irreplaceable. Most semistructured interview methods use an identical or similar interview given to the parent about the child. The way of handling these different sets of information (parent, child) about the same period of time (child's present episode of disorder) varies with different interviews. We prefer the method of arriving at summary ratings for each symptom by combining all sources of information, using clinical judgment (and sometimes joint interviews of both informants) in the case of major disagreements. As the majority of symptoms of major depression are inner and experiential, most clinical researchers now believe that a diagnosis of major depression should not be made or ruled out in children without interviewing the child himself. Although other types of assessment of childhood psychopathology have also been devised (self ratings, teacher ratings, parental checklist ratings from which "factors" or "dimensions" are statistically derived), their relationship to the diagnosis of major depression arrived at by semistructured interview and RDC or DSM-III criteria has either been found weak (27) or has not been rigorously tested. Thus at present, no method can be used to short circuit a proper semistructured interview.

The remarkable development of child psychiatric assessment in the last decade is, in our view, the main factor in the demise of "masked depression." Once proper assessments are done, a variety of other symptoms are found associated with major depression. These include symptoms of both emotional (8) and conduct disorders (28). Nevertheless, these are not masks, but associated psychiatric symptoms or diagnoses that sometimes may be the presenting problems or chief complaints (6).

For a rather detailed discussion of assessment of each symptom of major depression, the reader is referred to Puig-Antich et al (29) and Poznanski (30). Because of space limitations, only the assessment of a cardinal symptom during the child interview is described here.

Assessment of Depressive Mood

A child's negative answer to an inquiry on sadness is not equivalent to absence of depressive mood. We routinely ask for eight different labels for depressive mood: "sad, blue, down, low, very unhappy, empty, feel like crying, or having a bad feeling inside that is with you most of the time." Depressed prepubertal children can usually identify one of them (or sometimes several) as the persistent dysphoric feeling they have had no name for. Adolescents can usually be more articulate but it is also advisable to inquire about all eight labels. It is striking how many children report no sadness, but identify one of the other seven labels as present.

The duration and periodicity of depressive mood during the day and during the week should be assessed very carefully in order to differentiate relatively universal short-lived periods of sadness from true depressive mood. In children who report the coexistence of two or more of the seven labels, it is important to ask if the two (e.g. sadness and emptiness) occur together or separately. If separate, total duration should be the addition of the durations of each dysphoric mood. The younger the child is, the more imprecise the time estimates are likely to be. The use of standard time units (hours, etc) in our experience does not improve this imprecision because standard time units are frequently not clearly understood by the child. We find it much more useful to refer to other types of time units that mean something to the child: "the whole morning," "the whole afternoon until you go home," "from the time you get up to when you get to school," "from breakfast to lunch," "from dinner to the time you go to sleep," etc. When the child's time estimates are placed in the chronological structure of his or her average day as obtained from the parent, it is much easier to estimate duration of dysphoric mood. A good general way to inquire about duration is to ask about diurnal variation of mood: "Do you feel worse (more sad, empty, etc) in the morning or in the afternoon?" "At what time do you begin to feel better?" "Does this happen every day?" "Also on weekends?" The clinician must carefully assess *how long* the child felt worse. Some children will report that they feel worse in the morning, which for them means the short period between getting up and eating breakfast. This is not diurnal variation of mood. We require a regular period of at least 3 hours.

Lack of reactivity of dysphoric mood is a very important characteristic that helps to identify severity of the disorder (endogenous vs nonendogenous subtype). In children and adolescents with marked separation anxiety, separation situations may be a very specific trigger of sad mood. Thus, children with pathological separation anxiety may have feelings of sadness that occur only when separated from major attachment figures and never in their presence; we do not count this as a symptom of the depressive syndrome. If the child also feels dysphoric in the presence of the attachment figure for a substantial period of time and feels worse during separation, then we count this as a symptom of the depressive syndrome. The delineation of major depressive disorder from separation anxiety disorder is difficult because a significant proportion of children fit criteria for both diagnoses. A full discussion of this diagnostic problem is published elsewhere (31).

Most parents are able to report depressed mood in their depressed children. Frequently their report is based more on their empathic perception of the child's mood than on actual statements of the child, but, even so, we find that parental reports tend to agree with the child. Some parents, though, are remarkably insensitive, and our data tend to show that when disagreement occurs in prepuberty, the child is usually a better reporter. Some adolescents can be very threatened by admitting to persistent sadness or other feelings and, with tears in their eyes, will deny that they feel sad. In such cases the parental report, confirmed by the adolescent's behavior, is the best guide for clinical purposes.

Depressive mood is not sufficient for the diagnosis of major depression. The mood disturbance should be associated with at least 4 of the 8 symptoms characteristic of the depressive syndrome. These symptoms include appetite disturbance; sleep disturbance; loss of energy, fatigability, or tiredness; psychomotor agitation or retardation; feelings of excessive or inappropriate guilt; loss of interest or pleasure in usual activities; difficulty concentrating or thinking; and thoughts of death or suicide. In addition, there should be functional impairment in social or school performance and no concomitant signs of schizophrenia or of significant pediatric or neurological disease.

Once the depressive syndrome was systematically assessed we found that approximately half of our sample of prepubertal major depressive children fit adult RDC criteria for definite "endogenous" subtype (32). This subtype carries no etiological implications and it refers to the most severe symptom combination within the depressive disorders, including pervasive loss of interest or pleasure, diurnal variation of mood, lack of reactivity of mood to social positively reinforcing events, a different quality of mood than reaction to a loss, loss of appetite and/or weight, excessive guilt, psychomotor agitation or retardation, and early morning awakening.

Chambers et al (33) also found that about 40% of a sample of 58 prepubertal children with major depressive disorder fit criteria for psychotic subtype. The majority of these children presented auditory hallucinations consisting of a single voice talking to the child, while fully awake, the content of which was consistent with depressive mood (suicidal commands, derogatory statements), and which occurred within the time frame of the depressive episode and not outside it. In contradistinction to adult depressives, depressive delusions are very rare in prepuberty but not in adolescence. Strober et al (10), as well as our group, found the same subtypes among adolescent major depressives. It is of interest that at least in prepuberty endogenous and psychotic characteristics have psychobiological and treatment implications.

PSYCHOBIOLOGY OF PREPUBERTAL MAJOR DEPRESSION

The diagnosis of major depressive disorder in adults, especially the endogenous subtype, is associated with characteristic patterns of familial aggregation (34–36), polysomnography (37–41), neuroendocrine abnormalities (42–52), biochemical abnormalities (53), and long-term follow up (54, 55). It therefore stands to reason that children who present with a constellation of clinical symptoms fitting unmodified RDC or DSM-III criteria for major depressive disorder, may have a similar set of abnormal characteristics that differentiate them not only from normal children but also from nondepressed child psychiatric controls.

Familial Aggregation

The morbidity risks for major depressive disorder in first degree biological relatives of major depressive probands is between 0.18 (M. M. Weissman, personal communication) and 0.30 (T. Reich, personal communication) (both age corrected) if the proband is an adult, 0.35 (age corrected) if the proband is an adolescent (56), and 0.31 (before age correction) if the proband is prepubertal (J. Puig-Antich, unpublished data). Our data also indicate that first-degree biological relatives of prepubertal major depressives are also at high risk for alcoholism and antisocial personality, which have been at times conceptualized as part of "depressive spectrum disorder" (34–36). In addition, the morbidity risk for schizophrenia is extremely low in relatives of both prepubertal (J. Puig-Antich, unpublished data) and adolescent (56) major depressives. Mania is very rare among relatives of prepubertal depressives (J. Puig-Antich, unpublished data) but rather frequent in relatives of adolescent-onset depressives (56). Thus it appears that prepubertal, adolescent, and adult major depressives share rather similar pedigrees. Earlier age of onset is likely to correlate with more dense familial aggregation once all data are age corrected. Prepubertal-onset depressives are likely to be unipolar, while among adolescent-onset depressives bipolarity is found relatively frequently, not only in the patients' manic episodes but also in their family pedigrees. The density of prepubertal major depressives' pedigrees applies not only to major depression, but also to disorders that are frequently associated with, and which sometimes may be considered secondary complications of, affective disorders (28).

Cortisol Secretion

Mean 24-hour plasma cortisol concentrations are elevated in approximately 40% of adult endogenous depressives (44, 45). J. Puig-Antich et al (unpublished data) found that between 10 and 15% of prepubertal major depressives present this hypersecretory pattern. The others do not. Therefore, group comparisons do not turn up significant differences between depressives and controls, even if specific periods during the day are considered. Thus, although cortisol hypersecretion does exist in about 10% of prepubertal major depressives when studied during and after their depressive episode, the phenomenon has no value in discriminating between depressed and nondepressed children.

The low prevalence of the phenomenon in prepuberty may be due to age influences. In his adult endogenous depressive sample ($N=26$), Sachar found an interaction between age and cortisol hypersecretion. The older the depressive the more likely he or she was to hypersecrete cortisol (57). Prepubertal children may lie on the left side of the regression line. No 24-hour cortisol studies have been done in depressive adolescents. Data on this age group could help to clarify the relationship between age and cortisol hypersecretion in depressives.

The lack of group differences with 24-hour studies does not necessarily indicate that cortisol secretion in prepubertal depression is normal. It is clear that the low-dose dexamethasone suppression test (DST) identifies more adult endogenous depressives than the 24-hour studies, and that lack of suppression of cortisol secretion in the 24 hours following ingestion of 1 mg dexamethasone in adult samples (ages 18 to 85 years) does not vary with age (58). Consistent with the lack of age influences in adult depressive samples, Poznanski et al (59) reported that approximately two thirds of a small sample of prepubertal endogenous depressives were nonsuppressors in the 0.5-mg DST, while none of the cortisol cases escaped suppression. Conceivably dexamethasone suppression and spontaneous cortisol hypersecretion are mediated by different mechanisms.

Growth Hormone Secretion

Abnormalities of growth hormone (GH) secretion have been found in prepubertal depressives with two different experimental designs. Like their adult counterparts (46, 47) prepubertal endogenous depressives hyposecrete GH in response to insulin-induced hypoglycemia (60). GH-ITT hyposecretion occurs not only in endogenous prepubertal depressives but also in one third of nonendogenous depressives in the same age group. It is, therefore, more frequent than in adult depressives, a fact that may reflect both the severity of the illness when its onset is so early in life, and the virtual lack of circulating estrogens before puberty. Estrogens potentiate GH responses to most known stimuli (61, 62).

In addition, we have found that prepubertal major depressives, both endogenous and nonendogenous, secrete significantly more GH during sleep than normal and psychiatric nondepressed controls (63). Interestingly, there is little overlap between these two phenomena. Approximately 90% of our sample of prepubertal major depression can be identified by having at least one of these two GH secretion abnormalities. Work on sleep-related GH secretion is not sufficient yet to reach any conclusions regarding the presence or absence of an abnormality in adult major depressives.

It is of great interest that both GH abnormalities persist in prepubertal children with major depression, even after completely recovering from the depressive syndrome and being drug-free for at least one month (64, 65). These findings suggest that true markers of the trait may be identifiable, which could reduce phenotypic variation in future genetic studies and be useful in identifying children at risk and in future high-risk studies.

Overall, the neuroendocrine results so far tend to validate both the existence of prepubertal major depression and its similarity to adult major depression. Future work in this area promises to validate the disorder further, to lead to diagnostic tests for the condition, and perhaps to provide guidelines to clinicians regarding the solidity of apparent clinical recoveries and the appropriate timing for discontinuation of treatment.

Sleep Studies

In a large study of polysomnographic variables, Puig-Antich et al (66) found no significant differences among prepubertal major depressives during an episode, nondepressed neurotics, and normal children. The few significant differences (total sleep period and total sleep time) that occurred during the first night could be entirely attributed to adaptation effects in the neurotic group, and these differences had disappeared by the second night.

First REMP latencies were quite stable between 130 and 170 minutes in all four groups. Their percentages of stages 1, 2, 3, 4, and REM sleep showed no significant differences and no trends. Similarly, no differences appeared in sleep efficiency, number of minutes of body movement, number of awakenings, sleep latency, or REM density.

These findings on the sleep architecture of prepubertal depressives do not support the hypothesis that major depressive disorders are identical in prepuberty and in adulthood. Nevertheless, the negative findings in prepuberty are consistent with age effects on sleep architecture in both normals and depressives. Normative data across age groups indicate a progressive decrease with age in the percentage of delta sleep, first REMP latency, and sleep efficiency (67, 70). Coble et al (68) showed that the sleep architecture of middle-aged primary endogenous depressives differed from that of young adults with the same diagnosis on four variables. The older group presented higher REM density, lower first REMP latency, lower sleep efficiency, and fewer minutes of delta sleep. Ulrich et al (69) also reported a high negative correlation between age and first REMP latency during illness in adult primary endogenous depressives. It is conceivable that differences in the sleep patterns of adult depressives as compared with younger populations derive from an interaction between depressive illness and age. Thus, the lack of sleep findings in prepubertal major depressives could be due to maturational differences.

We also found that fully recovered drug-free prepubertal depressives show significantly shortened first REMP latencies as compared to both control groups, and also as compared to themselves before treatment during a depressive episode (71). Therefore, first REMP latency could also be a marker of trait.

In summary, familial aggregation and psychobiological findings in prepubertal major depressives are fairly consistent with adult depression data, when it exists. When the prepubertal and adult data for a marker of depressive illness differ, we invariably found that such markers showed strong age effects in adult depressive samples. Therefore, the initial hypothesis prompting our studies, namely, that prepubertal and adult depression were similar (or identical) disorders, has received considerable support.

TREATMENT

Psychopharmacology

During the last 12 years there have been reports of a variety of open studies in which antidepressant drugs were used to treat children diagnosed as depressed (72–78). In practically all studies, about 75% of the children were reported to have responded. Nevertheless, making conclusions from the cited studies is difficult for many reasons. All of the studies were uncontrolled, the diagnosis was made in clinical fashion, no semistructured interview protocols were used, no diagnostic criteria were specified, there were no indications of what specific symptoms had been observed, the length of the therapeutic trials was highly variable (from a few weeks to several months), and dosages were by and large low.

Recently, our group completed work on the possible effectiveness of imipramine in prepubertal children with major depressive disorder. They simultaneously conducted two studies in the same sample of children who fit the criteria for this diagnosis: (a) a five-week double-blind, placebo-controlled study of imipramine up to 5.0 mg/kg/day: and (b) a study of the relationship between steady-state plasma levels of imipramine plus desmethylimipramine and clinical response in children randomly assigned to the drug. Imipramine was administered in three daily doses, divided roughly equally. Dosage was increased to 5.0 mg/kg/day after a 12-day period. The dose was raised every third day in stepwise fashion from 0 to 1.5, 3.0, 4.0, and 5.0 mg/kg/day. Before each dose increase, electrocardiographic (ECG), blood pressure, and other clinical side effects were measured. If any of the following occurred, the dose either was not increased any further or was slightly decreased: (a) ECG changes induced by imipramine reached predetermined safety criteria (resting heart rate $>$ 130 per minute, PR interval $>$ 0.18, or QRS $>$ 130% of baseline); and/or (b) systolic blood pressure $>$ 145 or diastolic blood pressure $>$ 95 mmHg; and/or (c) unacceptable clinical side effects developed.

Analysis of the plasma level vs clinical response data at the end of the study (N=30) shows that responders had significantly higher plasma levels (IMI and DMI) than nonresponders, and that maintenance plasma levels over 155 ng/ml are associated with clinical response. In addition, prepubertal major depressives who had experienced depressive hallucinations during the current episode needed higher plasma levels to attain a clinical response of the depressive syndrome than did those children without psychotic symptoms. There was no evidence of a curvilinear relationship between plasma level and clinical response (79). This linearity is akin to findings in adult endogenous depressives (80, 81).

The double-blind study shows a 60% response rate for the group receiving placebo and a 60% response rate for the group receiving imipramine. Therefore, imipramine, administered up to 5.0 mg/kg/day with the cited safety criteria, does no better than placebo in inducing clinical response. However, when the group receiving imipramine is subdivided according to steady-state plasma level above and below 155 ng/ml, the response rate in the high plasma level subgroup is 100%, while in the low plasma level subgroup it is only 33%.

In summary, the effectiveness of imipramine in the treatment of prepubertal major depressive disorder does not receive final support from the studies. The data do suggest that plasma level may be a key variable in determining clinical response. As in adults, dose did not predict plasma level.

Two other ongoing studies of plasma level of tricyclic antidepressants in relationship to clinical response of prepubertal major depression are Geller's study of nortriptyline (82) and Preskorn's study of imipramine (83). Neither study is yet completed and conclusions are premature.

Psychosocial Interventions

The next question regarding treatment of prepubertal major depression is if psychotherapeutic techniques are necessary and effective in children with major depressions. There is little scientifically acceptable evidence supporting the effectiveness or lack of effectiveness of various child psychotherapies, parental counseling, and family therapy in prepubertal or adolescent major depression. Evidence is also lacking in most other childhood disorders where psychosocial interventions are thought to be the treatment of choice by many clinicians.

Recent studies of psychotherapy in adult depression reveal that interpersonal psychotherapy is helpful in improving the psychosocial functioning of patients in whom tricyclic antidepressants have induced and maintained improvement of depressive symptoms (84). The latency of detectable effects of such psychotherapies is of the order of several months to half a year.

In a controlled study, our group evaluated the interpersonal relationships of depressed children with a modification of the Maudsley Family Inventory, including measures of mother/child interactions and of peer relationships. Preliminary data indicate that mother/child relationships are markedly deficient in depressed children during illness when compared to normals and nondepressed neurotics. Similarly, depressed children, while ill, have markedly restricted peer relations. Compared to normals, nondepressed emotionally disturbed children are also impaired in their interaction with their mothers and in peer relations, but to a lesser degree than depressed children.

Obviously, the association between impaired social functioning and depression in children may be the result of either causing the other, or both may be caused by common antecedents.

Fourteen depressed children from the above group have been reexamined 3–4 months after clinical recovery from the depressive syndrome, and after being off imipramine for one month without relapse. After recovery, their peer relations were almost as impaired as during the illness. On the other hand, mother/child relationships had improved moderately, although depth of communication was still significantly worse than that of normals, and that of children with emotional disorders during their illness.

If confirmed when the study is completed, these findings are not compatible with an immediate effect of depression on interpersonal relations, but rather with a long-term effect, or with independent psychopathological complexes.

Such data will underscore the need to develop and test psychosocial interventions, especially those directed toward improving social skills, in prepubertal depressive children.

Literature Cited

1. Rie, H. E. 1966. Depression in childhood: a survey of pertinent contributions. *J. Am. Acad. Child Psychiatry* 4:653–86
2. Rutter, M., Hersov, L., eds. 1976. *Child Psychiatry: Modern Approaches.* London: Blackwell
3. Gleser, K. 1967. Masked depression in children and adolescents. *Am. J. Psychiatry* 21:565–74
4. Cytryn, L., McKnew, D. J. 1972. Proposed classification of childhood depressions. *Am. J. Psychiatry* 129:149–55
5. Pearce, J. B. 1977. Childhood depression. In *Child Psychiatry,* eds. M. Rutter, L. Hersov, p. 448. London: Blackwell
6. Kovacs, M., Beck, A. T. 1977. An empirical-clinical approach toward a definition of childhood depression. In *Depression in Childhood,* ed. J. G. Schulterbrandt, A. Raskin, pp. 1–25. New York: Raven
7. Cytryn, L., McKnew, D., Bunney, W. 1980. Diagnosis of depression in children: reassessment. *Am. J. Psychiatry* 137:22–25
8. Puig-Antich, J., Blau, S., Marx, N., et al. 1978. Prepubertal major depressive disorder: pilot study. *J. Am. Acad. Child Psychiatry* 17:695–707
9. Robbins, D. R., Alessi, N. E., Cook, S. C., Poznanski, E. O., Yanchyshyn, G. W. 1982. The use of the Research Diagnostic Criteria for depression in adolescent psychiatric inpatients. *J. Am. Acad. Child Psychiatry* 21:251–54
10. Strober, M., Green, J., Carlson, G. 1982. Phenomenology and subtypes of major depressive disorder in adolescents. *J. Affect. Dis.* 3:281–90
11. Puig-Antich, J. 1982. The use of RDC criteria for major depressive disorder in child and adolescent psychiatric patients. Editorial. *J. Am. Acad. Child Psychiatry* 21:291–93
12. Ling, W., Oftedal, G., Weinberg, W. A. 1970. Depressive illness in children presenting a severe headache. *Am. J. Dis. Child.* 120:122–24

13. Feighner, J. P., Robins, E., Guze, S. B., et al. 1972. Diagnostic criteria for use in psychiatric research. *Arch. Gen. Psychiatry* 26:57–61

14. Weinberg, W. A., Rutman, J., Sullivan, L., et al. 1973. Depression in children referred to an educational diagnostic center: diagnosis and treatment. *J. Pediatr.* 83:1065–72

15. Welner, Z., Welzer, A., McCray, M. D., et al. 1977. Psychopathology in children of inpatients with depression: a controlled study. *J. Nerv. Ment. Dis.* 164:408–13

16. Kupferman, S., Stewart, M. A. 1979. The diagnosis of depression in children. *J. Affect. Dis.* 1:213–17

17. Carlson, G. A., Cantwell, D. 1979. A survey of depressive symptoms in a child and adolescent psychiatric population. *J. Am. Acad. Child Psychiatry* 18:587–99

18. Carlson, G. A., Cantwell, D. 1980. Unmasking masked depression in children and adolescents. *Am. J. Psychiatry* 137:445–49

19. Spitzer, R. L., Endicott, J., Robins, E. 1978. Research Diagnostic Criteria: rationale and reliability. *Arch. Gen. Psychiatry* 35:773–82

20. American Psychiatric Association. 1980. *Diagnostic and Statistical Manual.* Washington, DC

21. Kovacs, M. 1982. *Long-term follow-up of nonpharmacologically treated depressed children.* Presented at Ann. Meet. Am. Psychiatr. Assoc., Toronto

22. Endicott, J., Spitzer, R. L. 1978. A diagnostic interview: the schedule for affective disorders and schizophrenia. *Arch. Gen. Psychiatry* 35:837–44

23. Orvaschel, H., Puig-Antich, J., Chambers, W. J., Tabrizi, M. A., Johnson, R. 1982. Retrospective assessment of child psychopathology with the Kiddie-SADS-E. *J. Am. Acad. Child Psychiatry* 21:392–97

24. Rutter, M., Graham, P. 1968. The reliability and validity of the psychiatric assessment of the child: the interview with the child. *Br. J. Psychiatry* 114:563–79

25. Herjanic, B., Campbell, W. 1977. Differentiating psychiatrically disturbed children on the basis of a structured interview. *J. Assoc. Child Psychol.* 5:127–34

26. Herjanic, B., Herjanic, M., Brown, F., et al 1975. Are children reliable reporters? *J. Assoc. Child Psychol.* 3:41–48

27. Carlson, G. A., Cantwell, D. P. 1982. Diagnosis of childhood depression: a comparison of DSM-III and Weinberg Criteria. *J. Am. Acad. Child Psychiatry* 21:247–50

28. Puig-Antich, J. 1982. Major depression and conduct disorder in prepuberty. *J. Am. Acad. Child Psychiatry* 21:118–28

29. Puig-Antich, J., Chambers, W. J., Tabrizi, M. A. The clinical assessment of current depressive episodes in children and adolescents: interviews with parents and children. In *Childhood Depression*, ed. D. Cantwell, G. Carlson. In press

30. Poznanski, E. O. 1982. The clinical characteristics of childhood depression. In *Psychiatry '82 Annual Review*, ed. L. Grinspoon, pp. 296–397. Washington, DC: Am. Psychiatr. Assoc. Press

31. Puig-Antich, J., Gittelman, R. 1980. Depression in childhood and adolescence. In *Handbook of Affective Disorders*, ed. E. S. Paykel. London: Churchill

32. Deleted in proof

33. Chambers, W. J., Puig-Antich, J., Tabrizi, M. A., Davies, M. 1982. Psychotic symptoms in prepubertal major depressives. *Arch. Gen. Psychiatry* 39:921–27

34. Winokur, G. 1979. Unipolar depression. *Arch. Gen. Psychiatry* 36:47–53

35. Winokur, G., Cadoret, R. J., Dorzab, J., et al. 1971. Depressive diseases. *Arch. Gen. Psychiatry* 24:135–44

36. Winokur, G., Morrison, J., Clancy, J., et al. 1973. The Iowa 500: familial and clinical findings favor two kinds of depressive illness. *Compr. Psychiatry* 14:99–106

37. Coble, P., Kupfer, D. J., Spiker, D. G., et al. 1980. EEG sleep and clinical characteristics in young primary depressives. *Sleep Res.* 9:165

38. Gillin, C., Duncan, W., Pettigrew, K. D., et al. 1979. Successful separation of depressed, normal and insomniac subjects by EEG sleep data. *Arch. Gen. Psychiatry* 36:85–90

39. Kupfer, D. 1976. REM latency: a psychobiological marker for primary depressive disease. *Biol. Psychiatry* 11:159–74

40. Vogel, G. W., Vogel, F., McAbee, R. S., et al. 1980. Improvement of depression by REM sleep deprivation. *Arch. Gen. Psychiatry* 37:247–53

41. Kupfer, D., Foster, F. G. 1979. EEG sleep and depression. In *Sleep Disorders: Diagnosis and Treatment*, ed. R. L. Williams, I. Karacan, pp. 163–203. New York: Wiley

42. Carroll, B. J., Curtis, G. C., Mendels, J. 1976. Neuroendocrine regulation in depression: I. Limbic system-adrenocortisol dysfunctions. *Arch. Gen. Psychiatry* 33:1039–44
43. Carroll, B. J., Curtis, G. C., Mendels, J. 1976. Neuroendocrine regulation in depression: II. Discrimination of depressed from nondepressed patients. *Arch. Gen. Psychiatry* 33:1051–58
44. Sachar, E. J. 1975. Neuroendocrine abnormalities in depressive illness. In *Topics in Psychoneuroendocrinology*, ed. E. J. Sachar, pp. 135–56. New York: Grune & Stratton
45. Sachar, E. J., Hellman, L., Roffwarg, H. P., et al. 1973. Disrupted 24-hour pattern of cortisol secretion in psychotic depression. *Arch. Gen. Psychiatry* 28:19–25
46. Gregoire, F., Branman, G., DeBuck, R., et al. 1977. Hormone release in depressed patients before and after recovery. *Psychoneuroendocrinology* 2:303–12
47. Gruen, P. H., Sachar, E. J., Altman, N., et al. 1975. Growth hormone responses to hypoglycemia in postmenopausal depressed women. *Arch. Gen. Psychiatry* 32:31–33
48. Laakman, G. 1979. Neuroendocrine differences between endogenous and neurotic depression as seen in stimulation of growth hormone secretion. In *Neuroendocrine Correlates in Neurology and Psychiatry*, ed. E. E. Miller, A. Agnoli, pp. 263–71. Amsterdam: Elsevier
49. Langer, G., Heinze, G., Reim, B., et al. 1976. Reduced growth hormone responses to amphetamine in endogenous depressive patients. *Arch. Gen. Psychiatry* 33:1471–75
50. Kirkegaard, C., Norlem, N., Lauridsen, U. B., et al. 1975. Protein stimulation test and thyroid function during treatment of depression. *Arch. Gen. Psychiatry* 32:1115–18
51. Prange, A. J. 1977. Patterns of pituitary responses to TRH in depressed patients. In *Phenomenology and Treatment of Depression*, ed. W. Fann, I. Karacan, A. D. Pokorny, R. L. Williams, pp. 1-16. New York: Spectrum
52. Takahasi, S., Kondo, H., Yoshimura, M., et al. 1974. Thyrotropin response to TRH in depressive illness. *Folia Psychiatr. Neurol. Jpn.* 28:355–65
53. Meltzer, H. Y., Arora, R. C., Baber, R., Tricou, B. J. 1981. Serotonin uptake in blood platelets of psychiatric patients. *Arch. Gen. Psychiatry* 38:1322–25

54. Angst, J., Felder, W., Frey, R. 1979. The course of unipolar and bipolar affective disorders. In *Origin, Prevention and Treatment of Affective Disorders*, ed. M. Schou, E. Stromegren, pp. 215–26. New York: Academic
55. Perris, C. 1968. The course of depressive psychoses. *Acta Psychiatry Scand.* 44:238–48
56. Strober, M., Burroughs, J., Salkin, B., Green, J. 1982. Ancestral secondary cases of psychiatric illness in adolescents with mania, depression, schizophrenia and conduct disorder. *J. Biol. Psychiatry*. In press
57. Asnis, G., Sachar, E. J., Halbreich, U., et al. 1981. Cortisol reaction in relation to age in major depression. *Psychosom. Med.* 43:235–42
58. Carroll, B. J., Feinberg, M., Greden, J. F., et al. 1981. A specific laboratory test for the diagnosis of melancholia: standardization, validation and clinical utility. *Arch. Gen. Psychiatry* 38:15–22
59. Poznanski, E. O., Carroll, B. J., Banegas, M. C., et al. 1982. The dexamethasone suppression test in prepubertal depressed children. *Am. J. Psychiatry* 139:321–23
60. Puig-Antich, J., Tabrizi, M. A., Davies, M., et al. 1981. Prepubertal endogenous major depressives hyposecrete growth hormone in response to insulin-induced hypoglycemia. *J. Biol. Psychiatry* 16:801–18
61. Frantz, A. G., Rabkin, M. T. 1965. Effects of estrogen and sex difference on secretion of human growth hormone. *J. Clin. Endocrinol. Metab.* 25:1470–80
62. Merimee, T. J., Feinberg, S. E. 1971. Studies of the sex-based variation of human growth hormone secretion. *J. Clin. Endocrinol. Metab.* 33:896–902
63. Puig-Antich, J., Goetz, R., Davies, M., et al. 1982. Growth hormone secretion in prepubertal major depressive children: II. Sleep related plasma concentrations during a depressive episode. Submitted
64. Puig-Antich, J., Davies, M., Halpern, F., et al. 1982. Growth hormone secretion in prepubertal major depressive children. III. Response to insulin induced hypoglycemia in a drug-free, fully recovered state. Submitted
65. Puig-Antich, J., Goetz, R., Davies, M., et al. 1982. Growth hormone secretion in prepubertal major depressive children: IV. Sleep-related plasma concentrations in a drug-free fully recovered clinical state. Submitted

66. Puig-Antich, J., Goetz, R., Hanlon, C., et al. 1982. Sleep architecture and REM sleep measures in prepubertal children with major depression during a depressive episode: a controlled study. *Arch. Gen. Psychiatry* 39:932–39
67. Williams, R. L., Karacan, I., Hursch, C. 1974. *EEG of Human Sleep: Clinical Applications,* pp. 37–47. New York: Wiley
68. See Ref. 37
69. Ulrich, R., Shaw, D.H., Kupfer, D. J. 1980. The effects of aging on sleep. *Sleep* 3:31–40
70. Gillin, J. C., Duncan, W. C., Murphy, D. C., et al. 1981. Age-related changes in sleep in depressed and normal subjects. *Psychiatry Res.* 4:73–78
71. Puig-Antich, J., Goetz, R., Hanlon, C., et al. 1982. Sleep architecture and REM sleep measures in prepubertal major depressives during recovery from the depressive syndrome in a drug-free state. *Arch. Gen. Psychiatry.* In press
72. Connell, H. M. 1972. Depression in childhood. *Depression, Child Psychiatry, Human Dev.* 4:71–85
73. Frommer, E. 1968. Depressive disorders of childhood. In *Recent development in affective disorders, Br. J. Psychiatry Spec. Publ.* No. 2. R.M.P.A., pp. 117–36, London
74. Kuhn, B., Kuhn, R. 1972. Drug therapy for depression in children. In *Depressive States in Childhood and Adolescence,* ed. A. L. Annel, pp. 163–203. New York: Wiley
75. Lelord, G., Etieene, T., Veauuy, N. 1972. Action de l'opripramol (G 33.040) dans les syndromes depress-

ifs de l'enfance et de l'adolescence. See Ref. 74
76. Lucas, A. R., Locket, H. J., Grimm, F. 1965. Amitriptyline in childhood depressions. *Dis. Nerv. Syst.* 26:105–10
77. Polvan, O., Cebiroglu, R. 1972. Treatment with psychopharmacologic agents in childhood depressions. See Ref. 74
78. Stack, J. J. 1972. Chemotherapy in childhood depression. See Ref. 74
79. Puig-Antich, J., Perel, J., Lupatkin, W., et al. 1982. Imipramine effectiveness in prepubertal major depressive disorders: I. Relationship of plasma levels to clinical response of the depressive syndrome. Submitted
80. Glassmann, A. H., Perel, J., Shostak, M., et al. 1977. Clinical implications of imipramine plasma levels for depressive illness. *Arch. Gen. Psychiatry* 34:197–204
81. Reisby, N., Gram, L., Bech, P., et al. 1977. Imipramine: clinical effects and pharmacokinetic variability. *Psychopharmacology* 54:263–72
82. Geller, B., Perel, J., Knitter, E., et al. 1982. Nortriptyline in major depressive disorder in children. Presented NCDEU Ann. Meet., Key Biscayne, Florida, June
83. Preskorn, S. H., Weller, E., Weller, R. 1982. Childhood depression: Imipramine levels and response. See Ref. 82
84. Weissman, M. M. 1978. Psychotherapy and its relevance to pharmacotherapy in the treatment of affective disorders: from ideology to evidence. In *Psychopharmacology: A Generation of Progress,* ed. M. A. Lipton, A. DiMascio, K. S. Killam, pp. 1313–21. New York: Raven

Ann. Rev. Med. 1983. 34:247–58

CANNABIS AND HEALTH

Reese T. Jones, M.D.

Drug Dependence Research Center, Langley Porter Psychiatric Institute,
University of California, San Francisco, San Francisco, California 94143

ABSTRACT

The effects of cannabis on health are not easy to summarize. What little is
known for certain and what can be inferred from an enormous but incomplete and imperfect literature is that cannabis under certain conditions is
harmful to health. Given the breadth and complexity of the issues, this very
selective review only considers health-related consequences where there was
consensus by two independent scientific review groups.

INTRODUCTION

Two independent scientific groups recently reviewed marijuana and health
considerations and issued reports (1, 2). Both concluded cannabis use has
significant health implications with the known and suspected health hazards enough to justify "serious national concern" (2). I had the good fortune
to participate in both reviews. This short review summarizes health considerations noteworthy in the deliberations of both review groups, yet not
always accurately discussed in newspapers or short summaries in the scientific literature.

Brief reviews of the consequences of using cannabis engender dissatisfac-
tion in many readers. The complex pharmacology of cannabis is so comin-
gled with social-political-cultural issues that summary statements are
inflammatory to some, no matter what their persuasion. Those readers
should seek more complete reviews (1, 2) or, better yet, go to original
sources. If in places I paraphrase material in the recent reports, it is because
it is difficult for me to separate my ideas from those of the groups. On the
other hand, I take the responsibility for any of the statements, misstate-
ments, or conclusions in this review. This review does not represent the
official opinions of either (1, 2) review group.

0066-4219/83/0401-0247$02.00

PHARMACOLOGY AND CHEMISTRY OF CANNABIS

A brief consideration of pharmacology and chemistry may help explain why so little is known with certainty about chronic cannabis use and health. The pharmacology is complex because cannabis is not a single drug but contains many biologically active chemicals (3). About 60 chemicals, termed cannabinoids, are unique to the cannabis plant. Very few of the cannabinoids have been studied well enough to characterize their individual pharmacology. Although delta-9-tetrahydrocannabinol (THC) accounts for most of the observable acute effects, interactions are likely and, because of the great variability in THC content and other cannabinoid content in plant material, must be considered.

In a laboratory, dose effect functions of THC are relatively well characterized. The intensity and spectrum of effects vary considerably with the cannabis preparation, the amount, the route, the frequency of prior use, and concurrent other drug use. These factors are rarely measured and never controlled in clinical studies outside a laboratory. The psychological and the physiological effects of the cannabinoids result from actions at multiple sites within the central nervous system and elsewhere. Specific, localized cannabis or THC receptors have not been identified. Many of the actions seem to be consistent with generalized membrane effects in biological systems. Much of what we know of cannabis from controlled laboratory studies is more accurately the pharmacology of THC, which, though probably similar, cannot provide a complete picture of cannabis effects. For example, the health consequences of smoked cannabinoids are likely to be quite different than the consequences of those orally ingested, yet much of the animal research, particularly chronic studies, must be done by the drug given parenterally or orally because of the complexity of smoking experiments in animals.

Perhaps the most significant characteristic of cannabis when considering health consequences is the long persistence of cannabinoid metabolites in the body and the related extreme lipid solubility (4). When inhaled, THC is absorbed rapidly. Peak blood levels occur about the time the cigarette is finished (5) and then decline very rapidly over the next hour to about 5–10% of their initial level. Subjective symptoms, physiologic and behavioral changes are measurable for about two to three hours, disappearing more slowly when compared to the rapid decline in blood levels. After oral ingestion, an equivalent dose of THC is absorbed more slowly and is markedly metabolized in its first pass through the liver, thus producing less intense intoxication and a longer latency of onset.

The rapid decline in THC blood levels and its major metabolites is due to two factors. The first, and probably most important, is the very high lipid solubility and protein binding of the cannabinoids (4). This leads to a rapid disappearance from blood into other tissues. The concentration of cannabinoids in other tissues, particularly in brain, has not been well studied in animals and not at all in humans. There is initially a rapid and complex metabolism, mostly in liver but possibly in other organs as well. The rapid metabolism to the 11-hydroxy metabolite of THC and to literally dozens of other metabolic products continues more slowly. Each metabolite probably has its own independent rate of elimination. In regular marijuana users, the terminal half-life of THC is about 19 or 20 hours (4). However, of greater significance for health considerations is that the half-life of metabolites is at least 50 hours or more. Thus, after a single dose of THC, up to 10–20% of the metabolites remain in the body one week later. Complete elimination of a single dose might take 30 days or more.

Thus, those clinical investigators reporting subtle cummulative effects of cannabinoids even in infrequent users (a few times a week or less) may be seeing some subtle consequence of metabolite accumulation and effects. The slow elimination of a drug or its metabolites, especially if they are not biologically active, does not necessarily lead to toxicity, but these characteristics make it impossible to dismiss as unlikely the many poorly documented reports of cumulative effects from relatively infrequent cannabis use.

Although their relevance to health considerations is not well understood, it is important to note that both tolerance and physical dependence manifested by withdrawal signs and symptoms can develop relatively rapidly (6). The tolerance that develops after only a few small doses can be marked and disappears rapidly. If tolerance should lead to higher or more frequent doses (as is probably the case with nicotine and alcohol), then many adverse consequences, e.g. respiratory changes associated with higher dosage, would be more likely to develop. Tolerance results from adaptive functional changes. The processes underlying these changes may have health consequences. The withdrawal signs and symptoms last a few days after a period of chronic intoxication. The abstinence phenomena resemble the restlessness, irritability, mild agitation, insomnia, and autonomic system disturbance that follows low doses of alcohol or sedative drugs given for a period of time. The intensity is similar to that experienced by one or two packs a day tobacco cigarette smokers who suddenly stop smoking. The relationship between drug-seeking and dependence is not understood for any drug. Any proposed relationship between cannabis use and dependence must be speculative.

EFFECTS ON NERVOUS SYSTEM FUNCTION

Psychiatric Effects of Cannabis Use

Anxiety, panic, and paranoid states are the most commonly reported short-term adverse psychological effects associated with cannabis use (2, 7, 8). They occur in clinical settings and in controlled laboratory settings. They are not uncommon and are partially determined by cannabis dose, adverse social settings, and relative inexperience. The symptoms last usually no longer than two to four hours, and are decreased by reassurance and supportive treatment. No specific drug treatment intervention is indicated. In clinical trials with THC, occasional dysphoric reactions characterized by disorientation, catatonia-like immobility, and mixed anxiety and sedation occur more often in older patients where the usual cannabis mood-altering effects seem unanticipated and unwelcome.

Many expected and predictable effects of cannabis are similar to a mild acute brain syndrome. As expected with any drug, the intoxication is more evident at higher (over 20 mg of THC) than at lower (under 10 mg of THC) doses. The mixed panic/anxiety/paranoid states and elements of acute brain syndrome are the most predictable adverse effects of cannabis intoxication. The health consequences, of course, are partially determined by the setting and by one's value system. The intoxicated user and an observer of the user might disagree on the consequences of cannabis intoxication. Such cases not infrequently turn up in emergency treatment clinics and, thus, are associated with some cost both as measured by the individual's discomfort and by utilization of treatment systems.

Longer-lasting cannabis effects, those persisting beyond the few hours of acute intoxication after a dose, are far more difficult to assess. An appropriate classification is not agreed upon. All the usual problems of assessing the validity and reliability of uncontrolled clinical reports muddle things. A cannabis-induced psychosis lasting from a few days to four or five weeks with symptoms of mental confusion, memory impairment, regressive and impulsive behavior, delusions, and perceptual distortions (7) has been described in many case reports over the years and from many countries. Its frequency is uncertain but probably low. It seems to be associated with frequent (multiple daily) doses and may be partially determined by preexisting mental illness.

The descriptions of long-lasting cannabis-induced psychoses are mostly in Eastern and middle Eastern medical literature, and thus are drawn from cultures where cannabis is used more frequently and at higher doses than is usual in the United States. Patients suffering from cannabis psychoses show more bizarre behavior, more violence and panic, and a relative absence of schizophrenic-like thought disorder, though, as judged by the case reports, sometimes the differences between schizophrenia and the cannabis psychoses blur.

Possible links between adverse reactions, schizophrenia, and affective disorders are suggested as more uncontrolled case reports appear. Some patients with a history of schizophrenia seem apt to develop acute schizophrenic-like psychoses after even modest amounts of cannabis. The clinical picture resembles schizophrenia, and the usual treatments for schizophrenia appear effective. Thus, the apparent confusion in older case reports between schizophrenia, cannabis-induced psychosis, and interactions between the cannabis and disease is not surprising.

Amotivation

Apathy, emotional blunting, lack of concern about the future, and a general loss of motivation persisting beyond the period of obvious intoxication has been described in some regular cannabis users (9). Many clinicians treating young marijuana users report that this constellation of symptoms is common. Improvement can follow several weeks of no cannabis use. The problem in determining cause and effect is that the amotivational syndrome is neither diagnostic of nor specific to chronic cannabis use. Its signs and symptoms are associated with chronic intoxication from a number of psychoactive, particularly sedative-hypnotic, drugs. Even non-drug-using adolescents or young adults show similar behaviors on occasion. Certainly, people who are more likely to develop the stigmata of the amotivational syndrome would be ill advised to use cannabis or any sedating drug.

Like amotivation, the term flashback also is deceptively oversimplified and perhaps has attracted undue attention. Flashbacks refer to the brief, spontaneous recurrence of a mental state, particularly perceptual phenomena, similar to that experienced during marijuana intoxication but occurring at some time after the last drug use. Flashbacks are not specific to cannabis or even to any drug use. The evidence is entirely from self-reports, mostly based on imprecise questionnaire surveys and case reports. No distinctive signs or tests document their occurrence. No pharmacological explanation fits. Systematic phenomenological analysis has been for the most part neglected and controlled studies are nonexistent (7).

Cannabis Effects on Behavior

Smoking a low to moderate dose of cannabis (about 20 mg of THC or less) produces a subjective sense of well-being, with relaxation, drowsiness, mild perceptual alterations, altered sense of time and distance, impaired recent memory, and inpaired coordination, particularly during complex perceptual motor tasks (10). The intoxication peaks immediately after smoking and lasts, at least in an objectively measurable way, for two to three hours after a single cigarette (5). With oral doses, the onset is slightly delayed and peak effects are less and perhaps last a little longer.

The health consequences of a mild intoxication, of course, depend on the setting, the demands on the individual, and a host of poorly understood constitutional factors. Probably for most cannabis consumers, an occasional period of mild intoxication is no more or no less behaviorally and psychologically hazardous than would be the effects of a few bottles of beer or a few glasses of wine unless the intoxicated person attempts to drive an automobile, fly an airplane, or to engage in complex and demanding intellectual, perceptual motor, or interpersonal tasks (10). Thus, even the expected and ordinary effects of cannabis intoxication can have or not have health consequences, depending on many considerations. The cumulative or chronic effects are unclear, but it is likely harmful ones exist. The acute effects are as predictable as with any psychoactive drug.

CARDIOVASCULAR AND RESPIRATORY SYSTEM

The cardiovascular effects of cannabis are among its most prominent and predictable ones (increased heart rate, decreased standing blood pressure, and increased supine blood pressure). The acute cardiovascular changes are of little consequence for users without cardiovascular disease. The tachycardia reflects mostly alterations in both sympathetic and parasympathetic activity to the cardiac pacemaker. The improved indices of cardiac performance are a consequence of the increase in heart rate. Diminished autonomic reflexes could be secondary to both central and peripheral cannabinoid effects. Most evidence suggests mainly central effects. With chronic cannabinoid administration, an increase in plasma volume seems causally related to the tolerance to orthostatic hypotension (11). The mechanisms responsible for retention of salt and water have not been explored.

The cannabis-induced increase in cardiac workload poses some risk to people with an abnormal heart or circulation, for example, patients with hypertension, cerebrovascular disease, and coronary atherosclerosis. The magnitude and incidence of risk is undetermined since cannabis smoking has largely been by younger adults relatively free of cardiovascular disease. When given to patients with coronary artery disease, smoked marijuana decreases exercise tolerance. Thus, a combination of cannabis effects increases the work of the heart in many ways and, when coupled with catecholamine stimulation, could lead to ill effects on the abnormal cardiovascular system. The magnitude of acute cardiovascular effects is as great as those produced by nicotine and tobacco smoking. Whether similar cardiovascular changes might follow after years of cannabis smoking cannot be answered now.

Respiratory System

Smoking cannabis, as with the inhalation of almost any substance if done frequently enough, over a long enough time will produce undesirable cellular and lung function alterations (8, 12). Regular and frequent smoking of cannabis produces inflammatory changes and what are often considered preneoplastic changes in airways similar to those produced by smoking tobacco (13). Cannabis smoke does not contain nicotine, but like tobacco it does have an equally complex aerosol of particles in a vapor phase that form what is commonly called tar. The mixture contains thousands of substances, including many of the same hydrocarbons suspected in tobacco tars to be associated with cancer causation (14). By weight, cannabis contains more tar than most tobaccos. Similar amounts of carbon monoxide can be delivered. Simple equations comparing the tar delivery of cannabis and tobacco cigarettes are bound to be misleading, no matter what the figures. Patterns of smoking cannabis and tobacco are different. THC and other cannabinoids have different effects in the body than nicotine and its metabolites, even though both have many shared effects.

The potential for smoked cannabis to produce bronchitis and functional changes of early obstructive pulmonary disease changes is clear. Confirmation of what may be increased cancer risk is not likely in the near future since marijuana has been heavily smoked in this country for considerably less than 20 years. Data have not been collected systematically in other countries with a longer history of heavy cannabis use. Even when they have, interactions with concurrent tobacco smoking and the fact that in many countries cannabis is mainly ingested rather than smoked are factors likely to keep the issue open. Increased risk is likely in those users (now the majority) who smoke cannabis and tobacco concurrently.

Given in single doses, THC or cannabis smoke produces a small, transient respiratory depression (15) along with bronchodilatation (16). The degree of depression is not enough to produce serious interactive effects with other respiratory depressants. The clinical utility of the bronchodilatation seems minimal.

The health consequences of paraquat-contaminated cannabis are the topic of recent medical and political debate. Large doses of paraquat taken by mouth or by aerosol unquestionably can cause pulmonary fibrosis. It damages many other organs we well, but most other effects are transitory. The evidence for injurious effects of paraquat, inhaled either through the spraying process or by smoking marijuana contaminated with paraquat, is too meager for any conclusions. It is unlikely that cannabis smokers would be exposed to amounts of paraquat large enough to produce acute lung damage. The consequences of chronic, low-grade exposure are unknown.

Paraquat and cannabis effects would be confounded. Most users would have only intermittent exposure given the relative rarity of paraquat-contaminated cannabis. A good guess from animal studies is that continued smoking of paraquat-contaminated cigarettes could produce lung injury, probably a diffuse interstitial fibrosis, and respiratory insufficiency (2).

Other contaminants are to be expected in plant material not always handled in the most sanitary way. At least one outbreak of salmonellosis was epidemiologically linked to marijuana use in the mid-West (17). Concern over aspergillosis, a common fungal contaminant of some cannabis, has been expressed (18, 19). This is of special significance in patients with compromised immune systems from chemotherapy treatments who are smoking cannabis for treatment purposes.

GASTROINTESTINAL EFFECTS

In humans, acute or subacute use of cannabis, particularly at high doses, may produce vomiting, diarrhea, and feelings of abdominal distress. Indirect evidence suggests that gastric emptying time may be prolonged and, in general, gut motility slowed enough to affect the absorption of certain drugs. For example, alcohol absorption may be delayed because it remains longer in the stomach when consumed along with cannabis. The antiemetic effects of cannabinoids are discussed in the section on therapeutic applications. They seem to be mainly central in origin.

CELLULAR TOXICITY AND CARCINOGENICITY

Cannabis and the cannabinoids have mutagenic and carcinogenic effects and impair biosynthesis of nucleic acids and proteins (20). Most of these effects have been best demonstrated with in vitro systems. The low water solubility of the cannabinoids and the common use of higher concentrations than are likely in living animals make the interpretation of in vitro experiments speculative when predicting health consequences.

Early reports of cannabis-induced chromosomal aberrations in general have not been replicated. Marijuana smoke produced chromosomal aberrations, hypoploidy, mutagenesis in bacteria as demonstrated by the Ames test (21), and impaired development in the second generation of offspring of treated animals. In humans, no cytogenetic abnormalities or mutagenic effects clearly and unambiguously attributable to cannabinoids have been identified. It is impossible to completely dismiss the in vitro and animal studies, even though the results are often inconsistent. However, as is the case with many other drugs, the clinical significance of most effects is not known and probably will only be determined by controlled studies of large human populations.

THE IMMUNE SYSTEM

Animal and in vitro studies all suggest that cannabinoids have a mild, transient immunosuppressant effect, both in vitro and in vivo (22). The effects are mild when compared with known immunosuppressant drugs. Evidence for immunosuppression in humans is contradictory. Some studies find mild and others no effects when comparing normals and chronic marijuana users. However, even weak immunosuppressant effects are important to specially predisposed individuals and may be of significance if the drug is used by large populations.

BIRTH DEFECTS AND TERATOGENICITY

Cannabis is clearly teratogenic at high doses in some species of animals (20). Thus far there is no evidence of obvious teratogenicity in the offspring of humans. The data are inadequate to document slowly developing or subtle functional impairments or a very low level of teratogenicity. Cannabinoids readily cross the placenta. Fetal metabolism and kinetics are unknown. Because of confounding influences of nutrition and other drug use, particularly tobacco and alcohol, it may be impossible to identify any specific role for cannabis.

As with other psychoactive drugs, lasting behavioral effects in the offspring have been noted, both in animals and in humans, when the mother is exposed to cannabis during pregnancy. In animals, these behavioral changes, most evident in learning, persist for many months (9). Human infants whose mothers used cannabis during pregnancy have increased tremor, startle, and altered visual responses, and perhaps abnormal cries, most evident in the immediate postpartum period. The gestational age was slightly shorter in these infants (23).

REPRODUCTIVE FUNCTION

Animal studies and in vitro studies suggest that cannabinoids can interfere with sex hormones and reproduction in a variety of ways (20). In animals and in some human studies, sperm number and motility are decreased during chronic cannabis use. In animals and inconsistently in humans, cannabinoids acutely lower gonadotropic secretion and testosterone concentrations. Whether the decreases in sperm number and motility or the hormonal changes have any effect on function and fertility is not known.

In female animals, acute administration of THC transiently inhibits functioning of the hypothalamic-pituitary-gonadal axes. Plasma LH and prolactin levels decrease, the preovulatory LH surge is suppressed, and esterus is delayed.

Chronic cannabinoid intake seems to impair reproductive function reversibly. Very few human studies have been reported. A single uncontrolled preliminary report claimed marijuana users were more often anovulatory or had an inadequate luteal phase when compared to a group of nonusers.

DRUG INTERACTIONS

Cannabis is usually consumed along with other drugs. It shares hepatic metabolic systems with many drugs, so interactions are likely at the drug metabolism level. Alcohol and phenobarbital can inhibit metabolism of THC, presumably by enzyme substrate competition. After a period of inhibition, if one drug is removed the increased enzyme activity can make for faster than expected metabolism of the remaining drug. When given simultaneously with other drugs, THC slows the metabolism of theophyllin, antipyrine, ethanol, and pentobarbital (24). Cannabidiol also inhibits metabolism of a variety of drugs normally metabolized by the hepatic enzyme systems. The interactions can be expected to be complex. THC administered orally has different effects on metabolism than does smoked cannabis, probably because a cannabis smoker is exposed to chemicals in smoke capable of interacting with other drugs differently than those an oral user is exposed to. In addition to drug interactions by shared metabolic pathways, THC could potentially interact with other drugs because of competition for available binding sites on plasma and tissue proteins. Finally, drug interactions occur by what appear to be functional mechanisms. These can be additive, leading to enhancement or prolongation of behavioral and psychological effects of CNS depressant drugs such as alcohol or barbiturates, along with the expected cross-tolerance. Thus far, cannabis has been shown to alter the effects of alcohol, barbiturates, nicotine, amphetamines, cocaine, phencyclidine, opiates, atropine, and chlorimipramine (12).

THERAPEUTIC USES OF CANNABIS

Cannabis, THC, and cannabidiol have been tried in preliminary studies as treatment for a variety of disorders (25). THC and cannabis are superior to placebo and about equal to prochlorperazine in treating the nausea and vomiting associated with cancer chemotherapies. Synthetic cannabinoid analogues, for example nabilone and levonantradol, seem to have equivalent potency and have a number of advantages over the crude cannabis compounds. The efficacy varies enough from study to study, as do the incidences of troublesome psychoactive and cardiovascular side-effects, so that it would be premature to accept cannabinoids as an established treatment.

The use of cannabinoids in treating glaucoma probably has received more attention in the media than deserved by the quality of scientific data. Thus far the clinical utility appears minimal. Psychoactive and cardiovascular side-effects are a major problem and even the specificity of the pressure-lowering effects is questioned (25, 26).

One of the more exciting observations is cannabidiol's potent anticonvulsant actions (27). Human studies thus far have not been well controlled and mechanisms of action are uncertain. Cannabidiol, having no psychoactive effects of its own, would offer advantages over cannabis or THC.

The antianxiety properties of both cannabis and the analogues do not seem to exceed those of existing anxiolytics and have the same associated side-effect problems. Although having mild and inconsistent analgesic effects, antibacterial and antiinflammatory, and a potential for decreasing muscle spasticity and possible applications in the treatment of asthma, support for all these therapeutic applications thus far is merely suggestive or less. The problems of side-effects and the development of tolerance to the therapeutic effects are such that it is extremely unlikely that cannabis given as plant material will have great therapeutic utility. However, the fact that the cannabinoids represent a class of drugs with a unique pharmacology offers promise for the identification of therapeutic agents with new modes of action. Although much effort has gone into this, no breakthroughs are immediately apparent (25).

ACKNOWLEDGMENTS

Supported in part by Grants No. DA00053 and DA01696 from the National Institute on Drug Abuse.

Literature Cited

1. Addiction Research Center/World Health Organization. 1981. *Report of Addiction Research Foundation/World Health Organization (ARF/WHO).* Conference on Adverse Health and Behavioral Consequences of Cannabis Use. Toronto: Addiction Research Center
2. National Academy of Science, Institute of Medicine. 1982. *Marijuana and Health: Report of a Study by a Committee of the Institute of Medicine.* Washington: National Academy Press
3. Turner, C. E., Elsohly, M. A., Boeren, E. G. 1980. Constituents of *Cannabis sativa* L. XVII. A review of the natural constituents. *J. Natural Prod.* 43:169–234
4. Hunt, C. A., Jones, R. T. 1980. Tolerance and disposition of tetrahydrocan-

nabinol in man. *J. Pharmacol. Exp. Ther.* 215:35–44
5. Ohlsson, A., Lindgren, J. E., Wahlen, A., Agurell, S., Hollister, L. E., Gillespie, H. K. 1980. Plasma delta-9-tetrahydrocannabinol concentrations and clinical effects after oral and intravenous administration and smoking. *Clin. Pharmacol. Ther.* 28:409–16
6. Jones, R. T. 1983. Cannabis tolerance and dependence. In *Adverse Health and Behavioral Consequences of Cannabis Use. Working Papers for the ARF/WHO Scientific Meeting. Toronto, 1981.* ed. K. O. Fehr, H. Kalant. Toronto: Addiction Research Foundation. In press
7. Negrete, J. C. 1983. Psychiatric effects of cannabis use. See Ref. 6, in press
8. Tennant, F. S. Jr. 1983. Clinical tox-

icology of cannabis use. See Ref. 6, in press

9. Fehr, K. O., Kalant, H. 1983. Long-term effects of cannabis on cerebral function: a review of the clinical and experimental literature. See Ref. 6, in press

10. Klonoff, H. 1983. Acute psychological effects of marihuana in man, including acute cognitive, psychomotor and perceptual effects on driving. See Ref. 6, in press

11. Benowitz, N. L., Jones, R. T. 1975. Cardiovascular effects of prolonged delta-9-tetrahydrocannabinol ingestion. *Clin. Pharmacol. Ther.* 18:287–97

12. Rosenkrantz, H. 1983. Cannabis, marihuana, and cannabinoid toxicological manifestations in man and animals. See Ref. 6, in press

13. Tennant, F. S., Guerry, R. L., Henderson, R. L. 1980. Histopathologic and clinical abnormalities of the respiratory system in chronic hashish smokers. *Substance Alc. Misuse* 1:93–100

14. Hoffmann, D., Brunnemann, K. D., Gori, G. B., Wynder, E. L. 1975. On the carcinogenicity of marijuana smoke. *Rec. Adv. Phytochem.* 9:63–81

15. Bellville, J. W., Swanson, G. D., Aqleh, K. A. 1975. Respiratory effects of delta-9-tetrahydrocannabinol. *Clin. Pharmacol. Ther.* 17:541–48

16. Tashkin, D. P., Shapiro, D. J., Frank, I. M. 1974. Acute physiologic effects of smoked marijuana and oral delta-9-tetrahydrocannabinol on specific airway conductance in asthmatic subjects. *Am. Rev. Resp. Dis.* 109:420–28

17. Schrader, J., Steris, C., Halpin, T. 1981. Salmonellosis traced to marijuana—Ohio, Michigan. *Ctr. Dis. Control Morbid. Mortal. Wkly. Rep.* 30:77–79

18. Llamas, R., Hart, D. R., Schneider, N. S. 1978. Allergic bronchopulmonary aspergillosis associated with smoking moldy marihuana. *Chest* 73:871–72

19. Kagen, S. L. 1981. Aspergillus: an inhalable contaminant of marihuana. *N. Engl. J. Med.* 304:483–84

20. Bloch, E. 1983. Effects of marihuana and cannabinoids on reproduction, endocrine function, development and chromosomes. See Ref. 6, in press

21. Wehner, F. C., van Rensburg, S. J., Thiel, P. G. 1980. Mutagenicity of marijuana and Transkei tobacco smoke condensates in the Salmonella/microsome assay. *Mutat. Res.* 77:135–42

22. Munson, A. E., Fehr, K. O. 1983. Immunological effects of cannabis. See Ref. 6, in press

23. Fried, P. A. 1982. Marihuana use by pregnant women and effects on offspring: an update. *Neurobehav. Toxicol.* 4, in press

24. Benowitz, N. L., Jones, R. T. 1977. Effects of delta-9-tetrahydrocannabinol on drug distribution and metabolism—antipyrine, pentobarbital, and ethanol. *Clin. Pharmacol. Ther.* 22:259–68

25. Milne, G. M., Johnson, M. R., Wiseman, E. H., Hutcheon, D. E., eds. 1981. *Therapeutic Progress in Cannabinoid Research.* Suppl. *J. Clin. Pharmacol.,* Aug.-Sep. 488 pp.

26. Merritt, J. C., Crawford, W. J., Alexander, P. C. 1980. Effect of marihuana on intraocular and blood pressure in glaucoma. *Ophthalmology* 87:222–28

27. Karler, R., Turkanis, S. A. 1981. Cannabinoids as potential antiepileptics. *J. Clin. Pharmacol.* 21:437S–48S

Ann. Rev. Med. 1983. 34:259–66

PSEUDOHYPOPARATHYROIDISM

Cornelis Van Dop, M.D., Ph.D., and Henry R. Bourne, M.D.

Departments of Pediatrics, Medicine, Pharmacology and the Cardiovascular Research Institute, University of California, San Francisco, California 94143

ABSTRACT

Pseudohypoparathyroidism includes a genotypically diverse group of syndromes of primary resistance to hormones whose actions are mediated by cyclic adenosine 3':5'-monophosphate. In most cases, clinical presentation results from resistance to actions of parathyroid hormone, while resistance to other hormones remains subclinical. The largest subgroup of patients with this disorder, characterized by a typical somatic phenotype termed Albright's hereditary osteodystrophy, exhibits generalized deficient activity of a membrane protein that couples hormone receptors to stimulation of adenylate cyclase. Phenotypic expression of the disease varies greatly between families, within families, and even during the clinical course of individual patients. Genetic transmission occurs via several distinct loci, which produce different patterns of inheritance.

Introduction

Forty years ago, Albright et al (1) described the first recognized disorder of primary hormone resistance, pseudohypoparathyroidism (PHP). This inherited disorder, initially thought to involve isolated resistance to parathyroid hormone, is now known to involve resistance to multiple hormones that utilize cyclic adenosine 3':5'-monophosphate (cAMP) as a second messenger. Recent evidence indicates that hormone resistance in many PHP patients is caused by partial deficiency of a membrane protein that couples hormone receptors to stimulation of adenylate cyclase, the enzyme that synthesizes cAMP from adenosine triphosphate (ATP). This evidence allows biochemical classification of subtypes of PHP and sheds new light on its pathogenesis, clinical variability, and mode of inheritance.

259

0066-4219/83/0401-0259$02.00

Historical Review

In 1942, Albright et al (1) described a syndrome, characterized by hypocalcemia and hyperphosphatemia, that resembled hypoparathyroidism—except that parenteral parathyroid extract did not elevate serum calcium concentration or increase urinary phosphate excretion. Albright postulated that the disease was caused by resistance to parathyroid hormone (PTH). These "pseudohypoparathyroid" patients exhibited short stature with moderate obesity, round face, and short fingers, a distinctive morphological phenotype now termed "Albright's hereditary osteodystrophy" (AHO). The apparent shortening of fingers is actually caused by shortening of the metacarpals (2).

In 1966, Tashjian et al (3) found elevated serum PTH in PHP, which indicated that low serum calcium could stimulate PTH secretion, although PTH was physiologically ineffective. Three years later, Chase et al (4) showed that exogenous PTH did not raise urinary excretion of cAMP in PHP patients, in contrast to normal or hypoparathyroid controls. Later studies showed that administration of a synthetic cAMP analog increases urinary phosphate excretion and raises serum calcium in PHP patients, as in normal subjects (5). Thus, the PHP defect is not due to resistance to cAMP. Rather, the defect involves reduced stimulation of cAMP synthesis by hormone. Patients with defective PTH-induced cAMP excretion are now classified as Type I because several "PHP, Type II" patients have been described, in whom resistance to the phosphaturic effect of PHT is associated with normal or increased PTH-induced urinary cAMP excretion (6).

Subsequently, Drezner & Burch (7) showed that adenylate cyclase in a kidney biopsy obtained from a PHP patient required additional guanosine triphosphate (GTP) to exhibit quantitatively normal stimulation by PTH. This finding suggested that PHP might be due to an abnormality of a guanine nucleotide-binding site associated with adenylate cyclase. Discovery of a guanine nucleotide-binding regulatory protein (8), called the N protein (9), that couples hormone receptors to adenylate cyclase (Figure 1) opened the way to biochemical exploration of the PHP phenotype. Two laboratories (10, 11) reported that erythrocytes of most PHP-I patients had only 50% of the N-protein activity found in erythrocytes of normal subjects. Later studies found deficient N-protein activity in platelets (12), fibroblasts (13), and virus-transformed lymphoblasts (14) of the same PHP-I patients. Erythrocytes (and other cells) of some PHP-I patients exhibit quantitatively normal N-protein activity. These patients are classified as PHP-Ib, to distinguish them from PHP-Ia patients, in whom erythrocyte N-protein activity is reduced. A more recent study directly documented that the N-protein defect in a PHP-Ia patient involves a PTH target organ, the kidney. This study (R. W. Downs, personal communication) found reduced N-protein activity in erythrocytes and membrane extracts of the kidney biopsy of the patient previously described by Drezner & Burch (7).

Associated Endocrinologic Abnormalities

Prior to the discovery of decreased N-protein activity in PHP-I, several reports indicated that some PHP patients were clinically hypothyroid, while others exhibited subtle (usually subclinical) resistance to thyrotropin (15, 16), antidiuretic hormone (17), and gonadotropins (18, 19). The apparently generalized nature of the N-protein defect in PHP-Ia predicts that these patients will show resistance to multiple hormones whose effects are mediated by cAMP. Table 1 shows that this prediction has proven correct.

PHP-Ia patients often exhibit clinically significant hypothyroidism, which is usually mild. Most of these patients exhibit elevated basal serum thyrotropin (TSH) and an exaggerated TSH response to administration of thyrotropin-releasing hormone (TRH), which indicates primary resistance of the thyroid gland to TSH stimulation (15, 16). Responsiveness to other hormones in PHP-Ia patients is usually sufficient to prevent clinically significant disease, although careful studies can reveal reduced responses—e.g. reduction of the plasma cAMP response to glucagon (20, 21) or mild impairment of urinary concentration upon water deprivation (10).

Some of the observations listed in Table 1 will require further investigation before firm conclusions can be made. Two laboratories reported decreased responsiveness of plasma prolactin to administration of TRH or phenothiazines in PHP-I (18, 22), whereas a third laboratory reported normal prolactin responses (21). In addition, it is not clear whether or not patients with the PHP-Ib phenotype are at risk of hypothyroidism (see Table 1).

Phenotypic Variability

Clinically, PHP-I patients can express a variety of distinct functional and morphologic abnormalities within a wide spectrum of severity. Assays of

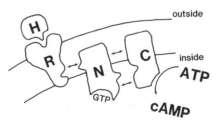

Figure 1   Components of hormone-sensitive adenylate cyclase in the plasma membrane. Hormone (H) binding to the receptor (R) induces GTP binding to the N protein (N). Following GTP binding, N protein activates the catalytic unit (C) of adenylate cyclase, which converts ATP to cAMP.

Table 1 Endocrine studies in intact patients

Hormone	Target organ	Response	Fraction of patients exhibiting abnormal response		Reference
			PHP-Ia	PHP-Ib	
TSH	thyroid gland	clinical hypothyroidism	4/5	2/5	10
			5/11	0/3	21
			6/10	4/4	27
			8/16	1/16	37
		exaggerated TSH response to TRH	4/4	0/1	21
			9/10	1/13	37
Gonadotropins	gonads	oligo-/amenorrhea	6/8	0/3	21
			9/13	0/12	37
		basal/stimulated plasma gonadotropins	1/4	0/3	21
			2/13	—	37
Glucagon	liver	plasma cAMP	5/5	2/6	20
			3/4	0/1	21
		plasma glucose	0/5	0/6	20
			0/4	0/1	21
ADH	kidney	urine concentration and plasma ADH after water deprivation	3/3	2/4	10
TRH	pituitary gland	prolactin	3/5	2/5	10
			0/12	0/11	37

N-protein activity in PHP-I have shed light on some sources of this variability.

Ten years after the original report of PHP, Albright et al (23) described varied morphologic findings in patients with chemical PHP (hypocalcemia and resistance to PTH), and reported a patient who was normocalcemic despite being resistant to the phosphaturic effect of parenteral parathyroid extract and who showed typical morphologic features of AHO. They named this variant of the syndrome "pseudo-pseudohypoparathyroidism" (PPHP). The designation of PPHP should now be discarded, in view of subsequent observations indicating that PHP and PPHP are in fact different manifestations of the same disease: (a) Families may include normo- and hypocalcemic members, all of whom exhibit AHO (24). (b) Patients with AHO and hypocalcemia may spontaneously become normocalcemic (25, 26). (c) In families with PHP-Ia, erythrocyte N protein is reduced equivalently in normo- and hypocalcemic family members with AHO while N-protein activity is normal in family members without AHO (27). Thus, variability in clinical presentation occurs not only within affected families, but also in the same patient at different times.

Radiologically, bone of PHP patients may present a picture consistent with normal calcium homeostasis, hypoparathyroidism, or even—in a small number of cases—hyperparathyroidism (28). Thus, bone in PHP patients may respond poorly or normally to the increased serum PTH. The reasons for this variability have not yet been determined; N-protein assays have not been systematically applied to subgroups of patients with different radiologic manifestations of the disorder.

Alterations in the vitamin D status of an individual PHP patient may introduce phenotypic variability. PTH stimulates 1-alpha-hydroxylation of 25-hydroxyvitamin D to form the biologically active form, 1-alpha,25-dihydroxyvitamin D (29). Some (30) but not all (31) cases of "classic PHP" exhibit deficient 1-alpha-hydroxylation of vitamin D. Vitamin D deficiency can produce apparent partial resistance to PTH (32, 33), and vitamin D administration restores serum calcium and urinary phosphate to normal in PHP. Based on these observations, it is likely that the vitamin D status of an individual patient may determine the appearance of clinically significant hypocalcemia. In addition to this and other environmental factors, the genetic background of a PHP patient may alter phenotypic expression of defective N-protein activity, much as sickle/thalassemia hemoglobinopathy differs clinically from sickle cell disease, sickle cell trait, and thalassemia.

Finally, assays of erythrocyte N-protein activity clearly show that the presence of AHO in PHP-I patients correlates with the PHP-Ia phenotype, whereas PHP-Ib patients (those with normal erythrocyte N-protein activity) frequently show none of the manifestations of AHO (27).

Genetics

The rarity and variable severity of PHP-I make definition of its mode of inheritance difficult. Different investigators have proposed X-linked dominant (24), autosomal dominant (34), and autosomal recessive (35) transmission of the disorder. A recent review (36) concluded that no consistent pattern of inheritance can be defined, although most pedigrees are consistent with autosomal dominant inheritance. Determinations of N-protein activity show that inheritance of the biochemical defect in erythrocytes, like the clinical manifestations, can follow either an autosomal dominant or an autosomal recessive pattern (27). Thus at least two (genetically) distinct mechanisms can produce phenotypic N-protein deficiency and PHP-Ia.

PHP-Ib is clearly a different biochemical entity from PHP-Ia. The molecular defect in PHP-I patients with normal N-protein activity is undefined, and this disorder may be heterogenous. One reported PHP-Ib family showed an autosomal dominant pattern of inheritance (27).

Approach to the Patient

Before instituting therapy for possible PHP, a thorough physical examination and several serum PTH determinations with concomitant serum calcium, phosphate, and magnesium levels are mandatory. The diagnosis must be firmly established because it commits the patient to lifelong vitamin D therapy and monitoring of serum calcium, and because it establishes a risk of genetic transmission of the disease to offspring. For these reasons, serum 25-hydroxyvitamin D must be measured to exclude vitamin D deficiency as the cause of elevated PTH with hypocalcemia. If 25-hydroxyvitamin D is normal, the phosphaturic and urinary cAMP response to PTH(1–34), a synthetic, biologically active fragment of PTH that will probably soon be commercially available, will designate the patient as Type I or Type II. Results of these tests will reduce misdiagnosis of PHP and aid in genetic counseling. Assays of N protein in erythrocytes, currently available only on a research basis, may prove useful for genetic counseling and for early detection of the disease in infants who are genetically at risk.

Most patients with PHP are easily treated with dihydrotachysterol or 1-alpha,25-dihydroxyvitamin D. Vitamin D intoxication remains a serious complication of vitamin D therapy but the risk of this complication can be minimized by measuring serum calcium regularly and maintaining serum calcium between 8 and 9 mg/dl. Regular evaluation of thyroid function is necessary, in view of the high incidence of hypothyroidism in PHP (Table 1).

Summary

PHP is a genotypically diverse group of diseases that present with a similar phenotype—hypocalcemia and post-receptor resistance to the action of PTH. Phenotypic expression of these genetic defects varies greatly between families, within families, and even during the clinical course of individual patients. Further elucidation of the underlying biochemical abnormalities of the disease may lead to more specific therapy for the various subgroups of PHP.

Although PHP is a rare disease, continued thorough evaluation of affected patients and studies of their cells will lead to a better understanding of interactions between hormone receptors and adenylate cyclase, and to new insights into the intracellular action of cAMP.

ACKNOWLEDGMENTS

This work was supported by NIH grants (GM27800 and GM28310) and a grant from the March of Dimes. C. Van Dop is supported by the Johnson & Johnson Institute for Pediatric Service.

Literature Cited

1. Albright, F., Burnett, C. H., Smith, P. H., Parsons, W. 1942. Pseudo-hypoparathyroidism—an example of "Seabright-Bantam Syndrome." Report of three cases. *Endocrinology* 30:922–32
2. Steinbach, H. L., Young, D. A. 1966. The Roentgen appearance of pseudohypoparathyroidism (PH) and pseudopseudohypoparathyroidism (PPH). Differentiation from other syndromes associated with short metacarpals, metatarsals, and phalanges. *Am. J. Roentgenol. Ther. Nucl. Med.* 97:49–66
3. Tashjian, A. H. Jr., Frantz, A. G., Lee, J. B. 1966. Pseudohypoparathyroidism: assays of parathyroid hormone and thyrocalcitonin. *Proc. Natl. Acad. Sci. USA* 56:1138–42
4. Chase, L. R., Melson, G. L., Aurbach, G. D. 1969. Pseudohypoparathyroidism: defective excretion of 3',5',-AMP in response to parathyroid hormone. *J. Clin. Invest.* 48:1832–44
5. Bell, N. H., Avery, S., Sinha, T., Clark, C. M. Jr., Allen, D. O., Johnston, C. Jr. 1972. Effects of dibutyryl cyclic adenosine 3',5'-monophosphate and parathyroid extract on calcium and phosphorus metabolism in hypoparathyroidism and pseudohypoparathyroidism. *J. Clin. Invest.* 51:816–23
6. Drezner, M., Neelon, F. A., Lebovitz, H. E. 1973. Pseudohypoparathyroidism Type II: a possible defect in the reception of the cyclic AMP signal. *N. Engl. J. Med.* 289:1056–60
7. Drezner, M. K., Burch, W. M. Jr. 1978. Altered activity of the nucleotide regulatory site in the parathyroid hormone sensitive adenylate cyclase from the renal cortex of a patient with pseudohypoparathyroidism. *J. Clin. Invest.* 62:1222–27
8. Ross, E. M., Gilman, A. G. 1977. Reconstitution of catecholamine-sensitive adenylate cyclase activity: interaction of solubilized components with receptor-replete membranes. *Proc. Natl. Acad. Sci. USA* 74:3715–19
9. Johnson, G. L., Kaslow, H. R., Farfel, Z., Bourne, H. R. 1980. Genetic analysis of hormone-sensitive adenylate cyclase. In *Advances in Cyclic Nucleotide Research*, ed. P. Greengard, G. A. Robison 13:1–38. New York: Raven. 342 pp.
10. Farfel, Z., Brickman, A. S., Kaslow, H. R., Brothers, V. M., Bourne, H. R. 1980. Defect of receptor-cyclase coupling protein in pseudohypoparathyroidism. *N. Engl. J. Med.* 303:237–42
11. Levine, M. A., Downs, R. W. Jr., Singer, M., Marx, S. J., Aurbach, G. D., Spiegel, A. M. 1980. Deficient activity of guanine nucleotide regulatory protein in erythrocytes from patients with pseudohypoparathyroidism. *Biochem. Biophys. Res. Commun.* 94:1319–24
12. Farfel, Z., Bourne, H. R. 1980. Deficient activity of receptor-cyclase coupling protein in platelets of patients with pseudohypoparathyroidism. *J. Clin. Endocrinol. Metab.* 51:1202–4
13. Bourne, H. R., Kaslow, H. R., Brickman, A. S., Farfel, Z. 1981. Fibroblast defect in pseudohypoparathyroidism Type I: reduced activity of receptor-cyclase coupling protein. *J. Clin. Endocrinol. Metab.* 53:636–40
14. Farfel, Z., Abood, M. E., Brickman, A. S., Bourne, H. R. 1982. Deficient activity of receptor-cyclase coupling protein in transformed lymphoblasts of patients with pseudohypoparathyroidism, Type I. *J. Clin. Endocrinol. Metab.* 55:113–17
15. Marx, S. J., Hershman, J. M., Aurbach, G. D. 1971. Thyroid dysfunction in pseudohypoparathyroidism. *J. Clin. Endocrinol. Metab.* 33:822–28
16. Werder, E. A., Illig, R., Bernasconi, S., Kind, H., Prader, A., Fischer, J. A., Fanconi, A. 1975. Excessive thyrotropin response to thyrotropin-releasing hormone in pseudohypoparathyroidism. *Pediatr. Res.* 9:12–16
17. Brickman, A. S., Weitzman, R. E. 1977. Renal resistance to arginine vasopressin in pseudohypoparathyroidism. *Clin. Res.* 26:164A
18. Shapiro, M. S., Bernheim, J., Gutman, A., Arber, I., Spitz, I. M. 1980. Multiple abnormalities of anterior pituitary hormone secretion in association with pseudohypoparathyroidism. *J. Clin. Endocrinol. Metab.* 51:483–87
19. Wolfsdorf, J. I., Rosenfield, R. L., Fang, V. S., Kobayashi, R., Razdan, A. K., Kim, M. H. 1978. Partial gonadotrophin-resistance in pseudohypoparathyroidism. *Acta Endocrinol. (Copenhagen)* 88:321–28
20. Brickman, A. S., Carlson, H. E., Raghavan, S., Williams, A., Katz, M., Levin, S. R. 1981. Glucagon resistance in pseudohypoparathyroidism. *Endocrinology* 108:177 (Suppl.)
21. Levine, M. A., Downs, R. W. Jr., Marx, S. J., Lasker, R. D., Aurbach, G. D., Spiegel, A. M. 1981. Clinical and biochemical features of pseudohypoparathyroidism. In *Hormonal Control of*

Calcium Metabolism, ed. D. V. Cohn, et al, pp. 95–101. Amsterdam: Excerpta Medica. 506 pp.

22. Carlson, H. E., Brickman, A. S., Bottazzo, G. F. 1977. Prolactin deficiency in pseudohypoparathyroidism. *N. Engl. J. Med.* 296:140–44

23. Albright, F., Forbes, A. P., Henneman, P. H. 1952. Pseudo-pseudohypoparathyroidism. *Trans. Assoc. Am. Physicians* 65:337–50

24. Mann, J. B., Alterman, S., Hills, A. G. 1962. Albright's hereditary osteodystrophy comprising pseudohypoparathyroidism and pseudo-pseudohypoparathyroidism with a report of two cases representing the complete syndrome occurring in successive generations. *Ann. Intern. Med.* 56:315–42

25. Palubinskas, A. J., Davies, H. 1959. Calcification of the basal ganglia of the brain. *Am. J. Roentgenol. Ther. Nucl. Med.* 82:806–22

26. Gershberg, H., Weseley, A. C. 1960. Pseudohypoparathyroidism and pregnancy. *J. Pediatr.* 56:383–86

27. Farfel, Z., Brothers, V. M., Brickman, A. S., Conte, F., Neer, R., Bourne, H. R. 1981. Pseudohypoparathyroidism: inheritance of deficient receptor-cyclase coupling activity. *Proc. Natl. Acad. Sci. USA* 78:3098–3102

28. Kidd, G. S., Schaaf, M., Adler, R. A., Lassman, M. N., Wray, H. L. 1980. Skeletal responsiveness in pseudohypoparathyroidism—a spectrum of clinical disease. *Am. J. Med.* 68:772–81

29. Kooh, S. W., Fraser, D., DeLuca, H. F., Holick, M. F., Belsey, R. E., Clark, M. B., Murray, T. M. 1975. Treatment of hypoparathyroidism and pseudohypoparathyroidism with metabolites of vitamin D: Evidence for impaired conversion of 25-hydroxyvitamin D to 1-alpha,25-dihydroxyvitamin D. *N. Engl. J. Med.* 293:840–44

30. Lambert, P. W., Hollis, B. W., Bell, N. H., Epstein, S. 1980. Demonstration of a lack of change in serum 1-alpha,25-dihydroxyvitamin D in response to parathyroid extract in pseudohypoparathyroidism. *J. Clin. Invest.* 66:782–91

31. Aksnes, L., Aarskog, D. 1980. Effect of parathyroid hormone on 1,25-dihydroxyvitamin D formation in Type I pseudohypoparathyroidism. *J. Clin. Endocrinol. Metab.* 51:1223–26

32. Stogmann, W., Fischer, J. A. 1975. Pseudohypoparathyroidism: disappearance of the resistance to parathyroid extract during treatment with vitamin D. *Am. J. Med.* 59:140–44

33. Metz, S. A., Baylink, D. J., Hughes, M. R., Haussler, M. R., Robertson, R. P. 1977. Selective deficiency of 1,25-dihydroxycholecalciferol: a cause of isolated skeletal resistance to parathyroid hormone. *N. Engl. J. Med.* 297:1084–90

34. Weinberg, A. G., Stone, R. T. 1971. Autosomal dominant inheritance in Albright's hereditary osteodystrophy. *J. Pediatr.* 79:996–99

35. Cedarbaum, S. D., Lippe, B. M. 1973. Probable autosomal recessive inheritance in a family with Albright's hereditary osteodystrophy and an evaluation of the genetics of the disorder. *Am. J. Hum. Genet.* 25:638–45

36. Drezner, M. K., Neelon, F. A. 1982. Pseudohypoparathyroidism. In *The Metabolic Basis of Inherited Disease*, ed. J. D. Stanbury et al. New York: McGraw-Hill. In press

37. Levine, M. A., Downs, R. W. Jr., Moses, A. M., Breslau, N. A., Marx, S. J., Lasker, R. D., Rizzoli, R. E., Aurbach, G. D., Spiegel, A. M. 1982. Resistance to multiple hormones in patients with pseudohypoparathyroidism and deficient guanine nucleotide regulatory protein. *Am. J. Med.* In press

Ann. Rev. Med. 1983. 34:267–81

PATHOGENESIS OF HYPERTHYROIDISM[1]

Inder J. Chopra, M.D., and David H. Solomon, M.D.

Department of Medicine, UCLA Center for the Health Sciences, University of California, Los Angeles, California 90024

ABSTRACT

Graves' disease is the most frequent cause of hyperthyroidism in the United States. It occurs predominantly in a genetically predisposed population. Autoimmune abnormalities constitute a major component of the disease. Immunoglobulins of patients with Graves' disease manifest a number of thyroid-targeted activities, including a thyroid-stimulating activity that is related to interaction of immunoglobulin G (IgG) with the TSH receptor. That hyperthyroidism in Graves' disease is caused by thyroid-stimulating IgGs is an attractive hypothesis but the evidence in favor of the hypothesis is still insufficient. A better alternative hypothesis is not available, however.

Introduction

The term hyperthyroidism may be defined as the clinical state resulting from supranormal concentrations of thyroid hormones in the circulation. It may be caused by any one of the following: (*a*) Graves' disease, (*b*) toxic multinodular goiter, (*c*) toxic solitary nodule ("hot" nodule), (*d*) ingestion of thyroid hormones (thyrotoxicosis factitia), (*e*) subacute thyroiditis, (*f*) chronic thyroiditis, (*g*) TSH-producing pituitary adenoma, (*h*) trophoblastic tumors (choriocarcinoma or hydatidiform mole), (*i*) thyroid carcinoma, or (*j*) struma ovarii.

In this presentation, we review only the pathogenesis of Graves' hyperthyroidism. We do so in order to focus on the disease most commonly responsible for hyperthyroidism and to simplify our task. It has been estimated that Graves' disease is the cause of a great majority of hyperthyroi-

[1]Supported by USPHS Grant AM16155 from the NIH.

267

dism in the US. Graves' disease is believed at present to be an autoimmune disease occurring in a genetically predisposed population. It is identified by one or more of the following three clinical syndromes: hyperthyroidism due to diffuse hyperplasia of the thyroid gland, infiltrative ophthalmopathy, and infiltrative dermopathy.

Autoimmunity

There is substantial evidence to suggest alterations in the immune system in Graves' disease. Sera of Graves' disease patients commonly contain immunoglobulins, (IgGs) that stimulate the thyroid gland of humans and experimental animals in vivo and in vitro (1–6), called thyroid-stimulating IgG (TSI) or thyroid-stimulating antibody (TSAb), and/or IgG that inhibits binding of thyrotropin (TSH) to thyroid membranes, called thyrotropin-binding inhibitory immunoglobulin (TBII). Antithyroglobulin and/or antimicrosomal antibodies are detectable in essentially all cases (7). Thymic hyperplasia, enlargement of lymph nodes and spleen, lymphocytosis, infiltration of the thyroid gland and retro-orbital tissues with lymphocytes and deposits of IgG, IgE, and IgM in the thyroid basement membrane are also features of the disease (8, 9). Additionally, Graves' disease frequently coexists with other autoimmune diseases including Hashimoto's thyroiditis, pernicious anemia, idiopathic adrenal insufficiency, myasthenia gravis, and systemic lupus erythematosus (see 8, 10–12 for reviews).

Table 1 examines the available evidence for autoimmunity in Graves' disease viewed in light of the postulates of Milgrom & Witebsky (13). Cell-mediated immunity as well as antibodies against thyroid elements are well documented in Graves' disease (7, 10). Lymphocytes of Graves' disease patients may stimulate, albeit modestly, bovine thyroid cells in vitro (14). Thyroid-stimulating IgGs are present in sera of most Graves' disease patients. It is suspected that the antigen for TSIs is the TSH receptor in the thyroid plasma membrane, but areas of the membrane close to the receptor may also be involved (15, 16). Some evidence is available to suggest that thyroid-stimulating antibodies may be produced by immunization of rabbits with thyroid plasma membranes (17). However, no data are available to suggest that clinical or pathological changes characteristic of Graves' disease are produced in experimental animals so immunized. There is at present no experimental model of persistent Graves' disease produced by infusion of Graves' sera. However, TSIs do go across the placenta from the mother to the fetus and appear responsible for the syndrome of neonatal thyrotoxicosis. Overall then, available information is quite suggestive that Graves' hyperthyroidism is an autoimmune disorder. However, more information is needed for one to be certain.

Table 1 Graves' disease: autoimmune pathogenesis

Milgrom-Witebsky postulate	Postulate satisfied	Evidence
Circulating antibody or cellular immune reaction in patients	yes	Thyroid-stimulating IgGs, antithyroglobulin, antimicrosomal antibody, cell-mediated immunity (1–7, 10)
A specific antigen in the affected tissue	yes	Microsomes, thyroglobulin, membrane, ? TSH-receptor (4, 7, 14)
Production of antibody in experimental animals by immunization with antigen	±	Some suggestive evidence is available for production of thyroid-stimulating IgGs (17)
Production of the disease in an immunized animal	no	No experimental model for Graves' disease is available
Passive transfer of the disease with serum or immunologically competent cells	±	Yes, if neonatal hyperthyroidism in the offspring of Graves' patients is due to placental transfer of thyroid-stimulating IgGs
		Although transient thyroid activation has been observed, persistent Graves' disease has not yet been produced by infusion of Graves' sera to normal subjects or experimental animals (18, 19)

Genetic Predisposition

Several lines of evidence suggest that genetic predisposition contributes importantly to the pathogenesis of Graves' disease and chronic (Hashimoto's) thyroiditis, another common disorder wherein autoimmunity plays an important role. Concurrence of Graves' disease and Hashimoto's thyroiditis is well documented in identical twins (20). In Graves' disease, the concordance rate is about 50% in monozygotic twins and about 9% in dizygotic twins of the same sex (11). In nonconcordant monozygotic pairs with Graves' disease, the euthyroid twin frequently has a goiter and positive antithyroid antibodies. Thyroid-stimulating IgG may also be demonstrated in the serum of a euthyroid twin of thyrotoxic patients (21). The genetic transmission of Graves' disease and Hashimoto's thyroiditis is thought to be polygenic and both diseases appear to be inherited equally from mother or father (22–26).

Incidence of Graves' disease was estimated to be 0.4% in the general population in a Danish study. It was increased about 20-fold in sisters and daughters of patients with Graves' disease. The incidence was increased to about nine times that in the general population in mothers and to about six times that in the general population even in second-degree relatives, such as maternal aunts. The incidence of Graves' disease in the male family members of the propositi did not differ significantly from that in the general population in this study (22). Others have also observed autoimmune thyroid disease much more commonly in women than in men. In a population survey in Whickham, located in Durham County close to Newcastle-upon-Tyne, England, the prevalence of established hyperthyroidism was 19 per 1000 women and 1.6 per 1000 men (27). Similarly, the prevalence of overt hypothyroidism was 14 per 1000 women and less than 1 per 1000 men. The prevalence of antithyroid antibodies was also about four-fold higher in women than in men (antithyroglobulin antibody, 3% vs 0.9%; antimicrosomal antibody 10.3% vs 2.7%). Additionally, the frequency of antithyroglobulin antibody increased with age in women from 1% below the age of 45 yr to 4.6% in the 45–54-yr age group and 7.4% at age 75 and above; there was no such increase in the incidence of antithyroid antibodies with age in men.

Both Graves' disease and Hashimoto's thyroiditis can present as a part of a multiple endocrine deficiency syndrome involving the adrenals, parathyroids, pancreas, and gonads. Gastric and cutaneous lesions, as well as mucocutaneous candidiasis, may accompany the endocrine disease. The common denominator of all these states appears to be organ-specific disorders of autoimmune origin. The various members of a family may suffer from similar as well as different components of the syndrome, which suggests that a genetic tendency may play an important part in the manifestations of the multiple endocrine deficiency syndrome (28).

While these several observations suggest that heredity contributes importantly to the pathogenesis of Graves' disease and Hashimoto's thyroiditis, the mechanisms responsible for the unusual propensity of some families for autoimmune thyroid disease are not clear at this time. A crucial finding was made by Grumet et al (28, 29), who discovered a supranormal frequency of a human leukocyte antigen in histocompatibility locus HLA-B8 in caucasian and HLA-BW35 in oriental patients with Graves' disease. Hence the susceptibility of Graves' relatives to the disease might be due to the inheritance of certain HLA antigens.

There is some evidence that, in humans, the locus for the antigens detected by mixed lymphocyte culture is nearer to the hypothetical "immune response gene" than are the other HLA loci. Recently, techniques were devised for serological diagnosis of D-related (or DRW) antigens that apparently correspond with the area of immune response genes on chromosome 6 (31, 32). Available data indicate that the frequency of DRW3 antigens is abnormal in Graves' disease to a much greater degree than HLA-B8. Farid et al (31) calculated that the risk of Graves' disease is increased by a factor of 2.81 if HLA-B8 is positive and by a factor of 6 if HLA-DRW3 is positive. They suggested that the susceptibility gene for

Graves' disease is in strong linkage disequilibrium with DRW3 and possibly with other DRW antigens (31, 32).

Searches for related genetic markers have unearthed a possible relationship between certain Gm allotypes (i.e. antigens on the heavy chain of IgG) and Graves' hyperthyroidism (33–35). However, the allotypic Gm markers commonly found in Graves' disease are also common in normal subjects, a finding that tends to detract from their significance. In any case, newer studies emphasize the linkage of susceptibility to Graves' hyperthyroidism within families to HLA and Gm allotypes (33–35).

Graves' Hyperthyroidism

Many theories have been considered to explain the mechanism of hyperthyroidism of Graves' disease. The reader is referred to Reference 12 for a recent detailed review. Only the issues popular in the last 25 years are considered here.

In the 1950s, hyperthyroidism in Graves' disease was suspected to be the result of a hyperfunctional pituitary elaborating increased amounts of thyrotropin (TSH). However, serum TSH and TSH response to thyrotropin-releasing hormone (TRH) were later found to be subnormal (rather than supranormal) in Graves' hyperthyroidism. That exogenous administration of thyroid hormones does not suppress thyroid function in Graves' disease, as it does normally, also suggested that factors other than pituitary TSH are responsible for the maintenance of hyperthyroidism (36, 37). Nonsuppressibility of thyroid function is correctly considered a hallmark of Graves' disease.

Subsequent studies examined the possibility that hyperthyroidism is caused by an intrinsic abnormality within the thyroid cell. However, thyroidal adenylate cyclase, 3',5',cyclic adenosine monophosphate (cAMP), and the components of the protein kinase system are all quite normal in Graves' disease (38). More recent studies show the cAMP content of Graves' thyroid glands to be supranormal (39). This is attributable to persistent stimulation of the gland by a circulating thyroid stimulator (*vide infra*) rather than to an intrinsic thyroid abnormality.

The possibility that an abnormal circulating thyroid stimulator is responsible for Graves' hyperthyroidism is certainly the most attractive hypothesis at this time. Adams & Purves (40) were the first to show the presence of a long-acting thyroid stimulator (LATS) in sera of Graves' disease patients. This activity was assayed routinely by the McKenzie assay in mice (41). LATS was subsequently characterized as an immunoglobulin G (42) and was generally considered the cause of Graves' hyperthyroidism until 1970, when many weaknesses in the hypothesis became evident. Thus, many patients with frank hyperthyroidism showed no LATS in their serum, while others with minimal or no hyperthyroidism showed large amounts of it. Furthermore, the prevalence of LATS in the serum of untreated hyperthyroid patients did not exceed 65% despite rigorous concentration procedures. While one could attribute these difficulties to the insensitivity of the bioassay, more damaging to the LATS hypothesis were the lack of correlation between either the presence or the level of LATS in serum of Graves' disease patients and the severity of the hyperthyroidism or the presence of nonsuppressibility of thyroid function (43, 44).

Since the idea of an abnormal thyroid stimulator as the cause of hyperthyroidism was basically attractive, investigators wondered whether the above-mentioned difficulties with the LATS hypothesis were related to the fact that LATS is measured by a bioassay in the mice and that the thyroid stimulator important in Graves' disease might be directed specifically at a human thyroid receptor. This line of reasoning led many groups to develop assay systems for detection of stimulators of the human thyroid in sera (and IgG) of Graves' disease patients. Several such stimulators were indeed documented. Discussion below examines the available evidence concerning their role in the pathogenesis of Graves' hyperthyroidism.

Human Thyroid-Stimulating Activity

Several different approaches have been undertaken to study the interaction between Graves' IgGs and the human thyroid plasma membrane and/or TSH receptor. These approaches led to several assay systems that detect thyroid-directed activities in Graves' IgGs, and several terms have been employed to describe the individual activities:

1. *Thyroid-stimulating IgGs:* This term is often used in a collective sense to describe a variety of thyroid-target activities in IgGs of Graves' disease patients.
2. *LATS-protector activity* (LPA) (2, 45): LPA is an activity in LATS-negative Graves' IgG that inhibits neutralization and presumably binding of LATS by human thyroid membranes.
3. *TSH-binding-inhibiting activity* (TBIA) (4, 46): This reflects the ability of Graves' IgG to inhibit binding of radioiodinated bovine TSH to human thyroid membranes. The terms TDA (TSH-displacing activity), TBII (TSH-binding inhibiting IgG) and TBIAb (TSH-binding inhibiting antibody) have also been used.
4. *Thyroid-stimulating activity* (TSA) (5, 6, 47–49): This term is used to describe the ability of Graves' IgGs to stimulate human thyroid adenyl cyclase or colloid droplet formation. HTS (for human thyroid stimulator) and TSAb (for thyroid-stimulating antibody) are additional terms that are used.

It was the demonstration of LPA that first made plausible the hypothesis that LATS is a mouse thyroid-stimulating activity of little direct relevance to human hyperthyroidism; the important immunoglobulin would be one that interacted with the *human* thyroid. LPA is demonstrated in the standard McKenzie bioassay by showing that a test IgG inhibits neutralization of a standard LATS preparation by human thyroid membranes. Whereas LATS is found in only about 30% of unconcentrated sera from patients with untreated Graves' disease, LPA can be demonstrated in 90% (2, 45, 50).

Infusion of LPA-positive, LATS-negative Graves' sera into normal subjects whose glands have been labeled with radioiodine enhances release of thyroidal radioiodine (18). Since we know now that LATS-negative Graves' sera may contain several thyroid-stimulating activities, it is unclear whether or not the phenomenon just described is due to LPA per se or another associated activity, e.g. TSA. Adams et al (51) reported a good correlation between LPA and thyroid radioiodine uptake. However, Shishiba et al (52) observed persistence of nonsuppressibility of thyroid radioiodine uptake even when LPA was undetectable in four Graves' disease patients rendered euthyroid by antithyroid drugs. Nonsuppressibility of thyroid function in the absence of detectable LPA was also observed by Solomon et al (50) in patients with euthyroid Graves' ophthalmopathy. These data may only mean that the sensitivity of LPA assay is insufficient. However, since the LPA assay detected LPA in 90% of patients with untreated Graves' disease, nonsuppressibility in Graves' disease may well result from factors other than circulating LPA. Findings of a study (50) showing that three of eight patients with euthyroid Graves' ophthalmopathy had LPA detectable in their serum supports this notion.

TSH-binding inhibiting activity (TBIA) of Graves' IgG has attracted much attention in the recent years. Its presence in Graves' IgG was first demonstrated by Smith & Hall (4) and Manley and co-workers (53). It is the general consensus now that TBIA is detectable in about 70% of patients with untreated Graves' disease (46, 54). It is difficult to improve upon the sensitivity of the assay by testing larger quantities of IgG because normal IgG interferes with the assay by inhibiting the binding of radioactive TSH to thyroid membranes (55). Furthermore, several non-IgG serum proteins that may contaminate IgG preparations also mimic the TBIA of Graves' IgG (55, 56). TBIA is not as specific for Graves' disease as LPA or LATS. It was detected in a low frequency in Hashimoto's thyroiditis, thyroid carcinoma, subacute thyroiditis, nodular goiter, and even in Addison's disease and juvenile diabetes mellitus (57–60).

TBIA correlates significantly with early (one-hour) thyroid ^{131}I uptake ($r = 0.67$) and early (30-min) ^{99m}Tc uptake ($r = 0.76$) (61, 62). Its levels usually fall during treatment of Graves' hyperthyroidism with antithyroid drugs or surgery (54). However, TBIA increases transiently in the first three months following treatment of hyperthyroidism with radioiodine (54).

Several studies examined TBIA in Graves' disease patients who underwent a course of antithyroid drugs (63–66). TBIA was detected in 91% of patients who relapsed; it was undetectable in 86% of those who remained in remission. However, McGregor et al (54) were dismayed with the reliability of TBIA as an indicator of the course of the disease in individual patients. They found that the course of the disease may be predicted more reliably if one measures both TBIA and HLA-DRW3. HLA-DRW3 was present in 16 (43%) of their 37 Graves' disease patients compared to 26% of 135 controls. Following a six-month course of carbimazole, 25 (68%) patients had relapsed and these included all 16 patients who were positive for HLA-DRW3. TBIA was detected in only 2 of these 16 patients. It was detected, however, in all of the remaining 9 patients who relapsed. Overall, TBIA was undetectable in 14 of 25 patients who relapsed and in all 12 patients who remained in remission during 12 months of observation following cessation of antithyroid drug therapy (54). The authors concluded that HLA-DRW3 invariably predicts relapse and that the presence of TBIA in HLA-DRW3-negative patients also predicts relapse.

The finding that TBIA may be negative in up to 56% (14 of 25) who relapse is disconcerting. It suggests the possibility that thyroidal hyperactivity and autononomy in Graves' disease are maintained by factors other than TBIA. Other studies also support this consideration. Schleusner et al (63) reported clearly detectable TBIA in three Graves' disease patients who had become euthyroid and normally suppressible following treatment with antithyroid drugs. Ozawa et al (46) described another similar case. These data seriously limit the significance of TBIA per se as the cause of Graves' hyperthyroidism. One could conceivably defend the causative role of TBIA, however, by considering that the lack of correlation between TBIA and nonsuppressibility in the above situations reflects the existence in some patients of excessive amounts of anti-TSH receptor antibodies that bind to the receptor but do not stimulate it. It must be recalled, however, that TBIA is detected by in vitro assays under quite unphysiological (e.g. hypotonic) conditions (4, 46). The possibility cannot be ruled out that the TBIA detected by the assay in general use may not even bind to the TSH receptor in vivo.

Study of thyroid-stimulating activity (TSA) in Graves' IgG is more pertinent to understanding of thyroidal autonomy and hyperactivity than that of LPA or TBIA, which pertain to the ability of Graves' IgG to bind to thyroid membranes. Human TSA in Graves' IgG was first described in 1973 by two independent groups. Onaya et al (47) and Shishiba et al (48) both observed that LATS-negative Graves' IgGs can stimulate formation of intracellular colloid droplets in human thyroid slices in vitro. Onaya et al also showed stimulation of thyroidal cAMP. Study of cAMP in human thyroid slices incubated with Graves' IgGs has been a popular assay for TSA in recent years (6, 67). A similar procedure has also been applied to crude thyroid plasma membranes (5), but it is less sensitive than the slice system. More recently, TSA has been studied using human thyroid cells in culture but the experience to date remains quite limited (68–70). Assay for TSA is actually impractical in studies using thyroid slices because each study requires fresh human tissue.

TSA may be detected in IgG of 80–92% of patients with untreated Graves' disease (6). There was little change in detectability of TSA during the first three months of antithyroid drugs in one study (6); in another, TSA disappeared very quickly within 4–6 weeks after initiation of therapy, regardless of T_3 suppressibility (67). In a study of 28 Graves' disease patients who received antithyroid drugs for a mean period of 26 months (range 4–48 months), Zakarija et al (6) found positive TSA in 12 cases and all relapsed during 0.25–10 months of follow-up. On the other hand, 13 of 16 who were without detectable TSA stayed in remission during 15–39 months (mean 26 months) of follow-up. Frequency of positive TSA is less in euthyroid Graves' ophthalmopathy than in untreated hyperthyroidism, but patients with positive TSA consistently show nonsuppressibility of thyroid function and/or subnormal thyrotropin response to thyrotropin-releasing hormone. Zakarija et al also reported on a modest experience with TSA in pregnancy. They observed that a high level of TSA consistently forecasts neonatal hyperthyroidism (6).

Few data are available on the relationship between TSA, on the one hand, and degree of hyperthyroidism, goiter size, or thyroidal nonsuppressibility, on the other hand. Nagataki and co-workers (67, 68) were impressed with the lack of relationship between TSA and nonsuppressibility. Surprisingly, they found nonsuppressibility of thyroid function to correlate better with TBIA than with TSA. Additionally, cAMP levels in thyroid glands of Graves' disease patients who had received 75 μg of T_3 daily for 5 days prior to surgery did not correlate significantly with levels of TSA in the serum (39, 68). Since thyroidal phosphodiesterase activity is essentially normal in Graves' disease, these data raise the possibility that factors other than TSA may have an important influence on the thyroidal adenylate cyclase activity in Graves' disease.

The cAMP-increasing activity of Graves' IgG is considered important because it may reflect thyroid-hormone-release-stimulating activity of the

IgG. However, recent direct studies of this activity cast some doubt on this relationship. Nagataki and co-workers (68) noted curious dissociations between the effects of Graves' IgG on cAMP concentrations and release of T_3 in short-term incubations of human thyroid slices. They observed that release of T_3 did not increase initially despite marked increases in thyroid cAMP concentrations. Release of T_3 did increase gradually and became significant only on the fourth and fifth days of incubation. Much still remains to be learned concerning the pathogenetic significance of circulating thyroid stimulators in Graves' hyperthyroidism. The situation is complicated by unavailability of a simple, practical, precise, and sensitive assay for measurement of thyroid stimulators and by the finding that some Graves' IgGs can actually inhibit thyroidal response to thyroid stimulators (5, 61).

Several investigators have attempted to determine whether the various thyroid-stimulating and/or TSH-binding-inhibiting activities in Graves' IgGs are the same or different. The results of the studies are conflicting and confusing. One problem is that each method of study has large methodologic errors, and correlation coefficients would be low even if all methods were actually measuring the effects of the same molecule. Additionally, studies of relationship of LATS with other human thyroid-directed activities of Graves' IgGs are complicated by the frequent undetectability of LATS. If LATS-positive cases are selected, there is a moderately strong correlation between LATS and TBIA (46) or TSA (5). However, studies indicate that TSA may become clearly undetectable while TBIA changes little in Graves' disease patients receiving treatment with antithyroid drugs, which suggests that TSA and TBIA are the activities of different IgGs that frequently coexist in Graves' disease. Others have postulated that Graves' IgGs represent a polyclonal response to immunization by a human thyroid antigen and that differences in levels of TSA and LATS activity in Graves' sera represent variations in the cross reaction of antihuman TSH-receptor antibody with nonhuman thyroid antigens (3). This consideration does not explain differences in levels of TSA and TBIA.

It should be emphasized that TBIIs are demonstrated by their ability to bind and TSAbs by their ability to stimulate. In some autoimmune systems (e.g. anti-insulin-receptor antibodies, anti-acetylcholine-receptor antibodies), the ability to bind and to stimulate are dissociable. The unifying concept is that all antireceptor antibodies bind to (or near) the receptor, but some can form an activating complex with the receptor while others cannot. If the latter occupy or alter enough of the active site, they become, of necessity, inhibitory or so-called blocking antibodies. Thus, a binding assay would be expected to identify both stimulatory and inhibitory antibodies against the TSH receptor or its neighbors, whereas a stimulation assay could only detect stimulatory antibodies. If many Graves' sera contain both types of antibodies, a great deal of the apparent failure of correlation among the various assay systems could be explained. This hypothesis suggests, further, that the precise antigenic specificity of these two types of antibodies might be different. For example, the stimulators might be directed at the active site of the TSH receptor, the site of hormone-receptor interaction, while the inhibitors might be directed at a different but closely linked molecule. If so, more precise binding assays, made feasible by the advent of monoclonal antibodies, might allow clear identification of the two types of thyroid-directed immunoglobulins.

In conclusion, available data concerning pathogenetic significances of circulating thyroid stimulators may be summarized as follows:

1. Graves' IgGs exhibit a variety of thyroid-targeted activities. Whether these activities are due to one or more than one IgG molecule is not known.
2. Graves' IgGs interact with thyroid plasma membranes in or close to the TSH receptor.
3. That hyperthyroidism in Graves' disease is initiated and sustained by the presence of IgG thyroid stimulators in circulation is an attractive hypothesis. However, the evidence presently available does not permit one to clearly associate circulating TSA and hyperthyroidism in a cause-and-effect manner.
4. Positive assays for TSA, TBIA, or LATS at the end of treatment with antithyroid drugs usually predict relapse of hyperthyroidism; negative assays usually correlate with persistence of remission. Prediction of the course of the disease may be further improved by measurements of HLA-DRW3. Patients with DRW3 generally relapse regardless of detection of TBIA (and presumably TSA).
5. High circulating TSA (and/or LATS or LATS-P) in maternal serum at term is usually associated with neonatal hyperthyroidism.
6. Further elucidation of the significance of thyroid-directed activities of Graves' IgG in pathogenesis of hyperthyroidism requires a simple, sensitive, precise, and practical assay for human TSA. Available assays do not meet those criteria.

Basis for Altered Immunity

If the underlying predisposition to Graves' disease is genetic, why doesn't the disease manifest itself fully right from birth and why is it the third or fourth decade of life before the incidence of disease reaches its peak? In other words, what is the factor (or factors) that ultimately triggers a break in tolerance to the TSH receptor? Several possibilities may be considered.

1. In a susceptible population there is a genetic predisposition to an abnormality in immune regulation that results in survival of a mutant clone of lymphoid cells directed against key self-antigens, e.g. the TSH receptor. Analysis of age-occurrence data suggests that the probability of events occurring that may precipitate a somatic mutation in lymphocytes changes little with age (71). The mutant lymphocytes may contribute to the disease by elaboration of thyroid-stimulating antibodies, secretion of lymphokines, cytotoxic effects, or a combination of these.
2. The somatic mutation referred to above is brought about by a viral infection (9).
3. There is a change in antigenic structure of some key structures (e.g. the TSH receptor) because of a genetic malfunction and/or an injury (e.g. viral infection) and this change invites an immune response from a normal immune system.
4. Certain antigens normally sequestered are released into circulation following an injury and stir up an immune response from normal immune mechanisms.

Stress is often cited as a precipitating factor of Graves' disease but the mechanism of its effect is not known. Volpe and co-workers (66) suggested that stress acts by increasing secretion of corticotropin-releasing factor, which in turn induces secretion of ACTH and cortisol. Glucocorticoids may inhibit lymphocytic functions, including T-suppressor cell function, and thus bring to full flower a latent deficiency in thyroid-antigen-specific T-suppressor function.

Conclusion

We have reviewed evidence that suggests Graves' disease occurs predominantly in a genetically predisposed population and that autoimmune abnormalities constitute a major component of the disease. Immunoglobulins of patients with Graves' disease manifest a number of thyroid-targeted activities, including thyroid stimulation that appears related to an interaction of IgG with the TSH receptor. That hyperthyroidism in Graves' disease is caused by thyroid-stimulating IgGs is an attractive hypothesis but the evidence in favor of it falls short of absolute proof. It is better than any alternative hypothesis available at present, however.

Literature Cited

1. McKenzie, J. M. 1968. Humoral factors in the pathogenesis of Graves' disease. *Physiol. Rev.* 48:252–310
2. Holmes, S. D., Dirmikis, S. M., Martin, T. J., Munro, D. S. 1979. Evidence that both long-acting thyroid stimulator and long-acting thyroid stimulator-protector stimulate the human thyroid gland, *J. Endocrinol.* 80:215–21
3. McKenzie, J. M., Zakarija, M. 1976. A reconsideration of a thyroid-stimulating immunoglobulin as the cause of hyperthyroidism in Graves' disease. *J. Clin. Endocrinol. Metab.* 42:778–81
4. Smith, B. R., Hall, R. 1974. Thyroid-stimulating immunoglobulins in Graves' disease. *Lancet* 2:427–31
5. Orgiazzi, J., Williams, D. E., Chopra, I. J., Solomon, D. H. 1976. Human thyroid adenyl cyclase stimulating activity in immunoglobulin G of patients with Graves' disease. *J. Clin. Endocrinol. Metab.* 42:341–54
6. Zakarija, M., McKenzie, J. M., Banovac, K. 1980. Clinical significance of assay of thyroid-stimulating antibody in Graves' disease. *Ann. Intern. Med.* 93: 28–32
7. Mori, T., Kriss, J. P. 1971. Measurements by competitive binding radioassay of serum antimicrosomal and antithyroglobulin antibodies in Graves' disease and other thyroid disorders. *J. Clin. Endocrinol.* 33:688–98
8. Solomon, D. H., Chopra, I. J. 1972. Graves' disease–1972. *Mayo Clin. Proc.* 47:803–13
9. Werner, S. C., Wegelius, O., Hsu, K. C. 1971. Immune responses in stroma and basement membranes of the Graves' disease thyroid (IgM, IgG, IgE, and complement). *Trans. Assoc. Am. Phys.* 84:139–42
10. Volpe, R., Farid, N. R., Von Westarp, C., Row, V. V. 1974. The pathogenesis of Graves' disease and Hashimoto's thyroiditis. *Clin. Endocrinol.* 3:239–61
11. Doniach, D. 1975. Humoral and genetic aspects of thyroid autoimmunity. *Clin. Endocrinol. Metab.* 4:267–85
12. Solomon, D. H., Kleeman, K. E. 1976. Concepts of pathogenesis of Graves' disease. *Adv. Intern. Med.* 22:273–99
13. Milgrom, F., Witebsky, E. 1962. Autoantibodies and autoimmune disease. *J. Am. Med. Assoc.* 181:706–16
14. Edmonds, M. W., Row, V. V., Volpe, R. 1970. Action of globulin and lymphocytes from peripheral blood of patients with Graves' disease on isolated thyroid cells. *J. Clin. Endocrinol. Metab.* 31:480–90
15. Pinchera, A., Fenzi, G., Vitti, P., Macchia, E., ToccaFondi, R., Baschieri, L. 1980. In *Endocrinology 1980*, ed. I. A. Cumming, J. W. Funder, F. A. O. Meldelsohn, pp. 126–29. Canberra: Australian Acad. Sci.
16. Solomon, D. H., Chopra, I. J. 1980. Is TSH a LATS-protector? Evidence suggesting different sites of binding of TSH and thyroid stimulating immunoglobulins (TSIs) in thyroid tissue. In *Thyroid Research VIII*, ed. J. R. Stockigt, S. Nagataki, pp. 717–20. Canberra: Australian Acad. Sci.
17. Ong, M., Malkin, D. G., Tay, S. K., Malkin, A. 1976. Activation of thyroid adenyl cyclase by antisera to thyroid plasma membrane preparations. *Endocrinology* 98:880–85
18. Adams, D. D., Fastier, F. N., Howie, J. B., Kennedy, T. H., Kilpatrick, J. A., Stewart, R. D. H. 1974. Stimulation of the human thyroid by infusion of plasma containing LATS protector. *J. Clin. Endocrinol. Metab.* 39:826–32
19. Knight, A., Adams, D. D. 1973. Infusion of LATS protector and LATS into monkeys. *Proc. Univ. Otago Med. Sch.* 51:11–13
20. Irvine, W. J., McGregor, A. G., Stuart, A. E., Hall, G. H. 1961. Hashimoto's disease in uniovular swines. *Lancet* 2:850–53
21. Jayson, M. I. V., Doniach, D., Benhamou-Glynn, N., Roitt, I. M., El Kabir, D. J. 1967. Thyrotoxicosis and Hashimoto's goiter in a pair of monozygotic twins with serum long-acting thyroid stimulator. *Lancet* 2:15–18
22. Bartels, E. D. 1941. *Heredity in Graves' disease.* Copenhagen: Munksgaard
23. Skillern, P. G. 1972. Genetics of Graves' disease. *Mayo Clin. Proc.* 47: 848–49
24. Hall, R., Stanbury, J. B. 1967. Familial Studies of autoimmune thyroiditis. *Clin. Exp. Immunol.* 2:719–25
25. Howell-Evans, A. W., Woodrow, J. C., McDougall, C. D. D., Chew, A. R., xstart Evans, W. R. 1967. Antibodies with families of thyrotoxic patients. *Lancet* one:636–41
26. Hall, R., Dingle P. R., Roberts, D. F. 1972. Thyroid antibodies: a study of first degree relatives. *Clin. Genet.* 3:319–24
27. Tunbridge, W. M. G., Evered, D. C., Hall, R., Appleton, D., Brewis, M., Clark, F., Grimley Evans, J., Youvd,

E., Bird, T., Smith, P. A. 1977. The spectrum of thyroid disease in a community: the Wickham survey. *Clin. Endocrinol.* 7:481–93
28. Blizzard, R. M., Chee, D., Davis, W. 1967. The incidence of adrenal and other antibodies in the sera of patients with iodiopathic adrenal insufficiency. *Clin. Exp. Immunol.* 2:19–30
29. Grumet, F. C., Payne, R. O., Konishi, J., Kriss, J. P. 1974. HL-A antigens as markers for disease susceptibility and autoimmunity in Graves' diseases. *J. Clin. Endocrinol. Metab.* 39:1115–19
30. Grumet, F. C., Konishi, J., Payne, R. O., Kriss, J. P. 1976. Association in Japanese of Graves' disease with HL-A specificity W5. In *Thyroid Research*, ed. J. Robbins, L. E. Braverman, pp. 376-79. New York: American Elsevier
31. Farid, N. R., Simpson, L., Noel, E. P., Barnard, J. M., Mandeville, R. P. 1978. A study of HLA-D-related (DRW) antigens in Graves' disease. Presented at 60th Ann. Meet. Endocrine Soc., June 14–16, Miami, Florida, p. 126, abstr. 103.
32. Moens, H., Farid, N. R. 1978. Hashimoto's thyroiditis is associated with HLA-DRW₃. *N. Engl. J. Med.* 299:133–34
33. Farid, N. R., Newton, R. M., Noel, E. P., Marshall, W. H. 1977. Gm phenotypes in autoimmune thyroid disease. *J. Immunogenet.* 4:429–32
34. Pepper, B., Noel, E. P., Farid, N. R. 1981. The putative antithyrotropin receptor antibodies of Graves' disease. *J. Immunogenet.* 8:89–100
35. Uno, H., Sasazuki, T., Tamai, H., Matsumoto, H. 1981. Two major genes, linked to HLA and Gm control susceptibility to Graves' disease. *Nature* 292:768–70
36. Werner, S. C., Spooner, M. 1955. A new and simple test for hyperthyroidism employing L-triiodothyronine and the twenty four hour I¹³¹ uptake method. *Bull. NY Acad. Med.* 31:137–45
37. Werner, S. C., Spooner, M., Hamilton, H. 1955. Further evidence that hyperthyroidism (Graves' disease) is not hyperpituitarism: effects of triiodothyronine and sodium iodide. *J. Clin. Endocrinol.* 15:715–23
38. Orgiazzi, J., Chopra, I. J., Williams, D. E., Solomon, D. H. 1975. Evidence for normal thyroidal adenyl cyclase, cyclic AMP-binding and protein-kinase activities in Graves' disease. *J. Clin. Endocrinol. Metab.* 40:248–55

39. Kuzuya, N., Uchimura, H., Ikeda, H., Chin, S. C., Hamada, N., Ito, K., Nagataki, S. 1980. Adenosine 3',5'-monophosphate concentrations and responsiveness to thyrotropin and thyroid-stimulating immunoglobulins in normal and Graves' thyroids. *J. Clin. Endocrinol. Metab.* 51:59–63
40. Adams, D. D., Purves, H. D. 1956. Abnormal responses in the assay of thyrotropin. *Proc. Univ. Otaga Med. Sch.* 34:11–12
41. McKenzie, J. M. 1958. The bioassay of thyrotropin in serum. *Endocrinology* 3:372–82
42. Kriss, J. P., Pleshakov, V., Chien, J. R. 1964. Isolation and identification of the long-acting thyroid stimulator and its relation to hyperthyroidism and circumscribed pretibial myxedema. *J. Clin. Endocrinol. Metab.* 24:1005–28
43. Chopra, I. J., Solomon, D. H., Johnson, D. E., Chopra, U. 1970. Thyroid gland in Graves' disease: victim or culprit? *Metabolism* 19:760–72
44. Chopra, I. J., Solomon, D. H., Limberg, N. P. 1970. Specific and nonspecific responses to the bioassay of long-acting thyroid stimulator. *J. Clin. Endocrinol. Metab.* 31:382–90
45. Adams, D. D., Kennedy, T. H. 1971. Evidence to suggest that LATS protector stimulates the human thyroid gland. *J. Clin. Endocrinol. Metab.* 33:47–51
46. Ozawa, Y., Maciel, R. M. B., Chopra, I. J., Solomon, D. H., Beall, G. N. 1979. Relationship among immunoglobulin markers in Graves' disease. *J. Clin. Endocrinol. Metab.* 48:381–87
47. Onaya, T., Kofani, M., Yamada, T., Ochi, Y. 1973. New in vitro tests to detect the thyroid stimulator in sera from hyperthyroid patients by measuring colloid droplet and cyclic AMP in human thyroid slices. *J. Clin. Endocrinol. Metab.* 36:859–66
48. Shishiba, Y., Shimuzu, T., Yoshimura, S., Shizume, K. 1973. Direct evidence for human thyroid stimulation by LATS-protector. *J. Clin. Endocrinol. Metab.* 36:517–21
49. Kendall-Taylor, P., Atkinson S. 1980. A biological method for the assay of TSAb in serum. See Ref. 16, pp. 763–66
50. Solomon, D. H., Chopra, I. J., Chopra, U., Smith, F. J. 1977. Identification of subgroups of euthyroid Graves' ophthalmophathy. *N. Eng. J. Med.* 296:181–86
51. Adams, D. D., Kennedy, T. H., Stewart, R. D. H. 1974. Correlation between long-acting thyroid stimulator protec-

tor level and thyroid ^{131}I uptake in thyrotoxicosis. *Br. Med. J.* 2:199–201

52. Shishiba, Y., Miyachi, Y., Takaichi, M., Ozawa, Y. 1978. LATS-protector activity in thyrotoxicosis measured by thyroidal intracellular colloid droplet formation. *J. Clin. Endocrinol. Metab.* 46:841–48

53. Manley, S. W., Bourke, J. R., Hawker, R. W. 1974. The thyrotropin receptor in guinea-pig thyroid homogenates; interaction with the long-acting thyroid stimulator. *J. Endocrinol.* 61:437–45

54. McGregor, A. M., Smith, B. R., Hall, R. 1980. Thyrotropin receptor antibodies. See Ref. 15, pp. 122–25

55. Beall, G. N., Chopra, I. J., Solomon, D. H., Kruger, S. R. 1978. Serum protein inhibition of thyrotropin binding to human thyroid tissue. *J. Clin. Endocrinol. Metab.* 47:967–73

56. Fenzi, G., Hashigume, K., Roudebush, C. P., DeGroot, L. J. 1979. Changes in thyroid-stimulating immunoglobulins during antithyroid therapy. *J. Clin. Endocrinol. Metab.* 48:572–76

57. Brown, R. S., Jackson, I. M. D., Pohl, S. L., Reichlin, S. 1978. Do thyroid-stimulating immunoglobulins cause nontoxic and toxic multinodular goiter? *Lancet* 1:904–6

58. Hall, R., Smith, B. R., Mukhtar, E. D. 1975. Thyroid stimulators in health and disease. *Clin. Endocrinol.* 4:213–30

59. Sugenoya, A., Kidd, A., Row, V. V., Volpe, R. 1979. Correlation between thyrotropin-displacing activity and human thyroid-stimulating activity by immunoglobulins from patients with Graves' disease and other thyroid disorders. *J. Clin. Endocrinol. Metab.* 48:398–402

60. Strakosoh, C. R., Joyer, D., Wall, J. R. 1978. Thyroid-stimulating antibodies in patients with autoimmune disorders. *J. Clin. Endocrinol. Metab.* 46:345–48

61. Endo, K., Kasagi, K., Konishi, J., Ikerubo, J., Okuno, T., Takeda, Y., Moui, T. Tarizuka, K. 1978. Determination and properties of TSH binding inhibitor immunoglobulins in patients with Graves' disease and Hashimoto's thyroiditis. *J. Clin. Endocrinol. Metab.* 46:734–39

62. Mukhtar, E. D., Smith, B. R., Pyle, G. A., Hall, R., Vice, P. 1975. Relation of thyroid-stimulating immunoglobulins to thyroid function and effect of surgery, radioiodine and antithyroid drugs, *Lancet* 1:713–15

63. Schleusher, H., Finke, R., Katulla, P., Wenzel, K. W., Meinhold, H., Roedler, H. D. 1979. Determination of thyroid-stimulating immunoglobulins (TSI) during the course of Graves' disease. A reliable indicator for remission and persistence of this disease. *J. Endocrinol. Invest.* 2:155–61

64. Davies, T. F., Yeo, P. P. B., Evered, D. C., Clark, F., Smith, B. R., Hall, R. 1977. Value of thyroid-stimulating antibody determinations in predicting short-term thyrotoxic relapse in Graves' disease. *Lancet* 1:1181–82

65. Teng, C. S., Yeung, R. T. T. 1980. Changes in thyroid-stimulating antibody activity in Graves' disease treated with antithyroid drug and its relationship to relapse: a prospective study. *J. Clin. Endocrinol. Metab.* 50:144–47

66. O'Donnell, J., Trokoudes, K., Silverberg, J., Row, V., Volpe, R. 1978. Thyrotropin displacement activity of serum immunoglobulins from patients with Graves' disease. *J. Clin. Endocrinol. Metab.* 46:770–77

67. Kuzuya, N., Chin, S. H., Ikeda, H., Uchimura, H., Ho, K., Nagataki, S. 1979. Correlation between thyroid stimulators and 3',5',3'-triiodothyronine suppressibility in patients during treatment for hyperthyroidism with thionamide drugs: comparison of assays by thyroid-stimulating and thyrotropin-displacing activities. *J. Clin. Endocrinol. Metab.* 48:706–11

68. Nagataki, S., Kubota, K., Hamada, S., Chiu, S. C., Kuzuya, N., Ikeda, H., Malda, M., Uchimura, H., Tamai, T., Kuma K., Ito, K. 1980. Abnormal thyroid stimulators in Graves' disease and their correlation with thyroid functional states. See Ref. 15, pp. 134–37

69. Stockle, G., Wahl., R., Seif, F. J. 1981. Micromethod of human thyrocyte cultures for detection of thyroid-stimulating antibodies and thyrotropin. *Acta Endocrinol. Copenhagen* 97:369–75

70. Rapoport, B., Takai, N. A., Filetti, S. 1982. Evidence for species specificity in the interaction between thyrotropin and thyroid-stimulating immunoglobulin and their receptor in thyroid tissue. *J. Clin. Endocrinol. Metab.* 54:1059–62

71. Volpe, R., Edmondo, M., Lamki, L., Clarke, P. V., Row, V. V. 1972. The pathogenesis of Graves' disease, a disorder of delayed hypersensitivity? *Mayo Clin. Proc.* 47:824–34

Ann. Rev. Med. 1983. 34:283–94

THE MEDICAL MANAGEMENT OF HORMONE-SECRETING TUMORS OF THE PITUITARY

J. A. H. Wass, M.D., M.R.C.P., and G. M. Besser, DSc., M.D., F.R.C.P.

Department of Endocrinology, St. Bartholomew's Hospital, West Smithfield, London, England EC1A 7BE

ABSTRACT

A great deal of knowledge is now available about the hypothalamic control of anterior pituitary function. This puts the medical treatment of pituitary tumors on a sound scientific footing. In addition, medical treatment may decrease the size of these tumors in some cases, as well as improve other pituitary functions.

INTRODUCTION

Several recent discoveries have revolutionized therapeutics in modern endocrinology. Radioimmunoassay (RIA) makes it possible, with a high degree of specificity and precision, to measure circulating levels of a wide variety of peptide hormones. Secondly, prolactin has been discovered to exist as a separate entity in man, and RIA reveals that hyperprolactinemia is a common cause of hypogonadism in both sexes. The almost simultaneous discovery of a group of drugs functioning as long-acting dopamine agonists that can suppress elevated prolactin levels to normal has resulted in their widespread application and the successful treatment of hyperprolactinemic symptoms.

Furthermore, the discovery of abnormal growth hormone regulation in acromegaly and the paradoxical fall in growth hormone (GH) levels that occurs in acromegalic patients given dopamine agonists allows this group of drugs to be used successfully in the treatment of acromegaly.

283

0066-4219/83/0401-0283$02.00

This review deals only with tumors secreting prolactin, growth hormone, and adrenocorticotrophic hormone (ACTH.) Medical management of these tumors, particularly of the former two, has become commonplace; tumors secreting the glycoprotein hormones, thyroid-stimulating hormone (TSH,) luteinizing hormone (LH,) and follicle-stimulating hormone (FSH) are exceedingly rare.

PHYSIOLOGY

The control of prolactin secretion is unique among the anterior pituitary hormones in that it is under the predominantly inhibitory control of the hypothalamus. It is now widely recognized that dopamine is the most important substance inhibiting prolactin secretion (1). Thyrotrophin-releasing hormone (TRH) causes prolactin secretion but it is not clear whether or not this is the physiological prolactin-releasing factor.

Growth hormone is also under the influence of two hypothalamic-releasing factors, the most important of which is GH-releasing factor. The structure of this is now known (31). GH-release-inhibiting hormone (somatostatin) was discovered in 1973 and is present in high concentrations in the hypothalamus but it is also found throughout the brain, nervous system, and gastrointestinal tract (2).

The control of growth hormone secretion by the anterior pituitary is complex, and a wide variety of pharmacological and physiological stimuli can alter it. The most important pharmacological agents are dopamine, noradrenaline, and serotonin. In normal subjects, dopamine or drugs that stimulate dopamine receptors increase GH secretion for a short duration. However, in acromegalic patients these drugs cause a paradoxical fall in growth hormone secretion (3).

ACTH is under the predominant control of corticotrophin-releasing factor (CRF); the molecular structure of this compound was recently described by Vale et al (4). Catecholamines are probably important in the control of CRF, thus L-dopa and drugs that release catecholamines inhibit stress-induced release of ACTH in dogs. 5-Hydroxytryptamine (serotonin) has long been implicated in the control of ACTH secretion. There is little doubt that it is excitatory to the release of CRF but it may act via a cholinergic interneuron. It is also probable that different neurotransmitters may affect the various causes of ACTH secretion differently. Thus cholinergic and serotoninergic mechanisms appear to be involved in the circadian release of ACTH, and the stress-induced responses may have cholinergic and adrenergic or dopaminergic components, the latter of which may be inhibitory (5). Inhibitory endogenous opiate influences are also important, recently discovered, physiological modulators of secretion of CRF and therefore of ACTH (6).

MANAGEMENT

Prolactinomas

The symptoms of prolactin-secreting pituitary tumors relate mostly to hyperprolactinemia but local symptoms, particularly headache, visual field defects, and, more rarely, symptoms of cavernous sinus compression, may occasionally occur. It is usual for men to present later with bigger tumors presumably because their symptoms are less well defined. Up to 80% of females experience galactorrhea, but this sign may also be seen in normoprolactinemic females. The most frequent symptom is a disturbance of menstruation. Amenorrhea is most common, but all menstrual abnormalities have been reported; even normal periods may occur in which the luteal phase is inadequate thus causing infertility. Some patients note low libido and dyspareunia, symptoms related to estrogen deficiency. Men present with a decrease in libido or potency, so that this symptom should always be evaluated before psychogenic impotence is diagnosed.

The most common cause of hyperprolactinemia is a pituitary adenoma, but a number of other problems must first be excluded. Hypothalamic disease may interfere with the secretion of prolactin-inhibiting factor, and large pituitary tumors including those not primarily secreting prolactin may compress the pituitary stalk. Drugs acting on dopamine receptors alter prolactin secretion. Dopamine antagonists like the phenothiazines chlorpromazine or haloperidol; domperidone and metoclopramide; false transmitters like methyl dopa; and dopamine-depleting agents like reserpine may all cause hyperprolactinemia. Estrogens stimulate the lactotrophs, elevating serum prolactin, and this accounts for the increase in size of the pituitary during pregnancy. Lastly, hypothyroidism may be associated with hyperprolactinemia presumably because hypothalamic TRH levels are raised and TRH also stimulates prolactin secretion (7).

Therapy for hyperprolactinemia aims to reduce or remove the tumor mass, to preserve anterior pituitary function, and to reduce elevated levels of prolactin to normal thus reversing the associated symptoms of hypogonadism.

The diagnosis of large prolactinomas presents no difficulty. Once other causes of hyperprolactinemia are excluded, a small pituitary tumor is the most likely etiology. These microadenomas are more difficult to diagnose, particularly because there is considerable controversy about the significance of minor abnormalities of the pituitary fossa on x ray (8). The use of recent generation CT scanning of the pituitary fossa makes diagnosis of microadenomas more reliable. Levels of prolactin over 2000 mU/liter (or 100 ng/ml) nearly always indicate a prolactinoma, but these tumors can be present in patients with lower circulating values.

Medical therapy has a clear role in the treatment of small and large tumors. It can be used either on its own as primary therapy or as an adjunct in the treatment of patients with big pituitary tumors whose levels of prolactin are not adequately normalized by surgery or pituitary irradiation.

Most experience in the medical management of prolactinomas has been gained with bromocriptine, an ergot alkaloid that is a long-acting dopamine agonist. This drug suppresses prolactin for between 8 and 12 hours because it stimulates dopamine receptors present on the prolactin-secreting cells of the pituitary gland. If bromocriptine is given in a dose of 2.5 mg every 8 hours, prolactin levels become normal in the majority of patients; a small group, usually with very large tumors or very high levels of prolactin require higher doses of between 15 and 60 mg per day. As a result of lowering prolactin, galactorrhea ceases and menstruation and ovulation return (9). In 80% of patients this occurs within two months. In men, symptoms also improve rapidly and potency and libido return shortly after starting bromocriptine. In either sex, normal gonadal function fails to return only in the rare patient with persisting gonadotrophin deficiency.

A number of patients with prolactinomas desire fertility. Before treating these patients with bromocriptine, it is important to consider the risk of tumor enlargement during pregnancy, which may cause chiasmal compression and visual field defects. This has been reported to occur in 5% of patients with microadenomas and 25% with macroadenomas (10). In view of these risks, therefore, prior treatment with surgery or external pituitary irradiation is advisable in patients with a clearly abnormal pituitary fossa (11). Worldwide experience with ovulation induction in hyperprolactinemic women using bromocriptine indicates that it is not teratogenic.

Bromocriptine must be carefully administered in order to avoid side-effects at the start of treatment. These consist of nausea, vomiting, and postural hypotension. They are usually avoided by beginning therapy with half a tablet (1.25 mg) last thing at night taken in bed during a snack. The patient then remains supine overnight. The tablets are always taken with food and increased every 3 to 7 days by 1.25 mg until the patient is taking 2.5 mg three times daily. Though any initiating side-effects are usually transient, there is a very small group of patients who cannot tolerate bromocriptine because of nausea or persistent headache. Long-term side-effects on this dose of bromocriptine are rare and no serious side-effects have been reported in patients who have been taking the drug continuously for over 10 years.

The results of bromocriptine therapy must be compared with those of surgery. Transfrontal surgery rarely cures big pituitary tumors secreting prolactin because of the technical difficulties involved in totally removing the tumor. However, the results of transsphenoidal hypophysectomy for microadenoma may be different. Cure has been reported in 60% of patients. Smaller tumors seem more amenable to successful surgery (12); however, medical treatment is effective in 95% of this group of patients without surgery. The major risk of surgical treatment is hypopituitarism and this is particularly pertinent in a group of young females desiring fertility. In contrast, during bromocriptine therapy, pituitary function does not worsen and may improve.

External pituitary irradiation has also been used in the treatment of hyperprolactinemia (13). It is clear that this arrests tumor growth, prevents further enlargement during subsequent pregnancies, and gradually decreases the circulating levels of prolactin. However, it may take between 5 and 10 years to become effective and few series have been reported that adequately document the effect of radiotherapy on prolactin-secreting pituitary tumors or pituitary function.

The choice of therapy for prolactinomas depends on the size of the tumor, the presence of local complicating factors, the degree of elevation of the prolactin and the expertise that is locally available. In all but the largest tumors compressing local structures, a case may now be made for giving medical treatment with bromocriptine, which in a large proportion of patients will suppress prolactin levels to normal and cause a resumption of normal gonadal function without the risk of causing hypopituitarism.

Acromegaly

The symptoms of acromegaly are well described and are usually related either to the local or endocrine effects of the tumor or the metabolic effects of growth hormone. Only rarely does local expansion of the tumor cause symptoms. Patients with acromegaly require early treatment because their life expectancy is decreased by cardiovascular and cerebrovascular disease related to hypertension and diabetes mellitus and by respiratory disease (14). Furthermore, morbidity, particularly from facial appearances and osteoarthritis, can be considerable.

The goals of therapy are the same as those for prolactin-secreting tumors, but they are harder to achieve because medical or surgical therapy rarely results in completely normal circulating levels of growth hormone. In comparing the effects of reported treatments of acromegaly, it must be remembered that there is regrettably no accepted definition of "cure." We believe it best to measure GH levels repeatedly throughout a day of normal activity to reflect the usual exposure of the tissues to growth hormone. Doing this it is clear that in normal subjects growth hormone is only rarely detectable, so a "cure" can only in reality be accepted with mean daily GH values of under 2 mU/liter (1 ng/ml). Unfortunately, many workers have measured growth hormone only during the unphysiological stimulus of oral glucose or have taken single basal levels in the morning.

The standard methods for treating acromegaly are radiotherapy and surgery. Radiotherapy is most effectively given from a linear accelerator using three portals of entry at no more than 200 roentgens (r) a day up to a total tumor dose of 4500 r. Results with this mode of therapy are good and 80% of patients may be cured, but GH levels may take up to 10 years to become normal and a small proportion of patients become hypopituitary (15). Yttrium-90 and proton-beam irradiation are available in a few specialized centers but the long-term statistics seem no better than with conventional external pituitary irradiation.

Surgery may be carried out either via the transfrontal or transsphenoidal routes. Transfrontal surgery rarely cures acromegaly. Transsphenoidal surgery, on the other hand, may cure acromegaly (particularly if the tumor is a microadenoma) and postoperatively 65% of patients have levels of 10 m U/liter or less (16). However, acromegalics rarely have microadenomas and, particularly with larger tumors, post-surgical hypopituitarism occurs in 25%. The incidence of recurrence after successful surgery is at present unclear.

A number of medical treatments for acromegaly have been tried. Bromocriptine is now the most widely used. The basis of its use in acromegaly stems from the observation of Liuzzi et al (17), who in 1972 showed a paradoxical fall in growth hormone levels of acromegalic patients given the dopamine agonist L-dopa. Unfortunately L-dopa has only a short duration of action. Bromocriptine was first described in 1974 to cause prolonged suppression of growth hormone. In vitro work showed that it directly inhibits anterior pituitary GH secretion. A number of other drugs with dopamine agonist actions also suppress growth hormone in acromegaly: lisuride, piribedil, metergoline, lergotrile, pergolide, and CU32–085 (Sandoz). Because the widest experience has been gained with bromocriptine, this drug, the first effective medical therapy for acromegaly, is discussed in more detail.

It is clear that the suppressive actions of bromocriptine on circulating growth hormone are shorter than those on prolactin, and last about 6 hours. For this reason it is essential to give bromocriptine 4 times daily in divided doses. The usual dose varies from 20 to 30 mg daily but we regularly use up to 60 mg daily in divided doses every 6 hours (18).

Growth hormone levels on bromocriptine do not, except in the minority of patients, fall to normal; only 20% of patients have mean GH levels during the day of less than 10 mU/liter. In 70% of patients, however, GH levels decrease and there follows marked metabolic improvement. Hyperprolactinemia is present in 35% of patients and is abolished together with the associated hypogonadism. Glucose intolerance, which is present in about 30% of acromegalics before treatment, improves in the majority and became normal in 65% of patients in one series (18). The effects on GH secretion depend on the presence of bromocriptine: GH levels rise and carbohydrate tolerance worsens if the drug is withdrawn. Unfortunately, it is not possible to predict the patients who will respond to bromocriptine using any pretreatment test.

Clinical symptoms improve in more than 90% of patients and hand and foot sizes decrease, facial appearances improve, headaches are relieved, and sweating usually ceases. In addition to these subjective effects, objective changes in ring size occur in 80% and hypertension, which occurs in 40% of acromegalics, improves in 40% of these.

A number of groups have noted and tried to explain the discrepancy between the clinical and biochemical benefits of bromocriptine in acromegaly. It is possible that the nature of circulating GH changes. It has been shown that the most biologically active, monomeric form of the hormone is reduced proportionally greater than the less biologically active, oligomeric forms; this accounts for inactive clinical acromegaly in the presence of detectable immunoreactive GH. It is also possible that the drug may produce part of its clinical and biochemical effect by a peripheral action not involving GH. Lastly, there is a group of patients in whom somatomedin-C levels decrease but in whom GH levels do not change; thus a direct effect on somatomedin C by bromocriptine may explain this phenomenon (19).

As in the therapy of prolactinomas, bromocriptine must be started slowly and taken with food. Initially a daily dose of 10 mg is achieved and the patient is reassessed clinically and biochemically. Further increments are made until no more clinical or metabolic improvement occurs or until side-effects are seen.

With careful initiation of therapy, however, side-effects are rare. It is clear, looking at the different groups of patients, that these are less common in patients with acromegaly than in those with prolactinomas. There are two groups of side-effects: the initiating side-effects of nausea, vomiting, and postural hypotension described earlier, which disappear with time, and the chronic side-effects, which are seen only with the higher-dose therapy used in acromegaly. The most common of these is constipation, which is related to the stimulation of dopamine receptors in the gastrointestinal tract. It is easily treated with bulk fiber laxatives. Dyspepsia may also occur. Serious gastrointestinal bleeding from peptic ulcers has been reported but it is now clear that peptic ulceration does not occur more often in these patients than in others; in studies of gastric function in acromegalics before and during bromocriptine therapy, no change was seen in gastric acid secretion or gastrin responses to a standard mixed meal. Digital vasospasm has been reported with higher doses of bromocriptine but this also responds to dosage reduction. It is not ergotism and no patients developing ischemia or any trophic changes of the digits have been reported. Lastly, increased alertness was reported by some patients, but this is not a problem of clinical usage and many patients consider it an added benefit of therapy.

It is usual to treat acromegaly caused by an intrasellar tumor primarily either with external pituitary irradiation or surgery. To augment these ablative therapies, either if the effects of surgery are incomplete or during the interval until radiotherapy has achieved its full effects, bromocriptine should be used. Bromocriptine can be used alone in elderly patients who have acromegaly with complications or in patients who refuse ablative therapy.

The Effect of Bromocriptine on Pituitary Tumor Size

There is good clinical and radiological evidence that pituitary tumor size may be decreased by drugs that stimulate dopamine receptors. Bromocriptine appears to reduce prolactin secretion by reducing exocytotic events. Prolonged therapy also decreases the prolactin content of prolactinomas, so an effect on synthesis is also apparent. Other workers showed a decrease in DNA synthesis of rat prolactin-secreting tumors, and the mitotic activity of prolactin-producing cells induced by estrogens is also decreased by this drug. There is animal evidence that both GH and prolactin-producing tumors become smaller after treatment with ergot derivatives (20).

The first suggestion that bromocriptine could cause tumor regression came in 1975. Many have now demonstrated tumor size reduction on bromocriptine either by improvement in visual field defects or by radiological means (pneumoencephalography, CT scan, or metrizamide cisternography.) The majority of patients had prolactin-secreting tumors but tumor regression in patients with acromegaly was also demonstrated (21).

Tumor shrinkage may commence rapidly, within a few days sometimes, with resolution of headaches, field defects, and ocular palsies but responses are sometimes delayed for several weeks. Residual pituitary function, deficient before treatment, may return to normal (22).

Recently published trials suggest that 65% of massive prolactinomas with extrasellar extensions decrease in size after about three months of treatment (22). The frequency with which nonfunctioning tumors or those secreting GH respond is as yet not known.

Such effects are also reported in patients treated with another dopamine agonist, lisuride (23). Dopamine agonist therapy may therefore shrink the tumor and make it more amenable to cure by radiotherapy or surgery. In view of these recent findings, in prolactinoma patients presenting with large extrasellar extensions it is reasonable to attempt to reduce the size of the pituitary gland in order to obviate the need for surgery or to make surgery easier. This should clearly be carried out under carefully controlled conditions with regular visual acuity and field monitoring. If there is any deterioration in these parameters, surgery should be carried out urgently. The same course should be followed if at the end of a three-month trial period no improvement has occurred.

Cushing's Disease

Cushing's disease, or pituitary-dependent Cushing's syndrome, is characterized by excessive ACTH secretion from the pituitary usually from a small basophil adenoma. The symptoms and signs of Cushing's syndrome are well described.

Treatment of Cushing's syndrome aims to reduce circulating cortisol levels to normal. This includes a return to a normal circadian rhythm of cortisol and ACTH and normal dexamethasone suppressibility. The diagnosis and differential diagnosis of Cushing's disease are out of the scope of this review. However, treatment is clearly necessary as there is a 50% mortality at five years (24).

Treatment of pituitary-dependent Cushing's disease involves transsphenoidal selective removal of any pituitary microadenoma, or surgical or medical adrenalectomy. Surgical adrenalectomy in unprepared patients may have a high mortality and morbidity and it is more usual to prepare patients with florid Cushing's disease before operation with drugs that interfere with cortisol synthesis in the adrenal gland, particularly metyrapone or op'-DDD. ACTH secretion may be reduced either by surgical removal of the pituitary tumor, external pituitary irradiation, or medical therapy. Radiotherapy improved pituitary-dependent Cushing's syndrome in 46% of cases in one study (25). However, there may be a prolonged time gap between administration of radiotherapy and its effectiveness. It is, however, free of morbidity and no pituitary dysfunction occurs in patients who have been followed up long-term. It apppears more efficacious in children. Pituitary surgery cures between 66 and 85% of patients; however, there is a complication rate related to the surgery itself and to post-operative hypopituitarism (26).

Neurotransmitter therapy for Cushing's disease has recently been introduced. Because of the known excitatory effect of serotonin on CRF release, cyproheptadine, a serotonin antagonist, was introduced by Dr. Dorothy Krieger. In her hands, 24 mg a day given for between 2 and 3 months induced a laboratory and clinical remission in 50% of patients (27). These patients had a return of normal dexamethasone suppressibility and cortisol and ACTH periodicity. To date, patients have been treated for up to 18 months. Side-effects of hyperphagia and somnolence have appeared but usually disappeared spontaneously. There is one negative report by Tyrell et al (28), who treated 6 patients but for a shorter period of time and with lower doses than those used by Krieger. There is also one very brief report of improved visual fields in a patient with Nelson's syndrome treated by cyproheptadine (29). To date the treatment has not been widely adopted.

Two groups reported that a single dose of 2.5 mg of bromocriptine can lower ACTH levels in patients with Cushing's disease and Nelson's syndrome (30). We used a dose of 1.25 mg bd and normal circadian rhythm returned as did the cortisol response to hypoglycemia. On withdrawal, Cushing's disease recurred. It thus appears that certain patients respond well to bromocriptine and this is possibly related to depletion of central dopamine stores. We have given bromocriptine to many patients with Cushing's disease and only the minority of patients respond. There does not appear, at present, to be any way in which these patients can be predicted.

Neurotransmitter therapy has not been widely adopted in the treatment of pituitary-dependent Cushing's disease. At present it must remain the second line of therapy when other treatment options are exhausted, largely because of side-effects or inconsistency of response.

SUMMARY

It is clear that medical therapy of prolactinomas has revolutionized the management of this common endocrine disorder. Bromocriptine specifically suppresses elevated prolactin levels without altering other pituitary hormone secretion, which thus allows normal feedback mechanisms to operate. The majority of prolactinomas decrease in size and medical therapy does not carry the risk of hypopituitarism that other treatments do.

In acromegaly, bromocriptine reduces GH levels in the majority of patients though not to normal. Usually it should not be used alone but either while waiting for the effects of radiotherapy to take hold or in cases where surgery is unsuccessful.

Bromocriptine therapy is expensive and it is to be hoped that the future will bring cheaper drugs that suppress prolactin and growth hormone secretion and that have a higher therapeutic ratio and a longer duration of action. In the treatment of Cushing's disease, further medical therapies will undoubtedly become available when the neuropharmacological control of corticotrophin-releasing factor is more fully understood.

Literature Cited:

1. MacLeod, R. M. 1976. Regulation of prolactin secretion. In *Frontiers in Neuroendocrinology,* ed. L. Martini, F. Ganong. 4:169–94. New York: Raven
2. Wass, J. A. H. 1982. Somatostatin and its physiology in man in health and disease. *Clinical Neuroendocrinology,* ed. L. Martini, G. M. Besser, 2:359–95. New York: Academic
3. Chiodini, P. G., Liuzzi, A., Botalla, L., Cremascoli, G., Silvestrini, F. 1974. Inhibitory effect of dopaminergic stimulation on growth hormone release in acromegaly. *J. Clin. Endocrinol. Metab.* 38:200–6
4. Vale, W., Spiess, J., Rivier, C., Rivier, J. 1981. Characterization of a 41-residue ovine hypothalamic peptide that stimulates secretion of corticotropin and β-endorphin. *Science* 213:1394–97
5. Jones, M. T., Gillham, B., Di Renzo, G., Beckford, U., Holmes, M. C. 1981. Neural control of corticotrophin secretion. *Front. Horm. Res.* 8:12–43
6. Stubbs, W. A., Delitala, G., Jones, A., Jeffcoate, W. J., Edwards, C. R. W., Rees, L. H., Besser, G. M. 1978. Hormonal and metabolic responses to an enkephalin analogue in normal man. *Lancet* 4:1225–27
7. Thorner, M. O. 1977. Prolactin. *Clin. Endocrinol. Metab.* 6:201–22
8. Besser, G. M. 1976. The pituitary fossa —normal or abnormal? *Br. J. Radiol.* 49:652
9. Thorner, M. O., Besser, G. M., Hagen, C., McNeilly, A. S. 1974. Long-term treatment of galactorrhoea and hypogonadism with bromocriptine. *Br. Med. J.* 2:419–22
10. Bergh, T., Nillius, S. J., Wide, L. 1978. Clinical course and outcome of pregnancies in amenorrhoeic women with hyperprolactinaemia and pituitary tumors. *Br. Med. J.* 1:875–80
11. Thorner, M. O., Edwards, C. R. W., Charlesworth, M., Dacie, J. E., Moult, P. J. A., Rees, L. H., Jones, A. E., Besser, G. M. 1979. Pregnancy in patients presenting with hyperprolactinaemia. *Br. Med. J.* 2:771–74
12. Fahlbusch, R. 1981. Surgical treatment of pituitary adenomas. In *The Pituitary,* ed. C. Beardwell, G. L. Robertson, pp. 76–105. London: Butterworths
13. Sheline, G. E. 1981. Pituitary tumors: radiation therapy. See Ref. 12, pp. 106–74
14. Wright, A. D., Hill, D. M., Lowy, C., Russell Fraser, T. 1970. Mortality in acromegaly. *Q. J. Med.* 39:1–13
15. Easterman, R. C., Gorden, P., Roth, J. 1979. Conventional supervoltage irradiation is an effective treatment for acromegaly. *J. Clin. Endocrinol. Metab.* 48:931–40
16. Laws, E. R., Piepgras, P. G., Randall, R. V., Abboud, C. F. 1979. Neurosurgical management of acromegaly. *J. Neurosurg.* 50:454–61
17. Liuzzi, A., Chiodini, P. G., Botalla, L., Cremascoli, G., Silvestrini, F. 1972. Inhibitory effect of L-dopa on GH release in acromegalic patients. *J. Clin. Endocrinol. Metab.* 35:941–43
18. Wass, J. A. H., Thorner, M. O., Morris, D. V., Rees, L. H., Stuart Mason, A., Jones, A. E., Besser, G. M. 1977. Long-term treatment of acromegaly with bromocriptine. *Br. Med. J.* 1:875–78
19. Wass, J. A. H., Clemmons, D. R., Underwood, L. E., Barrow, I., Besser, G. M., Van Wyk, J. J. 1982. Changes in circulating somatomedin-C levels in bromocriptine treated acromegaly. *Clin. Endocrinol.* 17:369–77
20. Quadri, S. K., Lu, K. M., Meites, J. 1972. Ergot-induced inhibition of pituitary tumor growth in rats. *Science* 176:417–18
21. Wass, J. A. H., Thorner, M. O., Charlesworth, M., Moult, P. J. A., Dacie, J. E., Jones, A. E., Besser, G. M. 1979. Reduction of pituitary tumour size in patients with prolactinomas and acromegaly treated with bromocriptine with or without radiotherapy. *Lancet* 2:66–69
22. Wass, J. A. H., Williams, J., Charlesworth, M., Kingsley, D. P. E., Halliday, A. M., Doniach, I., Rees, L. H., McDonald, W. I., Besser, G. M. 1982. Bromocriptine in the management of large pituitary tumours. *Br. Med. J.* 284:1908–11
23. Chiodini, P., Liuzzi, A., Cozzi, R., Verde, G., Oppizi, G., Dallabonzana, D., Spelter, B., Silvestrini, G., Borghi, G., Luccarelli, G., Rainer, E., Horowski, R. 1981. Size reduction of microprolactinomas by bromocriptine or lisuride treatment. *J. Clin. Endocrinol. Metab.* 53:737–43
24. Krieger, D. T. 1982. In *Monographs in Endocrinology, Vol. 22, Cushing's syndrome,* p. 119–37. New York: Springer Verlag
25. Orth, D. N., Liddle, G. W. 1971. Results of treatment in 108 patients with Cushing's syndrome. *N. Engl. J. Med.* 285:243–47

26. Salassa, R. M., Laws, E. R., Carpenter, P. C., Northcutt, R. C. 1978. Transsphenoidal removal of pituitary microadenoma in Cushing's disease. *Mayo Clin. Proc.* 53:24–28
27. Krieger, D. T. 1982. Treatment of Cushing's disease and Syndrome. See Ref. 24, pp. 131–35
28. Tyrrell, J. B., Brooks, R. M., Forsham, P. H. 1976. More on cyproneptadine. *N. Engl. J. Med.* 295:1137–38
29. Hartwig, W., Kasperlic-Zalusk, A., Wilczynska, J., Migdalaska, B. 1976. Treatment of Nelson's syndrome with cyproheptadine. *N. Engl. J. Med.*

295:394
30. Lamberts, S. W. J., Klijn, J. G. M., De Quijada, M., Tinnermans, H. A. T., Uitterlinden, P., Kirkenhager, J. C. 1980. Bromocriptine in the medical treatment of Cushing's disease. In *Neuroactive Drugs in Endocrinology*, ed. E. E. Muller, pp. 371–82. Amsterdam: Elsevier, North-Holland
31. Guillemin, R., Brazeau, P., Böhlen, P., Esch, F., Ling, N., Wehrenberg, W. B. 1982. Growth hormone releasing factor from a human pancreatic tumor that caused acromegaly. *Science* 218:585–87

Ann. Rev. Med. 1983. 34:295–309

THE DIAGNOSIS OF DIABETES:
New International Classification and Diagnostic Criteria[1]

Peter H. Bennett, M.B., F.R.C.P., F.F.C.M.

Epidemiology and Field Studies Branch, National Institute of Arthritis, Diabetes, and Digestive and Kidney Diseases, Phoenix, Arizona 85014

ABSTRACT

The National Diabetes Data Group and the World Health Organization recently made recommendations concerning the classification of diabetes mellitus and proposed new diagnostic criteria. These recommendations are summarized and their bases elucidated. Certain discrepancies between the recommendations are apparent and the reasons for these and their resolution are discussed. The shortcomings and difficulties that remain are largely due to a lack of knowledge of the etiology and pathogenesis of the most common forms of diabetes. Wide acceptance of the proposals promises much greater uniformity in diagnosis and classification than has occurred before, and should enhance the comparability and applicability of research concerning diabetes nationally and internationally.

INTRODUCTION

The concepts of diabetes have changed considerably in recent years. Diabetes is now recognized to consist of a number of diseases characterized by chronic hyperglycemia. The need for a new classification and a redefinition of diagnostic criteria arises from the recent increases in knowledge of the genetics and molecular basis of some of these disorders, and of the epidemiology and natural history of the more frequent forms of diabetes. The new classification and criteria for diagnosis developed by the National Diabetes

[1]The US Government has the right to retain a nonexclusive royalty-free license in and to any copyright covering this paper.

Data Group and the World Health Organization are presented. Their justifications are reviewed and their shortcomings discussed.

Historical Background

Diabetes was originally considered to be a disease characterized by wasting and the passage of large amounts of sweet urine leading to death over the course of a few weeks or months. The name diabetes was introduced by Aretaeus, a Roman physician of the first century A. D. (1). At this time, and indeed up to the first quarter of this century, the presence of sweetness (and later sugar) in the urine was the hallmark of diagnosis.

Interest in the disease increased considerably in the latter part of the nineteenth century. In 1875 Bouchardat (2) recognized that, clinically, at least two forms of diabetes existed in man, one characterized by obesity and the other occurring usually in younger persons of even subnormal weight. Then in 1889, von Mering & Minkowski (3) showed that pancreatectomy could produce diabetes in the dog. This led to the concept that human diabetes was a disease of the pancreas. Further developments in clinical diabetes awaited the ability to measure the blood sugar or blood glucose level in a systematic and reliable manner. The subsequent discovery and isolation of insulin in 1921 (4), and its successful application to reduce hyperglycemia and prolong life in human diabetes, strengthened the concept that the underlying lesions were in the pancreas.

At this point fasting hyperglycemia was the *sine qua non* of diagnosis. In the 1920s the glucose tolerance test was first introduced as a research tool, and later it became widely adopted as a diagnostic method. In the latter part of the 1930s, diabetic retinopathy and diabetic nephropathy were recognized as specific complications, not only of subjects with diabetes who had received insulin therapy for a number of years, but also of persons with less severe degrees of hyperglycemia who had never received insulin. During the next two decades there was increasing recognition that both insulin-treated and non-insulin-treated diabetics frequently suffered from these and other less specific forms of vascular disease, and that vascular complications caused much more disability and premature death among diabetics than among nondiabetics. In the 1950s and 1960s interest in the earlier recognition of the disease, with the hope that earlier treatment would prevent development of the complications, led to the widespread adoption of the glucose tolerance test to detect the disease at an early stage and before the appearance of fasting hyperglycemia.

There were at the same time many attempts to refine the oral glucose tolerance test and to refine criteria for its interpretation. In general, values falling above the mean and two standard deviations of the level found in a selected population of healthy volunteers without a family history of diabetes were accepted as diagnostic of diabetes (5, 6). The glucose tolerance used and interpreted in this way led to the identification of asymptomatic subjects with abnormally high one- or two-hour postload glucose levels, but with normal fasting values, who were generally presumed to have early or mild diabetes. However, the use of the glucose tolerance test in epidemiological studies revealed that large proportions of the population were abnormal by such criteria, and that the proportion increased considerably with age, so that beyond 60 years of age more than half of the population could be considered to be abnormal (7). These observations, however, were at variance with other findings since both symptomatic diabetes and its specific complications were by no means so frequent. Furthermore, follow-up studies of those with abnormal glucose tolerance subsequently indicated that the majority of subjects with lesser degrees of glucose intolerance defined in this way did not show definite evidence of diabetes within the next 5–10 years, and a large proportion even reverted to normal over a period of time (8–10).

In the 1960s the concept of the pathogenesis of diabetes started to change from being only a disease associated with insulin lack, which had been generally assumed to be the case. While the nature of the lesion was not known, it had been generally accepted that some insufficiency of the Islets of Langerhans was the basis for all diabetes (11). This was most clear-cut for the so-called secondary diabetes, where pancreatic dysfunction due to conditions such as hemochromatosis and calcific pancreatitis could be identified. The introduction of the radioimmunoassay for insulin led to the realization that many diabetics had appreciable insulin levels and that many who had abnormal glucose tolerance, and who were therefore considered to be diabetic, responded to an oral glucose load with insulin levels even higher than those seen in normal controls (12, 13). This was particularly true among the obese with an onset of diabetes in adult life (14, 15). These observations eventually led to the concept that diabetes could result from resistance to the action of insulin, as well as from a lack of insulin (16). This finding contributed to the concept of the heterogeneity of diabetes.

In the meantime, the potential significance of impaired glucose tolerance in pregnancy became more widely recognized (17). While the potential complications of pregnancy in the insulin-requiring diabetic, e.g. an increased frequency of fetal and neonatal deaths and congenital malformations, had been recognized for many years, it was found that impaired glucose tolerance, sometimes manifest only during the third trimester of pregnancy, could lead to increased perinatal mortality and morbidity (18, 19). The term gestational diabetes was used to describe such circumstances.

Associations between diabetes and certain genetic markers in the human lymphocyte antigen (HLA) system, and subsequently with islet cell and other autoantibodies, led to further characterization of insulin-dependent diabetes (20, 21). These markers were not found in non-insulin-dependent diabetes; thus a further criterion for the separation of the two most frequent types of the disease became available. A large number of specific genetic syndromes accompanied by hyperglycemia were also described (20), and diabetes became a recognized complication of a number of therapeutic agents.

It became apparent, therefore, that the growth in knowledge of the etiology and pathogenesis demanded revision of both the classification and the diagnostic criteria for diabetes. In 1979 a workgroup of the National Diabetes Data Group (NDDG) suggested revised classification and diagnostic criteria (22), which subsequently were adopted in large part as recommendations of the World Health Organization (WHO) Expert Committee on Diabetes (23).

THE NEW CLASSIFICATION OF DIABETES

Previously, attempts had been made to classify diabetes as primary, idiopathic, "essential," or "genetic," while secondary diabetes was associated with specific endocrine causes, such as pancreatic destruction, or the use of certain drugs. Primary diabetes was then subclassified by the age of onset of the disease (juvenile, juvenile-onset, maturity- or adult-onset), by the therapeutic response (brittle, stable, etc), by the stage in natural history of the disease, or by the severity of the hyperglycemia (subclinical, latent, chemical, or overt). Some classifications were based on insulin requirements (insulin-deficient, insulin-resistant, insulin-requiring, etc), on the predisposition to develop ketosis (ketosis prone, ketosis resistant), or on the degree of glucose intolerance (borderline, chemical, overt). No unanimity of definition of these terms was ever achieved and no one classification system gained wide acceptance.

The most logical classification of the group of disorders that constitute diabetes mellitus would be based on knowledge of the pathogenesis of the disease, but in most instances this is not known. The extent of knowledge about the various forms of diabetes varies, so some can be categorized etiologically, whereas others are recognized only on the basis of their clinical characteristics. Thus, no classification, including the new scheme, is completely satisfactory.

The classification recommended by the NDDG (22) and subsequently adopted by the WHO Expert Committee on Diabetes (23) is shown in Table 1. It was designed so that the classes were mutually exclusive. A given individual can be categorized in only one class at a specific point in time, although classification can change with time as features of the disease emerge.

Table 1   Classification of diabetes mellitus and other categories of glucose intolerance

---

Diabetes mellitus (DM)

Insulin-dependent type (IDDM)—Type 1
Noninsulin-dependent type (NIDDM)—Type 2
   a. nonobese
   b. obese

Other types—Includes diabetes mellitus associated with certain other conditions and syndromes, e.g.
   1. pancreatic disease
   2. disease of hormonal etiology
   3. drug- or chemical-induced condition
   4. insulin receptor abnormalities
   5. certain genetic syndromes
   6. miscellaneous

Impaired glucose tolerance (IGT)

   a. nonobese
   b. obese
   c. impaired glucose tolerance associated with certain conditions and syndromes, e.g.

      1. pancreatic disease
      2. disease of hormonal etiology
      3. drug- or chemical-induced
      4. insulin receptor abnormalities
      5. certain genetic syndromes
      6. miscellaneous

Gestational diabetes (GDM)

Statistical risk classes (subjects with normal glucose tolerance but statistically increased risk of developing diabetes)

Previous abnormality of glucose tolerance
Potential abnormality of glucose tolerance

The scheme represents a consensus of the categories that, given present knowledge, were considered likely to be homogeneous, but it recognizes that future developments will almost certainly call for modifications. Detailed descriptions of each of the subgroups are given in the original publications (22, 23).

Satisfactory application of the classification scheme, however, depends on standardization of methods of diagnosis. It is hoped that the international acceptance of the classification scheme and the recommended diagnostic criteria (see below) will result in a more logical approach to the terminology relating to diabetes, provide appropriate designations for clinical application to subjects with diabetes and glucose intolerance, and lessen the confusion in the medical literature.

DIAGNOSTIC CRITERIA

Diabetes may present with one or more of the classical symptoms such as excessive thirst, polyuria, and weight loss, or sometimes coma. Glucose will be present in the urine and the diagnosis can be made on the basis of a blood glucose estimation without provocative tests. The WHO recommendation is that a random plasma glucose level >200 mg/dl, or a fasting venous plasma glucose concentration of 140 mg/dl or over on more than one occasion, are themselves sufficient to establish the diagnosis. If the fasting glucose level does not consistently exceed 140 mg/dl, or if doubt remains as to whether or not the subject has diabetes, then the only recourse to establish the diagnosis is to perform an oral glucose tolerance test, as measurements made under standardized conditions are necessary to confirm or refute the diagnosis.

There is universal agreement that the diagnosis should not be based on the presence of glucosuria alone, nor can it be excluded on the basis of urinalysis, because of the low sensitivity of the test.

In the past, the interpretation of diagnostic tests for diabetes was hindered by a lack of uniformity in procedures and in agreement on criteria for abnormality (24). Now a standardized method of performing the oral glucose tolerance test (OGTT) has emerged as the only formal provocative test recommended for the diagnosis of diabetes. Nevertheless, the OGTT is not necessary for diagnosis in the majority of patients.

Oral Glucose Tolerance Test

The WHO recommendations warn specifically against the overuse of the OGTT and commence by stating that fasting venous plasma glucose values of less than 100 mg/dl or random glucose values of less than 140 mg/dl are sufficient to exclude the diagnosis. Such values render the performance of the test unnecessary, as does the presence of consistently high glucose levels mentioned earlier.

PREPARATION FOR THE OGTT   The methods of preparation for the OGTT first communicated by the American Diabetes Association in 1969 were re-endorsed (25). Briefly, no formal dietary preparation is recommended unless less than 150 g of carbohydrate per day are being consumed, in which case three days of preparation with a diet containing at least this amount of carbohydrate is recommended. The test should be performed in the morning after an 8–16-hour fast during which only water is permitted. The test should be performed only on ambulatory subjects, and after any acute illness a considerable period of time should elapse before the test is performed. Smoking should not be permitted during the test and it should be borne in mind that many drugs and other factors may influence the test and that it may be desirable or necessary to stop these in order to facilitate interpretation of the test result.

GLUCOSE LOAD   A major development in recommendations concerning the conduct of the OGTT, made by both the NDDG and the WHO, was that an oral 75-g carbohydrate (glucose) load be used for adults, or a load of 1.75 g/kg ideal body weight (up to a maximum of 75 g) be used for children.

There were several reasons for this recommendation, including the desire to achieve international standardization and to avoid nausea, which is not infrequent with the 100-g glucose load often used in the United States previously. Both the NDDG and WHO groups also considered acceptable the commercially available carbohydrate loads containing corn starch hydrolysates—maltose and low-molecular-weight dextrans—which are rapidly hydrolyzed to glucose, but which produce less nausea. Because of osmotic effects on absorption, the 75-g carbohydrate load should be in 250–350 ml of water and should be consumed in 5–15 mintes.

BLOOD SAMPLES   A fasting blood sample, taken before giving the glucose load, and a two-hour blood sample were recommended by both groups. The NDDG also suggested that intermediate glucose determinations should be made at 30-minute intervals; the reason for such determinations is unclear other than a recommendation that one intermediate value (as well as the two-hour value) exceed the minimum diagnostic criteria for the two-hour value. This would virtually always occur except in the case of serious laboratory error or mislabeling of tubes.

It is generally believed that venous plasma provides the best specimen for determination of glucose values, although whole blood or capillary blood is acceptable provided the differences in the results are accounted for in interpreting the test. Whole-blood glucose determinations (except in anemia) are approximately 15% lower than the corresponding plasma values (26); the capillary values are about 8% higher than the whole-blood values after glucose loading (27).

METHODS OF GLUCOSE MEASUREMENT   Many methods are used to determine glucose concentrations in blood and serum. Many of these give satisfactory and equivalent results, including the o-toluidine method, glucose oxidase methods, hexokinase and glucose dehydrogenase, as well as the Somogyi-Nelson, autoanalyzer-ferricyanide, and neocuproine methods (28). Provided the blood specimens are obtained appropriately and it is clearly recognized whether plasma, serum, or whole-blood concentrations are being reported, interpretation of the laboratory results can be made according to the criteria described below. Although various test strips and glucose meters are available, they are designed primarily for glucose monitoring during treatment. The variability of the glucose measurements is greater than with the standard laboratory based glucose measurements so that their use for establishing the diagnosis of diabetes cannot be generally recommended.

Criteria for Interpretation of the OGTT

A major departure from most previous recommendations is the designation of two degrees of severity of glucose abnormality, reflected in the classification scheme presented earlier. The category of impaired glucose tolerance (IGT) describes subjects whose glucose tolerance is not unequivocally within normal limits and yet falls short of criteria currently believed necessary for the diagnosis of diabetes itself. The criteria recommended by both NDDG and WHO for the categorization of subjects with abnormal glucose tolerance are summarized in Table 2.

DIFFERENCES BETWEEN NDDG AND WHO CRITERIA   There are certain differences between the NDDG criteria and the WHO recommendations. In particular, the NDDG criteria for diabetes *and for IGT* require that the ½- or 1- or 1½-hour plasma glucose value exceed 200 mg/dl. This is not a requirement of the WHO criteria. This requirement creates an appreciable group of subjects with "nondiagnostic" glucose tolerance tests, many of whom would be classified as IGT by the WHO criteria.

Table 2 Diagnostic values for interpretation of the oral glucose tolerance test performed under standard conditions using a 75-g oral carbohydrate (glucose) load

Diagnosis	Venous plasma glucose concentration
Diabetes Mellitus	
Fasting and/or	$\geqslant 140$ mg/dl
2-hour value[a]	$\geqslant 200$ mg/dl
Impaired Glucose Tolerance	
Fasting · and	< 140 mg/dl
2-hour value[a]	140–199 mg/dl

[a]The NDDG criteria in addition required that the ½-hour or 1-hour or 1½-hour value exceed 200 mg/dl (see discussion in text).

A further discrepancy in the recommendations arises in relation to glucose tolerance testing in pregnancy. The NDDG recommends continued usage of the criteria proposed in 1964 by O'Sullivan & Mahan (29), and continuation of the use of the 100-g glucose load for such tests, whereas the WHO recommendation is to use the 75-g load and the same criteria and diagnostic labels as in the nonpregnant state. The WHO recommendation does note the special clinical significance of IGT in pregnancy, whereas the NDDG considers all glucose intolerance recognized for the first time during pregnancy and meeting the O'Sullivan & Mahan criteria as constituting gestational diabetes mellitus (GDM). Further discussion of this issue, however, is beyond the scope of this chapter.

DISCUSSION

Distinction Between IDDM and NIDDM

IDDM and NIDDM (sometimes referred to as Type I and Type II diabetes, respectively) can generally be distinguished on the basis of the clinical history.

On occasion, however, there will still remain difficulties in the certain assignment of an individual to one class, because inadequate information is available on the subject. In particular, the correct categorization of an individual who is receiving insulin and is nonobese, but who does not have a history of spontaneous ketosis, may be difficult. Furthermore, the evolution of IDDM and NIDDM are such that each at times may mimic the other in certain regards. If, however, the diagnostic information is inadequate or equivocal, it was recommended that the classification of an individual subject should be held in abeyance until more adequate diagnostic or clinical information is forthcoming.

Age of onset is not considered in the classification because it has been increasingly recognized that NIDDM occurs in young persons and IDDM can appear for the first time in older subjects. Nevertheless, the definition of insulin dependency presents some problems. Insulin dependency implies that insulin is needed to prevent spontaneous ketosis and, ultimately, death. In the absence of definitive information on an individual's propensity to develop ketosis, other factors, such as age of onset, obesity, presence or absence of islet cell antibodies, and clinical course, are likely to be influential in arriving at an appropriate designation.

A therapeutic decision for treatment with insulin to maintain a satisfactory blood sugar level, however, itself is not considered adequate evidence to categorize the subject as IDDM, and indeed many subjects with NIDDM eventually receive insulin treatment for this purpose. While some doubt may remain as to the correct classification in particular instances, classification in the light of the total clinical history is to be encouraged. Such a practice will likely result in further information on the natural history of these two major forms of diabetes.

The Significance of IGT

The introduction of the impaired glucose tolerance (IGT) category has a number of implications. First, it emphasizes that mild degrees of glucose intolerance have a different prognostic significance than the diagnosis of diabetes. Second, the use of the term IGT avoids many of the psychosocial and economic implications that a diagnosis of diabetes carries, and as such alleviates many problems for the physician and the patient, particularly if the impaired tolerance can be corrected. The variability of the glucose tolerance test is such that there is considerable imprecision in the interpretation of results falling in the range now described as IGT. While this group carries a greater than normal risk of ultimately developing diabetes, several recent population-based follow-up studies have shown that the risk of decompensation is in the range of 1–5% per year over a 5- or 10-year time span (8, 9, 30–32). Furthermore, the likelihood of developing the specific complications of diabetes is virtually nonexistent as long as glucose tolerance remains in this range (33–35). While there is some evidence that persons with IGT are at increased risk of developing nonspecific complications, such as coronary heart disease (36, 37), glucose intolerance of a degree less than that diagnostic of diabetes may not be an independent risk factor. In any event, the absolute risk is much lower, particularly in females, than in persons with unequivocal evidence of diabetes, in whom the frequency of coronary heart disease is at least twice that of the nondiabetic (38). The term IGT, however, is not intended to foster neglect of the abnormality on the part of the patient or physician. Rather it should be a reason to search actively for explanations of glucose intolerance and to act appropriately on these at a stage before progression to diabetes (if this is indeed the reason for the intolerance) and if possible to correct other factors, such as obesity, hyperlipemia, drug usage, other endocrine conditions, that may be responsible for it.

Both the WHO Expert Committee and the NDDG draw attention to the special significance of glucose intolerance in pregnancy. Although the recommendations concerning diagnostic criteria and labeling of glucose intolerance in pregnancy are at variance, both groups recognize the importance of special management of such pregnancies. It is the author's view that the WHO recommendation has merit, especially from the point of view of simplicity and symmetry, as well as reflecting some disagreement about its significance (39), but this view was not the consensus of a recent conference on this subject (19).

Indications for Performing an OGTT

In spite of reliance on the OGTT as the basis for the diagnosis of diabetes and IGT, the WHO Expert Committee warned against overusing the glucose tolerance test. In clinical practice the use of the glucose tolerance test in nonpregnant subjects should probably be restricted to circumstances where there is real doubt concerning the presence of diabetes. The WHO report states that random venous plasma glucose concentrations of <140 mg/dl and fasting plasma values of ≤100 mg/dl should be considered normal, whereas screening values of >120 mg/dl in the fasting and 150 mg/dl in the nonfasting state merit further attention. An elevated *fasting* plasma glucose level itself, if present on more than one occasion, is sufficient for the diagnosis of diabetes, and only in persons whose levels fall between 100 and 140 mg/dl fasting can a glucose tolerance test be reasonably justified for clinical purposes.

A further justification for the performance of a glucose tolerance test is pregnancy (19). All women should be screened for diabetes early in pregnancy, and it is recommended that all women *not already* recognized to have glucose intolerance by the 24–28th week of gestation also receive a glucose tolerance test at that time. Unless provocative tests are performed early in the third trimester, the diagnosis of GDM or IGT in pregnancy will not be recognized in the majority of women.

Other indications for the performance of a glucose tolerance test fall into the research area, where it may be important to make a definitive statement about the presence of normal or impaired glucose tolerance, or in diabetics to document the severity of the hyperglycemia in response to a standardized provocative test.

Prognostic Significance of Glucose Intolerance

The formulation and adoption of the new diagnostic criteria for diabetes and IGT resulted largely from the outcome of several prospective population-based studies of glucose tolerance (8–10, 30–35). In the past, many sets of criteria were proposed [West (40) lists 17 sets of criteria for interpreting the OGTT alone.] This resulted in a wide variation in diagnostic criteria used in practice by diabetologists (24). The difficulty in arriving upon agreed criteria occurs in large part because in most populations the distribution of glucose levels, fasting or following a glucose load, is unimodal with some skewing toward higher values. Consequently, no obvious cut-off point to distinguish between those with and without diabetes was apparent.

In the past decade, however, several populations have been described with extremely high frequencies of diabetes in which bimodal frequency distributions of glucose concentrations are seen (41, 42). The optimum plasma glucose cut-off points to separate the two subpopulations are considerably higher than those widely used during the past twenty years for the diagnosis of diabetes. They range from about 135–145 mg/dl for the fasting and from 200–250 mg/dl for the two-hour postload plasma values (43). These findings add further weight to the concept that previous cut-off points were set too low.

Follow-up studies of one such population (the Pima Indians) (35), and the follow-up of the Bedford and Whitehall study populations, where unimodal glucose distributions are found, show a high degree of agreement in that the development of diabetic retinopathy, one of the most specific and pathognomonic complications of diabetes, was essentially confined to those whose two-hour plasma glucose levels (or their equivalent) were over 200 mg/dl (33–35) and whose fasting plasma glucose concentrations were in excess of 135 mg/dl (35). These results confirmed an earlier inference, made on the basis of the bimodal frequency distribution, that only individuals falling in the hyperglycemic component were at risk of developing complications (41).

The prospective population studies also add information on the natural history of the milder forms of glucose intolerance. While the rates of decompensation to diabetes are substantial and significant (8–10, 30–32), they also show that the majority of such individuals either return (apparently spontaneously) to normal glucose tolerance or remain persistently impaired for many years (9, 30). In both of the latter circumstances the risk of developing other sequelae associated specifically with diabetes is extremely low (33–35). There appears to be no justification for labeling such persons as diabetic because their prognosis is very different from those who have unequivocal evidence of fasting hyperglycemia. This was a major reason for adopting the term IGT to classify these subjects.

Other Considerations

The decision to recommend the 75-g oral carbohydrate or glucose load for the performance of the oral glucose tolerance test has been interpreted by many as an arbitrary compromise between the European and American traditions where 50 g and 100 g, respectively, have been used for many years. In fact, such a recommendation was made as far back as 1964 (44). In the subsequent years there has been an increasing consensus that the 50-g load is not a maximum stimulus and that administration of the 100-g load is often associated with nausea and/or vomiting, which invalidates the test result. Furthermore, extensive experience with the 75-g load, especially when administered as a mixture of low-molecular-weight dextrans, maltose, and glucose, shows that this is palatable and only occasionally associated with vomiting. In any event, the size of the carbohydrate load within this range has only a moderate effect on the postload glucose determinations, but the effect influences the individual classification sufficiently often to require international agreement and standardization.

There has been considerable discussion on the question of age and its relationship to glucose tolerance, although there is no specific reference to this question in the recent recommendations. It was felt that there was not enough evidence that the prognosis of different degrees of glucose intolerance in the range now considered as the cut-off for diabetes varies sufficiently to justify recommending age-dependent criteria. Indeed, even the NDDG and WHO recommendations for the diagnosis of diabetes in children are identical to those in adults, except that for children a glucose load of 1.75 g/kg ideal body weight, up to a maximum of 75 g, is recommended.

Both the NDDG and WHO place major emphasis on the fasting and two-hour postload glucose determinations. There are several reasons for this. The intermediate values, e.g. the 30-minute and 60-minute values, tend to be more variable and less reproducible within an individual than either the fasting or the two-hour values (45). In addition, there are fewer data on the prognostic significance of the intermediate values, so that a choice of cut-off points becomes problematical. Furthermore, there is no evidence that the intermediate values enhance the prediction of complications of the disease to any appreciable degree over and above that of the fasting and two-hour values.

No other tests for the diagnosis of diabetes appear in the recommendations of either group. Although a variety of tests, ranging from the intravenous glucose tolerance test to the determination of muscle capillary basement membrane thickening, have been proposed for the diagnosis of diabetes, there is no consensus that any of these tests is superior to the fasting glucose determination or the OGTT. Certainly none of the others has gained wide acceptance for diagnostic purposes, although several remain useful tools for research into other questions.

CONCLUSIONS

The proposals by the NDDG and WHO for a standardized classification and diagnostic criteria for diabetes appear to have gained rapid acceptance by diabetologists in many parts of the world. Use of the classification and of these criteria will result in much greater uniformity in the field than has prevailed in the past. In particular, the characterization of patients in a consistent manner in reasearch will lead to a greater applicability of findings and increase the comparability of studies done in different centers, nationally and internationally. While the classifications have a number of recognized shortcomings, the WHO version was adopted after the NDDG proposals had been widely circulated and discussed. The WHO version, therefore, represents an even wider international consensus than the NDDG report. The WHO proposals are attractive insofar as they are somewhat less complicated to apply, and they circumvent a classification problem for a group of subjects who, by the NDDG criteria, would have noncategorizable (and, therefore, nondiagnostic) glucose tolerance test results. While the classification is far from ideal in that it is not based uniformly on etiology, it does represent a working classification based on contemporary knowledge. As the etiology and pathogenesis become further defined, revisions will certainly be necessary, but in the interim the new classification and criteria will provide much improved, practical, operational definitions of diabetes than have been previously available.

Literature Cited

1. Marble, A. 1971. Correct concepts of diabetes. In *Joslin's Diabetes Mellitus,* ed. A. Marble, P. White, R. F. Bradley, L. P. Krall, 1:1–9. Philadelphia: Lea & Febiger. 884 pp. 11th ed.
2. Bouchardat, A. 1883. *De la Glycosurie on Diabète Sucré.* Paris: Germer-Bailliere. 180 pp.
3. von Mering, J., Minkowski, O. 1889. Diabetes mellitus nach Pankreasextirpation. *Arch. Exp. Pathol. Pharmakol.* 26:371–87
4. Banting, F. G., Best, C. H. 1922. The internal secretion of the pancreas. *J. Lab. Clin. Med.* 7:251–66
5. Mosenthal, H. O., Barry, E. 1950. Criteria for an interpretation of normal glucose tolerance tests. *Ann. Intern. Med.* 33:1175–94
6. Fajans, S. S., Conn, J. W. 1959. The early recognition of diabetes mellitus. *Ann. NY Acad. Sci.* 82:208–18
7. Siperstein, M. D. 1975. The glucose tolerance test: a pitfall in the diagnosis of diabetes mellitus. *Adv. Intern. Med.* 20:297–323
8. Birmingham Diabetes Survey Working Party. 1976. Ten-year follow-up report on Birmingham Diabetes Survey. *Br. Med. J.* 2:35–37
9. Jarrett, R. J., Keen, H., Fuller, J. H., McCartney, M. 1979. Worsening to diabetes in men with impaired glucose tolerance ("borderline diabetes".) *Diabetologia* 16:15–30
10. O'Sullivan, J. B., Mahan, C. M. 1965. Blood sugar levels, glucosuria and body weight related to the development of diabetes mellitus. *J. Am. Med. Assoc.* 194:117–22
11. Kipnis, D. M. 1968. Insulin secretion in diabetes mellitus. *Ann. Intern. Med.* 67:891–901
12. Genuth, S. M., Bennett, P. H., Miller, M., Burch, T. A. 1967. Hyperinsulinism in obese diabetic Pima Indians. *Metabolism* 16:1010–15
13. Reaven, G., Miller, R. 1968. Study of the relationship between glucose and insulin responses to an oral glucose load in man. *Diabetes* 17:560–69
14. Chiles, R., Tzagouris, M. 1970. Excessive insulin response to oral glucose in obesity and mild diabetes. *Diabetes* 19:458–64
15. Bagdade, J. D., Bierman, E. L., Porte, D. 1967. The significance of basal insulin levels in the evaluation of the insulin response to glucose in diabetic and nondiabetic subjects. *J. Clin. Invest.* 46:1549–57
16. Reaven, G. M., Bernstein, R., Davis, B., Olefsky, J. M. 1976. Nonketotic diabetes mellitus: insulin deficiency or insulin resistance? *Am. J. Med.* 60:80–88
17. Gabbe, S. G., Lowensohn, R. I., Wu, R. Y., Guerva, G. 1978. Current patterns of neonatal morbidity and mortality in infants of diabetic mothers. *Diabetes Care* 1:335–39
18. O'Sullivan, J. B., Charles, D., Mahan, C. M., Dandrow, R. V. 1973. Gestational diabetes and perinatal mortality rate. *Am. J. Obstet. Gynecol.* 116:901–4
19. Symposium on Gestational Diabetes. 1980. *Diabetes Care* 3:399–501
20. Rotter, J. I., Rimoin, D. L. 1978. Heterogeneity in diabetes mellitus—update 1978. *Diabetes* 27:599–605

21. Irvine, W. J., ed. 1979. *The Immunology of Diabetes Mellitus.* Edinburgh: Teviot Sci.
22. National Diabetes Data Group. 1979. Classification of diabetes mellitus and other categories of glucose intolerance. *Diabetes* 28:1039–57
23. WHO Expert Committee on Diabetes Mellitus Second Report. 1980. *World Health Organization Tech. Rep. Ser. 646.* Geneva: WHO
24. West, K. M. 1975. Substantial differences in the diagnostic criteria used by diabetes experts. *Diabetes* 24:641–44
25. Committee on Statistics, American Diabetes Association. 1969. Standardization of the oral glucose tolerance test. *Diabetes* 18:299–310
26. Zalme, E., Knowles, H. C. 1965. A plea for plasma sugar. *Diabetes* 14:165–66
27. Annex 1. 1980. See Ref. 22, pp. 70–71
28. Cooper, G. R. 1973. Methods for determing the amount of glucose in blood. *CRC Crit. Rev. Clin. Lab. Sci.* August, pp. 101–45
29. O'Sullivan, J. M., Mahan, C. M. 1964. Criteria for the oral glucose tolerance test in pregnancy. *Diabetes* 13:278–85
30. Keen, H., Jarrett, R. J., McCartney, P. 1982. The ten-year follow-up of the Bedford Survey (1962–1972): glucose tolerance and diabetes. *Diabetologia* 22:73–78
31. O'Sullivan, J. B., Mahan, C. M. 1968. Prospective study of 352 young patients with chemical diabetes. *N. Engl. J. Med.* 278:1038–41
32. Bennett, P. H., Knowler, W. C., Pettitt, D. J., Lisse, J. R. 1980. The prognostic significance of the glucose tolerance test. In *Endocrinology 1980,* ed. I. A. Cumming, J. W. Funder, F. A. O. Mendelsohn, pp. 711–14. Amsterdam: Elsevier. 736 pp.
33. Al Sayegh, H., Jarrett, R. J. 1979. Oral glucose-tolerance tests and the diagnosis of diabetes: results of a prospective study based on the Whitehall Survey. *Lancet* 2:432–33
34. Jarrett, R. J., Keen, H. 1976. Hyperglycaemia and diabetes mellitus. *Lancet* 2:1009–12
35. Pettitt, D. J., Knowler, W. C., Lisse, J. R., Bennett, P. H. 1980. Development of retinopathy and proteinuria in relation to plasma glucose concentrations in Pima Indians. *Lancet* 2:1050–52
36. O'Sullivan, J. B. 1982. The epidemiology of cardiovascular disease and diabetes mellitus in perspective. *Mount Sinai J. Med.* 49:163–68
37. Stamler, R., Stamler, J., eds. 1979. Asymptomatic hyperglycemia and coronary heart disease: a series of papers by the International Collaborative Group. *J. Chron. Dis.* 32:683–828
38. Knowles, H. C. Jr., Meinert, C. L., Prout, T. E. 1976. Diabetes mellitus: The overall problem and its impact on the public. In *Diabetes Mellitus,* ed. S. S. Fajans, 2:11–32. DHEW Pub. No. (NIH) 76–854. Washington, DC: GPO. 361 pp.
39. Jarrett, R. J. 1981. Reflections on gestational diabetes mellitus. *Lancet* 2: 1220–22
40. West, K. M. 1978. *Epidemiology of Diabetes and Its Vascular Lesions,* pp. 94–95. New York: Elsevier. 579 pp.
41. Bennett, P. H., Burch, T. A., Miller, M. 1971. Diabetes in the Pima Indians. *Lancet* 2:125–28
42. Zimmet, P., Whitehouse, S. 1978. Bimodality of fasting and two-hour glucose tolerance distributions in a Micronesian population. *Diabetes* 27:793–800
43. Rushforth, N. B., Miller, M., Bennett, P. H. 1979. Fasting and two-hour postload glucose levels for the diagnosis of diabetes. *Diabetologia* 16:373–79
44. Pratt, J. W. 1964. *Conference on Methodological Approaches to Population Studies in Diabetes,* p. 206. Public Health Service (DHEW) Pub. No. 1486. Washington, DC: GPO. 232 pp.
45. Rushforth, N. B., Bennett, P. H., Steinberg, A. G., Miller, M. 1975. Comparison of the value of the two-hour and one-hour glucose levels of the oral GTT in the diagnosis of diabetes in Pima Indians. *Diabetes* 24:538–46

Ann. Rev. Med. 1983. 34:311–19

THE NOSOCOMIAL SPREAD OF RESPIRATORY SYNCYTIAL VIRAL INFECTIONS

Caroline Breese Hall, M.D.

Departments of Pediatrics and Medicine, University of Rochester Medical Center, Rochester, New York 14642

ABSTRACT

Respiratory syncytial virus is a regular winter visitor that is highly contagious among persons of all ages. It is the major nosocomial pathogen on infant and toddler wards, and has recently been recognized as also causing appreciable nosocomial illness in the elderly. Control of the spread of this virus has been difficult, but transmission appears to require close contact via large-particle aerosols or via fomites. Environmental conditions affect the survival of the virus on varying surfaces and skin, but self-inoculation after touching contaminated surfaces appears to be an important mode of transmission.

In the cold winter months of 1937 in the nurseries of two Minneapolis hospitals an outbreak of pneumonia occurred (1). Thirty-two infants, mostly between 4 and 12 weeks of age, developed pneumonia that tended to be widespread and severe: 28% of these babies died. These cases were carefully studied by John Adams, who showed the presence of cytoplasmic inclusions in the bronchial epithelium of all of the babies who died. These findings, plus the distinctive epidemiologic and clinical picture of these outbreaks, led Adams to suggest that the outbreak was caused by a virus. More than two decades later Adams and his colleagues described a markedly similar epidemic of lower respiratory tract disease in infants and this time were able to identify its cause as a newly discovered virus, respiratory syncytial virus (RSV) (2, 3). Adams then suggested, retrospectively, that this newly acknowledged virus, RSV, was also the agent of the earlier

311

nursery outbreaks that had been accompanied by such striking morbidity and mortality. These descriptions of epidemic pneumonitis occurring in nurseries 45 years ago are probably the first reports of a nosocomial outbreak from respiratory syncytial virus.

This agent, when discovered in the late 1950s, was initially given the sobriquet "CCA," the chimpanzee coryza agent, because it was initially recovered from a chimpanzee with a cold. However, over the ensuing years it was quickly recognized as the most important respiratory pathogen of infants and young children (4, 5). Despite this, and Adams' earlier description, the potential of RSV to cause nosocomial illness has only recently been recognized (6–8).

During a recent community outbreak of RSV in Rochester, New York, a number of young children were admitted to the infant and toddler ward with RSV lower respiratory tract disease. However, other children housed in this ward who had been hospitalized with other conditions also began developing respiratory illness, as shown in Figure 1 (7). Forty-five percent of these contact infants who had been hospitalized for at least 7 days, the time necessary to define an infection as nosocomial, became infected with

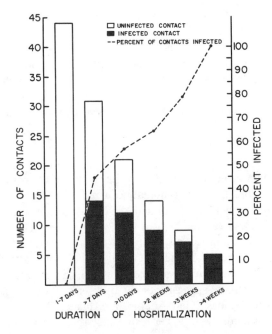

Figure 1   Number and percentage of contact infants acquiring nosocomial respiratory syncytial virus infection according to length of stay on a pediatric ward (7; reprinted by permission of the *New England Journal of Medicine.*)

RSV. Furthermore, the risk of nosocomial infection increased with each subsequent week of hospitalization. About a third of these children developed pneumonia or bronchiolitis, which significantly extended their hospitalization.

Why then has this nosocomial infection not been more commonly recognized? In part, this may be because nosocomial illness has traditionally been attributed to bacterial agents. There is much less awareness of viruses as nosocomial pathogens and facilities for making a quick viral diagnosis may not be available. Furthermore, colds and upper respiratory tract signs are so frequent in young children that they may be thought to be trivial, and their potential as a nosocomial hazard not appreciated.

Respiratory viral agents are actually the major causes of nosocomial infection on pediatric wards and differ from bacterial nosocomial pathogens in several important ways (9). Viral nosocomial infections, such as RSV, reflect the epidemiologic pattern of activity of the agent in the community, and therefore, those that occur in epidemics will be most frequent. Furthermore, the epidemiologic characteristics of these viral infections are similar, whether community or hospital acquired. The age predilection, type of illness, and seasonal occurrence are similar. In contrast to most bacterial nosocomial infections, those from respiratory viruses do not predominantly occur in the predisposed child, although the illness may be more severe in such children.

Certain distinctive traits of respiratory syncytial virus may explain why it is the major such nosocomial hazard. First, it causes yearly outbreaks of infection (10). It is also highly contagious, such that everyone experiences infection with RSV within the first several years of life (10–14). The morbidity arising each year among young children is, therefore, appreciable. In Washington, D.C., Parrott and colleagues (11) estimate that about half of the children will acquire RSV infection during the first epidemic they experience, and if acquired during the first year of life the infection will be manifest by a febrile pneumonitis in 40%. Furthermore, infection is not limited to young children, but repeated infections may occur throughout life (14–17). A susceptible population, therefore, is readily available, for immunity is of short duration, possibly lasting only months (14, 15). Severe lower respiratory tract involvement, pneumonia, and bronchiolitis, are, however, confined to the first several years of life. But during these initial years a child may have a second bout of RSV lower respiratory tract disease in the subsequent years' outbreak, which is as severe as the first (14).

Nosocomial infection from RSV thus reflects the patterns of community-acquired infection. On the ward, RSV is highly contagious, and susceptible populations of infants and staff are ever present. During a nosocomial RSV outbreak 20–45% of infants admitted for other reasons may acquire the infection nosocomially, and their illness is almost always symptomatic (6, 7, 18–21). Lower respiratory tract involvement occurs in 20–50% of these young children. In the rest, nosocomial infection is manifest by fever, otitis, and upper respiratory tract signs. In addition, RSV infection in this age group is accompanied by prolonged and abundant shedding of the virus from the respiratory tract, enhancing the potential spread of the virus (22).

Nosocomial outbreaks of RSV infection may also occur in neonatal units (19, 20, 23–25). In this setting nosocomial RSV infection may be even more difficult to recognize, but may be disastrous. In neonates, especially during the first several weeks of life, RSV infection may be atypical, lacking the classical signs of lower respiratory tract disease. The infection may be manifest by only such nonspecific signs as lethargy, irritability, and poor feeding (19). Upper respiratory tract signs may be present in less than a half of these infants. Apnea may also be a frequent sign. The resulting morbidity and mortality in these compromised infants has usually been high.

Nosocomial RSV infection is not confined to the children on the wards, but also readily involves the adult personnel (17, 19, 21). Up to 50% of the staff on these pediatric wards during an RSV outbreak will acquire RSV infection. About 80% of these illnesses are symptomatic. Most are manifest by upper respiratory tract illness, with or without fever, sometimes there is tracheobronchitis. However, even in these young, healthy adults RSV infection may be quite prolonged and accompanied by lower respiratory tract involvement that is clinically silent but results in abnormal pulmonary function for 6–8 weeks (26).

More recently RSV was noted to cause outbreaks of illness among the elderly and chronically ill who are institutionalized (27, 28). In this group of elderly adults, RSV infection may mimic an outbreak of influenza. The attack rate in one such nursing home reached 50%, and pneumonia occurred in 47% of those infected (28).

Controlling the nosocomial spread of RSV, however, has been a conundrum. The pattern of transmission of RSV on the wards during these outbreaks suggests that personnel might be important in the spread of the virus and that large open wards allow greater transmission than wards composed of smaller rooms (6–8, 18). A new hospital facility in Rochester with wards consisting of rooms with one to three beds allowed us to evaluate methods to control the spread of RSV during a community outbreak of RSV infection (18). The procedures listed in Table 1 were employed and monitored during the time RSV was active in the community. This decreased the number of nosocomial RSV infections in infants (19%), but had no effect on the prevention of nosocomial infection in the ward personnel. Despite these procedures, 56% of personnel became infected and 82% had symptomatic illness (18). Hence, such infection control procedures ap-

Table 1 Infection control procedures evaluated during a nosocomial outbreak of respiratory syncytial virus (RSV) infections on a pediatric ward (18)

1. Isolation or cohorting of RSV-infected infants	4. Cohorting of staff to RSV-infected infants
2. Handwashing	5. Isolation of high risk contact infants
3. Use of gowns on direct patient contact	6. Limitation of visitors

peared to affect the modes of transmission of the virus to the infants but not to the staff members.

Theoretically, RSV could be spread by one of three modes: (a) by large particles or droplets, (b) by self-inoculation after touching contaminated surfaces (fomites,) and (c) by small-particle aerosols. Inoculation of virus by large-particle aerosols or droplets appears feasible for most viruses if there is close contact, as these droplets can traverse only a few feet. Small-particle aerosols, on the other hand, may travel greater distances and not require close contact. The patterns of the nosocomial spread of RSV on the wards indicate that those personnel in close contact with infected babies were most likely to become infected, which suggests that either the first or second mode is operative. Spread by fomites, though, requires that the virus be stable in the environment for periods sufficient to allow transmission. Respiratory syncytial virus, however, is considered to be a labile virus. We, therefore, undertook a series of experiments to determine whether RSV would survive in the environment for sufficient periods to allow transmission by fomites (29).

Fresh secretions from infants admitted with RSV lower respiratory tract disease were allowed to contaminate a variety of surfaces around the infant's bed. We subsequently determined the amount of virus that could be recovered from these surfaces at various time periods, as shown in Figure 2 (29). Indeed, infectious virus could be recovered from a variety of surfaces. The length of time that RSV could survive on these surfaces was apparently influenced by the temperature, humidity, and type of surface. Nonporous surfaces such as countertops, glass and plastic provided an adequate stage for RSV to remain infectious for many hours and occasionally even for a day. Additional experiments showed that infectious virus could be transferred to and recovered from hands touching contaminated surfaces. Thus, fomite transmission and subsequent self-inoculation of RSV seemed feasible.

Which of the three possible modes of transmission occurred on hospital wards remained to be evaluated. During a recent outbreak of RSV infection we exposed young, healthy volunteers to RSV on the pediatric ward by one of three methods (30). The first group, called "cuddlers," were exposed to

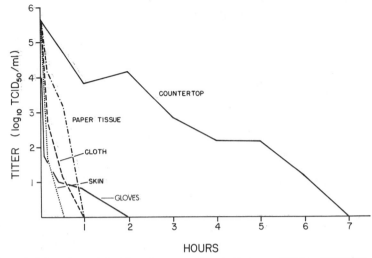

Figure 2 Mean titer and duration of recovery of respiratory syncytial virus (RSV) from skin (hands) and environmental surfaces that were contaminated with nasal secretions freshly obtained from infants hospitalized lower respiratory tract disease caused by respiratory syncytial virus (29; reprinted by permission of the University of Chicago Press.)

an infected infant by caring for the baby in the usual manner, which included feeding, bathing, and playing with the infant. The volunteers wore gowns but no masks or gloves. The second group, called "touchers," were exposed with the infant out of the room by touching surfaces contaminated with the baby's secretions and then subsequently touching the mucous membranes of their eyes or nose. The third group, called "sitters," were exposed to infected babies by sitting more than six feet from the infant's bed. These volunteers wore gowns, gloves but no masks, and were allowed to read but to touch nothing else. As shown in Figure 3, the cuddlers could potentially be exposed by any of the three routes of transmission, but the touchers and sitters could be exposed only by fomites or small-particle aerosols.

Infection occurred in the cuddlers and in the touchers, but not in the sitters. This, therefore, suggested that RSV could be spread not only by

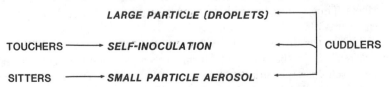

Figure 3 Possible modes of spread of respiratory syncytial virus and groups of subjects exposed by each route.

direct contact with large particles or droplets, but also by fomites and self-inoculation. The infection control procedures mentioned above thus may not protect staff members against self-inoculation when they inadvertently touch their eyes or nose while caring for an infant. However, these procedures if followed would diminish spread to other infants because hands are washed and gowns are changed between infants.

What infection control procedures should then be used? Would masks help? Masks affect only half of the possible portals of entry for RSV. Studies of experimental RSV infection show that infection from RSV appears to occur only when the virus is inoculated via the nose or eye, but not if it enters via the mouth (31).

Although the donning of gowns and masks are time-honored rituals for control of respiratory illnesses, their routine use appears to be of little additional benefit in the prevention of the spread of RSV (21, 32). During a recent RSV season, the rates of nosocomial infection in infants and in personnel on an infant and toddler ward were compared during two controlled periods when masks and gowns were and were not used. The rates of nosocomial infection were not significantly different in either the infants or personnel (21). Similarly, in Denver, use of gowns and masks were shown to have no effect on the rate of acquisition of upper respiratory tract infections by ward personnel (32).

For RSV, therefore, the infection control procedure that is probably of the most use is handwashing. Isolation and cohorting of infants to staff also seem advisable. However, during the midst of an RSV outbreak facilities may not allow individual isolation of infants admitted with respiratory disease. Rapid viral diagnostic techniques can be of great benefit at admission in guiding the cohorting or grouping of infants infected with the same agent (20).

In addition, infants at high risk for severe or complicated RSV infection should not be electively admitted to the pediatric wards during an RSV outbreak. If such children must be admitted, isolating them in a private room may help prevent them from acquiring RSV nosocomially. Currently, the children who appear to be in this high risk category include infants with congenital heart disease, immunosuppressed patients, and premature infants with pulmonary problems (33, 34). Over the past six years 37% of our infants hospitalized with congenital heart disease and RSV infection have died (33). Many of these infections were acquired nosocomially. The risk of severe or fatal disease appears particularly high in infants with congenital heart disease and pulmonary hypertension. Immunosuppressed patients are also at risk for acquiring RSV infection nosocomially (34, 35). In normal hosts, pneumonia from RSV infection is usually confined to the first three years of life. However, in the immunocompromised host of any age RSV infection may be manifest as pneumonia, which is frequently severe, generalized, and prolonged. Some children with malignancies have recurrent bouts of RSV pneumonia that appear to correlate with their chemotherapy and degree of immunosuppression. Immunocompromised adults may also be at risk for nosocomial RSV pneumonia introduced by staff or visitors. A recent report graphically illustrates this with the description of rapidly progressive, fatal pneumonia in an immunosuppressed man confined to a laminar airflow room (35). Epidemiologic information suggested he acquired RSV from his children who had visited him.

It is difficult to measure the impact of these nosocomial infections, particularly since most go unrecognized. RSV reaches its 25th birthday this year. But it has not come of age. Diagnostic means are not always readily available, and it remains recalcitrant to control by immunization. Perhaps these coming years will mark its maturing. An immunolologic profile may be drawn that will allow us to provide protection from this virus, which, if durable, will surpass the evanescent natural immunity. In the meantime, our awareness and understanding of RSV's often silent transmission may help limit its spread among the high risk hospitalized populations, both young and old.

Literature Cited

1. Adams, J. M. 1941. Primary virus pneumonitis with cytoplasmic inclusion bodies: a study of an epidemic involving thirty-two infants with nine deaths. *J. Am. Med. Assoc.* 116:925–33
2. Adams, J. M., Imagawa, D. T., Zike, K. 1961. Epidemic bronchiolitis and pneumonitis related to respiratory syncytial virus. *J. Am. Med. Assoc.* 176:1037–39
3. Adams, J. M., Imagawa, D. T., Zike, K. 1961. Relationship of pneumonitis in infants to respiratory syncytial virus. *Lancet* 81:502–6
4. Chanock, R. M., Finberg, L. 1957. Recovery from infants with respiratory illness of a virus related to chimpanzee coryza agent (CCA). II. Epidemiologic aspects of infection in infants and young children. *Am. J. Hyg.* 66:291–300
5. Chanock, R. M., Parrott, R. H. 1965. Acute respiratory disease in infancy and childhood: present understanding and prospects for prevention. *Pediatrics* 36:21–39
6. Gardner, P. S., Court, S. D. M., Brocklebank, J. T., et al. 1973 Virus cross-infection in pediatric wards. *Br. Med. J.* 2:571–75
7. Hall, C. B., Douglas, R. G. Jr., Geiman, J. M., et al. 1975. Nosocomial respiratory syncytial virus infections. *N. Engl. J. Med.* 293:1343–46
8. Sims, D. G., Downham, M. A. P. S., Webb, J. K. G., et al. 1975. Hospital cross-infection on children's wards with respiratory syncytial virus and the role of adult carriage. *Acta Pediatr. Scand.* 65:541–45
9. Hall, C. B. 1981. Nosocomial viral respiratory infections: perennial weeds on pediatric wards. *Am. J. Med.* 70:670–76
10. Glezen, W. P., Denny, F. W. 1973. Epidemiology of acute lower respiratory disease in children. *N. Engl. J. Med.* 288:498–505
11. Parrott, M. F., Kim, H. W., Arrobio, J. O., et al. 1973. Epidemiology of respiratory syncytial virus infection in Washington, DC. II. Infection and disease with respect to age, immunologic status, race, and sex. *Am. J. Epidemiol.* 98: 289–300
12. Brandt, C. D., Kim, H. W., Arrobio, J. O., et al. 1973. Epidemiology of respiratory syncytial virus infection in Washington, DC. III. Composite analysis of eleven consecutive yearly epidemics. *Am. J. Epidemiol.* 98:355–64
13. Parrott, R. H., Kim., H. W., Brandt, C. D., et al. 1974. Respiratory syncytial virus in infants and children. *Prev. Med.* 3:473–80

14. Henderson, F. W., Collier, A. M., Clyde, W. A. Jr., et al. 1979. Respiratory-syncytial-virus infections, reinfections and immunity: a prospective, longitudinal study in young children. *N. Engl. J. Med.* 300:530–34

15. Hall, C. B., Douglas, R. G. Jr. 1982. Reinfection and duration of immunity to respiratory syncytial virus. *Pediatr. Res.* 16:242A

16. Hall, C. B., Geiman, J. M., Biggar, R., et al. 1976. Respiratory syncytial virus infections within families. *N. Engl. J. Med.* 294:414–19

17. Berglund, B. 1967. Respiratory syncytial virus infection in families: a study of family members of children hospitalized for acute respiratory disease. *Acta Pediatr. Scand.* 56:395–404

18. Hall, C. B., Geiman, J. M., Douglas, R. G. Jr., et al. 1978. Control of nosocomial respiratory syncytial viral infections. *Pediatrics* 62:728–31

19. Hall, C. B., Kopelman, A. E., Douglas, R. G. Jr., et al. 1979. Neonatal respiratory syncytial virus infection. *N. Engl. J. Med.* 300:393–96

20. Mintz, L., Ballard, R. A., Sniderman, S. H., Roth, R. S., Drew, W. L. 1979. Nosocomial respiratory syncytial virus infections in an intensive care nursery: rapid diagnosis by direct immunofluourescence. *Pediatrics* 64:149–53

21. Hall, C. G., Douglas, R. G. Jr. 1981. Nosocomial respiratory syncytial virus infections: the role of gowns and masks on prevention. *Am. J. Dis. Child.* 135:512–145

22. Hall, C. B., Douglas, R. G. Jr., Geiman, J. M. 1976. Respiratory syncytial virus infections in infants: quantitation and duration of shedding. *J. Pediatr.* 89:11–15

23. Neligan, G. A., Steiner, H., Gardner, P. S., et al. 1970. Respiratory syncytial virus infection of the newborn. *Br. Med. J.* 3:146–47

24. Goldson, E. J., McCarthy, J. T., Welling, M. A., Todd, J. K. 1979. A respiratory syncytial virus outbreak in a transitional care nursery. *Am. J. Dis. Child.* 133:1280–82

25. Valenti, W. M., Clarke, T. A., Hall, C. B., Menegus, M. A., Shapiro. D. L. 1982. Concurrent outbreaks of rhinovirus and respiratory syncytial virus in an intensive care nursery: epidemiology and associated risk factors. *J. Pediatr.* 10:722–26

26. Hall, W. J., Hall, C. B., Speers, D. M. 1978. Respiratory syncytial virus infections in adults. Clinical, virologic, and serial pulmonary function studies. *Ann. Intern. Med.* 88:203–5

27. Mathur, U., Bentley, D. W., Hall, C. B. 1980. Concurrent respiratory syncytial virus and influenza A infections in the institutionalized elderly and chronically ill. *Ann. Intern. Med.* 93:49–52

28. Center for Disease Control. 1978. Respiratory syncytial virus—Missouri. *Morbid. Mortal. Wkly. Rep.* 26:351

29. Hall, C. B., Geiman, J. M., Douglas, R. G. Jr. 1980. Possible transmission by fomites of respiratory syncytial virus. *J. Infect. Dis.* 141:98–102

30. Hall, C. B., Douglas, R. G. Jr. 1981. Modes of transmission of respiratory syncytial virus. *J. Pediatr.* 99:100–3

31. Hall, C. B., Douglas, R. G. Jr., Schnabel, K. C., Geiman, J. M. 1981. Infectivity of respiratory syncytial virus by various routes of inoculation. *Infect. Immun.* 33:779–83

32. Murphy, D., Todd, J. K., Chao, R. K., Orr., I., McIntosh, K. 1981. The use of gowns and masks to avoid respiratory illness in pediatric hospital personnel. *J. Pediatr.* 99:746–50

33. MacDonald, N. E., Hall, C. B., Suffin, SC., Alexson, C., Harris, P. J., Manning, J. A. 1982. Respiratory syncytial virus infection in infants with congenital heart disease. *N. Engl. J. Med.* 307:397–400

34. Hall, C. B., MacDonald, N. E., Klemperer, M. K., Ettinger, L. J. 1981. Respiratory syncytial virus in immunocompromised children. *Pediatr. Res.* 15:613

35. Crane, L. R., Kish, J. A., Ratanatharathorn, V., Merline, J. R., Raval, M. F. T. 1981. Fatal syncytial virus pneumonia in a laminar airflow room. *J. Am. Med. Assoc.* 246:366–68

Ann. Rev. Med. 1983. 34:321–35

FALCIPARUM MALARIA:
The Urgent Need for Safe
and Effective Drugs

Karl H. Rieckmann, M.D.

Division of Tropical Medicine, University of New Mexico Medical Center,
Albuquerque, New Mexico 87131

ABSTRACT

The spread of multidrug-resistant strains of *Plasmodium falciparum* poses
an increasing threat to the effective treatment and prophylaxis of malaria.
Recent advances in determining the drug sensitivity of malaria parasites
should promote the more rational use of standard or alternative antimalarials in areas with emerging or well-established drug resistance. The use of
currently available alternative drugs is usually associated with more problems than that of the standard, synthetic antimalarials. Safe and effective
drugs, capable of being administered as a single-dose or short-course treatment, are urgently needed to control the adaptable malaria parasite.

INTRODUCTION

Malaria continues to be a major health problem in many tropical and
subtropical areas of the world. The disease affects more than 200 million
people each year, and it is anticipated that the global malaria situation will
deteriorate further in the foreseeable future. Resistance of malaria parasites
to antimalarial drugs is spreading rapidly. In many areas of the American,
Asian, and Pacific regions, malaria no longer responds adequately to 4-
aminoquinolines, such as chloroquine, which have been the cornerstone for
the treatment and prophylaxis of malaria for the past three decades. In the
absence of any meaningful preventive measures, chloroquine resistance also
appears to be becoming firmly established in East Africa and will undoubtedly extend to the rest of Africa. Chloroquine resistance currently affects
Plasmodium falciparum, the only one of the four species of human plas-

321

0066-4219/83/0401-0321$02.00

modia that frequently kills its host. The more benign species, *P. vivax, P. ovale,* and *P. malariae,* have retained their susceptibility to chloroquine; in fact, the overall treatment of infections with these three species has not changed appreciably during the past two decades.

Parasites of *P. falciparum* are also becoming resistant to alternative or "second-line" drugs or combinations of drugs. In many parts of South America and Southeast Asia, for example, malaria infections are no longer cured after the administration of Fansidar®. This fixed drug combination of sulfadoxine, a long-acting sulfonamide, and pyrimethamine, a folate antagonist, is the main alternative to chloroquine in most countries afflicted with malaria. Furthermore, the old "standby," quinine, is now no longer able to cure a disturbingly large number of falciparum infections. There are, nevertheless, a few other drugs that can be used in the treatment and prophylaxis of drug-resistant malaria. Unfortunately, they all have either limited antimalarial activity or appreciable toxic side-effects. They also have to be taken at frequent intervals over a long period of time; this raises practical problems in many rural endemic areas with limited medical personnel and facilities. Furthermore, none of these alternative drugs can be recommended for use by pregnant women, a segment of the population particularly vulnerable to malaria.

This review focuses upon (*a*) methods developed to monitor the rapid change in the drug susceptibility of malaria parasites; (b) alternatives to the use of chloroquine in the treatment and prophylaxis of malaria; and (c) new antimalarial drugs.

ASSESSMENT OF PARASITE SUSCEPTIBILITY TO DRUGS

The treatment and prophylaxis of falciparum malaria should be based on information concerning the susceptibility of malaria parasites to various drugs. The lack of adequate information and the accompanying confusion regarding appropriate treatment and prophylaxis have been responsible for many deaths. Until recently, it was difficult to determine parasite susceptibility to various drugs routinely. Although the susceptibility of *P. falciparum* to antimalarial drugs, especially chloroquine, has been successfully determined in vitro by numerous investigators under laboratory and field conditions (1–6), the original in vitro test (7) had some disadvantages that limited its widespread application. More recently, a microtest was developed by which the susceptibility of parasites to chloroquine and other antimalarials can be determined more readily (8). As this test requires the collection of only 50–100 μl of blood, the specimens are collected by finger prick rather than by venipuncture. This makes it easier to carry out susceptibility testing in young children. The test is based on the inhibition of parasite growth by effective concentrations of a drug during 24–48 hours of uninterrupted incubation. The period of incubation depends on the maturity of ring forms of *P. falciparum* at the start of incubation. The effect of drugs is determined by microscopically examining cultures after incubation and noting the extent to which the formation of normal schizonts or parasite reinvasion of erythrocytes has been inhibited.

The microtest has been simplified further (9). The inhibition of parasite growth by various drugs can now be determined visually and no longer requires the preparation of blood films or the use of a microscope. By adding a mixture of sodium hydroxide and sodium chloride to cultures at the end of incubation, one can observe a dark precipitate in the control wells of the microculture plate, presumably caused by interaction between the alkali and the malaria pigment produced during the maturation of rings to schizonts. In the presence of effective concentrations of a drug such as chloroquine, quinine, or mefloquine, the precipitates are not observed because rings are unable to mature to pigment-containing schizonts.

The availability of well-standardized test kits now provides a convenient way of determining the susceptibility of parasites to antimalarial drugs.[1] In fact, a routine drug sensitivity test should be performed before any patient with falciparum malaria is started on antimalarial therapy. Treatment can then be modified, if necessary, after the results of the test become available. The test kits can also solve the problem of obtaining reliable information regarding parasite susceptibility to antimalarials in various endemic areas of a country. Although limited testing for chloroquine susceptibility has been carried out under the auspices of the World Health Organization (10), adequate information about the prevalence and degree of resistance to chloroquine and other drugs is rather sparse or outdated in most malarious countries (11).

Under such circumstances, it is difficult to formulate effective prophylactic and treatment regimens to be used against *P. falciparum* acquired in such areas. For example, our ignorance of the status of parasite drug sensitivity to chloroquine and proguanil in many parts of Africa creates somewhat of a dilemma in recommending appropriate chemoprophylaxis for temporary residents or visitors to that area (12). Far more important, though, are the human suffering and the social and economic impact of drug-resistant malaria on the permanent residents of malarious areas. In his opening address to the Interregional Workshop on Drug-resistant Malaria, 10 August 1981, the Minister of Health for Malaysia, Mr. Y. B. Tan Sri Chong Han Nyan, stated: "We now face a new anxiety . . . the emergence of the drug-resistant malaria parasite . . . The malarial parasite does not

[1] Test kits are available from TropMed Resources, P.O. Box 4921, Albuquerque, NM 87196, USA.

recognize political or geographical boundaries. With the rapid development of this whole region, and the increasing mobility of our total population, we have to widen our horizons ... We cannot afford the wastage of human energy caused by this debilitating disease, especially when it affects our rural people, whose social and economic betterment is of priority concern to us all." This eloquent statement emphasizes the urgent need to meet the challenge of drug resistance whenever and wherever it develops. The first step in meeting this challenge is to constantly monitor the spread, extent, and severity of drug resistance. This should no longer be a problem, even in the most remote rural areas, now that a field incubator not requiring a conventional source of electricity is available to culture malaria parasites (13) and that drug susceptibility tests can be determined without the use of a microscope (9). By having up-to-date information available to them, health authorities can institute appropriate countermeasures to deal with the rapidly changing spectrum of parasite response to various antimalarial drugs.

ALTERNATIVES TO CHLOROQUINE

Quinine and Quinidine

The well-established use of quinine in the treatment of malaria declined after the introduction of synthetic antimalarials, especially after chloroquine became widely available about 30 years ago. Chloroquine has far fewer toxic side-effects, is considerably cheaper, and is administered over a shorter period of time than quinine. With the emergence of chloroquine-resistant strains, quinine, although far from being an ideal antimalarial, was reintroduced for the treatment of falciparum malaria. In fact, it is still regarded as the most efficacious drug available for terminating acute attacks in nonimmune individuals infected with chloroquine-resistant malaria (14). Although quinine has proven to be uniformly effective in bringing the infection under control rapidly, it does not always produce radical cure of falciparum malaria. Soon after quinine's reintroduction in the 1960s, recrudescences of parasitemia were observed after 7–10 days of treatment (15–17). Parasites were also observed to become less susceptible to quinine after exposure to it (18). More recently, it has become obvious that, despite its clinical efficacy, quinine is incapable of preventing breakthroughs in an increasing number of falciparum infections. For example, about one third of 50 patients in Thailand were not cured after 7 days of quinine therapy (19).

Quinidine, the d-isomer of quinine, was used occasionally for treating human malaria in the 1930s (20). A recent study by White et al (21) showed that all 14 patients infected with falciparum malaria were cured after they received 30 mg of quinidine/kg/day for seven days. No significant side-effects were observed during the course of treatment. The authors pointed out that 72% of patients living in this area are cured after a seven-day course of treatment with quinine followed by a single dose of sulfadoxine-pyrimethamine. Although further investigations are needed to evaluate the efficacy and toxicity of this drug regimen, the results of this study suggest that quinidine may prove to be superior to quinine for treating multidrug-resistant infections of *P. falciparum*. Although it is as expensive as quinine, quinidine is more readily available than quinine in many countries, thereby preventing any undue delay in instituting treatment of acutely ill patients.

Amodiaquine

Amodiaquine, a 4-aminoquinoline drug similar to chloroquine, was observed to be more effective than chloroquine in individuals infected with falciparum malaria (22). Although treatment with amodiaquine promptly cleared fever and parasitemia in infections showing little response to chloroquine, radical cure was never observed after the use of amodiaquine. However, addition of a slower-acting drug, such as tetracycline, to the treatment regimen cured patients of their infections (see below.) It is not known at present whether amodiaquine is more effective than chloroquine in the prophylaxis of chloroquine-resistant malaria.

Sulfonamide-Pyrimethamine Combinations

Various combinations of sulfonamides and pyrimethamine were introduced in the mid-1960s as alternatives to quinine for treating chlorquine-resistant infections (23–26). The components of such drug combinations act at different points along the folate metabolic pathway of the parasite and thereby potentiate each other's antimalarial activity. These drug combinations, when used alone, acted too slowly to terminate acute attacks of falciparum malaria in nonimmune individuals. However, when they were administered together with standard courses of quinine, there were fewer recrudescences of parasitemia after treatment.

In many endemic areas, sulfonamide-pyrimethamine drug combinations were used without concurrent quinine medication. Administration of a single dose of a sulfadoxine-pyrimethamine combination, marketed under the trade name Fansidar, was effective in curing most falciparum infections, and it was gradually adopted as the standard treatment for uncomplicated cases of *P. falciparum* in endemic areas with chloroquine-resistant malaria.

The single-dose treatment was a practical and convenient means of handling the situation in areas where limited medical personnel and facilities are available. During the past two to three years, it has become increasingly obvious that Fansidar is losing its effectiveness against *P. falciparum* in some areas of South America, Southeast Asia, and the Pacific (27–30). This is a particularly disturbing development because an alternative single-dose or short-course therapy to replace Fansidar is just not available at the present time. In Thailand, even a seven-day supplementary course of quinine failed to cure about one fifth of 32 patients treated with Fansidar (19).

Fansidar is also being used in Asia and South America for prophylaxis against chloroquine-resistant falciparum malaria (11, 31). Quite recently, with mounting evidence that chloroquine-resistant parasites are widely dispersed in East Africa, it has been recommended that this drug combination be used in that part of the world, too (12). As Fansidar is often ineffective in suppressing vivax malaria (32, 33), it is advisable to take chloroquine concurrently for prophylaxis against *P. vivax*. The addition of chloroquine to the suppressive drug regimen should also delay the emergence of Fansidar-resistant parasites and effectively suppress chloroquine-sensitive parasites of *P. falciparum* in persons with "host-failure" to Fansidar prophylaxis (23, 34, 35).

Fansidar cannot be used during pregnancy, by nursing mothers, or by infants less than two months of age because pyrimethamine is teratogenic in laboratory animals and because the use of sulfonamides has been associated with neonatal jaundice. Its use is also contraindicated for persons who are allergic to sulfonamides. Toxic manifestations associated with long-term Fansidar prophylaxis, alone or in combination with chloroquine, have not yet been determined. In one study, however, leucopenia (but not agranulocytosis) was observed in 11% of individuals who received the currently recommended weekly suppressive dose of Fansidar for 4–19 months (36). It is, therefore, advisable to perform a routine hematological examination every three to four months on people who are on long-term prophylaxis. One should also be aware that severe bone marrow depression can be induced by patients who take too many tablets of Fansidar (containing more than 200 mg of pyrimethamine) in an attempt to get rid of their symptoms (personal observations.) Fortunately, folinic acid (leucovorin, citrovorum factor) can reverse this adverse side-effect of pyrimethamine (37) apparently without interfering with its antimalarial activity (38, 39). If these findings are confirmed by further studies, and if all antifolate effects of pyrimethamine are reversed by folinic acid, pregnant women could be given pyrimethamine and folinic acid simultaneously without fear of any teratogenicity.

Sulfone-Antifolate Drug Combinations

The need for adequate protection against chloroquine-resistant falciparum malaria led to the evaluation of various sulfones (40–46). As observed with sulfonamides, the antimalarial activity of a sulfone could be potentiated by the addition of a folate antagonist (e.g. pyrimethamine, chloroguanide) even when parasites were resistant to the antifolates (43, 46).

The most widely used sulfone-antifolate combination is Maloprim®, a fixed dapsone-pyrimethamine combination. The ingestion of this drug combination once a week has been recommended as an alternative to the weekly dose of Fansidar for the suppression of chloroquine-resistant falciparum malaria (11, 47). However, the short pharmacological half-life of dapsone (about 25 hours) means that pyrimethamine is the only component of this drug combination that persists for the entire week. It was therefore suggested that Maloprim be taken twice a week so that parasites would always encounter adequate blood levels of both components of the drug (48). However, the total weekly dose of dapsone would then be comparable to that at which agranulocytosis has been observed to develop in a few individuals taking the drug on a daily basis (44,49). Further information concerning the prophylactic efficacy and long-term toxicity of Maloprim is required before any definite recommendations can be made regarding optimum intervals between drug administration.

When dapsone is administered on a daily basis, it is often given in combination with proguanil (chloroguanide), another folate antagonist (44). Although antimalarial doses of proguanil have far fewer side-effects than pyrimethamine, the suppressive activity of proguanil alone is inadequate against many chloroquine- or pyrimethamine-resistant strains of *P. falciparum*. However, as observed with other antifolates, its activity against the blood stages of *P. falciparum* is undoubtedly potentiated by sulfones or sulfonamides. As such potentiation may also extend to the pre-erythrocytic tissue stages of *P. falciparum* (50), it is possible that dapsone (at doses below those at which agranulocytosis has been observed) in combination with proguanil might be an effective causal prophylactic in areas with drug-resistant falciparum malaria.

Sulfone-antifolate drug combinations can be suitable chemoprophylactic substitutes for Fansidar for individuals who are allergic to sulfonamides and who have no cross-hypersensitivity to sulfones. However, as is the case with sulfonamides, sulfones exert little effect against the blood stages of *P. vivax* (41, 51), and their effectiveness against *P. ovale* and *P. malariae* is not yet defined. Chloroquine should, therefore, be included in the prophylactic regimen in areas where parasites of these plasmodial species are not adequately suppressed by pyrimethamine or proguanil.

Antibiotics

During the 1950s, three tetracyclines were found to exert some activity against human malaria (52–54). Because the clearance of fever and parasitemia after treatment with these drugs was slower than that observed with other antimalarials such as chloroquine or quinine, antibiotics were not considered to be of significant value in the treatment of malaria infections (55).

With the subsequent development of multidrug-resistant infections of *P. falciparum*, the value of tetracyclines as antimalarial agents was reappraised in the early 1970s. It was found that most chloroquine-resistant infections could be cured by 7–10 days of treatment with tetracycline (56, 57). Tetraycline appeared to exert no appreciable influence on the level of parasitemia or the clinical condition of patients during the first few days of treatment; clearance of parasites and abatement of symptoms were usually observed only between the fourth and seventh day after the start of treatment. Because of the slow action of tetracycline, a rapidly acting blood schizontocide, such as quinine or amodiaquine, was adminstered at the start of the treatment course. Subsequent field studies in Thailand confirmed the value of using such drug combinations against chloroquine-resistant falciparum malaria (58, 59). It is encouraging that, despite the diminishing efficacy of quinine and Fansidar, 10-day courses of tetracycline continue to cure falciparum infections in Thailand (19).

Newer and more expensive tetracyclines—doxycycline and minocycline—also exert a marked activity against multidrug-resistant strains of *P. falciparum* (60, 61). As with tetracycline, these drugs must be given in conjunction with a rapidly acting blood schizontocide to ensure prompt clearance of symptoms and parasites. Both of these tetracyclines can be administered less frequently (every 12–24 hours) and at lower doses than tetracycline because of their more complete intestinal absorption and their longer serum half-lives. Antimalarial studies with both drugs were, in general, carried out at higher doses than those used at present for the treatment of bacterial infections. However, a few patients who received lower-than-recommended doses of minocycline (only 100 mg daily for seven days) were also cured of their falciparum infections. As the incidence of side-effects associated with the use of these antibiotics (e.g. gastrointestinal distress, colitis, vestibular dysfunction with minocycline) appears to rise at the higher dose levels, further studies are urgently needed to determine the minimum doses of doxycycline and minocycline necessary to achieve radical cure of falciparum infections. If lower doses of these drugs prove to be effective, the cost of treatment might eventually approach that of a course of tetracycline. The advantages of doxycycline and minocycline are that these drugs can be taken at less frequent intervals than the other tetracyclines, they are absorbed more reliably in the presence of food, and they can be used to treat patients who have concurrent disease. Furthermore, doxycycline may induce fewer changes in the intestinal flora than tetracycline, and minocycline may produce fewer phototoxic reactions than do other tetracyclines.

The potential value of the tetracyclines in antimalarial therapy is somewhat limited by the duration of the course of treatment. Since three- to five-day courses have been associated with a high proportion of treatment failures (56, 60, 62), the duration of treatment cannot be less than 7–10 days. Many patients will fail to complete such a long course of treatment unless it is given under medical supervision. As this is not feasible in most malarious rural areas, there will be many recurrences after the use of tetracyclines.

It has recently been suggested that the tetracycline antibiotics be used, in a limited way, as prophylactic agents in areas where both chloroquine- and Fansidar-resistant strains of *P. falciparum* are prevalent (11). Although tetracyclines exert a marked causal prophylactic activity (57, 61), they should be used judiciously. The likelihood of transferring resistance, by R plasmids, between serious endemic pathogens of the same or unrelated bacterial species is a legitimate concern. However, since tetracyclines are already being used indiscriminately in many malarious countries to treat or suppress a multitude of other infections, it is unlikely that their limited use for malaria prophylaxis would affect the prevalence of drug-resistant bacteria.

The long-term use of tetracyclines (for prophylaxis) or, for that matter, their short-term use (for treatment) may be associated with appreciable toxic side-effects. Gastrointestinal intolerance is not uncommon. The overgrowth of yeasts or bacteria resistant to the tetracyclines can also be induced by the use of tetracyclines. Yet, prolonged courses of tetracycline, widely prescribed for the treatment of acne vulgaris, have surprisingly not been associated with overwhelming overgrowth of drug-resistant bacteria and yeasts or any other significant toxic side-effects (63). This may not necessarily be the case, however, for individuals in malarious areas whose overall health and nutritional status may not be as good as that of acne patients, most of whom are otherwise healthy young people. Hepatotoxicity is another serious side-effect, observed particularly in individuals with impaired renal function and in pregnant or postpartum women. The well-known discoloration of children's teeth associated with the use of tetracyclines can be prevented by not administering these drugs during the latter half of pregnancy and the first eight years of life. However, in the absence of safe and effective alternative antimalarials, these drugs should be used without hesitation if the life of a pregnant woman or young child is threatened.

Another antibiotic, clindamycin, has been used to cure chloroquine-resistant infections of falciparum malaria (64–66). Because clindamycin acts slowly, it was given in combination with quinine; however, the combined administration of both drugs often created unacceptable upper gastrointestinal side-effects. As clindamycin was given at doses two or three times higher than those recommended for the treatment of bacterial infections, it is possible that lower doses, given after three days of quinine, might reduce the incidence of this side-effect. Clindamycin does not produce many of the side-effects observed after administration of the tetracyclines and can be used in patients with mild to moderate impairment of renal function. On the other hand, the relatively high frequency of antimicrobial-associated colitis, observed in North America and Europe after administration of clindamycin, is a deterrent to the current use of this drug. Recent advances in understanding the etiology of antimicrobial-associated colitis (67) may eventually render clindamycin more acceptable for the treatment of falciparum malaria.

The extensive distribution of antibiotics as prophylactic drugs, no matter how safe or effective, should be avoided because these are the only commercially available drugs still universally effective against *P. falciparum*. Although the development of resistance by rodent malaria parasites to minocycline and clindamycin appears to be slower than to other antimalarials (68), *P. falciparum* will develop resistance to the antibiotics if their widespread use is not discouraged. Resistance might be acquired by the transfer of R plasmids from one organism to another (as in Gram-negative bacteria) or by genetic mutation and subsequent selection through drug pressure. If it is shown that mutations are the predominant mechanism by which parasites acquire resistance to antibiotics, the use of appropriate drug combinations might prevent or delay the emergence of drug-resistant strains.

NEW ANTIMALARIAL DRUGS

The serious problem created by the scarcity of effective antimalarial agents emphasizes the need for new drugs. Unfortunately, there is only one such drug in an advanced stage of clinical testing. This is mefloquine, a quinolinemethanol compound developed by the US Army Antimalarial

Drug Development Program (69, 70). Initial clinical studies with mefloquine showed that a single dose of this drug exerted a marked and prolonged activity against multidrug-resistant strains of *P. falciparum* (71, 72). Its remarkable antimalarial activity was confirmed by subsequent field studies (73, 74). No serious side-effects were observed during these studies. The extended field trials of mefloquine being conducted under the auspices of the World Health Organization will further determine the safety and efficacy of this drug. If unacceptable side-effects are observed, mefloquine could conceivably be replaced by one of six aminoalcohols that possess significant antimalarial activity and that, at the same time, might be better tolerated than mefloquine (70). It is, however, unlikely that any of these potential substitutes would be effective against strains that might develop resistance to mefloquine (70). The emergence of mefloquine resistance could be retarded by using it in combination with other drugs. This would involve further extensive studies to ensure that such drug combinations are safe, particularly in view of the slow elimination of mefloquine from the body. It may not be possible, though, to resist the mounting pressure for a new single-dose treatment in many areas where Fansidar is no longer effective. Let us hope that this valuable drug will not lose its therapeutic edge too soon.

Another drug, qinghaosu, is arousing considerable interest as a possible blood schizontocide against drug-resistant malaria (75). It is derived from the medicinal herb, *Artemisia annua,* which has been used for malaria therapy in China for about 2000 years. Qinghaosu and its derivatives represent an entirely novel chemical class of antimalarial compounds, and it has already been used successfully in the treatment of chloroquine-resistant falciparum infections (76). The potential of this drug and its derivatives as antimalarial agents will have to await the results of further safety and efficacy studies.

The rapid rate at which once-reliable antimalarial drugs are losing their efficacy is one of the main problems facing tropical medicine today. New drugs are not available to replace existing ones because of the enormous cost and complexity of identifying and developing new antimalarials. The search for new drugs will be even slower if there is little prospect of protecting such drugs from a fate similar to that which is overtaking the older antimalarials. Increased knowledge concerning all aspects of the development, spread, and prevention of drug resistance by malaria parasites is of vital importance for the continued development of new drugs and for preserving and improving the efficacy of existing antimalarial drugs.

Literature Cited

1. Peters, W., Seaton, D. R. 1971. Sensitivity of *Plasmodium falciparum* to chloroquine in Africa. *Ann. Trop. Med. Parasitol.* 65:267–69
2. Rieckmann, K. H., Lopez-Antunano, F. J. 1971. Chloroquine resistance of *Plasmodium falciparum* in Brazil detected by a simple *in vitro* method. *Bull. WHO* 45:157–67
3. Colwell, E. J., Phintuyothin, P., Sududee, N., Bonjapong, W., Neoypatimanondh, S. 1972. Evaluation of an *in vitro* technique for detecting chloroquine resistant falciparum malaria in Thailand. *Am. J. Trop. Med. Hyg.* 21:6–12
4. Ebisawa, I., Fukuyama, T., Kawamura, Y. 1976. Additional foci of chloroquine-resistant falciparum malaria in East Kalimantan and West Irian, Indonesia. *Trop. Geogr. Med.* 88:349-54
5. Palmer, T. T., Townley, L. B., Yigzaw, M., Armstrong, J. C. 1976. Chloroquine sensitivity of *Plasmodium falciparum* in Ethiopia. II. Results of an *in vitro* test. *Am. J. Trop. Med. Hyg.* 25:10–13
6. Sucharit, P., Harinasuta, T., Chongsuphajaisiddhi, T., Tongprasroeth, N., Kasemsuth, R. 1977. *In vivo* and *in vitro* studies of chloroquine-resistant malaria in Thailand. *Ann. Trop. Med. Parasitol.* 71:401–5
7. Rieckmann, K. H., McNamara, J. V., Frischer, H. Stockert, T. A., Carson, P. E., Powell, R. D. 1968. Effects of chloroquine, quinine and cycloguanil upon the maturation of asexual erythrocytic forms of two strains of *Plasmodium falciparum in vitro*. *Am. J. Trop. Med. Hyg.* 17:661–71
8. Rieckmann, K. H., Sax, L. J., Campbell, G. H., Mrema, J. E. 1978. Drug sensitivity of *Plasmodium falciparum*. An *in-vitro* microtechnique. *Lancet* 1:22–23
9. Rieckmann, K. H. 1982. Visual *in vitro* test for determining the drug sensitivity of *Plasmodium falciparum*. *Lancet* 1:1333–35
10. Wernsdorfer, W. H., Kouznetzov, R. L. 1980. Drug-resistant malaria—occurrence, control, and surveillance. *Bull. WHO* 58:341–52
11. Centers for Disease Control. 1982. Prevention of malaria in travelers 1982. *Morbid. Mortal. Wkly. Rep.* 31:15–285 (Suppl.)
12. Centers for Disease Control. 1982. Revised recommendations for malaria chemoprophylaxis for travelers to East Africa. *Morbid. Mortal. Wkly. Rep.* 31:328–30
13. Eastham, G. M., Rieckmann, K. H. 1981. Field incubator for measuring drug susceptibility of *Plasmodium falciparum*. *J. Trop. Med. Hyg.* 84:27–28
14. Canfield, C. J. 1982. Malaria. In *Current Therapy*, ed. H. F. Conn, 1:39–40. Philadelphia: Saunders. 1016 pp. 28th ed.
15. Powell, R. D., Brewer, G. J., DeGowin, R. L., Alving, A. S. 1964. Studies on a strain of chloroquine-resistant *Plasmodium falciparum* from Viet Nam. *Bull. WHO* 31:379–92
16. DeGowin, R. L., Powell, R. D. 1965. Drug resistance of a strain of *Plasmodium falciparum* from Malaya. *Am. J. Trop. Med. Hyg.* 14:519-28
17. Legters, L. J., Wallace, D. K., Powell, R. D., Pollack, S. 1965. Apparent refractoriness to chloroquine, pyrimethamine, and quinine in strains of *Plasmodium falciparum* from Vietnam. *Mil. Med.* 130:168–76
18. McNamara, J. V., Rieckmann, K. H., Frischer, H., Stockert, T. A., Carson, P. E., Powell, R. D. 1967. Acquired decrease in sensitivity to quinine observed during studies with a strain of chloroquine-resistant *Plasmodium falciparum*. *Ann. Trop. Med. Parasitol.* 61:386–95
19. Reacher, M., Campbell, C. C., Freeman, J., Doberstyn, E. B., Brandling-Bennett, A. D. 1981. Drug therapy for *Plasmodium falciparum* malaria resistant to pyrimethamine-sulfadoxine (Fansidar.) A study of alternate regimens in Eastern Thailand. 1980. *Lancet* 2:1066–69
20. Sanders, J. P. 1935. Treatment of malaria with a short course of quinidine. *Am. J. Trop. Med.* 15:651–60
21. White, N. J., Looareesuwan, S., Warrell, D. A., Chongsuphajaisiddhi, T., Bunnag, D., Harinasuta, T. 1981. Quinidine in falciparum malaria. *Lancet* 2:1069–71
22. Rieckmann, K. H. 1971. Determination of the drug sensitivity of *Plasmodium falciparum*. *J. Am. Med. Assoc.* 217:573–78
23. Chin, W., Contacos, P. G., Coatney, G. R., King, H. K. 1966. The evaluation of sulfonamides, alone or in combination with pyrimethamine, in the treatment of multi-resistant falciparum malaria. *Am. J. Trop. Med. Hyg.* 15:823–29
24. Bartelloni, P. J., Sheehy, T. W., Tigertt, W. D. 1967. Combined therapy for

chloroquine-resistant *Plasmodium falciparum* infection: concurrent use of
long-acting sulphormethoxine and
pyrimethamine. *J. A. Med. Assoc.*
199:173–77
25. Harinasuta, T., Viravan, C., Reid, H. A.
1967. Sulphormethoxine in chloroquine-resistant falciparum malaria in
Thailand. *Lancet* 1:1117–19
26. Powell, R. D., DeGowin, R. L.,
McNamara, J. V. 1967. Clinical experience with sulphadiazine and pyrimethamine in the treatment of persons experimentally infected with chloroquine-
resistant *Plasmodium falciparum. Ann.
Trop. Med. Parasitol.* 61:396–408
27. DeSouza, J. M. 1980. *Abstr. Int. Congr.
Trop. Med. Malar., 10th, Manila, Phil-
ippines,* p. 270 (Abstr. 431.) Quezon
City: P. B. Press
28. Harinasuta, T., Bunnag, D., Pini-
pongse, S. 1980. See Ref. 27, p. 282
(Abstr. 454)
29. Darlow, B., Vrbova, H., Stace, J., Hey-
wood, P., Alpers, M. 1980. Fansidar-
resistant falciparum malaria in Papua
New Guinea. *Lancet* 2:1243
30. Hurwitz, E.S., Johnson, D., Campbell,
C.C. 1981. Resistance of *Plasmodium
falciparum* malaria to sulfadoxine-
pyrimethamine (Fansidar) in a refugee
camp in Thailand. *Lancet* 1:1068–70
31. World Health Organization. 1982. Information on malaria risk for international travelers. *Wkly. Epidemiol. Rec.*
57:91–94
32. Doberstyn, E. B., Teerakiartkamjorn,
C., Andre, R. G., Phintuyothin, P., Noeypatimanondh, S. 1979. Treatment of
vivax malaria with sulfadoxine-pyrimethamine and with pyrimethamine alone.
Trans. R. Soc. Trop. Med. Hyg. 73:
15–17
33. Darlow, B., Vrbova, H., Gibney, S., Jol-
ley, D., Stace, J., Alpers, M. 1982. Sulfadoxine-pyrimethamine for the treatment of acute malaria in children in
Papua New Guinea. II. *Plasmodium
vivax. Am. J. Trop. Med. Hyg.* 31:10–13
34. Trenholme, G. M., Williams, R. L.,
Frischer, H., Carson, P. E., Rieckmann,
K. H. 1975. Host failure in treatment of
malaria with sulfalene and pyrimethamine. *Ann. Intern. Med.* 82:219–23
35. Williams, R. L., Trenholme, G. M.,
Carson, P. E., Frischer, H., Rieckmann,
K. H. 1975. Acetylator phenotype and
response of individuals infected with a
chloroquine-resistant strain of *Plasmodium falciparum* to sulfalene and
pyrimethamine. *Am. J. Trop. Med. Hyg.*
24:734–39

36. Muto, T., Ebisawa, I., Mitsui, G. 1971.
Malaria in Laos. II. Peripheral leucocyte counts during long-term administration of combined folic inhibitors
(pyrimethamine with sulformethoxine
or sulfamonomethoxine.) *Jpn. J. Exp.
Med.* 41:459-70
37. Frenkel, J. K., Hitchings, G. H. 1957.
Relative reversal by vitamins (p-
aminobenzoic, folic, and folinic acids)
of the effects of sulfadiazine and pyrimethamine on *Toxoplasma,* mouse and
man. *Antibiot. Chemother.* 7:630–38
38. Hurly, M. G. D. 1959. Administration
of pyrimethamine with folic and folinic
acids in human malaria. *Trans. R. Soc.
Trop. Med. Hyg.* 53:410–11
39. Tong, M. J., Strickland, G. T., Votteri,
B. A., Gunnig, J. J. 1970. Supplemental
folates in the therapy of *Plasmodium
falciparum* malaria. *J. Am. Med. Assoc.*
214:2330–33
40. DeGowin, R. L., Eppes, R. B., Carson,
P. E., Powell, R. D. 1966. The effects of
diaphenylsulfone (DDS) against chloroquine-resistant *Plasmodium falciparum. Bull. WHO* 34:671–81
41. Rieckmann, K. H. 1967. A new reposi-
tory antimalarial agent, CI–564, used in
a field trial in New Guinea. *Trans. R.
Soc. Trop. Med. Hyg.* 61:189–98
42. Clyde, D. F., Rebert, C. C., McCarthy,
V. C., Daukins, A. T., Cucinell, S. A.
1970. Diformyl diaminodiphenyl sulfone (DFD) as an antimalarial in man.
Mil. Med. 135:527–36
43. Lucas, A. O., Hendrickse, R. G.,
Okubadejo, O. A., Richards, W. H. G.,
Neal, R. A., Kofie, B. A. K. 1969. The
suppression of malarial parasitaemia by
pyrimethamine in combination with
dapsone or sulphormethoxine. *Trans.
R. Soc. Trop. Med. Hyg.* 63:216–29
44. Black, R. H. 1973. Malaria in the Australian army in South Vietnam. Successful use of a proguanil-dapsone combination for chemoprophylaxis of chloroquine-resistant falciparum malaria.
Med. J. Aust. 1:1265–70
45. Pearlman, E. J., Thiemanun, W., Cas-
taneda, B. F. 1975. Chemosuppressive
field trials in Thailand. II. The suppression of *Plasmodium falciparum* and
Plasmodium vivax parasitemias by a
diformyldapsone-pyrimethamine combination. *Am. J. Trop. Med. Hyg.*
24:901–9
46. Ponnampalam, J. T., Seow, C. L., Roy,
O. S. 1976. A comparative study of the
efficacy of chloroquine and a combination of dapsone and pyrimethamine in
the prophylaxis of malaria in Peninsular

Malaysia. *J. Trop. Med. Hyg.* 79: 220–25
47. Bradley, D. J., Mackay, D. M., Southgate, B. A., Peters, W., Woodruff, A. W., Bryceson, A. D. M., Cook, G. C., Hall, A. P., Gilles, H. M., Morgan, H. V., Bruce-Chwatt, L. J., Berrie, J. R. H., Noah, N. 1981. Malaria prevention in travelers from the United Kingdom. *Br. Med. J.* 283:214–18
48. Woodruff, A. W., Ridley, D. S., Harries, J. R., Tomkins, A. M, Hall, A. P., Rowland, H. A. K., Heaf, P. J. D. 1980. Prophylaxis of malaria. *Lancet* 2:1079
49. Ognibene, A. J. 1970. Agranulocytosis due to dapsone. *Ann. Intern. Med.* 72:521–24
50. Rieckmann, K. H., Willerson, D. Jr., Carson, P. E. 1971. Drug potentiation against pre-erythrocytic stages of *Plasmodium falciparum*. *Trans. R. Soc. Trop. Med. Hyg.* 65:533–35
51. Rieckmann, K. H., Brewer, G. J., Powell, R. D. 1968. Effects of diaphenylsulphone (Dapsone) against *Plasmodium vivax* of South West Pacific origin. *Trans. R. Soc. Trop. Med. Hyg.* 62: 649–53
52. Cooper, W. C., Coatney, G. R., Imboden, C. A. Jr., Jeffery, G. M. 1949. Aureomycin in experimental Chesson strain vivax malaria. *Proc. Soc. Exp. Biol. Med.* 72:587–88
53. Imboden, C. A. Jr., Cooper, W. C., Coatney, G. R., Jeffery, G. M. 1950. Studies in human malaria. XXIX. Trials of aureomycin, chloramphenicol, penicillin, and dihydrostreptomycin against the Chesson strain of *P. vivax*. *J. Natl. Malar. Soc.* 9:377–80
54. Ruiz-Sanchez, F., Ruiz-Sanchez, A., Naranjo-Grande, E. 1956. The treatment of malaria with tetracycline. *Antibiot. Med. Clin. Ther.* 3:193–96
55. World Health Organization. 1961. Chemotherapy of malaria. *WHO Tech. Rep. Ser.,* No. 226, p. 16
56. Rieckmann, K. H., Powell, R. D., McNamara, J. V., Willerson, D. Jr., Kass, L., Frischer, H., Carson, P. E. 1971. Effects of tetracycline against chloroquine-resistant and chloroquine-sensitive *Plasmodium falciparum*. *Am. J. Trop. Med. Hyg.* 20:811–15
57. Rieckmann, K. H., Willerson, W. D. Jr., Carson, P. E., Frischer, H. 1972. Effects of tetracycline against drug-resistant falciparum malaria. *Proc. Helminthol. Soc. Wash.* 39(Special Issue):339–47
58. Colwell, E. J., Hickman, R. L., Intraprasert, R., Tirabutana, C. 1972. Mino-cycline and tetracycline treatment of acute falciparum malaria. *Am. J. Trop. Med. Hyg.* 21:144–49
59. Colwell, E. J., Hickman, R. L., Kosal, S. 1972. Tetracycline treatment of chloroquine-resistant falciparum malaria in Thailand. *J. Am. Med. Assoc.* 220: 684–86
60. Clyde, D. F., Miller, R. M., DuPont, H. L., Hornick, R. B. 1971. Antimalarial effects of tetracycline in man. *J. Trop. Med. Hyg.* 74:238–42
61. Willerson, D. Jr., Rieckmann, K. H., Carson, P. E., Frischer, H. 1972. Effects of minocycline against chloroquine-resistant falciparum malaria. *Am. J. Trop. Med. Hyg.* 21:857–62
62. Chin, W., Intraprasert, R. 1973. The evaluation of quinine alone or in combination with tetracycline and pyrimethamine against falciparum malaria in Thailand. *Southeast Asian J. Trop. Med. Public Health* 4:245–49
63. Ad Hoc Committee on the Use of Antibiotics in Dermatology. 1975. Systemic antibiotics for treatment of acne vulgaris: efficacy and safety. *Arch. Dermatol.* 111:1630–36
64. Miller, L. H., Glew, R. H., Wyler, D. J., Howard, W. A., Collins, W. E., Contacos, P. G., Neva, F. A. 1974. Evaluation of clindamycin in combination with quinine against multidrug-resistant strains of *Plasmodium falciparum*. *Am. J. Trop. Med. Hyg.* 23:565–69
65. Clyde, D. F., Gilman, R. H., McCarthy, V. C. 1975. Antimalarial effect of clindamycin in man. *Am. J. Trop. Med. Hyg.* 24:369–70
66. Hall, A. P., Doberstyn, E. B., Nanakorn, A., Sonkom, P. 1975. Falciparum malaria semi-resistant to clindamycin. *Br. Med. J.* 2:12–14
67. George, W. L., Sutter, V. L., Goldstein,, A. J. C., Ludwig, S. L., Finegold, S. M. 1978. Aetiology of antimicrobial-agent-associated colitis. *Lancet* 1:802–3
68. Jacobs, R. L., Koontz, L. C. 1976. *Plasmodium berghei*: development of resistance to clindamycin and minocycline in mice. *Exp. Parasitol.* 40:116–23
69. Canfield, C. J., Rozman, R. S. 1974. Clinical testing of new antimalarial compounds. *Bull. WHO* 50:203–12
70. Canfield, C. J. 1980. Antimalarial aminoalcohol alternatives to mefloquine. *Acta Trop.* 37:232–37
71. Rieckmann, K. H., Trenholme, G. M., Williams, R. L., Carson, P. E., Frischer, H., Desjardins, R. E. 1974. Prophylactic activity of mefloquine hydrochloride

(WR 142490) in drug-resistant malaria. *Bull WHO* 51:375–77

72. Trenholme, G. M., William, R. L., Desjardins, R. E., Frischer, H., Carson, P. E., Rieckmann, K. H., Canfield, C. J. 1975. Mefloquine (WR 142490) in the treatment of human malaria. *Science* 190:792–74

73. Doberstyn, E. B., Phintuyothin, P., Noeypatimanondh, S., Terrakiartkamjorn, C. 1979. Single-dose therapy of falciparum malaria with mefloquine or pyrimethamine-sulfadoxine. *Bull. WHO* 57:275–79

74. Pearlman, E. J., Doberstyn, E. B., Sudsok, S., Thiemanun, W., Kennedy, R. S., Canfield, C. J. 1980. Chemosuppressive field trials in Thailand. IV. The suppression of *Plasmodium falciparum* and *Plasmodium vivax* parasitemias by mefloquine. *Am. J. Trop. Med. Hyg.* 29:1131–37

75. Jiang, J.-B., Li, G.-Q., Guo, X.-B., Kong, Y. C., Arnold, K. 1982. Antimalarial activity of mefloquine and qinghaosu. *Lancet* 2:285–88

76. Qinghaosu Antimalaria Coordinating Research Group. 1979. *Chin. Med. J.* 92:811–16

Ann. Rev. Med. 1983. 34:337–58

URETHRAL INFECTIONS IN MEN AND WOMEN[1]

Edward S. Wong, M.D., and Walter E. Stamm, M.D.

Department of Medicine, University of Washington, Seattle, Washington 98195

ABSTRACT

Gonococcal and nongonococcal urethritis (NGU) remain the two most common sexually transmitted diseases seen in males in developed countries (1, 2). The past decade has witnessed important developments in these diseases, including the emergence of penicillinase-producing *Neisseria gonorrhoeae* (3, 4), the recognition of *Chlamydia trachomatis* (5–8) and *Ureaplasma urealyticum* (6, 9, 10) as etiologic agents of NGU, a clearer understanding of the spectrum of illness caused by these agents, and the use of newer therapeutic regimens. In both sexes, these agents can either cause mucosal urogenital tract infection (urethritis, cervicitis) or spread contiguously or hematogenously to produce epididymitis, endometritis, pelvic inflammatory disease or disseminated gonococcal infection. In this paper we review important advances in the epidemiology, pathogenesis, diagnosis, and treatment of urethral infections in men and women, emphasizing particularly the acute urethral syndrome in women.

URETHRAL INFECTION IN MEN

Gonorrhea

In the United States, the yearly incidence of gonorrhea increased at a constant rate from 1957 until 1976 when the number of reported cases plateaued at approximately 1 million (1, 2, 11). Since 1978, there has been an actual decline in the number of reported cases, a trend that experts attribute mainly to the efficacy of public health programs (1, 11). This decline is remarkable since it occurred despite changing sexual mores, an

[1]The US Government has the right to retain a nonexclusive royalty-free license in and to any copyright covering this paper.

increasing population of young sexually active adults, and widespread use of oral contraceptives, all factors that probably promote the spread of infection (12–14). In the US, gonorrhea is most commonly reported among young, poor, black, unmarried, sexually active individuals living in urban centers (1, 12, 14). A slight male predominance is noted among reported cases of gonorrhea, with a male to female ratio of 1.5 : 1 (11). This inequality in the sexes may, however, be due to artifacts in case-finding and reporting (14). Men and women between the ages of 20 and 24 have the highest attack rate (1, 11). Teenagers from 15 to 19 years old have the second highest attack rate but are the age group with the largest number of reported cases (11, 15). The prevalence of gonorrhea appears to be strongly affected by sexual preference. In a prospective study of urethral infection in unselected males presenting to a sexually transmitted disease (STD) clinic, *N. gonorrhoeae* was isolated from 12% of heterosexual men, but 29.6% of homosexual men (16).

Most European countries report a much lower rate of infection than the US. In England, the yearly incidence of gonorrhea is approximately 120 cases per 100,000 population, four to five times lower than the rate in the US (17). This rate has remained stable for the past five years. Data on the incidence of gonorrhea in developing countries are sparse, but studies in select populations in Africa and Asia suggest high endemicity of gonorrhea with prevalence rates ranging from 3% to over 18% (17–19).

A development that likely contributed to the increasing incidence of gonorrhea is the gradual emergence of relative antibiotic resistance to penicillin. In the 1950s, over 99% of gonococcal strains tested had minimal inhibitory concentrations (MICs) of less than 0.06 μg/ml (20). By 1969, more than 65% of strains of gonococci similarly tested exhibited MICs > 0.06 μg/ml (21). Sparling and colleagues showed that the low-level resistance to penicillin is chromosomally mediated and is most likely due to series of mutations that have altered surface permeability of the gonococcus to penicillin (22). Low-level antibiotic resistance eventually necessitated higher doses of antibiotics to reliably cure infections and undoubtedly contributed to treatment failures and spread of disease. This trend, while continuing in Africa, Southeast Asia, and the South Pacific, appears to be reversing itself in the US. Analysis of surveillance data collected by the Centers for Disease Control (CDC) shows that from 1972 to 1975 there was a twofold increase in the number of strains of gonococci with MICs $\leqslant$ 0.03 μg/ml (23, 24).

In 1976, the CDC identified isolates of *N. gonorrhoeae* that were highly resistant to the usual therapeutic dose of penicillin (25). In contrast to chromosomally mediated low-level resistance, which could be overcome by larger doses of penicillin, antibiotic resistance in these isolates was plasmid-mediated and complete (26–28). Two different plasmids (3.2 and 4.4 megadaltons respectively) that code for penicillinase production have been identified (26–28). In DNA homology experiments, these plasmids share base sequences with plasmids from *Hemophilus influenzae* and gram-negative enteric organisms (27, 28). In mating experiments, plasmids have been successfully transfered to recipient gonococci (28). These studies suggest that penicillinase-producing *N. gonorrhoeae* (PPNG) most likely arose by way of conjugation with other gram-negative organisms carrying the resistance plasmid for penicillinase.

The first cases of PPNG in this country were seen in 1976 in servicemen returning from abroad (25). In 1979, 27 countries in Europe, Asia, Oceania, and North America reported cases of PPNG to the World Health Organization (29). Prevalence studies showed that PPNG constituted from 10 to 30% of all gonococcal isolates in parts of Asia and Africa (29, 30). In the US, despite the periodic importation of PPNG into the country, the number of cases detected by a national surveillance system remained low (approximately 15–20 cases per month) through 1979 (4, 29, 30). This limited spread has been attributed to prompt tracing and treatment of contacts, although the possibility of spontaneous loss of the plasmid in the absence of intensive antibiotic pressure has also been suggested (4, 29, 31). Beginning in the third quarter of 1980, however, the number of cases of PPNG reported to the CDC increased tenfold, largely as a result of urban outbreaks in Los Angeles, California, Shreveport, Louisiana, and the state of Washington (31–33). Using auxotyping and serogrouping by coagglutination as epidemiologic tools in their investigation of outbreaks in Louisiana and Washington, Handsfield and co-workers concluded that these epidemics resulted from spread of imported strains rather than from transmission of R plasmids to indigenous gonococci (31). They also found no evidence that spontaneous loss of plasmids played a role in ending the outbreaks and attributed containment to intensive public health efforts.

TRANSMISSION   Asymptomatically infected individuals of both sexes or those with atypical symptoms and signs are responsible for most of the transmission of gonorrhea. Women were once thought to be the major reservoir of infection in the community because of the erroneous concept that the majority of women infected with gonorrhea were asymptomatic (1, 2). This concept arose as a result of early studies conducted in STD clinics where men attended voluntarily because of symptoms and women were seen because of contact tracing (34, 35). This method of case-finding results in a bias toward symptomatic men and women not sufficiently symptomatic to seek treatment spontaneously. In studies assessing gonorrhea cases outside of STD clinics, the presence of symptoms in newly infected women and their absence in male partners of these patients is amply documented.

Not every contact of an infected partner develops gonorrhea. The risk of acquiring infection is affected by the frequency and nature of sexual contact, the sex of the infected index case, intrinsic susceptibility to infection (i.e. previous infections may confer strain-specific immunity) and perhaps other factors. Wiesner & Thompson (1) estimated the prevalence of infection among female consorts of infected men to be 50–70% whereas only 20–30% of male sex partners of infected women developed infection. Others, however, found the prevalence of infection after exposure to be higher and nearly equal regardless of sex (14, 36, 37). Comparisons between studies are difficult because parameters that affect the rate of transmission, such as sexual habits, frequency of coitus, and the prevalence of gonorrhea in each study population, differ.

Transmission of gonorrhea among homosexual men resembles that seen in heterosexuals in that asymptomatic individuals serve as the major reservoir for the organism. Anorectal gonorrhea is often asymptomatic, with only an estimated 3–10% developing tenesmus, purulent discharge, or rectal bleeding (1, 2). Oropharyngeal gonorrhea is also largely asymptomatic, although this site is believed not to be an important reservoir. At present, there is little information on the rate of transmission of gonorrhea between homosexual contacts.

CLINICAL MANIFESTATIONS   The frequency of asymptomatic infection is low among men attending STD clinics, but has been reported to be as high as 60% in studies that have screened sexually active males or examined contacts of women with symptomatic infections (38–40). The true incidence of asymptomatic gonorrhea in men is therefore not known with certainty and varies with the population studied. In the general population, however, the best estimate is that between 2 and 10% of infected men never become symptomatic (2).

N. gonorrhoeae preferentially infects columnar and transitional epithelium; acute anterior urethritis is the most common manifestation of infection. The usual incubation period is 3–5 days, followed by rapid onset of dysuria and purulent urethral discharge. Jacobs & Kraus (41) found that 71% of 185 men with gonococcal urethritis had both dysuria and discharge, while 27% complained of discharge only and 2% had dysuria alone. Similar signs and symptoms have been described in other series (2, 42).

Gonococcal urethritis can ascend and infect the epididymis. Clinically, epididymitis presents as unilateral scrotal pain, swelling, and tenderness, with or without fever. Such men often have simultaneous urethritis, although it may be asymptomatic. Harnish and co-workers isolated *N. go-*

norrhoeae from the urethra in 7 of 24 men presenting with acute idiopathic epididymitis (43). Berger and associates, however, were unable to isolate *N. gonorrhoeae* from any men with acute epididymitis (44). In a study of 167 men with gonococcal urethritis prospectively followed, Stamm et al (16) found no cases of gonococcal epididymitis. These studies suggest that while epididymitis may complicate gonococcal urethritis, it is likely to be an infrequent event if effective antimicrobial therapy has been given.

About 1–3% of patients with gonococcal infections of the urethra, rectum, or pharynx will disseminate the organism hematogenously, which gives rise to the syndrome of disseminated gonococcal infection (DGI) (45, 46). Early in the course of disease, patients develop an asymmetrical polyarticular arthritis or tenosynovitis involving the wrists, knees, ankles, and small joints of the hand or feet and typical skin lesions that are small in number (3–20) and located on the extremities (45, 46). Left untreated, a septic monoarticular arthritis may develop that is clinically indistinguishable from other pyogenic arthritides. Host characteristics that are epidemiologically associated with an increased risk of DGI include female sex, pregnancy, menstruation, deficiency of the late components of the complement system, and primary oropharyngeal infection (2, 44–47). Characteristics of gonococcal strains associated with DGI include increased sensitivity to penicillin (48), nutritional requirements for arginine, hypoxanthine, and uracil (Arg⁻ Hyx⁻ Ura⁻ auxotype) (49), and resistance to the bactericidal activity of normal human serum (50).

DIAGNOSIS   In men with symptomatic urethritis, the gram-stained smear of urethral exudate is an excellent, quick, and reliable laboratory method for diagnosing gonorrhea. Jacobs & Kraus (41) demonstrated that smears with typical gram-negative diplococci (GND) located within polymorphonuclear leukocytes have a high sensitivity (90%) and specificity (98%) in diagnosing gonorrhea when compared to culture results. Smears with typical GND located extracelluarly or atypical GND with rare extracellular typical GND were also noted, which on culture were positive for *N. gonorrhoeae* in 75 and 21% of the cases, respectively. These results suggest that unless typical intracellular GND are found, in which case the smear is diagnostic and culture is optional, all other situations require culture confirmation of diagnosis. Other published studies reported sensitivities of genital smears to range from 83 to 95% and specificities from 95 to 99% (51–53). These differences likely reflect variability in collecting and reading the smears or in the sensitivity of the culture system used. One recent study demonstrated a 17% difference in sensitivity and a 45% difference in specificity between the most and least experienced technician interpreting the slides (53). Urethral smears are not generally useful in screening for gonorrhea among asymptomatic men in whom the expected frequency of infection is low; in this situation, cultures are generally required (40).

Serologic diagnosis of gonococcal infection is presently an area of active research (54). The sensitivity, specificity, and predictive value of serologic tests such as detection of gonococcal antibodies to pili antigens by quantitative radioimmunoassay or detection of cell-associated soluble antigen complex by latex agglutination have been too low for serodiagnosis to be diagnostically useful (55, 56). The major problems with serodiagnosis appear to be the persistence of antibody from past infection and cross-reactivity with other neisseria species.

Culture for *N. gonorrhoeae* remains the gold standard for diagnosis. Confirmation is usually based upon colonial morphology, gram stain, the oxidase test, and sugar fermentation reactions. The sensitivity of cultures for gonorrhea can be influenced by a number of factors, including techniques used in obtaining cultures, loss of viability during transport (use of holding media), and inhibition by selective media (57, 58). Modified Thayer-Martin media, presently the most widely used selective medium because of its relative ease of preparation and low cost, contains the antibiotics vancomycin (3 μg/ml), colistin (7.5 μg/ml), nystatin (12.5 μg/ml), and trimethoprim (5 μg/ml). Between 0.3 and 30% of gonococcal isolates may not grow on this medium because of inhibition by vancomycin (53, 59, 60). In areas where vancomycin-sensitive gonococci are prevalent, use of a nonselective media, such as enriched chocolate agar, would minimize misdiagnosis. Such areas can be identified by periodically culturing gonococci on both selective and nonselective media or by monitoring culture results from specimens that contain typical GND on urethral smear.

TREATMENT   Guidelines for the treatment of uncomplicated gonorrhea were recently updated by the Centers for Disease Control (Table 1; 61). A notable change is the recommendation for combination chemotherapy (ampicillin or amoxicillin plus probenecid as a single dose, followed by tetracycline for 7 days) in heterosexual men and women with uncomplicated anogenital gonorrhea. The combined regimen offers single-dose therapy that is more than 90% effective in uncomplicated gonorrhea (23) with additional coverage for coexisting chlamydial infection (see the following section on nongonococcal chlamydial urethritis). Overall, the prevalence of coinfection with chlamydia is 15–25% of heterosexual men with gonorrhea but less than 2% of homosexual men with gonorrhea (5–8, 16). In gay men, in whom coinfection with chlamydia is less of a consideration, and in whom rectal and pharyngeal gonococcal infection often occur, aqueous procaine penicillin G (APPG) remains the therapy of choice for gonorrhea (61, 62).

Table 1 Therapy of uncomplicated gonococcal infections in adults[a]

1. Ampicillin, 3.5 g, or amoxicillin, 3.0 g, either with 1 g probenecid by mouth, in a single dose, PLUS tetracycline HCl: 0.5 g by mouth 4 times a day for 7 days
2. Tetracycline HCl: 0.5 g by mouth 4 times a day for 7 days
3. Ampicillin, 3.5 g, or amoxicillin, 3.0 g, either with 1 g probenecid by mouth in a single dose[b]
4. Aqueous procaine penicillin G (APPG): 4.8 million units injected intramuscularly at two sites, with 1 g probenecid by mouth[c]

[a] Adapted from CDC guidelines (61).
[b] Not recommended for pharyngeal infection.
[c] Preferred regimen in homosexual men.

Sexual partners of patients with gonorrhea should be evaluated, cultured, and epidemiologically treated because of their high risk of acquiring infection. All persons with culture-proven gonorrhea should have follow-up cultures 4–7 days after completion of therapy. Treatment failures are most likely due to reinfection, but infection with PPNG should be ruled out. Because of the latter possibility, CDC recommends that treatment failures be re-treated with spectinomycin, 2.0 g intramuscularly (61). Recently, the first case of PPNG resistant to spectinomycin was reported (63). Such patients can be treated with cefoxitin (2.0 g in a single intramuscular injection), with probenecid (1.0 g orally), or with trimethoprimsulfamethoxazole (9 tablets orally daily for 3 days) (63).

VACCINE The emergence of PPNG and spectinomycin-resistant gonococci has renewed interest in the development of a gonococcal vaccine. The major antigenic fractions of the gonococcus include the outer membrane complex, which consists of three proteins; pili; and lipopolysaccharide (endotoxin) (64–69). Of these, the principal outer membrane protein (POMP) and pili are viewed as candidates for a vaccine. Pili appear to determine virulence by promoting adherence of gonococci to human epithelial cells and by inhibiting phagocytosis by human macrophages. Both effects are blocked by the presence of antibodies to pili (68, 69). Pili have two components: a larger repeating subunit that is antigenically similar in all pili, and a smaller subunit that exhibits antigenic heterogeneity (65). Two recently published phase 1 vaccine trials demonstrated that the pili vaccine is both well tolerated and immunogenic, producing antibody that blocks adherence and enhances phagocytosis of homologous organisms (69, 70). However, because of the large number of gonococcal strains with antigenically dissimilar pili, a pili vaccine may not be feasible.

The POMP of the outer membrane complex appears to have less antigenic heterogeneity than pili (71). Thus far POMP is being further characterized and a vaccine has not been produced. Buchanan et al observed that women with recurrent salpingitis were less likely to be reinfected with gonococci of the same POMP serogroup, which suggests the development of protective antibodies and the potential usefulness of POMP vaccine in preventing systemic infections (50).

Nongonococcal Urethritis

Nongonococcal urethritis (NGU), as the name implies, is defined as urethritis from which *N. gonorrhoeae* is not isolated. In developed countries, NGU is at least as common as gonorrhea in men attending STD clinics and up to 3 to 10 times more common in men seen by private physicians and at student health centers (2, 8). Epidemiologic studies show that a higher proportion of urethritis is due to NGU than to gonorrhea among whites, men of higher socioeconomic status, and heterosexuals (8, 16, 72). Of 1221 patients screened for urethral infections at an STD clinic, 5.2% of homosexual men but 14% of heterosexual men had positive urethral cultures for *C. trachomatis* (16). In the United Kingdom, where this condition is a reportable disease, NGU continues to rise at an incidence rate of approximately 10% per year, in contrast to gonorrhea, which has declined in incidence (2, 72).

ETIOLOGY   NGU does not have a single etiology but is a clinical syndrome with multiple etiologies. Although Koch's postulates have not been specifically fulfilled, the evidence is persuasive that *C. trachomatis* causes up to 50% of the NGU in heterosexual men (2, 5, 6, 8). Evidence for the role of *Ureaplasma urealyticum* in NGU is not as convincing but this organism is believed to be responsible for 20–25% of NGU (2, 9). The cause for the remaining 20–30% of NGU cases is not known. *Herpes simplex* virus, *Trichomonas vaginalis*, and *Candida albicans* are believed to be infrequent causes of NGU (< 5%) (2). *Gardnerella vaginalis*, *Mycoplasma hominis*, *Corynebacterium genitalum*, *C. pseudogenitalum*, coliform bacteria, and commensal bacteria of the urethra and perineum have not been causally associated with urethritis (2, 6, 73).

Cultural and serologic studies, antimicrobial trials, and animal experimentation established that *C. trachomatis* is a causative agent in NGU. *C. trachomatis* was isolated from 30–50% of men with NGU compared to 0–5% of control subjects without urethritis (5, 6, 73). When female partners of chlamydia-positive and chlamydia-negative men with NGU were evaluated, 60–75% of the former and 0–10% of the latter had chlamydial cervicitis, a pattern consistent with sexual transmission of *C. trachomatis* (5, 74, 75). Serum IgM antichlamydial antibody is found frequently in chlamydia-positive men with NGU but rarely in culture-negative men with NGU (6). In therapeutic trials, agents with antichlamydial activity, such as sulfisoxazole, were more effective in producing a clinical response in chlamydia-positive men than were placebo or agents with little antichlamydial activity, such as spectinomycin (76, 77). Elimination of chlamydia in these studies coincided with resolution of symptoms. In animal studies, inoculation of *C. trachomatis* into the urethra of monkeys resulted in clinical urethritis and the development of antichlamydial antibodies (78).

Ureaplasma urealyticum was first isolated from men with NGU by Shepard in 1954 (79). Over 30 studies have since been published that compare the isolation rate of ureaplasma in men with and without NGU. The role of ureaplasma in NGU was recently reviewed (80, 81) by Taylor-Robinson and Csonka, who concluded that these studies did not convincingly show that ureaplasma caused NGU. Approximately one half of the studies demonstrated a significantly higher isolation rate in patients with NGU than in control subjects, but the other studies did not (81). They attributed this failure to demonstrate a clear association between NGU and ureaplasma to the difficulty in properly matching controls for sexual experience, an important determinant of the prevalence of colonization with ureaplasma. Other methodologic problems with isolation studies include the failure to do quantitative cultures for ureaplasma, failure to exclude the presence of other pathogens that can cause urethritis, and grouping of first episode and later episode cases of NGU. Two groups recently demonstrated an association between ureaplasma and NGU but only when men with chlamydial urethritis were excluded from the analysis and when first NGU episodes were studied using quantitative cultures (6, 82).

Differential antibiotic therapy studies provide additional evidence to implicate ureaplasma in NGU. Aminocyclitols (streptomycin and spectinomycin), which are active against ureaplasma, produced a clinical response in men with chlamydia-negative, ureaplasma-positive urethritis (77). Ford & Smith (83) and Stimson et al (10) reported cases of persistent urethritis unresponsive to tetracycline therapy from whom tetracycline-resistant ureaplasma were isolated. In the first report, the symptoms improved when the patient was treated with erythromycin.

Clinical Features

The clinical features of NGU resemble those of gonorrhea but are less florid and begin more gradually after a longer incubation period (41). Jacobs & Kraus found that patients with NGU presented with dysuria and urethral discharge less frequently than patients with gonorrhea (38 versus 78% respectively) (41). Single symptoms—dysuria alone or discharge only—were noted in 15 and 47% of men with NGU, compared with 2 and 27% in men with gonococcal urethritis. On examination, both quantitative and qualitative differences in the character of the urethral discharge were noted.

Discharge was more often absent or demonstrable only after penile strip-ping in NGU, and, when present, was usually described as mucoid (41). In gonorrhea, the discharge was usually spontaneous, often copious, and puru-lent in appearance (2, 41). Stamm and associates similarly found less severe signs and symptoms in NGU than in gonorrhea (16). In addition, they noted a difference in the presentation of chlamydia NGU in heterosexual versus homosexual men. In their study population of men attending a STD clinic, 72% of heterosexual men but only 35% of homosexual men with chlamydial-positive NGU complained of discharge or dysuria. Sixty-three percent of heterosexual men but only 27% of homosexual men exhibited a discharge upon examination. The observed differences between the two populations is as yet unexplained.

As in gonorrhea, complications of chlamydial urethritis probably arise from contiguous spread of infection. Berger et al studied 23 men with acute epididymitis and found *C. trachomatis* to be the most common etiologic agent in young men (44). Positive cultures from the urethra or an epididy-mal aspirate, or a four-fold rise in antichlamydial antibody titers, incrimi-nated *C. trachomatis* in 11 of 35 men less than 35 years of age. The remaining 10 men, who were over 35 years old, had coliform infections and usually had a history of urologic disease or instrumentation. An association between chlamydial urethritis and nonbacterial prostatitis is postulated by Mardh and associates (84), who noted that men with chronic prostatitis had a higher prevalence of antichlamydial antibodies than did control subjects. In a subsequent study, however, the same group could not incriminate chlamydia as an etiologic agent in 53 men with nonbacterial prostatitis (85). Thus, the role of chlamydia in prostatitis is unclear and requires further study. Reiter's syndrome (urethritis, conjunctivitis, arthritis, and character-istic mucocutaneous lesions) or inflammatory arthritis or tenosynovitis ["sexually acquired reactive arthritis" (SARA)] have been observed to oc-cur following or concurrently with *C. trachomatis* genital infections (86). Serologic studies in men with Reiter's syndrome indicate a high prevalence of antichlamydial antibodies (86), but the incidence of this disease following chlamydial infections of the urogenital tract is not known with certainty. The histocompatibility antigen HLA-B27 occurs more frequently in pa-tients with Reiter's syndrome and SARA (63–96%) than in normal controls (4–8%) (86–88) and appears to confer a tenfold increased susceptibility toward SARA (89).

DIAGNOSIS   Practically, the diagnosis of NGU usually rests upon docu-mentation of urethritis and the exclusion of gonococcal infection. Most clinicians do not have access to cultures for *C. trachomatis* or *U. urealyti-cum*. A gram-stained smear of urethral exudate is useful in confirming the presence of urethritis. Bowie and associates showed that a smear with abnormal leukocytosis ($\geqslant$ 4 PMNs per field in five 1000X fields), even without symptoms, compared favorably with examination of the first-voided urine sediment for demonstrating abnormal pyuria ($\geqslant$ 15 PMNs per field in five 400X fields) and correlated with the presence of chlamydial urethritis by culture or serology (90). However, Stamm and associates found that nearly a third of men with positive chlamydial cultures lacked abnormal leukocytosis on examination of a urethral gram stain (16). In a study by Desai & Robson (91), abnormal pyuria ($\geqslant$ 15 PMNs/HPF of centrifuged urine) appeared to have a better correlation (89%) with positive urethral cultures for *C. trachomatis* than the gram stain.

As previously noted, gonococcal infection can be excluded on the basis of a negative examination for typical intracellular GND (ICGND). In one study, failure to find ICGND on urethral gram stain correlated with the diagnosis of NGU in 98% of the cases, i.e. only 2% urethral specimens with negative smears grew *N. gonorrhoeae* (41). When urethral smears are equivocal, a culture is required to exclude gonorrhea.

TREATMENT   Before *C. trachomatis* was shown to cause NGU, empiric trials with tetracyclines showed them to be effective therapy (92, 93). In vitro studies subsequently confirmed that the tetracyclines are highly active against *C. trachomatis* (94, 95), as are rifampin, the macrolides, sulfonamides, and clindamycin. Clinical trials demonstrated that tetracycline hydrochloride, doxycycline, minocycline, triple tetracycline, erythromycin, trimethoprim-sulfamethoxazole, and rosaramicin all achieve cure rates of 85–95% in men with chlamydial NGU (76, 78, 92, 96, 97). Sulfonamides, while active against chlamydia, have little activity against ureaplasma (77) and therefore are not the drugs of choice against NGU. Tetracycline hydrochloride is active against most ureaplasma and, because of its low cost and efficacy, has become the most widely used antibiotic in the treatment of NGU. The recommended duration of therapy ranges from 7 to 21 days. Bowie and associates recently compared a 21-day course of minocycline with a 7-day course and found that the prolonged therapy had no greater efficacy or prevention of recurrence of symptoms (98).

RECURRENT OR PERSISTENT NGU   Despite appropriate antimicrobial therapy, a sizable percentage of patients with NGU have persistent symptoms or have recurrence. Handsfield and associates found the 6 of 35 (17%) chlamydia-positive men redeveloped symptoms of NGU within 1 to 6 weeks of completion of therapy (96). Of 20 men who were recultured at time of persistence or recurrence, none was found to be chlamydia-positive. Among NGU patients whose initial urethral cultures were chlamydia-negative, an even higher number (14 of 30, 47%) redeveloped symptoms of urethritis at follow-up. Bowie et al (98) similarly found that the rate of recurrence or persistence depended on the organism initially present in the urethra: 19% of men from whom *C. trachomatis* was initially isolated developed persistent or recurrent NGU, compared to 39% recurrence or persistence in men without chlamydia. Similarly, the rate of recurrence or persistence was lower if *U. urealyticum* was initially isolated (26%) than when *U. urealyticum* was not (42%). The highest rate of recurrence or persistence was found among men from whom neither *C. trachomatis* nor *U. urealyticum* had been isolated (52%).

The etiology of persistent or recurrent NGU is not known. Generally, repeat cultures for chlamydia at the time of follow-up for recurrent symptoms have been negative (96, 98). *U. urealyticum* has been isolated from the urethra in 21% of such men but not any more frequently than from men whose NGU responded to therapy (98). In a recent prospective study, Wong, Stamm, and co-workers extensively cultured 60 men who had persistent NGU despite at least two recent courses of antibiotics, but they were unable to incriminate any etiologic agent (99). They additionally sought evidence for prostatic involvement by ultrasound and quantitative leukocyte analysis of expressed prostatic secretion and found abnormalities suggestive of prostatitis in 40%. Despite prolonged courses of antibiotics (up to 3 weeks), 30–60% of men with recurrent symptoms failed to respond to therapy. Thus, the etiology, pathophysiology, and management of persistent or recurrent NGU remain an enigma.

URETHRITIS IN WOMEN

Unlike urethritis in men, urethritis in women rarely produces frank urethral discharge. Instead, complaints of dysuria and/or frequency predominate. Recent studies indicate that urinary symptoms are one of the most common reasons for young women to seek a physician's care. Nearly 25% of women attending STD clinics cite dysuria as a major complaint, and, in general practice settings, symptoms of dysuria appear with equal or even greater frequency (100, 101). A community-based study in England suggested that more than 20% of adult women experience at least one episode of dysuria annually. In this study, dysuria was equally common in women aged 18–70, but younger women more often sought medical care because of their symptoms (101).

Etiology and Pathogenesis

Noninfectious causes of urethritis symptoms have been advanced, including hormonal, traumatic (related to intercourse), anatomic, psychological, allergic, or chemical (related to foodstuffs, alcohol, caffeine, or urinary concentration) etiologies, but little proof for these causations exists and current evidence indicates that the majority of women with acute dysuria and frequency have infections of the urethra, vagina, or bladder. However, the relative proportion of cases attributable to vaginitis remains uncertain (Figure 1) and probably varies depending upon the population studied (102). In a group of younger women seen in a hospital outpatient department, Komaroff et al (102) found that 60% of women who complained of dysuria appeared to have vaginitis as a cause for their urinary symptoms. Thus although the presence of dysuria is less common in women with vaginitis than in women with urethritis or cystitis, in many populations of young women the prevalence of vaginitis may exceed the prevalence of urinary tract infection by severalfold, thus making vaginitis the most common cause of dysuria in such populations.

Of dysuric women without vaginitis, about 50–60% have significant bacteriuria in a midstream urine specimen and thus have cystitis as the cause of their symptoms. The remaining one third of women have the acute urethral syndrome (defined as dysuria and frequency without significant bacteriuria) and based upon recent investigations can be subdivided into three groups (Figure 1): those with bladder and/or urethral infection due to coliforms or staphylococci; those with sterile pyuria, often due to chlamydial or gonococcal infection; and those with no pyuria, who usually have no demonstrable infection (103, 104). Simultaneous vaginitis, urethri-

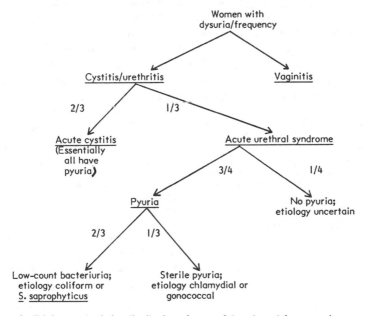

Figure 1 Etiology and relative distribution of cases of dysuria and frequency in women.

tis, and cystitis in various combinations doubtlessly occurs, but the frequency of such coinfection has not been carefully defined. The other noninfectious etiologies mentioned above may be more important in women with chronic dysuria and frequency, or in those with acute dysuria who have no evidence of pyuria or infection.

Table 2 outlines the etiologic agents most commonly responsible for acute urethritis-like symptoms in women. Vaginitis results from infection with *Trichomonas vaginalis*, *Candida albicans*, or *Gardnerella vaginalis* (in association with anaerobic vaginal organisms, the apparent cause of nonspecific vaginitis). It has not been established whether these vaginitis-causing organisms produce dysuria because they also infect the urethra (producing an actual urethritis in some women) or because they cause sufficient vulvar and labial inflammation such that burning urination results from urine passing over these infected areas. Komaroff reported that women with dysuria due to vaginitis usually experienced external labial burning rather than internal dysuria (102). However, all three vaginitis-causing agents can be readily cultured from the urethra of women with vaginal discharge and symptoms of dysuria and frequency, which suggests that an acutal urethritis may well occur in some women. In women with trichomonas infection, this may actually be associated with pyuria or pus cells seen on a urethral gram stain (105).

Among women without vaginitis, dysuria and frequency result from two other major groups of etiologic agents: the sexually transmitted, urethritis-causing organisms *Chlamydia trachomatis* and *Neisseria gonorrhoeae* and the nonsexually transmitted uropathogens *Escherichia coli*, *Staphylococcus saprophyticus*, and Klebsiella (105). Both *C. trachomatis* and *N. gonorrhoeae* cause dysuria, frequency, and pyuria (the acute urethral syndrome) in women in much the same way that nongonococcal and gonococcal urethritis result from urethral infection with these organisms in men (75, 103, 106).

Table 2 Etiologic agents responsible for dysuria and frequency in women

Site of infection	Etiologic agents(s)	Clinical characteristics
Vaginitis	*T. vaginalis, C. albicans, G. vaginalis*	External dysuria; associated vaginal discharge, odor, itching; no hematuria, urgency, or frequency
Urethritis	*C. trachomatis, N. gonorrhoeae, Herpes simplex* virus	Internal dysuria; sexually active patient, recent new partner, no hematuria; sterile pyuria; more gradual onset
Cystitis	*E. coli, S. saprophyticus,* Klebsiella	Internal dysuria, sudden onset, suprapubic, pain, gross hematuria, previous urinary tract infections

Thus these infectious agents are transmitted sexually and the urinary symptoms result from urethral infection. *E. coli*, *S. saprophyticus* (a staphylococcal species characterized by negative coagulase production and in vitro resistance to novobiocin), and Klebsiella cause nonsexually transmitted infection usually involving both the urethra and the bladder. In cases where $\geqslant 10^5$ bacteria/ml can be isolated from urine, the term cystitis has been used, while women with $< 10^5$ bacteria/ml have been said to have the acute urethral syndrome. Both groups typically exhibit pyuria. This distinction probably has little value, since cases with $< 10^5$ and $\geqslant 10^5$ bacterial/ml cannot be distinguished clinically or by laboratory tests other than quantitative urine culture, and since pathogenesis in both instances does not appear to involve sexual transmission. Instead, these infections result from the establishment of persistent periurethral and vaginal colonization with coliforms, with subsequent ascending infection of the bladder and, in some cases, kidneys. The pathogenesis of *S. saprophyticus* urinary infection is probably similar but has not yet been extensively studied; sexual transmission may also occur. Precisely why some women experience frequent coliform infections while others do not has not been established. Two prevailing and not necessarily mutually exclusive hypotheses are that:

1. Women with recurrent cystitis have unique periurethral or vaginal epithelial cells that support attachment of coliform bacteria more avidly than comparable cells from women without recurrent cystitis (107). This unique susceptibility may result from an inability to produce local antibody or perhaps from a lack of specific, competing anaerobic or aerobic flora that inhibit coliform growth.
2. Women with recurrent cystitis have fecal coliform strains that exhibit specific virulence properties (pili, other attachment organelles, hemolysins, or perhaps other factors) resulting in an enhanced ability to cause cystitis (108).

Initial genital infection with *Herpes simplex* virus (HSV) produces dysuria in 10% of women but most often can be readily diagnosed by the presence of typical herpetic lesions on the vulva and/or cervix and by associated adenopathy. Rarely, these lesions appear after the onset of dysuria, which makes initial diagnosis difficult. *Ureaplasma urealyticum*, *Mycoplasma hominis*, and cytomegalovirus, lactobacilli, and anaerobes have not been shown to play a causative role in acute urethral syndrome.

Diagnosis

In evaluating women with acute dysuria and frequency, the etiologic agents previously outlined should all be considered. Factors favoring the diagnosis of vaginitis include an associated history of recently increased or changed vaginal discharge, vaginal odor, vaginal or labial itching, or previous recurrent vaginitis. In most instances, women with vaginitis as the cause of burning urination describe their dysuria as external (that is, occurring as urine passes over the labia). They generally lack associated symptoms of urgency, frequency, suprapubic pain, or hematuria. In the sexually active woman with dysuria and frequency, particularly with the historical factors noted above, a pelvic examination should be performed and potential causes of vaginitis evaluated by physical examination, determination of vaginal fluid pH, and wet preparation and KOH microscopy. Whether a vaginal exam should be performed in all women with dysuria remains debatable. Komaroff and colleagues suggested that in women with internal dysuria and none of the above-mentioned symptoms suggesting vaginitis, a pelvic exam was rarely helpful and could be omitted (102). However, since other sexually transmitted pathogens such as *C. trachomatis* and *N. gonorrhoeae* are important causes of dysuria, a strong argument could be made for performing a vaginal examination in all sexually active women with acute dysuria and frequency.

After excluding vaginitis, the clinician should next consider the other two etiologic categories outlined above, namely, urethritis-causing pathogens (*C. trachomatis* and *N. gonorrhoeae*) and urinary pathogens (coliforms and *S. saprophyticus*). Although these two groups cannot be clearly distinguished on clinical grounds alone, suprapubic pain, gross hematuria, or a history of previous urinary tract infection suggests the latter group. In these women, abrupt onset of symptoms generally occurs and the patient has usually experienced symptoms for only one to four days before seeking medical care. Laboratory data consistent with coliform infection includes the presence of abnormal pyuria, accompanied by hematuria in about 50% of cases. When coliform or staphylococcal organisms are present in bladder urine in quantities $\geqslant 10^5$ bacteria/ml, they can readily be seen in a gram stain of unspun urine, confirming the diagnosis. However, in cases of the acute urethral syndrome when bacteria are present in lesser quantities, the gram stain will be negative and the urine culture becomes critical for etiologic diagnosis. In such women with a clinical presentation typical of cystitis but with 10^1–10^4 coliforms in urine, the diagnosis of acute urethral syndrome due to coliforms should be regarded as highly probable, with isolation of even these lower quantities of bacteria being confirmatory. However, particular care should be exercised in obtaining clean-voided specimens in these patients to minimize contamination of the cultured urine with low quantities of perineal or fecal coliforms. In some patients, specimens obtained by urethral catheterization or suprapubic aspiration may be the only means of accurately distinguishing "low count" coliform infection from a contaminated specimen.

Infection with *C. trachomatis* or *N. gonorrhoeae* occurs most commonly in young, sexually active women who have recently changed sex partners. A history of a partner with recent gonococcal or nongonococcal urethritis may also be obtained. Women with acute dysuria and frequency due to chlamydial infection usually lack urgency, hematuria, or suprapubic pain and give a history of a gradual onset of illness and 7–21 days of symptoms before seeking medical attention. Examination may reveal mucopurulent cervicitis and many polymorphonuclear leukocytes but not gonococci upon examination of a cervical gram stain. The urinalysis typically shows pyuria, no hematuria, and no coliforms on gram stain of unspun urine. Women with gonococcal urethritis and/or cervicitis also tend to have suprapubic pain or hematuria, but may exhibit an illness of more abrupt onset. A cervical gram stain will show intracellular gram-negative diplococci in about 50% of women and, as with chlamydia, pyuria and/or pus cells on gram stain should be demonstrable.

If available, chlamydial cultures of both the urethra and cervix should be obtained in women with sterile pyuria. A thin, calcium-alginate swab should be used for the former and a plastic-shafted swab for the latter, with care taken in both cases to obtain many epithelial cells. In instances where chlamydial cultures are not available, the presence of sterile pyuria (that is, pyuria associated with neither coliforms nor *S. saprophyticus*) and a negative gonococcal culture in a woman with acute dysuria and frequency and clinical features typical of chlamydial infection suggest the latter as the etiologic agent. It should be emphasized that simultaneous infection with more than one of these agents may well occur.

In women without demonstrable pyuria, it has usually not been possible to demonstrate an infectious agent responsible for acute dysuria and frequency.

Treatment

Women with chlamydial infection should be treated with tetracycline, 500 mg P.O. q.i.d. for 7 days. Effective alternative regimens include 7–14 days of doxycycline or trimethoprim-sulfamethoxazole (TMP-SMX). In potentially pregnant women, erythromycin (500 mg P.O. q.i.d. for 14 d) should be utilized. Several effective regimens are available for women with coliform or staphylococcal infection of the urethra and/or bladder as a cause for their dysuria and frequency. In women with uncomplicated cystitis, single-dose therapy with ampicillin (3.5 g orally), amoxicillin (3 g orally), or TMP-SMX (4 single-strength tablets all at once, orally) have been successfully utilized. These regimens appear as effective as 7–10-day regimens of ampicillin, sulfamethoxazole, nitrofurantoin macrocrystals, or trimethoprim-sulfamethoxazole in standard doses used for urinary tract infections (109). Single-dose therapy should be utilized only in reliable patients who will return for post-treatment cultures and/or persisting or recurrent symptoms. It should not be used in women with urologic abnormalities, symptoms of pyelonephritis, or when dysuria and frequency have been present for more than ten days (110). Women with acute urethral syndrome due to coliforms or staphylococci, like women with cystitis, also benefit from antimicrobial therapy, although few regimens have yet been studied. It seems likely, in view of the similarities between these women and those with cystitis in terms of clinical picture and pathogenesis, that the same regimens used for acute cystitis will work well in women with urethral syndrome due to coliforms or *S. saprophyticus*.

In most patients, the clinician will want to initiate therapy before the etiologic diagnosis is known. In this circumstance, the presence or absence of pyuria plays a critical role. In women with pyuria, infection can nearly always be demonstrated, and empiric treatment is thus reasonable. When clinical and epidemiologic factors, as well as laboratory data, favor coliform or staphylococcal infection, single-dose or traditional 7–10-day therapy with the regimens outlined above for urinary tract infection should be utilized. When the same type of information favors gonococcal or chlamydial infection, tetracycline should be chosen until culture results are available. In women with sterile pyuria, tetracycline should also be utilized. In women without pyuria, few data indicate that antimicrobial therapy should be utilized. These women should be treated with pyridium to relieve symptoms, and asked to return in 48 hours if symptoms do not resolve. In most cases, symptoms will resolve. If they do not, another examination and evaluation for pyuria and etiologic agents should be undertaken.

The efficacy of urologic procedures such as urethral dilatation, urethrotomy, and others for treatment of acute urethral syndrome has not been established in controlled trials and, since most women have demonstrable infection, they should be avoided. Their role in treating recurring or prolonged dysuria also needs further evaluation.

Literature Cited

1. Wiesner, P. J., Thompson, S. E. 1980. Gonococcal diseases. DM 26:1–44
2. Handsfield, H. H. 1978. Gonorrhea and nongonococcal urethritis. Recent advances. *Med. Clin. North. Am.* 62:925–43
3. Philips, I. 1976. Beta-lactamase-producing penicillin-resistant gonococcus. *Lancet* 2:656–57
4. Siegel, M. S., Thornsberry, C., Biddle, J. W., O'Mara, P. R., Perine, P. L., Wiesner, P. S. 1978. Penicillinase-producing *Neisseria gonorrhoeae:* results of surveillance in the United States. *J. Infect. Dis.* 137:170–75
5. Holmes, K. K., Handsfield, H. H., Wang, S. P., et al. 1975. Etiology of nongonococcal urethritis. *N. Engl. J. Med.* 292:1199–1205
6. Bowie, W. R., Wang, S. P., Alexander, E. R., et al. 1977. Etiology of nongonococcal urethritis: evidence for *Chlamydia trachomatis* and *Ureaplasma urealyticum. J. Clin. Invest.* 59:735–42
7. Oriel, J. D., Reeve, P., Thomas, B. J., et al. 1975. Infections with chlamydia

group A in men with urethritis due to *Neisseria gonorrhoeae. J. Infect. Dis.* 131:376–82

8. Schachter, J. 1978. Chlamydial infections. *N. Engl. J. Med.* 298:428–35
9. McCormack, W. M., Braum, P., Lee, Y. H., et al. 1973. The genital mycoplasmas. *N. Engl. J. Med.* 288:78–89
10. Stimson, J. B., Hale, J., Bowie, W. R., Holmes, K. K. 1981. Tetracycline-resistant *Ureaplasma urealyticum*: a cause of persistent nongonococcal urethritis. *Ann. Intern. Med.* 94:192–94
11. VD Fact Sheet. 1976. Center for Disease Control, Bureau of State Services, Venereal Disease Control Division, Atlanta, Georgia. HEW Publ. No. (CDC) 77–8195
12. Wiesner, P. J., Holmes, K. K. 1975. Current view of the epidemiology of sexually transmitted diseases in the United States. In *Genital Infections and Their Complications,* ed. D. Danielson, L. Juhlin, P. A. Mardh, pp. 15–24. Stockholm: Almquist & Wiksell
13. Darrow, W. W. 1975. Changes in sexual behavior and venereal diseases. *Clin. Obstet. Gynecol.* 18:255
14. Rein, M. F. 1977. Epidemiology of gonococcal infections. In *The Gonococcus,* ed. R. B. Roberts, pp. 1–31. New York: Wiley
15. Wallace, H. M. 1971. Venereal disease in teenagers. *Clin. Obstet. Gynecol.* 14:432
16. Stamm, W. E., Koutsky, L., Jourden, J. L., Brunham, R., Holmes, K. K. 1981. Prospective screening for urethral infection with *Chlamydia trachomatis* and *Neisseria gonorrhoeae* in men attending a clinic for sexually transmitted diseases. *Clin. Res.* 29:51A
17. Arya, O. P. 1981. Epidemiology of gonorrhea. In *Recent Advances in Sexually Transmitted Diseases.* ed. J. R. W. Harris, pp. 35–48. New York: Churchill Livingstone
18. Arya, O. P., Taber, S. R. 1975. Correlates of venereal disease and fertility in rural Uganda. World Health Organization Document, *WHO/VDT/75, 400*
19. Arya, O. P., Nsanzymuhire, H., Taber, S. R. 1973. Clinical, cultural, and demographic aspects of gonorrhea in a rural community in Uganda. *Bull. WHO* 49:587–95
20. Reyn, A., Kormer, B., Bentzon, M. W. 1958. Effects of penicillin, streptomycin, and tetracycline on *Neisseria gonorrhoeae* isolated in 1944 and 1957. *Br. J. Vener. Dis.* 34:227

21. Martin, J. E., Lester, A., Price, E. V., et al. 1970. Comparative study of gonococcal susceptibility to penicillin in the United States, 1955–1969. *J. Infect. Dis.* 122:459
22. Sparling, P. R., Sarubbi, F. A. Jr., Blackman, E. 1975. Inheritance of low-level resistance to penicillin, tetracycline, and chloramphenicol in *Neisseria gonorrhoeae. J. Bacteriol.* 134:740–49
23. Kaufman, R. E., Johnson, R. E., Jaffe, H. W., et al. 1976. National gonorrhea therapy monitoring study: treatment results. *N. Engl. J. Med.* 294:1–4
24. Jaffe, H. W., Biddle, J. W., Thornsberry, C. et al. 1976. National gonorrhea therapy monitoring study: in vitro antibiotic susceptibility and its correlation with treatment results. *N. Engl. J. Med.* 294:5–9
25. Center for Disease Control. 1976. Penicillinase-producing *Neisseria gonorrhoeae. Morbid. Mortal. Wkly. Rep.* 25(33):261
26. See Ref. 3
27. Elwell, L. P., Roberts, M., Mayer, L. W., Falkow, S. 1977. Plasmid-mediated beta-lactamase production in *Neisseria gonorrhoeae. Antimicrob. Agents. Chemother.* 11:528–33
28. Eisenstein, B. I., Sox, T., Biswasg, G., Blackman, E., Sparling, P. F. 1977. Conjugal transfer of the gonococcal penicillinase plasmid. *Science* 195:998–1000
29. Center for Disease Control. 1979. Penicillinase-producing *Neisseria gonorrhoeae*—United States, worldwide. *Morbid Mortal. Wkly. Rep.* 28:85–87
30. Center for Disease Control. 1982. Global distribution of penicillinase-producing *Neisseria gonorrhoeae* (PPNG). *Morbid. Mortal. Wkly. Rep.* 31:1–3
31. Handsfield, H. H., Sandstrom, E. G., Knapp. J. S., et al. 1982. Epidemiology of penicillinase-producing *Neisseria gonorrhoeae* infections. Analysis by auxotyping and serogrouping. *N. Engl. J. Med.* 306:950–54
32. Center for Disease Control. 1980. An outbreak of penicillinase-producing *Neisseria gonorrhoeae*—Shreveport, Louisiana. *Morbid. Mortal. Wkly. Rep.* 29:241–43
33. Center for Disease Control. 1980. Penicillinase-producing *Neisseria gonorrhoeae*—Los Angeles, California. *Morbid. Mortal. Wkly. Rep.* 29:541–43
34. Lucas, J. B., Price, E. V., Thayer, T. D., et al. 1967. Diagnosis and treatment of gonorrhea in the female. *N. Engl. J. Med.* 276:1454–59

35. Pariser, H. 1972. Asymptomatic gonorrhea. *Med. Clin. North Am.* 56:1127
36. Lycke, E., Lowhagen, G., Hallhagen, G., Johannisson, G., Ramsted, T. K. 1980. The risk of transmission of genital *Chlamydia trachomatis* infection is less than that of genital *Neisseria gonorrhoeae*. *Sex Transm. Dis.* 7:6–10
37. Felton, W. F. 1972. How infectious is gonorrhea? *Br. Med. J.* 4:431
38. Gilstap, L. C., Herbert, W. H. P., Cunningham, G., et al. 1977. Gonorrhea screening in male consorts of women with pelvic infection. *J. Am. Med. Assoc.* 238:965–66
39. Portnoy, J., Mendelson, J., Clecner, B., et al. 1974. Asymptomatic gonorrhea in the male. *Can. Med. Assoc. J.* 110:169
40. Handsfield, H. H., Lipman, T. O., Harnish, J. P., Tronca, E., Holmes, K. K. 1974. Asymptomatic gonorrhea in men. Diagnosis, natural course, prevalence, and significance. *N. Engl. J. Med.* 290:117–23
41. Jacobs, N. F., Kraus, S. J. 1975. Gonococcal and nongonococcal urethritis in men. Clinical and laboratory differentiation. *Ann. Intern Med.* 82:7–12
42. Holmes, K. K. 1974. Gonococcal infection: clinical, epidemiology and laboratory perspectives. *Adv. Intern. Med.* 19:259–85
43. Harnish, J. P., Berger, R. E., Alexander, E. R., et al. 1977. Etiology of acute epididymitis. *Lancet* 1:819–21
44. Berger, R. E., Alexander, E. R., Monda, G. D., et al. 1978. *Chlamydia trachomatis* as a cause of acute "idiopathic" epididymitis. *N. Engl. J. Med.* 298:301–4
45. Handsfield, H. H. 1975. Disseminated gonococcal infection. *Clin. Obstet. Gynecol.* 18:131–34
46. Holmes, K. K., Counts, G. W., Beaty, H. N. 1971. Disseminated gonococcal infection. *Ann. Intern Med.* 74:979–93
47. Petersen, B. H., Graham, J. A., Brookes, G. F. 1976. Human deficiency of the eighth component of complement. The requirements of C8 for *Neisseria gonorrhoeae* bactericidal activity. *J. Clin. Invest.* 57:283–90
48. Wiesner, P. J., Handsfield, H. H., Holmes, K. K. 1973. Low antibiotic resistance of gonococci causing disseminated infection. *N. Engl. J. Med.* 288:1221–22
49. Knapp, J. S., Holmes, K. K. 1975. Disseminated gonococcal infections caused by *Neisseria gonorrhoeae* with unique nutritional requirements. *J. Infect. Dis* 132:204–8
50. Schoolnick, G. K., Buchanan, T. M., Holmes, K. K. 1976. Gonococci causing disseminated gonococcal infection are resistant to the bactericidal action of normal human sera. *J. Clin. Invest.* 58:1163–73
51. Juhlin, J., Krook, G. 1965. Problems in diagnosis, treatment and control of gonococcal infections. I. A comparison of direct microscopy and culture. *Acta Dermatol. Venereol.* 45:142–47
52. Dans, P. E., Judson, F. 1975. The establishment of a venereal disease clinic. II. An appraisal of current diagnostic methods in uncomplicated urogenital and rectal gonorrhea. *J. Am. Vener. Dis. Assoc.* 82:7–12
53. Goodhart, M. E., Ogden, J., Zaidi, A. A., Kraus, S. J. 1982. Factors affecting the performance of smear and culture tests for the sectection of *Neisseria gonorrhoea*. *J. Am. Vener. Dis. Assoc.* 9: 63–69
54. Sandstrom, E., Danielsson, D. 1975. A survey of gonococcal serology. See Ref. 12, pp. 253–59
55. Dans, P. E., Rothenberg, R., Holmes, K. K. 1977. Gonococcal serology: how soon, how useful, and how much? *J. Infect. Dis.* 135:330–34
56. Holmes, K. K., Buchanan, T. M., Adam, J. L., Aschenbach, D. A. 1978. Is serology useful in gonorrhea? A critical analysis of factors influencing serodiagnosis. In *Immunobiology of Neisseria gonorrhoeae*, ed. G. F. Brooks, E. C. Gotschlich, K. K. Holmes, W. D. Sawyer, F. E. Young, pp. 370–76. Washington, DC: Am. Soc. Microbiol.
57. Kraus, S. J. 1979. Culture methods of *Neisseria gonorrhoeae*. *Arch. Androl.* 3:343–49
58. Mehaffey, M. A., Cook, E. C., Griffin, C. W. 1979. Proficiency testing summary analysis for *Neisseria gonorrhoeae*. Atlanta: Center for Disease Control
59. Cross, R. C., Hager, M. B., Neibaur, R., et al. 1971. VCN-inhibited strains of *Neisseria gonorrhoeae*. *Health Serv. Mental Health Admin. Health Rep.* 86:940–42
60. Windall, J. J., Hall, M. M., Washington, J. A., et al. 1980. Inhibitory effects of vancomycin on *Neisseria gonorrhoeae* in Thayer-Martin medium. *J. Infect. Dis.* 142:775
61. Centers for Disease Control. 1982. Sexually transmitted diseases: treatment guidelines. *Morbid. Mortal. Wkly. Rep.* 31:355–605
62. Wiesner, P. J., Tronca, E., Bonnin, P., et al. 1973. Clinical spectrum of pharyn-

geal gonococcal infection. *N. Engl. J. Med.* 288:181
63. Centers for Disease Control. 1981. Spectinomycin-resistant penicillinase-producing *Neisseria gonorrhoea*—California. *Morbid. Mortal. Wkly. Rep.* 30:221–22
64. Johnston, H. K. H., Gotschlich, E. C. 1974. Isolation and characterization of the outer membrance of *N. gonorrhoeae. J. Bacteriol.* 119:250–57
65. Buchanan, T. M. 1975. Antigenic heterogeneity of gonococcal pili. *J. Exp. Med.* 141:1470–75
66. Kellog, D. S. Jr., Cohen, I. R., Norins, L. C., Schrocter, A. L., Reising, G. 1968. *Neisseria gonorrhoeae.* II. Colonial variation and pathogenicity during 35 months in vitro. *J. Bacteriol.* 96:596–605
67. Swanson, J. 1973. Studies on gonococcus infection. IX. Pili: their role in attachment of gonococci to tissue culture cells. *J. Exp. Med.* 137:571–89
68. Dilworth, J. A., Hendley, J. D., Mandell, G. L. 1975. Attachment and digestion of gonococci by human neutrophils. *Infect. Immun.* 11:512–16
69. Tramont, E. C. 1981. Gonococcal pilus vaccine: studies of antigenicity and inhibition of attachment. *J. Clin. Invest.* 68:881–88
70. Siegel, M. S., Olsen, D., Critchlow, C., Buchanan, T. M. 1982. Gonococcal pili: safety and immunogenicity in humans and antibody function in vitro. *J. Infect. Dis.* 145:300–10
71. Johnston, K. H., Holmes, K. K., Gotschlich, E. C. 1976. The serologic classification of *N. gonorrhoeae.* I. Isolation of the outer membrane complex responsible for serologic specificity. *J. Exp. Med.* 143:741–58
72. Wiesner, P. J. 1977. Selected aspects of the epidemiology of nongonococcal urethritis. In *Nongonococcal Urethritis and Related Infections,* ed. D. Hobson, K. K. Holmes, pp. 9–14 Washington, DC: Am. Soc. Microbiol.
73. Bowie, W. R., Pollack, H. M., Forsyth, P. S., et al. 1977. Bacteriology of the urethra in normal men and men with nongonococcal urethritis. *J. Clin. Microbiol.* 6:482–88
74. Dunlop, E. M. C., Jones, B. R., Darougar, S. 1972. Chlamydia and nonspecific urethritis. *Br. J. Vener. Dis.* 2:575–77
75. Paavonen, J. 1979. *Chlamydia trachomatis*-induced urethritis in female partners of men with nongonococcal urethritis. *Sex. Transm. Dis.* 6:69–71

76. Paavonen, J., Lousa, M., Saikka, P., Vartianinen, E., Kanerva, L., Lassus, A. 1980. Treatment of NGU with trimethoprim-sulphadiazine and with placebo. A double blind partner controled study. *Br. J. Vener. Dis.* 56:101
77. Bowie, W. R., Alexander, E. R., Floyd, J. F., et al. 1976. Differential response of chlamydial and ureaplasma—associated urethritis to sulphafurazole (sulfisoxazole) and aminocyclitols. *Lancet* 2:1276–78
78. Diagiacomo, R. F., Gale, J. L., Wang, S. P., Kiviat, M. D. 1975. Chlamydial infection of the male baboon urethra. *Br. J. Vener. Dis.* 51:310–13
79. Shepard, M. C. 1954. The recovery of pleuropneumonia-like organisms from Negro men with and without nongonococcal urethritis. *Am. J. Syphilis, Gonorrhea, Vener. Dis.* 38:113–24
80. Taylor-Robinson, D., McCormack, W. M. 1980. Medical progress: the genital mycoplasmas. *N. Engl. J. Med.* 302: 1003–10, 1063–67
81. Taylor-Robinson, D., Csonka, G. W. 1981. Laboratory and clinical aspects of mycoplasma infections of the human genitourinary tract. See Ref. 17, pp. 151–86
82. Wong, J. L., Hines, P. A., Brasher, M. D., Rogers, G. T., Smith, R. F., Schachter, J. 1977. The etiology of nongonococcal urethritis in men attending a venereal disease clinic. *Sex. Transm. Dis.* 4:4–8
83. Ford, D. K., Smith, J. R. 1974. Nonspecific urethritis associated with a tetracycline-resistant T-mycoplasma. *Br. J. Vener. Dis.* 50:373–74
84. Mardh, P. A., Colleen, S., Holmquist, B. 1972. Chlamydia in chronic prostatitis. *Br. Med. J.* 4:361
85. Mardh, P. A., Ripa, K. T., Coleen, S., Treharne, J. D., Darougar, S. 1978. Role of *Chlamydia trachomatis* in nonacute prostatitis. *Br. J. Vener. Dis.* 54:330–34
86. Kousa, M., Saikku, P., Richmonds, S., Lassus, A. 1978. Frequent association of chlamydial infections with Reiter's syndrome. *Sex. Transm. Dis.* 5:57
87. Brewerton, D. A., Nichols, A., Oates, J. K., et al. 1973. Reiter's disease and HL-A27. *Lancet* 2:996–98
88. Morris, R., Metzger, A. L., Bluestone, R., et al. 1974. HLA-AW27—a clue to the diagnosis and pathogenesis of Reiter's syndrome. *N. Engl. J. Med.* 290: 554–56
89. Keat, A. C., Maini, R. N., Nkwazi, G. C., Pegrum, G. D., Ridgeway, G. L.,

Scott, J. T. 1978. Role of *Chlamydia trachomatis* and HLA-B27 in sexually acquired reactive arthritis. *Br. Med. J.* 1:605–7

90. Bowie, W. R. 1978. Comparison of gram stain and first-voided urine sediment in diagnosis of urethritis. *Sex. Transm. Dis.* 5:39–42

91. Desai, K., Robson, H. 1982. Comparison of the gram-stained urethral smear and first-void urine sediment in the diagnosis of nongonococcal urethritis. *Sex. Transm. Dis.* 9:21–25

92. Holmes, K. K., Johnson, D. W., Floyd, T. M. 1967. Studies in venereal disease. III. Double-blind comparison of tetracycline hydrochloride and placebo in treatment of nongonococcal urethritis. *J. Am. Med. Assoc.* 202:138–40

93. Willcox, R. R. 1972. Triple tetracycline in the treatment of nongonococcal urethritis. *Br. J. Vener. Dis.* 48:137–40

94. Ridgeway, G. L., Owen, J. M., Oriel, J. D. 1976. A method for testing the antibiotic susceptibility of *Chlamydia trachomatis* in a cell culture system. *J. Antimicrob. Chemother.* 2:71–76

95. Kuo, C., Wang, S. P., Grayston, J. T. 1977. Antimicrobial activity of several antibiotics and a sulfonamide against *Chlamydia Trachomatis* organisms in organ culture. *Antimicrob. Agents Chemother.* 12:80

96. Handsfield, H. H., Alexander, E. R., Wang, S. P., Pederson, A. H. B., Holmes, K. K. 1976. Differences in the therapeutic response of chlamydia-positive and chlamydia-negative forms of nongonococcal urethritis. *J. Am. Vener. Dis. Assoc.* 2:5–9

97. Oriel, J. D., Ridgway, G. L., Tchamouroff, S. 1977. Comparison of erythromycin stearate and oxytetracycline in the treatment of non-gonococcal urethritis. *Scott. Med. J.* 22:375

98. Bowie, W. R., Alexander, E. R., Floyd, J. F., Stimson, J. B., Holmes, K. K. 1981. Therapy for nongonococcal urethritis double-blind randomized comparison of two doses and two durations of minocycline. *Ann. Intern. Med.* 95:306–11

99. Wong, E. S., Stamm, W. E., Hooton, T. M., Cole, B., Hill, C., Holmes, K. K. 1982. Persistent nongonococcal urethritis (NGU). *Conf. Antimicrob. Agents Chemother., 22nd, Miami, Fla.* Prog. Abstr. Intersci.

100. Brunham, R., Irwin, B., Stamm, W. E., Holmes, K. K. 1981. Epidemiological and clinical correlates of *Chlamydia trachomatis* and *Neisseria gonorrhoeae* infection among women attending a clinic for sexually transmitted diseases. *Clin. Res.* 29:474

101. Waters, W. E., Elwood, P. C., Asscher, A. W., Abernethy, M. 1970. Clinical significance of dysuria in women. *Br. Med. J.* 2:754–57

102. Komaroff, A. L., Pass, T. M., McCue, J. D., Cohen, A. B., Hendricks, T. M., Friedland, G. 1978. Management strategies for urinary and vaginal infections. *Arch. Intern. Med.* 138:1069–73

103. Stamm, W. E., Wagner, K. F., Amsel, R., et al. 1980. Causes of the acute urethral syndrome in women. *N. Engl. J. Med.* 303:409–15

104. Stamm, W. E., Running, K., McKevitt, M. et al. 1981. Treatment of the acute urethral syndrome. *N. Engl. J. Med.* 304:956–58

105. Wallin, J. E., Thompson, S. E., Zaidi, A., Wong, K. 1981. Urethritis in women attending an STD clinic. *Br. J. Vener. Dis.* 57:50–54

106. Curran, J. W. 1977. Gonorrhea and the urethral syndrome. *Sex. Transm. Dis.* 4:119–21

107. Schaeffer, A. J., Jones, J. M., Dunn, J. K. 1981. Association of in-vitro *Escherichia coli* adherence to vaginal and buccal epithelial cells with susceptibility of women to recurrent urinary tract infection. *N. Engl. J. Med.* 304:1062–66

108. Svanborg-Eden, C., Hanson, L. A. 1978. *Escherischia coli* pili as possible mediation of attachment to human urinary tract epithelial cells. *Infect. Immun.* 21:229

109. Kunin, C. M. 1981. Duration of treatment of urinary tract infections. *Am. J. Med.* 71:849–54

110. Stamm, W. E. 1980. Single-dose treatment of cystitis. *J. Am. Med. Assoc.* 244:591–92

Ann. Rev. Med. 1983. 34:359–66

PERCUTANEOUS DISSOLUTION OF RENAL CALCULI

Stephen P. Dretler, M.D., and Richard C. Pfister, M.D.

Departments of Urology and Radiology, Massachusetts General Hospital and Harvard Medical School, Boston, Massachusetts 02114

ABSTRACT

The use of percutaneous nephrostomy catheters has allowed access to intrarenal urinary calculi for dissolution. Renacidin is the successful agent for dissolving struvite stones. THAM-E is the most effective agent for the intrarenal dissolution of cystine stone. Calcium oxalate stones are still resistant to dissolution techniques.

Chemolysis of renal calculi by direct irrigation is not a new idea. As early as 1932 Keyser attempted dissolution of stones by retrograde infusion (1), and in 1943 Howard Suby and Fuller Albright (2) introduced Suby's solution for the dissolution of renal calculi. However, the techniques of dissolution were not accepted. There were no antibiotics and infection was common. Furthermore, indwelling small-bore ureteral catheters obstructed with debris could not be placed accurately at the site of the stone and were not useful in instances of obstruction. More recently, nephrostomy tubes have been placed at surgery so that postoperative dissolution of remaining fragments could be performed. This has the obvious disadvantage of requiring open surgery.

The use of percutaneous nephrostomy (PCN) for dissolution does not require surgery or anesthesia; allows use of large bore (8–12 F) catheter(s) (high perfusion rates, infrequent obstruction); permits positioning of a second catheter to facilitate outflow in the presence of obstruction or a sequestered stone; provides direct access with accurate catheter positioning; and avoids the epididymitis, cystitis, and irritation of an indwelling bladder catheter. Experience with the technique of placement of PCN catheters has allowed the concept of direct, primary dissolution of renal calculi to be actualized.

359

0066-4219/83/0401-0359$02.00

Technique of Percutaneous Nephrostomy and Stone Irrigation

The technique of PCN was described by Pfister & Newhouse (3). The skin of the back is prepared with antiseptic solution and local anesthesia given. Under ultrasonic or fluoroscopic guidance the renal pelvis is punctured with a 22 gauge needle via a posterior approach. The collecting system is then opacified by injecting contrast media through the needle; continued injection provides a persistent image of the collecting system as a target for the trocar-cannula unit and serves to keep an unobstructed collecting system distended to facilitate puncture. A pencil-point hollow-bore trocar with overlying cannula is advanced toward the collecting system until urine flow signals successful entry; the trocar is removed, a catheter is inserted through the cannula into the renal pelvis, and the cannula is withdrawn over the catheter. The tip of the catheter is guided so that the infused solvent will flow onto the stone. A second catheter is placed in instances of outflow obstruction to allow maximal contact of solution and stone and permits irrigation at low pressure (Figure 1).

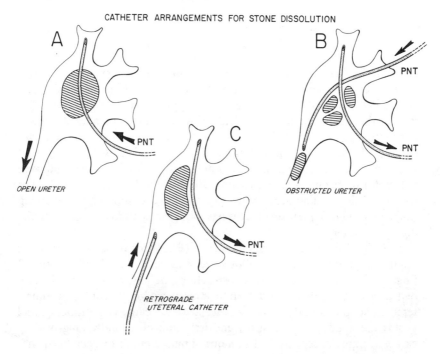

Figure 1 Schematic representation of various percutaneous nephrostomy (PNT) catheter arrangements for irrigation inflow and outflow routes during stone dissolution (from Ref. 4).

After waiting 24 hours to allow the puncture site to seal, irrigation is started with saline at 30 ml/hr and slowly increased to 120 ml/hr or a rate that can be tolerated without flank pain or elevation of intrarenal pressure above 25 cm H_2O. Three-way valves are incorporated into the system to ensure that the 25 cm H_2O limit is not exceeded. Once the infusion is working properly and the urine is sterile, the solvent appropriate for the stone type may be infused. Abdominal roentgenograms and nephrosto-grams are done periodically to assess the progress of dissolution. All patients receive broad spectrum antibiotics before, during, and for ten days after completion. The indications, special precautions, results, and discussion of this method for each stone type are presented below.

Magnesium-Ammonium-Phosphate Calculi (Struvite)

The $CaPO_4$-$MgNH_4PO_4$-$6H_2O$ calculi occur primarily in patients with urea-splitter infection and, although they comprise only 10–15% of calculi, probably represent 20–25% of those that require surgery. Because of the chronic nature of the primary disease process, patients with this stone type are prone to multiple recurrences. The presumptive diagnosis of struvite calculi is made by clinical history or prior stone analysis. The patients chosen for dissolution therapy are those who would otherwise require surgery because of pain, infection, obstruction, or progressive renal damage (4). The solvent used for dissolution is Renacidin® (Guardian Chemical Company, Hauppauge, Long Island, NY 11787).

Renacidin is a multi-electrolyte solution that provides hydrogen ion and citrate to form soluble complexes with the phosphate (phosphoric acid) and calcium (calcium citrate) components of the calculus. Early in its use (1962), complications prompted the FDA to withdraw approval for use within the kidney. However, further study has shown that if the urine is sterile, intrarenal pressures kept below 25 cm H_2O and phosphate and magnesium levels monitored, Renacidin may be safely used (5). However, informed consent, peer approval, and close observation are necessary for use of this drug in the kidney.

We have perfused Renacidin via PCN tube in 23 kidneys with struvite calculi that would otherwise have had immediate surgical intervention. In 16 kidneys the stone(s) was totally dissolved and no surgery was necessary (Figure 2). Stones in 2 of these 16 kidneys recurred in the subsequent 1–5 years. Each of two other patients had a small fragment remaining and this was extracted intact during other surgical procedures on the urinary tract; however, direct renal surgery was avoided. One of the 23 failed to dissolve at all and was subsequently found to be calcium oxalate. Another, initially thought to have been totally dissolved, was noted to have a fragment

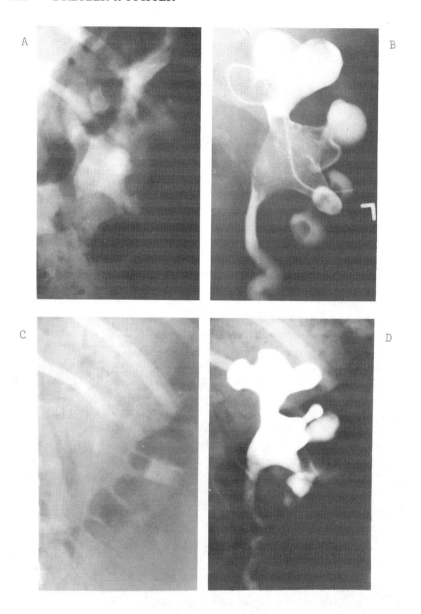

Figure 2 Dissolution of struvite staghorn calculus. (*Top left*) Plain film of large stone. (*Top right*) Percutaneous catheter enters lower kidney and its tip lies in the upper calyx; the ureter is unobstructed. (*Bottom left*) Plain film and (*Bottom right*) nephrostogram two weeks later shows complete dissolution of the calculus (From Ref. 13).

remaining on follow-up study. Five kidneys had remaining fragments that failed to dissolve; one required surgery. In all of the 23 kidneys that would have had surgery when initially seen, only two have required renal exploration.

The time interval from the onset of irrigation to the end of solvent infusion (including periods of cessation because of flank pain, fever, positive culture, serum PO_4, magnesium, or creatinine abnormalities) ranged from 6 to 45 days. Daily urine culture and measurement of serum magnesium, phosphate, and creatinine were performed. Although the dissolution time was sometimes long, all patients who were otherwise well were able to leave the hospital and resume normal activities immediately.

The technique of PCN with Renacidin irrigation is an effective method of chemolysis of struvite calculi and is an alternative to surgery for selected patients under controlled conditions.

Uric Acid Calculi

Uric acid calculi make up 8–10% of all stones but because they are amenable to dissolution techniques are rarely cause for surgical intervention. Nonobstructing uric acid calculi may be treated with high fluid intake (> 2000 cc/day), allopurinol, and oral alkalinization. Experience with medical treatment indicates that 80% may be expected to successfully dissolve over a 4–16-month period (6).

Oral alkalinization is based on the fact that at urine pH 5.75 only half the uric acid exists in the ionized (soluble) form. At pH 7 almost all uric acid exists as the soluble monosodium urate. However, the urine of patients who form uric acid stones is notoriously difficult to alkalinize, and large doses of sodium bicarbonate or potassium citrate and/or acetazolamide often are necessary and may result in edema, hypertension, potassium intoxication, or precipitation of calcium salts (acetazolamide). Therefore, the idea of direct renal instillation of solvent was born of necessity.

Techniques for direct dissolution include retrograde placement of ureteral catheters (7, 8) and percutaneous nephrostomy (3, 9). Solvents used are 0.1 M $NaHCO_3$ and THAM (10) (tris[hydroxymethyl]aminomethane). THAM-E (pK 7.84) is a stronger base than bicarbonate (pK 6.10). The resulting increase in pH is not significant enough to warrant the use of this agent instead of bicarbonate to speed the dissolution process. Laboratory studies, as yet unpublished, show the uric acid calculi dissolve significantly faster with THAM-E than with straight bicarbonate.

The time required for direct dissolution by bicarbonate or THAM-E infusion ranges from three days to two weeks. There have been no reported complications; however, attention must be directed toward maintaining sterile urine and keeping perfusion pressure below 25 cm H_2O.

When a patient presents with an asymptomatic uric acid stone, oral dissolution by sodium bicarbonate and allopurinol is the method of choice. If sodium or potassium intoxication is a problem, direct dissolution is preferred. When a symptomatic or obstructing stone occurs, or an asymptomatic stone is present and growing within the kidney and unresponsive to oral alkali, then an infusion of bicarbonate or THAM-E by percutaneous nephrostomy is the simplest, fastest, most effective method of therapy.

Cystine

Nonobstructing, asymptomatic cystine calculi may be treated with high fluid intake, alkali, and penicillamine with the expectation that, if carried out for one year, 40% of calculi will dissolve, 20% will decrease in size by one third, and the remainder will show either no change or stone growth (11). Prior to the use of chemolysis via PCN, symptomatic or obstructing cystine calculi required surgery.

Recently, using a saline solution with 60 ml of 20% N-acetyl-L-cysteine (Mucomyst®, Mead-Johnson Laboratories, Evansville, IN 47721) and 300 meq of bicarbonate per liter (12), we attempted dissolution via PCN of five cystine staghorn calculi. Three were successfully dissolved in 4–6 weeks (Figure 3), one had a 30% reduction in size (unexplained failure) and required surgical removal, and the fifth did not change with irrigation and was found at surgery to be coated with a 2-mm shell of calcium oxalate. All patients successfully treated resumed normal life activity immediately upon discharge. There were no complications.

Acetylcysteine cleaves the cystine disulfide bond, thus reducing the dimer, cystine, to the more soluble monomer, cysteine. That this reduction is the mechanism of action for dissolution and not the increase in solubility from the added bicarbonate is suggested by amino acid chromatography performed on the effluent. Chromatography revealed little or no residual urine cystine. Although it could be argued that bicarbonate dissolved the stone and acetylcysteine converted it once in solution, the poor results of bicarbonate on cystine stone dissolution make this an unlikely explanation.

Acetylcysteine is also not designated for use within the kidney; therefore, informed patient consent, peer approval, and close observation are required. All previously noted precautions observed during PCN and dissolution must be followed.

Recently, we have used THAM-E with a pH of 10.2 instead of acetylcysteine for the dissolution of cystine calculi. In our limited experience with three patients, the THAM-E appears to dissolve the cystine calculi at a

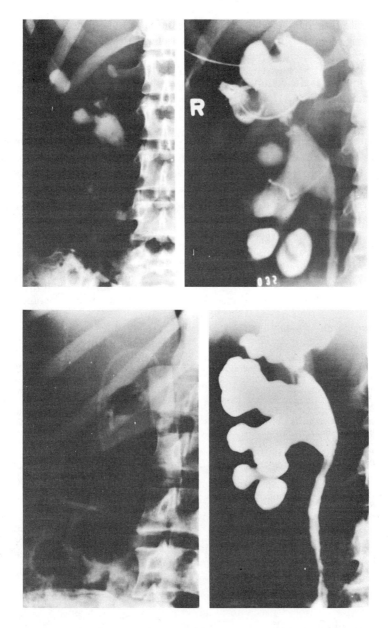

Figure 3   Dissolution of cystine stones. (*Top left*) Preliminary film shows multiple pyelocaly-ceal and ureteral calculi. (*Top right*) Two 8F nephrostomy catheters placed percutaneously for low pressure irrigation. (*Bottom left*) Follow up plain film and (*Bottom right*) nephrosto-gram demonstrates total dissolution of all calculi.

faster rate than acetylcysteine. The infusion of THAM-E may become the treatment of choice. It is still undergoing clinical testing.

Calcium Oxalate

Although this is the commonest stone type, there is no available agent that will safely dissolve it.

Summary

The increasing expertise with which PCN can be placed has facilitated more aggressive chemolysis of renal and ureteral calculi. All patients who undergo treatment may be expected to have mild intermittent flank discomfort, occasional hematuria, and sometimes extended hospitalization. Despite these considerations, all patients here described have provided informed consent and have chosen the technique of PCN and dissolution as an alternative to surgery.

More effective solutions are desirable so that the period of hospitalization is decreased. Additionally, further experience is necessary to determine the most appropriate and efficacious situations in which to recommend its use. PCN for dissolution of renal calculi is an idea whose time has come.

Literature Cited

1. Keyser, L., Scherer, P., Claffey, L. W. 1947. Studies in the dissolution of urinary calculi: report of clinical aspects. *Trans. Am. Assoc. Genitourinary Surg.* 39:173–88
2. Suby, H. I., Albright, F. 1943. Dissolution of phosphate urinary calculi by the retrograde induction of a citrate solution containing magnesium. *N. Engl. J. Med.* 228:81
3. Pfister, R. C., Newhouse, J. H. 1979. II. Percutaneous nephrostomy and other procedures. *Radiol. Clin. North Am.* 17:351–63
4. Dretler, S. P., Newhouse, J. H., Pfister, R. C. 1979. Renal stone dissolution via percutaneous nephrostomy. *N. Engl. J. Med.* 300:341–43
5. Nemoy, N. J., Stamey, T. A. 1971. Surgical, bacteriological and biochemical management of "infection stones." *J. Am. Med. Assoc.* 215:1470
6. Uhlir, K. 1970. The peroral dissolution of renal calculi. *J. Urol.* 104:239
7. Freiha, F. S., Hemady, K. 1976. Dissolution of uric acid stones: An alternative to surgery. *Urology* 8:334
8. Hardy, B., Klein, L. 1976. *In situ* dissolution of ureteral calculus. *Urology* 8 (5):444
9. Spataro, R. F., Linke, C. A., Barbaric, Z. L. 1978. The use of percutaneous nephrostomy and urinary alkalinization in the dissolution of obstructing uric acid stones. *Radiology* 129:629
10. Gordon, M. R., Carrion, H. M., Politano, V. A. 1978. Dissolution of uric acid calculi with THAM irrigation. *Urology* 12(4):393
11. Smith, L. 1977. Clinical features and management of cystinuria. *Proc. Mayo Clin.* 52:533
12. Smith, L., Lange, P. 1980. Dissolution of cystine calculi by acetylcysteine via percutaneous nephrostomy. *Urology* 13 (4):422
13. Pfister, R. C., Yoder, I. C., Newhouse, J. H. 1981. Percutaneous uroradiologic procedures. *Sem. Roentgenol.* 16: 135–51

Ann. Rev. Med. 1983. 34:367–75

SUBARACHNOID HEMORRHAGE[1]

Roberto C. Heros, M.D., and Nicholas T. Zervas, M.D.

Massachusetts General Hospital, Boston, Massachusetts 02114

ABSTRACT

Subarachnoid hemorrhage (SAH) is an important cause of death and serious morbidity, accounting for about 10% of all cases of stroke. In spite of recent advances in the surgical treatment of aneurysms and arteriovenous malformations (AVMs), the overall morbidity associated with SAH has changed little over the last several decades. A greater awareness by the medical community of the warning signs of SAH is essential in effectively reducing the morbidity associated with this illness. With modern surgical techniques, most aneurysms and many AVMs can be obliterated safely and effectively if detected early, before they result in a major SAH.

INTRODUCTION

Spontaneous subarachnoid hemorrhage (SAH) accounts for approximately 10% of all cases of stroke. If trauma is excluded, about 75% of the cases of SAH are due to rupture of an intracranial aneurysm. Cerebral arteriovenous malformations (AVMs) account for approximately another 10%, and the remainder are due to a variety of other conditions and, in many instances, no etiology can be found. In North America and Europe, the annual incidence of SAH is approximately 15 per 100,000 population. There are approximately 30,000 new cases of SAH in the United States each year. Of these patients, about 40% die or become permanently disabled as a result of the initial hemorrhage and another 20–30% will die as a result of a future hemorrhage if left untreated (1, 4). It is clear then, that major efforts continue to be necessary in order to reduce the morbidity and mortality associated with SAH.

[1]This study was partially supported by National Institute Health Grant NS 10828.

367

DIAGNOSIS

The best way to reduce the high morbidity and mortality of SAH is to detect and eradicate the lesions responsible before they produce a major hemorrhage. With high-resolution CT scanning and intravenous digital subtraction angiography, it should be possible to detect most intracranial aneurysms of significant size (>7 mm) and essentially all AVMs. Individuals at high risk of harboring such lesions probably should be screened by these noninvasive methods. Such individuals include the members of families in which more than one person is known to have an intracranial aneurysm. In addition, screening should be carried out in patients with diseases that predispose to the formation of intracranial aneurysms, such as fibromuscular dysplasia, polycystic kidneys, or coarctation or hypoplasia of the aorta, or diseases associated with defects in vascular walls, such as Ehlers-Danlos and Marfan's syndromes and pseudoxanthoma elasticum (1).

Greater awareness among the medical community of warning signs of aneurysmal rupture is of paramount importance. Almost 50% of all major SAHs due to ruptured aneurysms are preceded by warning symptoms. Most of these symptoms fall into one of two major groups. The first group consists of symptoms such as localized head pain, diplopia (particularly from paresis of the oculomotor nerve), and visual defects that can be attributed to aneurysmal expansion. The second group of symptoms is thought to be caused by "minor leaks" and consists of generalized headache, which can last several hours or days and is frequently accompanied by nausea, neck pain, back pain, malaise, and photophobia. These patients can be identified by the alert physician who takes seriously a patient who presents with a history of an unusually severe headache without a previous history of migraine, frequent headaches, or psychosomatic complaints. A lumbar puncture will show evidence of fresh subarachnoid bleeding in these patients. The importance of recognizing these warning signs lies in the fact that when an aneurysm is diagnosed before a major rupture, it can be surgically eliminated with minimal morbidity using modern microsurgical techniques (1, 2).

Most major first hemorrhages from AVMs occur without antecedent symptoms. However, a substantial number of AVMs produce seizures and, occasionally, intractable headaches before they result in a major SAH. Less frequently, they can produce a progressive neurologic syndrome from dysfunction in the general area of the brain where they are located. This is thought to be due to ischemia, which results when the AVM "steals" blood from surrounding tissue. Dementia can also occur, though rarely, as a result of this phenomenon. In essentially all of these cases, a properly enhanced CT scan will be diagnostic. An occasional patient with otherwise typical "migraine headaches" will be found to have an AVM, which will most commonly be located in the occipital lobe. Of course, migraine is too common a disorder to subject every patient with it to a CT scan, especially if there is a typical family history and if the patient has a longstanding history of migraine headaches. If the syndrome is somewhat atypical, however, and especially if there is no family history of migraine, it may be worthwhile to perform a CT scan on such a patient when first seen.

Once a major SAH has occurred, one usually has little problem recognizing it, especially when the patient presents alert and without major focal neurologic deficits. The initial symptom is usually a severe headache of precipitous onset or sudden transient loss of consciousness followed by headache. The headache is frequently described as "explosive," "crushing," "the worst in my life," etc. Signs of meningeal irritation such as photophobia and nuchal rigidity develop several hours after the onset of the SAH and may be absent if the patient is seen soon after the hemorrhage. Subhyaloid hemorrhages (irregular blots of blood on the most superficial layer of the retina) are almost pathognomonic of SAH when seen on funduscopic examination in a patient without focal neurologic deficits complaining of extremely severe headache of sudden onset.

The diagnosis is more difficult when the patient presents in coma or with major focal neurologic deficits. If subhyaloid hemorrhages are seen in such patients and there is no history of head trauma, SAH must be suspected and will be confirmed in about 50% of the cases. Most patients presenting in coma or with decreased level of consciousness and major neurologic deficits, however, will probably have suffered either a major ischemic stroke or an intracerebral hemorrhage rather than a SAH. The same applies to the alert patient who presents with major focal neurologic deficits. Because of their location within the brain parenchyma, AVMs, as contrasted with aneurysms, can result in a localized intracerebral hemorrhage, which will produce focal neurologic deficits at times unaccompanied by symptoms of diffuse SAH such as generalized headache and meningeal irritation.

When a patient is diagnosed as having had a SAH, a CT scan should be obtained as soon as possible after admission. The initial CT scan should be done without contrast material to identify and localize blood in the subarachnoid space. This is followed by a CT scan with contrast, which will usually identify the lesion responsible for the bleeding. Early cerebral angiography is not necessary unless early surgery is planned or the patient has an intracerebral hematoma that may require prompt surgical evacuation. When the problem is due to a ruptured aneurysm, surgery is usually deferred for 8 to 12 days and, in that case, cerebral angiography should be carried out just before surgery since many surgeons will prefer to defer surgery if cerebral vasospasm is found in the arteriogram. When the patient deteriorates during the preoperative period, again, the CT scan is most helpful in revealing the cause of the deterioration.

NATURAL HISTORY

The natural history of asymptomatic, incidental, unruptured aneurysms is not well known, but it has been estimated that they rupture at a rate of approximately 3% per year. This risk, of course, goes on year after year so that a young individual found to have an incidental intracranial aneurysm has almost an even chance of having a major SAH over the next 20–30 years of life.

There is even less certainty about the natural history of AVMs, but a few studies of patients with untreated AVMs followed over a number of years suggest that patients who have never bled have approximately a 25% chance of experiencing a major hemorrhage within 15–20 years. If the AVM has already bled, there is a risk of about 25% that another hemorrhage will occur within the next five years. If the patient has bled twice, then there is approximately a 25% chance that he or she will bleed again within a year of the last hemorrhage. Of these hemorrhages, about one fourth are fatal or disabling.

The natural history of ruptured intracranial aneurysms is better known. Approximately 20% of these patients die before ever reaching a hospital. Of those that do reach medical attention, about 30% die during the next several days to months as a result of the initial hemorrhage or its complications. If the aneurysm is left untreated, about one third of the patients that recover from the initial hemorrhage die as a consequence of recurrent bleeding. This incidence of rebleeding, of course, decreases with time so that by the end of two weeks the chance of a recurrent hemorrhage within the next six months is only about 10%. Even at the end of six months, however, a patient who has recovered from an initial rupture continues to have about a 3% chance of suffering another hemorrhage each year (3).

MANAGEMENT

Arteriovenous Malformations

The treatment of SAH from an AVM must be considered separately from that of SAH secondary to a ruptured intracranial aneurysm. In the former case, the SAH is rarely severe enough to cause the serious complications described in the section on aneurysms. As stated earlier, AVMs are almost always located within the substance of the brain so that, even though they do result in some degree of SAH, the major bleeding usually occurs within the substance of the brain. Also, AVMs have less chance of rebleeding during the immediate period after a hemorrhage than do aneurysms, even though they continue to have a steady chance of rebleeding over the next months and years, as indicated above. Therefore, elaborate precautions to protect these patients from an immediate recurrent hemorrhage are not necessary. The main consideration, then, consists of deciding whether the AVM should be treated and, if so, by which method. An understanding of the natural history of these lesions, grossly oversimplified above, is essential to this consideration. Each one of these lesions is different from the last one and, therefore, must be considered on a highly individual basis. The treatment of choice, whenever feasible, is surgical excision. Today this treatment is possible for the majority of cerebral AVMs and can be carried out with relative safety, using modern microsurgical techniques. There are a number of malformations, however, that, because of their critical location or because of their enormous size, cannot be excised surgically with safety. Some of these lesions, particularly the smaller ones, respond favorably to specialized types of radiotherapy such as proton beam therapy and highly collimated gamma irradiation. These forms of treatment are available only in a few centers. Another therapeutic modality that is becoming increasingly available is that of embolization of the AVM by selective catheterization of the feeding arteries and injection of different substances into the nidus of the malformation. This form of therapy can also be used in conjunction with surgical resection and has made it possible to completely obliterate some lesions that otherwise would have been very difficult to treat surgically (9, 10).

Aneurysms

GENERAL MEASURES   The patient with a recent SAH from a ruptured aneurysm should be nursed in a quiet environment designed to prevent stress and excitement with their attendant abrupt increases in systemic arterial pressure. This is done to reduce the chance of rebleeding, which is very high during the first two or three weeks. We routinely prescribe anticonvulsants to minimize the chance of a seizure. The use of steroids is reserved for patients with evidence of significant increase in intracranial pressure. Today, it is felt that the blood pressure should be kept at approximately normal levels. When patients present with significant hypertension, a gradual careful lowering of the blood pressure is in order. If signs of cerebral ischemia develop, however, all antihypertensive medications should be withdrawn and, in fact, artificial hypertension should sometimes be induced, as described below.

SYSTEMIC COMPLICATIONS   The SAH associated with a ruptured aneurysm frequently results in widespread hypothalamic dysfunction. This is not surprising in view of the fact that most intracranial aneurysms occur in the circle of Willis in close proximity to the hypothalamus. The hypothalamic disturbance can usually be characterized as overactivity of the sympathetic axis and overstimulation of both the adrenal cortex and the medulla. This can result in typical electrocardiographic changes such as peaked P waves, short P-R intervals, long Q-T segments, large U waves, and peaked T waves. At times, more overt arrhythmias and frank subendocardial ischemia and infarction can occur. These effects correlate highly with the levels of circulating catecholamines and, in fact, these changes can be produced experimentally by injection of catecholamines in high doses. The arrhythmias and ischemic changes must be treated as if they were of primary cardiac origin since indeed their hemodynamic effects are identical.

Electrolyte disturbances are also frequent after SAH. Again, they are usually the result of hypothalamic dysfunction, but can also be compounded by other factors including iatrogenic overhydration or dehydration. Of the electrolyte disturbances seen after SAH, hyponatremia is the most common. The hyponatremia seen after SAH is usually associated with decreased serum osmolarity and increased urinary sodium and osmolarity, as would be expected with inappropriate secretion of ADH. However, these patients are usually found to have a decreased total blood volume and, therefore, need to be treated with a combination of water restriction to correct the hyponatremia and colloid or blood replacement to replenish the intravascular volume and maintain adequate cerebral perfusion (4).

Other systemic problems that develop in these patients, such as respiratory and septic complications, must be treated in the usual manner. An exception to this is venous thrombosis and its attendant risk of pulmonary embolism. This problem is seen frequently in these patients because of the prolonged bed rest and the frequent use of antifibrinolytic agents. The usual treatment for this condition is, of course, anticoagulation, but patients with a recent SAH cannot be anticoagulated for fear of inducing rebleeding. Therefore, less satisfactory mechanical forms of treatment must be relied upon, such as caval plication or insertion of an umbrella.

NEUROLOGIC COMPLICATIONS   When a patient with a ruptured aneurysm who has recovered from the initial hemorrhage deteriorates neurologically, and systemic causes such as electrolyte disturbances or fever have been eliminated, we are usually left with three major causes of deterioration: (a) hydrocephalus, (b) rebleeding, and (c) vasospasm. Hydrocephalus oc-

curs frequently after SAH. It can be acute and severe if the initial hemorrhage ruptures into the ventricle. These patients require immediate
ventricular drainage. More frequently, the hydrocephalus occurs gradually
and, in these instances, it is usually communicating in nature and related
to blockage of the subarachnoid pathways and interference with reabsorption of the cerebrospinal fluid by the blood in the subarachnoid space. This
form of hydrocephalus frequently resolves spontaneously, but occasionally
it necessitates a permanent shunting procedure.

Rebleeding continues to be a major problem after initial recovery from
a SAH. Antifibrinolytic agents have been used now for over 10 years in an
effort to reduce the rate of rebleeding from ruptured aneurysms. There has
been a multitude of studies designed to prove or disprove their effectiveness
in this setting. The results of the studies have been mixed with some showing significant benefit and others showing no benefit at all. We feel that the
studies showing a benefit have in general been slightly better designed and
have had a greater statistical power than the other studies and, on this basis,
we continue to use epsilon-aminocaproic acid routinely in patients with
SAH due to a ruptured aneurysm (5).

Vasospasm is currently the most important cause of morbidity and mortality in the patient who has recovered from an initial SAH. About 20–30%
of patients with SAH will develop delayed ischemic neurologic symptoms
that cannot be attributed to hydrocephalus or rebleeding. The deterioration
usually occurs between the fourth and the twelfth days after the initial
hemorrhage. These patients invariably show angiographic evidence of
severe narrowing of the intracranial vessels supplying the areas of the brain
responsible for the symptoms. The syndrome may resolve gradually over a
period of a few days or it may progress relentlessly to coma and death within
a period of hours or days. A number of therapies such as vasodilators, alpha
and beta blockers, calcium antagonists, and prostaglandin inhibitors have
been tried, but none has yet been conclusively found to be beneficial. Augmentation of cerebral perfusion pressure by expansion of intravascular
volume, vasopressors, cardiac stimulants, and reduction of intracranial
pressure, seems to be the only effective measure widely used in the treatment
of vasospasm today (6).

Although few advances have been made in the treatment of vasospasm,
some progress is evident in our understanding of its etiology and our ability
to predict which patients will become symptomatic from it. It seems clear
that the blood clot around the vessels in the base of the brain is responsible
for vasospasm and, with an early CT scan, this blood clot can be identified
and quantified with accuracy. In those patients predicted to be at high risk
of developing vasospasm by the early CT scan (patients with thick localized

blood clots in the basal cisterns), our practice is to maintain an expanded intravascular volume with regular infusions of colloid in an effort to keep the cerebral perfusion pressure elevated. We also use systemic reserpine in low doses and oral kanamycin in an effort to reduce the concentration of catecholamines and serotonin in platelets, since there has been some experimental evidence to the effect that such substances may play a role in vasospasm. This form of prophylactic therapy was of benefit in a double-blind control study carried out in our institution.

SURGICAL THERAPY   One of the most important aspects of the surgical therapy of aneurysms is the timing of surgery. During the early years of direct intracranial surgery for aneurysms, surgeons learned that early surgery (within the first week) carried a very high morbidity and mortality. During this time, the brain is usually swollen and retraction is difficult and vasospasm, if present, may be exacerbated. For this reason, most surgeons learned to defer surgery for at least 8–10 days after SAH. Lately, however, there has been a shift in some centers, particularly in Japan, toward early surgery (within 72 hours after SAH) (8). It has been argued that, even though early surgery carries a higher morbidity, the prevention of vasospasm by washing out the subarachnoid clots and of rebleeding by clipping the aneurysm, more than compensate so that the overall case management morbidity and mortality are decreased. There is still insufficient data to evaluate the results of modern early surgery. At present, we continue to defer surgery for 10–12 days in all patients except those who present after a relatively minor hemorrhage and are alert, without neurologic deficit, and without severe meningeal irritation. However, we await with interest the results of a large international cooperative study on the timing of aneurysm surgery currently being conducted (1).

With new advances such as the operating microscope, safer anesthetic techniques, and, particularly, better selection of patients for surgery, the results of modern intracranial aneurysm surgery have improved significantly. From a mortality of approximately 30–35% about 15 years ago, some neurosurgeons are now reporting combined morbidity and mortality rates of under 10%. Aneurysms that were previously inoperable such as most basilar aneurysms and many giant aneurysms, can now be approached with considerable safety by experienced surgeons (1, 7).

Literature Cited

1. Drake, C. G. 1981. Management of cerebral aneurysm. *Stroke* 12:273–83
2. Waga, S., Ohtsubo, K., Handa, H. 1975. Warning signs in intracranial aneurysms. *Surg. Neurol.* 3:15–20
3. Alvord, E. C. Jr., Thorn, R. B. 1977. Natural history of subarachnoid hemorrhage: early prognosis. *Clin. Neurosurg.* 24:167–75
4. Wilkins, R. H. 1981. Update—subarachnoid hemorrhage and saccular intracranial aneurysms. *Surg. Neurol.* 15:92–101
5. Ramirez-Lassepas, M. 1981. Antifibrinolytic therapy in subarachnoid hemorrhage caused by ruptured intracranial aneurysms. *Neurology (Minneapolis)* 31:316–22
6. Heros, R. C., Zervas, N. T., Negoro, M. 1976. Cerebral vasospasm. *Surg. Neurol.* 5:354–62
7. Sundt, T. M. Jr., Kobayashi, S., Fode, N. C., Whisnant, J. P. 1982. Results and complications of surgical management of 809 intracranial aneurysms in 722 cases. *J. Neurosurg.* 56:753–65
8. Mizukami, M., Kawase, T., Usami, T., Tazawa, T. 1982. Prevention of vasospasm by early operation with removal of subarachnoid blood. *Neurosurgery* 10:301–7
9. Stein, B. M., Wolpert, S. M. 1977. Surgical and embolic treatment of cerebral arteriovenous malformations. *Surg. Neurol.* 7:359–69
10. Wilson, C. B., U, H. S., Dominque, J. 1979. Microsurgical treatment of intracranial vascular malformations. *J. Neurosurg.* 51:446–54

Ann. Rev. Med. 1983. 34:377–90

RIGHT VENTRICULAR INFARCTION[1]

Robert Roberts, M.D., and Alon T. Marmor, M.D.

Cardiovascular Division, Baylor College of Medicine, Houston, Texas 77030

ABSTRACT

Right ventricular (RV) infarction, once considered rare, is now recognized as common in patients with inferior infarction. It usually involves the posterior wall of the right ventricle and seldom the anterior right ventricle. There is concomitant transmural injury to the posterior wall of the left ventricle and interventricular septum. Severe RV dysfunction may be associated with cardiogenic shock, and conventional treatment may be deleterious. Avoidance of diuretics and administration of fluids is associated with a much better prognosis. Hemodynamic monitoring is necessary and the diagnosis should be confirmed by radionuclide assessment. Exclusion of tamponade and constrictive pericarditis by echocardiography is often essential.

Introduction

Right ventricular infarction, until recently, received very little attention clinically and was observed infrequently at necropsy. In post-mortem studies from 1932 through 1970 (1–5), with the exception of the study by Bean (6), the observed incidence varied from 5 to 18% in patients dying from myocardial infarction. With the increased emphasis on ischemic heart disease and more detailed post-mortem examinations, a much higher incidence has been observed in the past decade. Harnarayan et al (7) in 1970 observed RV involvement in 85% of patients dying from cardiogenic shock. In 1974, Erhardt (8) reported that RV infarction was observed at necropsy in 43% of patients with inferior infarction. In a series by Isner & Roberts (9) in 1978, 50% of patients with posteroseptal infarction had RV involvement.

[1]Supported in part by National Institues of Health SCOR in Ischemic Heart Disease grant number HL 17646.

377

Similar findings were observed by Ratliff & Hackel (10) in 1980. Clinical recognition of RV infarction remains difficult, but with the advent of the Swan-Ganz catheter and radionuclide techniques, right ventricular infarction is now recognized to be a common occurrence in the setting of inferior infarction.

Pathology

From the outset it should be stated that infarction localized on the ECG as inferior, namely, exhibiting changes in leads II, III, and AVF, is referred to as posterior by the pathologist. Infarction high in the posterior wall, referred to clinically as true posterior, is also referred to as posterior by the pathologist. RV infarction, as a result of coronary artery disease is seldom observed except in association with concomitant left ventricular infarction (8–10). It is almost always transmural involving the posterior wall of the right ventricle with varying degrees of extension to the lateral and anterior free walls. Concomitant damage involves the posterior wall of the left ventricle (inferior infarction) and almost always transmural involvement of the posterior interventricular septum (9). RV involvement is usually contiguous with LV damage. However, whether or not the right ventricle is involved does not depend on the extent of damage in the left ventricle (10). RV infarction is seldom observed with anterior infarction. Infrequent detection of RV subendocardial infarction at necropsy may represent simply the selection of patients with more severe disease.

Severe coronary stenosis from atherosclerosis is observed consistently in the proximal right coronary artery and there is usually disease of the left anterior descending and circumflex arteries. In one study, the incidence of recent coronary thrombi was 80% in patients with RV involvement as opposed to only 30% in patients without RV involvement (10). Whether or not this represents a general phenomenon remains to be determined.

Pathogenesis

To understand the development of ischemia or infarction in the right ventricle, it is helpful to discuss briefly the coronary vascular anatomy, which is reviewed by Farrer-Brown (11), Erhardt (8), Rotman et al (12), and Wade (13). In the majority of human hearts (90%), the right coronary artery is the dominant vessel, giving rise to the posterior descending branch (PDB). The free wall of the right ventricle is supplied by the right coronary artery (RCA) except for the anterior margin, which is supplied by branches from the left anterior descending coronary artery (LAD). The lateral margin of the right ventricle is supplied by the marginal branch of the RCA. In addition, the anterior portion of the free wall of the right ventricle is also supplied by the LAD and the conus branch, which in most hearts arises from the aorta and in the remainder is a proximal branch of the RCA.

The PDB of the RCA supplies the posterior walls of the left and right ventricles. The anterior two thirds of the interventricular septum derives its blood supply primarily from the LAD with some potential collateral supply from the RCA. The posterior one third is from the LAD and the PDB of the RCA. The apical portion is supplied solely from the LAD. In about 10% of human hearts the PDB arises from the circumflex, but the right ventricle is still predominately supplied by the RCA. The distribution of the intramural arteries of the right ventricle are the same as the left ventricle, namely, long penetrating vessels to the endocardium and short branching vessels to the epi- and mid-myocardium. The right atrium is supplied solely from the right coronary artery and the AV node by the RCA in 90% of the cases. The anterior papillary muscle of the tricuspid valve is supplied by both the right and left coronary vessels, whereas the posterior is supplied solely by the RCA.

Since coronary atherosclerosis occurs predominately in the proximal portions of the extramural vessels, the distribution of the damage in the right ventricle observed at necropsy is somewhat expected. As stated previously, right ventricular infarction occurs as a result of right coronary artery obstruction and always occurs in association with concomitant left ventricular damage. Infarction involves the posterior wall (inferior) of the left ventricle together with posterior involvement of the right ventricle and seldom involves the anterior free wall of the right ventricle. The available blood supply to the anterior RV free wall from the right coronary artery, the LAD, and the conus branch may in part explain the sparing of this portion of the right ventricle. Posterior interventricular septal involvement is almost always seen with RV infarction. It is reasonable to assume that, because of the rich collateral blood supply that may be available to the right ventricle from the left coronary artery, the extent of RV involvement will depend somewhat on the degree of obstruction in the left coronary tree as well as that present in the RCA. It is also not surprising that we have observed some anterior involvement of the right ventricle in patients with anteroseptal infarction (14).

The observation at necropsy that RV infarction is almost always transmural (9), although subendocardial has also been observed (8), may in part be related to the very thin wall of the right ventricle (13). Of course, the other possibility is that subendocardial involvement represents a less severe form, which would preclude a high incidence at necropsy. Pericarditis tends to be very common with RV infarction, in keeping with transmural involvement (13). It has been stated that right atrial infarction is common, but there is very little substantial data (13). It is also stated that the posterior papillary muscle of the tricuspid valve is commonly involved.

Prior to the recent interest in RV infarction, several reasons were proposed (8, 13), which have since been discarded, to account for its supposedly low incidence. Despite the presently observed increased incidence of RV infarction, it appears less common than the LV infarction; yet severity and frequency of atheroma in the right and left coronaries is the same. Involvement of the posterior wall appears to be almost as frequent as that of the left ventricle, but involvement of the anterior wall is clearly much less frequent. The lower intracavitary pressure of the right ventricle and the much lower work load probably do to some extent protect the right ventricle, but the rich collateral blood supply from the LAD and conus arteries probably plays a dominant role in protecting the anterior right ventricular wall. Infarction of the right ventricle appears to result from right coronary artery obstruction, which leads to decreased perfusion to the posterior wall of the right ventricle and septum via the PDB. Clinical evidence suggests that RV involvement is the rule rather than the exception in patients with electrocardiographic evidence of inferior infarction (15). Infarction of the anterior wall of the right ventricle is very uncommon; however, if both the RCA and the LAD are severely obstructed, infarction may occur (8).

Hemodynamics

In the past, RV dysfunction did not receive specific attention in the management of myocardial infarction since it was argued that the right ventricle was a volume conduit, and thus, even if severely injured would not markedly impair cardiac function. This notion was reinforced by results from studies by Starr et al (16), Bakos (17), and Kagan (18), who observed that damaging the right ventricle of the dog by cauterization did not significantly increase systemic venous pressure. These results were further emphasized by Rodbard & Wagner (19) showing that pulmonary blood flow could be maintained even with exclusion of the right ventricle.

However, in a more recent experimental study by Guiha et al (20), cauterization of the right ventricle resulted in only a slight increase in right ventricular end-diastolic pressure but dysfunction was present as manifested by the reduced pressure gradient between the left and right atria. With progressive volume loading, a paradoxical right-to-left ventricular pressure gradient developed. Thus, it was concluded that cauterization of the free wall of the right ventricle produced RV dysfunction, but was not catastrophic as long as intravascular volume was adequately maintained. These studies involved isolated damage to the free wall of the right ventricle without concomitant left ventricular damage. In the clinical situation of inferior infarction, there is concomitant posterior right and left ventricular damage with septal involvement, which may explain the more severe dysfunction observed in man.

Since the hemodynamic description of RV infarction by Cohn et al (21), it has been recognized that severe RV dysfunction can occur in patients with inferior infarction. Several studies emphasize the hemodynamic manifestations of RV dysfunction in patients with inferior infarction (22–25). RV failure occurring secondary to LV failure, as with anterior infarction, is usually associated with a ratio of left-to-right ventricular end-diastolic pressure of about 3 to 1. When RV dysfunction occurs as a result of RV infarction despite concomitant LV impairment, this ratio is reduced (15, 24, 25). In cases of predominant RV dysfunction, there is equalization of right and left atrial pressures, with elevated systemic venous pressure. The contour of the right atrial pressure tracing consists of a steep y-descent, its depth exceeding that of the x-descent, and a diastolic dip-plateau pattern referred to as the square-root sign in keeping with reduced right ventricular compliance. This diastolic dip-plateau pattern is also observed in the RV pressure tracing. As observed by Guiha et al (20) in the dog, this pattern becomes more apparent with volume loading (see Figure 1).

The diagnosis of RV dysfunction due to RV infarction, based on hemodynamics, still overlaps considerably that of impairment secondary to left ventricular failure. In an attempt to provide a specific and sensitive hemodynamic criterion of primary RV dysfunction, Lopez-Sendon et al (26) analyzed the hemodynamic findings on 22 patients with RV infarction. Equalization of right and left atrial pressures, while very specific for RV dysfunction, had a sensitivity of only 45%. Similarly the noncompliant pattern of a y-descent greater than the x-descent, with a diastolic dip-plateau contour, was highly specific but had a sensitivity of only 54%. In an attempt to develop an all-embracing criterion for primary RV dysfunction, the authors propose the following: a right atrial pressure of 10 mm Hg that is either greater than, equal to, or 1–5 mm lower than the pulmonary occlusive pressure. The authors found this criterion to have a sensitivity of 73% and a specificity of 100%. The difficulty of identifying primary RV dysfunction is inherent in the fact that there is always concomitant LV impairment, which may cause secondary RV failure. In the authors' experience, this proposed hemodynamic criterion is quite useful and provides a practical guideline in identifying and treating concomitant left and right ventricular dysfunction. It should be emphasized that this criterion will be more evident with volume loading but may be significantly modified if the patient is being treated with diuretics or inotropic agents. The hemodynamic pattern observed in RV dysfunction, particularly when a noncompli-

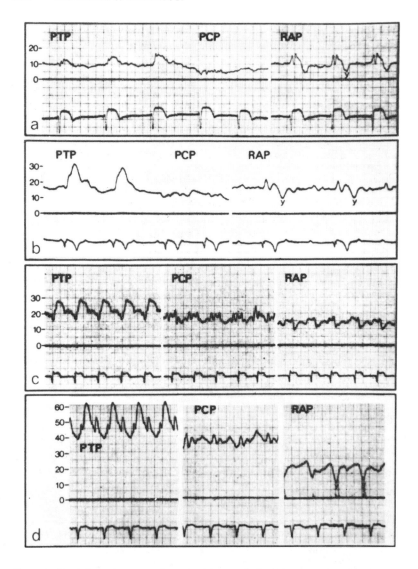

Figure 1 Hemodynamic patterns in acute right ventricular infarction. *(a)* Pulmonary trunk pressure (PTP) is reduced, right atrial pressure (RAP) is higher than pulmonary capillary pressure (PCP), and a severe noncompliant pattern is present, as indicated by the square-root sign. *(b)* The PTP difference is normal and RAP exceeds PCP. In this patient, a severe noncompliant pattern is also present. *(c)* PTP difference is normal, and RAP is slightly lower than PCP. In this patient, the noncompliant pattern is absent. *(d)* PCP is higher than RAP and a severe noncompliant pattern is the only finding to suspect right ventricular infarction. Reproduced with permission from *Circulation* (see Ref. 26, p. 522).

ant pressure pulse contour is present, must be differentiated from constrictive pericarditis, cardiac tamponade, pulmonary emboli, and restrictive cardiomyopathies.

Clinical Features

The diagnosis of right ventricular infarction is very difficult from clinical examination alone. The diagnosis of RV infarction associated with coronary artery disease should be suspected in any patient presenting with electrocardiographic evidence of inferior or posterior infarction. The clinical features, in patients with severe predominant RV dysfunction, are striking. The patient presents with inferior infarction having Q-waves or ST-segment elevations in leads II, III, and AVF, with elevated jugular venous pressure, prominent a-wave, steep y-descent, Kussmaul's sign, hypotension, absence of pulmonary edema, and on occasions a paradoxical pulse (27, 28). Predominant RV dysfunction, however, is uncommon and probably occurs in less than 5% of the cases of RV infarction. In the authors' experience lack of decrease in the level of jugular venous pressure on inspiration is very common and occurs in the majority of patients with inferior infarction, which presumably reflects decreased compliance of the right atrium and ventricle. A prominent a-wave is often present even when the jugular venous pressure is not elevated, particularly if the patient is hypovolemic as is common with inferior infarction. A steep y-descent may be observed without elevated jugular venous pressure. RV dyskinesis may be palpated over the precordium. The presence of right-sided S3 or S4 sounds may help, but it is often difficult to determine if they come from the right or left ventricle. Occasionally, right-sided papillary muscle dysfunction may give rise to a systolic murmur that varies with respiration in keeping with tricuspid regurgitation. Frequently, the signs of RV dysfunction may not be evident until the patient undergoes volume loading. Nevertheless, even when the signs are florid, diagnosing RV infarction solely on clinical grounds must be done with caution.

Diagnosis

One must consider the clinical features, electrocardiographic manifestations, and hemodynamic manifestations in conjunction with radionuclide assessment. The ECG usually shows evidence of inferior or true posterior infarction. Erhardt et al (29), using a right-sided chest lead in the midclavicular line of the fifth intercostal space, detected ST-segment elevation in 25% of survivors and 50% of the 18 patients who died with RV infarction. Post-mortem correlation studies showed that 25% or more involvement of the right ventricle was necessary to produce ST segment elevation.

Others propose the use of an intraventricular unipolar electrogram (30) or body surface isopotential maps (31).

Wackers et al (32), using both thallium-201 and ^{99m}Tc-PYP myocardial scans, showed right ventricular infarction in 37% of patients with inferior infarction despite very little evidence of RV dysfunction, indicating the diagnostic insensitivity of hemodynamic criteria. RV infarction may be diagnosed with the use of pyrophosphate or thallium-201 imaging alone, but this lacks the necessary sensitivity and specificity. Recently, the use of radionuclide ventriculograms to assess regional wall motion abnormalities has become the more conventional technique for diagnosing RV infarction. Rigo et al (33) and Sharpe et al (34) used gated blood pool images to detect right ventricular infarction in 43 and 40%, respectively, of patients with inferior infarction. A later study by Reduto et al (35), using the first-pass methods, observed an incidence of 50%. In 42 consecutive patients with acute infarction, blood pool images were obtained 48 hours after onset of infarction and repeated again around 10 days. We showed a persistent regional defect in the right ventricle of essentially all patients with inferior infarction (36) (Figure 2). At present we recommend the routine use of gated blood pool imaging with ^{99m}Tc-labelled red blood cells to diagnose RV infarction and to assess RV dysfunction when suspected. Echocardiography may show a dilated or enlarged right ventricle, but it is very important to exclude tamponade if suspected. It should also be stated that a steep y-descent, seen frequently in RV infarction, is seldom seen in cardiac tamponade.

Constrictive pericarditis, however, may be confused with the noncompliant hemodynamic pattern of right ventricular infarction and should be assessed further by both hemodynamic and radionuclide studies. If pulmonary emboli are suspected, then a lung scan is indicated. Restrictive cardiomyopathy can usually be excluded on the basis of enzymatic evidence of myocardial infarction.

Management and Treatment

Important in the management of patients with infarction is to have a high index of suspicion for right ventricular dysfunction, particularly in patients with inferior infarction. When suspected, a catheter should be placed to monitor hemodynamics and cardiac output, but, if facilities do not permit, a fluid challenge with careful monitoring of vital signs is warranted. An important part of therapy is to avoid diuretics and administer fluids to maintain adequate right and left ventricular filling pressures. However, there is a tendency to push fluids until the pulmonary artery occlusive pressure has increased to 15–20 mmHg. If this rule is followed, all too frequently this results in excessive fluid administration and pulmonary

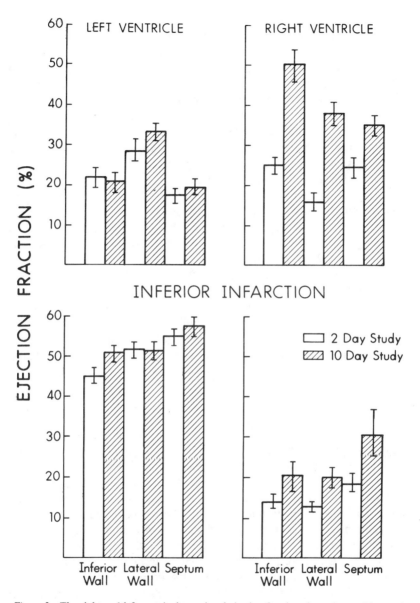

Figure 2   The right and left ventricular regional ejection fractions in patients with anterior and inferior myocardial infarction showing the changes between the initial study, done within 48 hours after admission *(open bars)*, and the second study, done at day 10 *(hatched bars)*. The height of each bar represents the mean and the vertical bar the standard error of the mean. Persistent regional inferior dysfunction was observed in the right ventricle in patients with inferior infarction. Reproduced with permission from *Circulation* (see Ref. 15).

edema ensues. The endpoint to be followed in assessing fluid requirements should be cardiac output; if adequate output can be achieved with a low wedge pressure, it is all the better and no attempt should be made to further increase the filling pressure. If cardiac output cannot be maintained with fluids, inotropic agents and peripheral vasodilators must be considered. Nitrates should be avoided because of venodilatation, which may attenuate venous return and further compromise cardiac output. Low-dose nitroprusside may decrease impedance to the left ventricle and increase cardiac output, but, if venodilatation occurs, cardiac output may decrease. It may be better to use a vasodilator that is predominantly active on the arterioles such as hydralazine. We have had good results with dobutamine, which provides good inotropic support with arterial vasodilatation (37). Dobutamine is recommended over dopamine because of the alpha vasoconstricting effect of the latter. Secondly, if dobutamine is administered such that the heart rate does not increase by more than 10%, it does not enhance myocardial ischemia (38). It may be advantageous to administer dobutamine in combination with a vasodilator; others have used balloon counterpulsation (39). Conventional therapy such as oxygen and anti-arrhythmic drugs must be maintained as in patients with acute infarction. Morphine administration to relieve pain should be monitored carefully because of venodilatation. The results of fluid administration with an inotropic agent have been encouraging in patients with cardiogenic shock and predominant RV dysfunction (21, 27, 37).

Prognosis

There are too few studies available to assess prognosis in patients with predominant right ventricular dysfunction. Preliminary studies suggest that with appropriate therapy the acute prognosis is much better than in patients with predominant left ventricular failure. In one series (23) an acute mortality of only 40% was reported for cardiogenic shock occurring in association with predominant RV dysfunction. It has been recognized for some time that acute mortality is much lower in patients with inferior, as opposed to anterior, infarction. We reported on the acute and long-term prognosis in 249 patients with transmural myocardial infarction, of which 130 were inferior (36). The acute mortality was 12% in patients with inferior and 23% in patients with anterior infarction (Figure 3). This difference was maintained in the subsequent three to four years, as shown in Figure 4. Contrary to our expectation, infarct size estimated enzymatically was similar in the two groups. The possibility that more CK is released into the plasma per gram of necrosis from the right than from the left ventricle was excluded on the basis of subsequent studies performed in the dog (40).

We postulated at that time, because of a decreased ratio of left-to-right ventricular pressure (36), that RV infarction was much more common than previously appreciated in patients with inferior infarction, which has since been confirmed (15). We also postulated that the lower mortality associated with inferior infarction was due to a sharing by both ventricles of the total myocardial damage, resulting in a lessening of the hemodynamic impact to any one ventricle. It may be more explicitly stated as follows: suppose the total infarct size is 30 grams, which in anterior infarction is essentially all in the LV, but with inferior infarction 20 g may be in the LV and 10 g in the right; one may thus expect the hemodynamic impact to be less. There are perhaps other reasons why patients with inferior infarction do better, and more studies are required to further elucidate the less harmful effects of inferior, relative to that of anterior, infarction.

ACKNOWLEDGMENTS

The authors wish to thank Jean Epstein and Sheryl Butler for preparation of the manuscript.

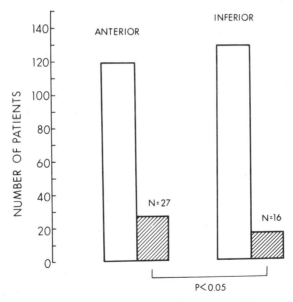

Figure 3 The mortality in patients with anterior infarction was 23% versus only 12% in patients with inferior infarction, which was statistically significant at the 0.05 level. Reproduced with permission from *Circulation* (see Ref. 41).

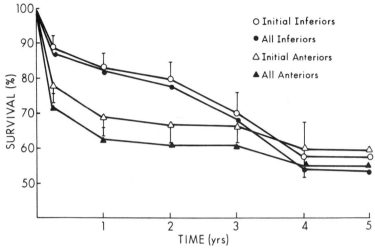

Figure 4 Shown here is the difference in the long-term prognosis between anterior and inferior infarction. The actuarial survival curves are indicated for patients with *(solid circles and triangles)* and without *(open circles and triangles)* previous infarction. As is illustrated, survival is much better in patients with inferior as opposed to anterior infarction, with or without previous infarction. At the end of three years, survival is similar in part because of the small number of patients and possibly recurrent infarction. Reproduced with permission from *Circulation* (see Ref. 41).

Literature Cited

1. Lisa, J. R., Ring, A. 1932. Myocardial infarction or gross fibrosis. *Arch. Intern. Med.* 50:131
2. Appelbaum, E., Nicholson, G. H. B. 1934–35. Occlusive diseases of the coronary arteries. *Am. Heart J.* 10:662
3. Feil, H., Cushing, E. H., Hardesty, J. T. 1938. Accuracy in diagnosis and localization of myocardial infarction. *Am. Heart J.* 15:721
4. Wartman, W. B., Hellerstein, H. K. 1948. The incidence of heart disease in 2000 consecutive autopsies. *Ann Intern. Med.* 28:41
5. Wood, P. 1956. *Diseases of the Heart and Circulation.* London: Eyre & Spottiswoode. 2nd ed.
6. Bean, W. 1938–39. Infarction of the heart III. Clinical course and morphological findings. *Ann. Intern. Med.* 12:71
7. Harnarayan, C., Bennett, M. A., Pentecost, B. L., Brewer, D. B. 1970. Quantitative study of infarcted myocardium in cardiogenic shock. *Br. Heart J.* 32:728

8. Erhardt, L. R. 1974. Right ventricular involvement in acute myocardial infarction. *Eur. J. Cardiol.* 1:441
9. Isner, J. M., Roberts, W. C. 1978. Right ventricular infarction secondary to coronary heart disease. *Am. J. Cardiol.* 42:885
10. Ratliff, N. B., Hackel, D. B. 1980. Combined right and left ventricular infarction: pathogenesis and clinicopathologic correlations. *Am. J. Cardiol.* 45:217
11. Farrer-Brown, G. 1968. Vascular pattern of myocardium of right ventricle of human heart. *Br. Heart J.* 30:679
12. Rotman, M., Ratliff, N. B., Hawley, J. 1974. Right ventricular infarction: a haemodynamic diagnosis. *Br. Heart J.* 36:941
13. Wade, W. G. 1959. The pathogenesis of infarction of the right ventricle. *Br. Heart J.* 21:545
14. Mukharji, J., Rudge, R. E., Poole, K., Croft, C., Thomas, L. J., Strauss, H. W., Roberts, R., Raabe, D. S., Braunwald, E., Willerson, J. T. 1982. Late sudden death following acute myocardial in-

farction: importance of combined presence of repetitive ventricular ectopy and left ventricular dysfunction. *Clin. Res.* 30:208

15. Marmor, A., Geltman, E. M., Biello, D. R., Sobel, B. E., Siegel, B. A., Roberts, R. 1981. Functional response of the right ventricle to myocardial infarction: dependence on the site of left ventricular infarction. *Circulation* 64:1005

16. Starr, I., Jeffers, W. A., Meade, R. H. 1943. The absence of conspicuous increments of venous pressure after severe damage to the right ventricle in the dog with a discussion of the relation between clinical congestive failure and heart disease. *Am. Heart J.* 26:291

17. Bakos, A. C. 1950. The question of the function of the right ventricular myocardium: an experimental study. *Circulation* 1:724

18. Kagan, A. 1952. Dynamic responses of the right ventricle following extensive damage by cauterization. *Circulation* 5:816

19. Rodbard, S., Wagner, D. 1949. By-passing the right ventricle. *Proc. Soc. Exp. Biol. Med.* 71:69

20. Guiha, N. H., Limas, C., Cohn, J. N. 1974. Predominant right ventricular dysfunction after right ventricular destruction in the dog. *Am. J. Cardiol.* 33:254

21. Cohn, J. N., Guiha, N. H., Broder, M., Limas, C. 1974. Right ventricular infarction. *Am. J. Cardiol.* 33:209

22. Cohn, J. N. 1979. Right ventricular infarction revisited. *Am. J. Cardiol.* 43:666

23. Coma-Canella, I., Lopez-Sendon, J., Garmalo, C. 1979. Low output syndrome in right ventricular infarction. *Am. Heart J.* 98:613

24. Coma-Canella, I., Lopez-Sendon, J. 1980. Ventricular compliance in ischemic right ventricular dysfunction. *Am. J. Cardiol.* 45:555

25. Jensen, D. P., Goolsby, J. P., Oliva, P. B. 1978. Hemodynamic pattern resembling pericardial constriction after acute inferior myocardial infarction with right ventricular infarction. *Am. J. Cardiol.* 42:858

26. Lopez-Sendon, J., Coma-Canella, I., Gamallo, C. 1981. Sensitivity and specificity of hemodynamic criteria in the diagnosis of acute right ventricular infarction. *Circulation* 64:515

27. Raabe, D. S., Chester, A. C. 1978. Right ventricular infarction. *Chest* 73:96

28. Lorell, B., Leinbach, R. C., Pohost, G. M., Gold, H. K., Dinsmore, R. E., Hutter, A. M., Pastore, J. O., DeSanctis, R. W. 1979. Right ventricular infarction. Clinical diagnosis and differentiation from cardiac tamponade and pericardial constriction. *Am. J. Cardiol.* 43:456

29. Erhardt, L. R., Sjogren, A., Wahlberg, I. 1976. Single right-sided precordial lead in the diagnosis of right ventricular engagement in inferior myocardial infarction. *Acta Med. Scand. Suppl.* 560

30. Varriale, P., Niznik, J. 1978. Unipolar ventricular electrogram in the diagnosis of right ventricular ischemic injury. *Pace* 1:335

31. Sugiyama, S., Wada, M., Sugenoya, J., Toyoshima, H., Toyama, J., Yamada, K. 1977. Diagnosis of right ventricular infarction: experimental study through the use of body surface isopotential maps. *Am. Heart J.* 94(4):445

32. Wackers, F. J. T., Lie, K. I., Sokole, E. B., Res, J., Van der Schoot, I. B., Durrer, D. 1978. Prevalence of right ventricular involvement in inferior wall infarction assessed with thallium 201 and technetium-99m pyrophosphate. *Am. J. Cardiol.* 42:358

33. Rigo, P., Murray, M. Taylor, D. R., Weisfeldt, M. L., Kelly, D. T., Strauss, H. W., Pitt, B. 1975. Right ventricular dysfunction detected by gated scintiphotography in patients with acute inferior myocardial infarction. *Circulation* 52:268

34. Sharpe, D. N., Botvinick, E., Shames, D. M., Schiller, N. B., Massie, B. M., Chatterjee, K., Parmley, W. W. 1978. The noninvasive diagnosis of right ventricular infarction. *Circulation* 57:483

35. Reduto, L. A., Berger, H. J., Cohen, L. S., Gottschalk, A., Zaret, B. L. 1978. Sequential radionuclide assessment of left and right ventricular performance after acute transmural myocardial infarction. *Ann. Intern. Med.* 89:441

36. Marmor, A., Geltman, E., Biello, D. R., Sobel, B. E., Siegel, B. A., Roberts, R. 1981. Functional response of the right ventricle to myocardial infarction: dependence on the site of left ventricular infarction. *Circulation* 64(5):1005

37. Clark, G., Strauss, H. D., Roberts, R. 1980. Dobutamine versus furosemide in the treatment of cardiac failure due to right ventricular infarction. *Chest* 77:220

38. Gillespie, T. A., Ambos, H. D., Sobel, B. E., Roberts, R. 1977. Effects of dobutamine in patients with acute myo-

cardial infarction. *Am. J. Cardiol.* 39:588

39. Haffajee, C. I., Ockene, I. S., Dalen, J. E. 1978. Cardiogenic shock due to right ventricular infarction. *Chest* 74(5):601

40. Ishikawa, Y., Marmor, A., Sobel, B. E., Roberts, R. 1982. Release of creatine kinase from right compared to the left ventricle: implications regarding flow-dependence of release and estimates of infarct size. *Clin Res.* 30:194A

41. Strauss, H. D., Sobel, B. E., Roberts, R. 1980. The influence of occult right ventricular infarction on enzymatically estimated infarct size, hemodynamics, and prognosis. *Circulation* 62:503–8

Ann. Rev. Med. 1983. 34:391–412
Copyright © 1983 by Annual Reviews Inc. All rights reserved

EXERCISE AND CORONARY HEART DISEASE

Nancy A. Rigotti, M.D., Gregory S. Thomas, M.D., M.P.H., and Alexander Leaf, M.D.

Massachusetts General Hospital, Boston, Massachusetts 02114; and Harvard Medical School, Boston, Massachusetts 02115

ABSTRACT

The epidemiologic evidence examining the effect of physical activity on the development and course of coronary heart disease is reviewed. This evidence indicates that physically active individuals have a lower incidence of myocardial infarction and mortality from coronary disease. While there is no documentation that an exercise program following myocardial infarction will significantly increase patient survival, exercise does increase functional capacity, lessen angina pectoris, and improve self-image in patients with coronary heart disease. Possible mechanisms for the beneficial effects of exercise are considered.

INTRODUCTION

By any measurement made, be it population surveys or sales of running shoes, it is clear that interest in physical activity has risen dramatically over the past three decades. This has been accompanied by a popular belief that physical fitness will increase longevity and, in particular, protect against coronary heart disease (CHD), the leading cause of death in the US (1). In this review, we examine the evidence relating regular exercise to the prevention of coronary heart disease.

Repetitive endurance aerobic exercise, such as walking, jogging, swimming, rowing, or bicycling, is the type of activity believed to have a beneficial cardiovascular effect. Isometric, muscle-building exercises do not confer such benefits. When aerobic exercise is carried out at sufficient intensity, frequency, and duration, predictable cardiovascular, metabolic,

391

and muscular changes occur that allow an individual to perform more work within the aerobic range. Collectively these changes are referred to as the "training effect." This effect is achieved by aerobic exercise of at least 20 minutes three times weekly, sustained at an intensity sufficient to keep an individual's pulse at 70% of maximal heart rate (estimated by subtracting the individual's age from 220).

Whether or not these effects of exercise are associated with the prevention of coronary heart disease is the question we review. We examine the evidence for a beneficial effect of aerobic exercise on the risk of developing coronary heart disease and on survival following myocardial infarction. We conclude by considering the physiologic effects of exercise and how they might mediate a protective effect on coronary heart disease.

PRIMARY PREVENTION OF CORONARY HEART DISEASE

The evidence that physical activity can prevent the development of CHD comes from epidemiologic studies of large populations, in whom the incidence or prevalence of CHD is correlated with activity level. Over the past thirty years, an extensive epidemiological literature has accumulated; it has been reviewed in detail in a series of articles by Froelicher (2–6) and others (7–12). The results of these studies are mixed. Direct comparisons between studies are difficult because of wide variability in study design, outcome measures, and methods of assessing physical activity. Methodologic problems make both positive and negative findings difficult to interpret.

Most of the early evidence, reported from 1950 to 1970, came from two types of studies. Retrospective case control studies compared the activity of patients with CHD to that of healthy controls, while cross-sectional studies compared the prevalence of CHD in active and sedentary members of a population. The results of such studies are subject to distortion by many potential biases. Data from prospective cohort studies, in which active and sedentary groups are observed over time for the development of CHD, are less subject to bias. By their design, such studies provide a higher quality of evidence for determining whether or not a causal relationship exists between exercise and the prevention of CHD. The bulk of such studies have been published since 1970. The strongest evidence for a causal relationship between inactivity and CHD would be derived from an experimental trial in which healthy sedentary individuals, randomly allocated to exercise and control groups, would be observed for the development of CHD. No such definitive study has been successfully completed. Therefore, this review focuses on the results of prospective cohort studies, giving the most weight to those of soundest methodology.

Regardless of design, all studies must contend with the problem that physical activity is more difficult to quantify in large populations than blood pressure or serum cholesterol. Most early studies considered only activity at work and inferred activity levels from job title. Energy expenditure was assumed to be comparable among all workers in the same job classification. This assumption was rarely tested by direct observation and was found to be incorrect in the one case in which it was examined (13). In many cases the activity gradient between the most and least active job classifications was so narrow that the range of activity levels within a job classification might approach the range between job classifications. Recognition of this problem led to other methods of activity assessment, most commonly an interview or questionnaire concerning an individual's current or previous level of physical activity. Few studies attempted to validate the instruments used, and at least one found reproducibility to be poor (14). The imprecision of many questionnaires allows only very gross distinctions to be made in the activity levels of populations. Studies of job activity also ignored the contribution of leisure time activity, which became more significant as work became more sedentary.

This imprecision in the measurement of activity and the small gradient of activity in a sedentary population minimize the chance of detecting any true relationship between exercise and CHD. This may account for negative findings in some studies. Bias in the other direction, toward overstating such a relationship, derives from confounding variables and self-selection, problems inherent in nonrandomized studies.

An observed association of inactivity and CHD will be overstated if other factors independently predisposing to a higher risk of CHD occur more commonly in the inactive group. Known CHD risk factors such as hypertension, hypercholesterolemia, obesity, and smoking frequently cluster in sedentary groups and may serve to confound results. However, such factors may not act as confounders because they do not increase the risk of CHD independent of activity: exercise alters weight, blood pressure, and serum lipids, and may alter smoking habits. Without a randomized study it is impossible to determine whether a clustering of risk factors in the sedentary group is independent of, or the result of, exercise. Another problem, self-selection, refers to an individual's choice of sedentary work or recreational activity based on factors also predisposing to higher CHD risk. Individuals who are less healthy may choose less physically demanding jobs, while those who develop initial symptoms while holding jobs requiring substantial physical activity may transfer to more sedentary work before the diagnosis of CHD is made. Both the initial self-selection of jobs and the so-called "premorbid job transfer" to sedentary work result in a bias toward finding a higher prevalence of CHD in sedentary occupational groups. Selection bias is a particular problem in studies where physical activity is assessed only from the last job held.

Retrospective Studies

The observations that stimulated further examination of a possible link between physical activity and CHD were reported by Morris and colleagues (15) in 1953. Studying records of London bus drivers and conductors, they found that conductors had 70% of the age-adjusted incidence of CHD and only half the rate of myocardial infarction (MI) and CHD mortality of drivers (15). Although no attempt was made to directly measure physical activity, it was assumed that the conductors, who collected tickets on double-decker buses, were more active than drivers. This presumed difference in activity was proposed as a possible explanation for the difference in disease rates. Morris et al found a similar result in a study of British postal workers: the presumably more active postmen had lower CHD rates than did sedentary clerks and supervisors (15).

These initial studies did not address the problems of confounding or self-selection. Conductors were subsequently found to have smaller girths (16), lower blood pressures, and lower serum cholesterol levels (17) than drivers, which suggests that the unequal distribution of these established risk factors, rather than activity, might account for differences in CHD incidence. Since young recruits for the two jobs differed in weight and skinfold thickness even before employment (18), it appeared that the smaller girth of conductors was a consequence of self-selection rather than job activity. Morris subsequently corrected for the difference in girth and still observed a lower CHD mortality among conductors (19).

Morris' work attracted wide attention to the role of exercise, and many studies examining CHD rates in diverse populations followed. In the years before 1970, most focused on activity at work and used retrospective, case control study design. Although most confirmed Morris' work, results were mixed and methodological problems common.

Among studies of occupational activity assessed by job title, higher activity levels at work correlated with lower CHD risk in retrospective studies of US postal workers (20) and railmen (21), North Dakota farmers and nonfarmers (14), and English and Israeli workers (22–24), but not in South African railmen (25). Prevalence studies in Evans County, Georgia (26), and a Chicago gas company (27) also reported an inverse relationship between work activity and CHD. Finnish lumberjacks had fewer ST abnormalities on ECG compared to their presumably more sedentary neighbors (28) on cross-sectional study. Two small case control studies, from Canada (29) and Sweden (30), reported no difference in prior activity between MI survivors and healthy controls, but a larger study of men insured by a New

York insurance plan reported higher morbidity and early mortality from MI among those reporting lower habitual activity on and off the job (31, 32). While some of these studies attempted to control for the bias of job transfer (20, 23) and other risk factors, problems of self-selection cannot be excluded in case control studies.

Prospective Studies

Prospective studies in 17 population groups have been reported since 1964, the bulk since 1970. Recent studies have been more careful to measure risk factors, minimize self-selection, and assess activity levels more precisely. Most documented a link between activity and the incidence of CHD.

Whether the possible beneficial effects of exercise are due solely to a reduction in known cardiovascular risk factors, e.g. the effects on plasma cholesterol levels, or whether lack of exercise is itself an independent risk factor is not known. From a clinical standpoint such a distinction is academic and not relevant.

The first prospective studies considered only occupational activity measured by job title. In a five-year follow-up of the London busmen reported previously, Morris found that drivers had 1.8 times the CHD incidence of conductors (17). However, as stated above, drivers had higher blood pressures and serum cholesterol levels and this might have explained the observed difference in disease incidence. Whether this difference resulted from self-selection or was the consequence of differences in physical activity is uncertain. Similar results were reported for a large cohort of Italian railroad workers followed for five years (33). Four prospective studies of occupational activity defined by job title—Los Angeles civil servants (34), US railmen (13), and Chicago gas (27) and electrical (35) company workers—found no protection in more active groups. Initial prevalence studies in two of these populations (21, 27) had demonstrated a relationship between work activity and CHD that was not confirmed by prospective observation. Low gradients of occupational activity and failure to consider leisure activity have been invoked as explanations for these negative results (9).

The inverse relationship between activity measured by job title and CHD, observed in the prevalence study of Evans County, Georgia (26), was partly confirmed in a seven-year follow-up. An occupational gradient in CHD incidence was observed among farmers and between farmers and nonfarmers, but not between active and sedentary nonfarming groups (36). The authors suggest that this reflects a need for a high threshold of work activity for CHD protection.

Strong evidence for a protective role of job-related physical activity comes from a 22-year prospective study of over 3000 San Francisco longshoremen followed by Paffenbarger and colleagues (37–41). They reported a significantly lower risk of fatal MI and sudden death in those men whose work activity required a heavy energy expenditure, estimated at over 8500 kcal per week (38). This difference persisted after correction for seven CHD risk factors by multiple logistic analysis, which indicates that the protective effect of activity was independent of such factors (41). Precision in classification of work activity was enhanced by direct measurement of oxygen consumption of workers in various job classes and by annual reclassification of workers transferring to new jobs.

Selection bias was minimized in two ways. Union rules requiring that all entering longshoremen do heavy work for at least five years suggested that all had good cardiovascular health at entry. Nevertheless, it is possible that those who subsequently changed to less active work were the relatively weaker of this group. Second, in an attempt to minimize the effect of transfers to less active work because of illness, men were classified according to the job held six months before death.

Thus, union rules and the investigators' sophisticated methodology and analysis allowed for minimization of potential sources of bias. The high work activity of the group minimized the potentially contaminating effect of unmeasured leisure time activity. The wide activity gradient between least and most active groups maximized the opportunity to detect differences. The positive findings of this study provide very strong evidence for a causal role for exercise in protection from CHD.

As work activity has become more sedentary, exercise during leisure time has become a larger fraction of total physical activity. Investigators have used questionnaires or interviews to include recreational exercise in overall activity assessment.

Morris and colleagues (42) investigated the leisure time activity of a group of middle-aged British civil servants whose sedentary office jobs were considered to contribute little to overall activity. A questionnaire distributed on a random Monday requested detailed accounts of activity on the previous Friday and Saturday. Defining vigorous exercise as that requiring an estimated peak output of 7.5 kcal per minute for a total of one hour over the two-day sampling period, they found that the relative risk of developing CHD for men reporting vigorous activity was decreased by one third over the subsequent two to four years (42) and by one half over eight years of follow-up (43). No correlation was observed with low intensity exercise or with any estimate of total activity time. The finding appeared to be independent of smoking, weight, and family history of CHD. Vigorous exercise also correlated with fewer ST abnormalities and fewer ectopic beats on a resting ECG done two years after the initial activity assessment (44).

Among prospective studies assessing both occupational and leisure activity, data from Framingham (45), Finland (46), Norway (47), Harvard alumni (48), and the American Cancer Society (49) support a protective role for exercise. Studies in Sweden (50) and Puerto Rico (51) also report a protective effect of exercise but one that is not independent of other risk factors. No protective effect was seen in the Seven Countries Study (52).

Paffenbarger and co-workers followed a large cohort of Harvard University alumni who entered college between 1916 and 1950 (48). College records were searched to assess student activity levels, while adult exercise habits were surveyed in 1962 by a questionnaire inquiring about stairs climbed, blocks walked, and sports played daily. From this, an index of weekly energy expenditure was devised. Over the subsequent ten years the incidence of MI among alumni with a weekly energy expenditure of over 2000 kcal was half that of their more sedentary classmates. The protective effect was independent of smoking, hypertension, obesity, diabetes, or family history of CHD. Paffenbarger eliminated much of the potential self-selection bias of nonrandomized studies by comparing ex-varsity athletes with their less athletic classmates. He reasoned that if a lower CHD risk was due to superior endowment rather than to exercise, then varsity athletes, with a presumably superior genetic endowment, should be protected regardless of adult activity habits. In fact, athletes were at a low risk for CHD only if they had continued vigorous activity into adulthood. Furthermore, a low risk of MI was associated with a physically active adulthood regardless of student activity level, which implied that recent exercise was the predictive variable.

In the Framingham study, a questionnaire assessing overall activity found the population to be highly sedentary (45, 53). Despite the small gradient of activity, CHD mortality and total CHD incidence after 14 years were inversely related to a physical activity index in men (45). Though independent of age, blood pressure, smoking and cholesterol, the effect of activity was weaker than these other risk factors, perhaps because even the maximal level of exercise attained in the population was so small. Among women, exercise was not an independent predictor of CHD mortality, perhaps because the activity gradient, already small among the men, was even less in women. In a recently reported study from Eastern Finland, low activity as assessed by job classification was associated over a seven-year follow-up period with a 1.5-fold risk of MI in men and 2.4-fold risk in women, even after standard CHD risk factors were taken into account (46). Again exercise was a weaker predictor of MI than hypertension, smoking, or serum cholesterol. Leisure time activity alone did not correlate with CHD mortality, but the effects of inactivity at work and leisure were additive in increasing the risk of MI.

Beneficial effects of exercise have been observed in other prospective studies. A study of over one million Americans, sponsored by the American Cancer Society, documented a higher CHD morality over six years in those individuals reporting their activity level as low (49). A similar six-year study in Norway showed a positive correlation of inactivity and CHD mortality (47), but did not control for risk factors. Physical activity was included in an investigation of CHD risk factors in men born in 1913 and living in Göteborg, Sweden, in 1963 (50). Over the subsequent eight years CHD risk correlated with activity at leisure but not at work, consistent with the higher fitness levels found in those active in leisure time compared to those active at work. On multivariate analysis exercise was not found to be an independent risk factor. A 2.5-year follow-up of a Puerto Rican population reported that the slight increase in CHD found in urban males who were sedentary was not independent of the effect of serum cholesterol (51). On the other hand, one large study of populations in seven countries found no relationship between the five-year incidence of CHD and habitual physical activity (52).

Daily caloric intake per kilogram body weight has been used as an indirect index of physical activity under the assumption that individuals consuming more calories per kilogram have a higher energy expenditure because of greater activity. Increased caloric intake per kilogram body weight has been inversely related to the incidence of CHD in populations in Honolulu, Puerto Rico, and Framingham (54), and in England (55).

The evidence cited so far, derived from nonintervention studies, supports the hypothesis that physical inactivity is a risk factor for the development of CHD. There is, however, no direct evidence available to determine whether the adoption of exercise habits by individuals without coronary disease will alter the incidence of the disease. Such data must be obtained from a randomized intervention trial, requiring the random assignment of a large number of individuals to exercise and control groups and the maintenance of long-term adherence to regular exercise habits. An adequate test would require a large-scale, long-term effort. Two published intervention studies were not able to test the hypothesis because long-term compliance with an exercise program could not be obtained. In a study by Ilmarinen & Fardy (56) of Finnish men with CHD risk factors, exercise and control groups differed neither in exercise habits nor the incidence of MI or angina three years after an 18-month training program, despite an initial improvement in fitness by the exercise group. A pilot study in the US suffered such a high initial dropout rate that a national trial of exercise for primary prevention was deemed not feasible (57). Problems of cost and compliance make the successful accomplishment of a large-scale intervention trial unlikely.

Amount and Type of Exercise for Coronary Protection

The amount and intensity of exercise required for CHD protection is uncertain, although it appears that achievement of a training effect is a necessary minimum. It is not clear whether progressive increases in activity correlate with increased coronary protection or whether a threshold is reached, beyond which increasing activity yields little additional protection. It appears from the Harvard alumni study (48) that for the same level of physical activity, the more intense the exercise the greater the benefit, but the differences are not large or definite. The work of Morris and colleagues is consistent with this idea; vigorous exercise correlated with lower CHD incidence, while less vigorous activity did not (42).

EFFECT ON SURVIVAL
AFTER MYOCARDIAL INFARCTION

Survival

Epidemiologic studies examining the effect of exercise training on recurrent myocardial infarction and death in persons who have survived a first heart attack are inconclusive. Randomized clinical trials have been beset with problems. Many subjects randomized to the exercising group dropped out of their prescribed program while many control subjects began exercising on their own—the so-called cross-over problem. Investigators have also had difficulty attracting as many subjects as they had initially planned. These problems, combined with the overall decrease in CHD mortality occurring in the United States and elsewhere, have left investigators with numbers large enough to show some improvement in mortality in the exercising group but not large enough to be statistically significant. Four randomized clinical trials have been undertaken.

Wilhelmsen and his colleagues in Sweden undertook the first large-scale clinical trial on this subject when they randomized 315 patients with myocardial infarction into exercise training and control groups (58). Of those who were randomized into the exercising group and began training, 40% had dropped out by the end of their first year. During the first four years after myocardial infarction, 28 patients died in the experimental group and 35 died in the control group. This difference was not statistically significant.

The National Exercise and Heart Disease Project in the United States yielded another nonsignificant benefit in survival for the exercising group (59). Among 651 subjects randomized after MI into supervised exercise and control groups, 4.6% of the exercising group died over the three-year follow-up period compared to 7.3% of the controls. Cross-over between groups was a problem; 23% of the exercise group was not exercising either in or out of the program at the end of two years, while 31% of the controls had adopted exercise habits. Sample size was also a problem. The investigators originally estimated that 4200 participants would be desirable, but the actual number of subjects enrolled was only 651. Combining this with the decreasing CHD mortality rate, statistical significance could only have been obtained if the effect of exercise on mortality was substantially greater than the 39% decrease they found.

The on-going Ontario Exercise-Heart Collaborative Study has had problems similar to those discussed above. No benefit from exercise has been observed during the first 20 months of the 48-month trial (60–62).

A controlled, though not randomized, clinical trial of post-MI patients in Finland found coronary mortality to be 10% in the exercising group and 14.5% in the control group in follow-up periods of 31.5 and 26.5 months respectively (63). With 380 subjects, this difference did not prove to be significant.

Kallio and his co-workers (64) reported results from the World Health Organization trial in 1979. They did find a significant benefit in the exercising group. Cumulative overall mortality over three years was 21.8% in the exercise group compared to 29.9% in the control group. However, exercise was only one of the interventions in the multifactorial risk factor reduction program for the experimental group; diet alteration and psychosocial counseling were chief components as well. Furthermore, a higher percentage of the exercising group was receiving beta-adrenergic antagonist medication by the end of the study (45% vs 27%). The experimental group had received their medical care from the program staff, while the control group had utilized their own physicians during the three-year period.

In addition to these intervention trials, data are available from a prospective observational study of Harvard alumni, in which Paffenbarger and his colleagues followed 782 men with a history of MI or angina pectoris over 12 to 16 years (48, 65). Those alumni who expended fewer than 2000 kcal weekly on leisure time exercise were at 42% greater risk of subsequent fatal heart attack than those men who expended more than 2000 kcal on these activities. This difference was not statistically significant. It is also possible that those men with less extensive CHD may have been overrepresented in the more active group and thus be expected to be at lower risk for fatal heart attack.

Physical activity was also among the factors assessed in the Coronary Drug Project in which the effect of clofibrate and niacin were examined in the post-MI population (66). Those individuals whose activity was characterized as moderate or vigorous on entry had a five-year total mortality of 14.4% compared to 23.8% in those individuals whose physical activity was rated as light. This difference, subjected to chi-square analysis, is significant.

However, as in the Harvard alumni population, persons with more extensive CHD may have been overrepresented in the less physically active group.

In sum, epidemiologic studies have not provided a definitive answer to the question of whether exercise training favorably affects survival after myocardial infarction. Trends in the available data do seem to indicate that a beneficial effect is present, but it has not been demonstrated in a conclusive fashion.

Cardiac Rehabilitation

While the effect of exercise training on mortality after MI can be debated, the beneficial effects of exercise in the rehabilitation of cardiac patients is clear. A wide range of studies found exercise training to increase substantially the ability of these patients to tolerate physical activity. The best measure of this ability is an individual's oxygen consumption at peak exercise ($\dot{V}_{O_2}$max). This may be directly measured via gas analysis or calculated from an individual's performance on a maximal exercise test (67).

Exercise training appears to increase functional capacity primarily by inducing changes not in the heart itself but in the periphery, specifically altering the peripheral vascular system and oxygen transport at the muscular level. These peripheral changes allow the heart to do less work at any given workload. The workload on the heart is best determined by myocardial oxygen consumption, which can be estimated by measuring the product of the heart rate and blood pressure (68). This rate-pressure product (RPP) at any given workload decreases after training in patients with CHD (69–73). A similar effect is found in healthy individuals after training. One of the chief peripheral effects of training is the enhanced oxygen uptake of the periphery. This was demonstrated by the increased arterio-mixed venous oxygen concentration difference (A-V$_{O_2}$) seen in most of the studies that examined this (74–77); one study, however, failed to show such an effect (78).

Investigations of the specific cardiac effects of training after MI or in patients with angina pectoris yield conflicting results. While a single study found exercise training to increase the RPP at peak exercise (79), others have not (73, 80–83). Training does, however, seem to increase stroke volume at rest (78) and with exercise, either submaximal (74) or maximal (84). One might expect radionuclide studies of left ventricular ejection fraction to clarify the effect of training on contraction of nonischemic and ischemic myocardium, but early studies have again produced mixed results. While some investigators found an increase in ejection fraction at rest (85, 86) most did not (71, 73, 87, 88). Jensen and his associates found an increase in ejection fraction measured at submaximal exercise but found no change in ejection fraction at rest (89). Among four studies of ejection fraction at maximal exercise, two found an increase (73, 90) and two did not (86, 89). Patterson and his colleagues (74) point out that changes in resting and exercise ventricular preload and afterload induced by exercise may confound the ability of measurements of ejection fraction to assess myocardial pump function accurately.

The effect of training on perfusion to areas of ischemic myocardium is also controversial. Using ^{201}Th imaging pre- and post-training to assess changes in perfusion, Froelicher and his associates found improved perfusion at the same heart workload as measured by RPP (85), Verani and co-workers found no effect (86), and Charuzi and colleagues found improvement in some patients and worsening in others (80).

Exercise has a therapeutic role for reduction of symptoms in patients with angina pectoris. The peripheral effects of training allow the patient with angina to perform more exercise prior to reaching the threshold, measured by the RPP, at which angina develops. Whether training increased the actual RPP at which angina develops is controversial. Measuring ischemia by the development of anginal pain or ST depression, Kellerman et al (70), Nolewajka et al (87), and Detry & Bruce (91) found no increase in the RPP threshold for angina after training, while Eshani et al (79), Redwood et al (92), and Sim & Neill (93) did find such an increase. In two similar studies, Kattus et al (94) and Cooksey et al (95) found an increase in exercise performed prior to the onset of angina but neither specifically compared the RPP at which angina developed pre- and post- exercise training.

Two studies examined the effect of training on atherosclerosis directly via coronary artery catheterization before and after exercise training. Neither Nolewajka et al (87) nor Lee et al (88) found an improvement in atherosclerosis after exercise programs of 7 and 18 months, respectively.

Preliminary data does indicate that regular exercise by post-MI patients is of some benefit on psychological parameters. In the National Exercise and Heart Disease Project, all 651 patients underwent a six-week low-level training program prior to randomization into long-term training and control groups. Patients reported a decrease in depression with a concomitant increase in anxiety after the training period, as assessed by the Katz Adjustment Scale (96). In the same study, however, wives of the patients reported husbands to be less depressed and less anxious. In a study of 44 post-MI patients with initially high depression scores on the Minnesota Multiphasic Personality Inventory (MMPI), Kavanagh and his colleagues found a decrease in scores after a 16- to 18-month training program (97). Naughton and associates also found a decrease in MMPI depression scores after training, but among their 14 subjects the difference was not significant (98). This improvement in mood may be related to exercise-induced changes in endogenous opioid peptides, such as the rise in plasma levels of beta-endorphin reported by Carr and colleagues (99).

The effect of exercise training on the rehabilitation of patients following coronary artery bypass graft (CABG) surgery has just begun to be evaluated. Of three studies reported, all found an increase in functional capacity as measured by $\dot{V}_{O_2}$max estimates (100–102). Comparing CABG patients to post-MI patients, Hartung & Rangel (100) found little difference between the two groups in the functional improvements that occurred with training.

CARDIOVASCULAR RESPONSE TO EXERCISE

Possible Mechanisms of Protection

Are there known metabolic and hemodynamic effects of regular aerobic exercise that might lead one to anticipate a reduction in CHD risk? There are two means by which exercise might reduce risk. Exercise could decrease atherogenesis or it could act to minimize the clinical ischemic sequelae resulting from atherosclerotic vessels. A true distinction between the two possibilities requires anatomic rather than epidemiologic evidence. Autopsy studies could provide such evidence in humans, but, to date, methodologic problems preclude firm conclusions (103, 104).

Animal studies provide another source of anatomic evidence. A recent definitive study in primates by Kramsch and colleagues (105) demonstrated that regular aerobic training could retard atherogenesis as well as minimize the tissue effects of what atherosclerosis occurred, even in the presence of an atherogenic diet and high serum cholesterol levels in both trained and untrained monkeys. Exercised monkeys had larger coronary arteries, less extensive atherosclerosis, and fewer signs of ischemia than unexercised monkeys. In this study exercise training began well before introduction of the atherogenic diet. Whether exercise begun along with, or after, an atherogenic diet would have a similar protective effect was not examined.

Other animal studies, reviewed elsewhere (5, 106), demonstrated an increase in coronary artery diameter, collateral circulation, and capillary-to-muscle-fiber ratio, all of which may increase myocardial perfusion. Whether such effects occur in humans and whether improved perfusion can develop in the presence of fixed arterial lesions is not known.

Clinical evidence in man indicates that exercise may also minimize the consequences of atheromata by decreasing thrombotic and arrhythmic events and allowing the myocardium to tolerate ischemia better. The increased fibrinolysis in response to an occlusive stimulus reported in trained individuals (107) may decrease thrombotic consequences leading to MI. The decrease in sympathetic tone occurring with training (95) may play a role in reducing serious arrhythmias. This protection may be mediated by a decrease in the number of beta-adrenergic receptors observed after training (108).

While the effect of exercise on improving perfusion is sketchy, evidence supporting a decreased myocardial oxygen demand in trained individuals is strong. Training results in a lower oxygen consumption required for any submaximal workload, reflected in a lower blood pressure, heart rate, and their product, the RPP. The result is a better functional tolerance of narrowed coronary arteries.

Effect of Exercise on Coronary Risk Factors

There is considerable evidence that exercise favorably alters risk factors in individuals without clinically evident CHD. Prevalence studies have often observed lower blood pressure (109–112), weight (109, 110, 113), serum cholesterol (109, 110, 114), and triglycerides (110, 111, 114, 115) and less smoking (109, 111, 113) among the more active or more fit individuals. Such an association might be the result of exercise, but could also be found if individuals with low risk factor levels chose to be more active. A randomized assignment of healthy but sedentary individuals to a control or exercise program would be the ideal means of avoiding selection bias.

The effect of an exercise program on participants' total serum cholesterol is controversial. Studies reporting a fall in cholesterol (116–118) may be confounded by accompanying weight loss. Other studies report no change (56, 57, 119–123). More consistent changes have been observed for the proportion of cholesterol carried by high density lipoprotein (HDL), which epidemiological evidence suggests may be a more powerful predictor of CHD than total cholesterol (124). Levels of HDL-cholesterol are consistently higher in athletes or active individuals than in sedentary persons (111, 113–115); in one study they correlated with weekly running mileage (125). Exercise training uniformly increases levels of HDL-cholesterol in men, usually accompanied by a fall in LDL-cholesterol (116–118, 121–123). Women may respond differently; three studies reported no significant change in HDL- or LDL-cholesterol following exercise training (116, 123, 126). Triglyceride levels fall almost uniformly with regular exercise (116, 117, 119–123, 127).

The evidence about the effect of exercise training on resting blood pressure is not conclusive (128, 129). Small but significant decreases in systolic and diastolic blood pressure were reported in some uncontrolled prospective studies (130, 131). Controlled studies are few and sample sizes small. One study observed a fall in blood pressure with exercise, but only the decrease in systolic blood pressure was significantly different from controls (120). Two others reported no change from controls (56, 57). Studies generally report a greater effect in hypertensive than normotensive individuals (120, 130, 131). Even small decreases in blood pressure may be sufficient to have a prophylactic value, as suggested by recent observations of decreased mortality in mild borderline hypertensives who experienced only a small reduction in blood pressure with treatment (132).

It has been suggested that adopting regular exercise habits may induce individuals to improve other health habits, such as diet and cigarette smoking. Cross-sectional studies consistently report a lower smoking rate and a higher prevalence of former smokers in more active individuals compared with inactive controls (109, 111, 113). However, prospective studies in healthy people are few and have not documented any significant decline in smoking among individuals adopting exercise habits (56, 57, 108, 116, 120).

Exercise in diabetic patients improves glucose tolerance and reduces insulin requirement, probably by increasing insulin binding in peripheral muscle (133, 134).

Effect on Risk Factors in Patients with Coronary Heart Disease

The effect of exercise training on risk factors for coronary artery disease among patients who already have CHD has, with one significant exception, not been substantial. That exception, the increase in HDL-cholesterol seen with training, was demonstrated in two studies. Erkelens and fellow workers (135) found a significant increase in HDL-cholesterol, from 35.2 to 40.0 mg/dl, among 18 CAD patients in the first week of training with little change from that result over the full six-month training period. Confounding factors, including total cholesterol, triglycerides, body weight, triceps skinfold measurement and alcohol consumption, did not change over the same period. Among another 18 patients studied by Hartung and his colleagues, a significant increase in HDL-cholesterol, from 40.9 to 47.1 mg/dl, was observed over a three-month training period without a change in total cholesterol (136). The subjects did experience, however, a significant decrease in weight (1.2 kg) and body fat.

Of five studies (135, 137–140) examining the effect of training on total cholesterol, only one (137) found a significant decrease after training. Among four studies (100, 139–141) examining systolic and one (141) examining diastolic blood pressure of CAD patients, none found a change with training. Training reduced obesity in patients with CHD in four studies (100, 136, 141, 142) but not in another (135).

While the presumed mental and physical transformation into athleticism seen during exercise training in CHD patients might be expected to improve health habits such as cigarette smoking, little work has been done in this area. In a study of over 500 patients who entered the Toronto Rehabilitation Centre program, Kavanagh & Shephard (139) found only a slight drop in the prevalence of smoking after training, although many continuing smokers claimed substantial reductions in the number of cigarettes smoked. Palatsi (63) found no difference in smoking habits between the exercise and control groups in his study of 380 patients.

SUMMARY AND CONCLUSIONS

Numerous epidemiologic studies, retrospective and prospective, have examined the relationship of physical activity of populations on the job and/or at leisure to the incidence, prevalence, or mortality from coronary heart disease. *The findings support the view that physically active persons suffer a lower incidence of heart attacks and associated mortality;* an inverse relationship holds between CHD and physical activity. The documented physiological effects of exercise and the reduction in some known risk factors associated with habitual repetitive endurance aerobic exercise heightens the expectation of this favorable consensus.

These epidemiologic studies are, however, flawed by many problems including difficulty in quantifying levels of physical activity actually performed, self-selection of sedentary lifestyles by less healthy individuals, changing levels of activity by individuals because of disease, confounding independent variables, difficulty confirming the diagnosis of CHD, the small gradient in physical activity within some populations, and cross-over problems. Unfortunately, the logistical obstacles to an adequate randomized prospective intervention trial in normal subjects make the performance of a definitive study unlikely. Such an adequate trial has been made for only one of the conventional coronary risk factors, hypertension (131); no randomized studies have proven the benefit of a reduction in smoking or hypercholesterolemia on the mortality of coronary disease.

In patients with coronary heart disease the effects of exercise on the progression of atherosclerosis or the incidence of morbidity and mortality from CHD is not known. The intervention trials conducted have been inadequate to test the hypothesis of a beneficial effect. The opportunity seems at hand to utilize new noninvasive technology for determining the structure and function of the cardiovascular system in before-and-after intervention studies to assess the effects of exercise and of reduction in other risk factors on the progression of atherosclerosis. Definitive answers regarding the benefit or lack of benefit of exercise may be forthcoming in a shorter time than with large population epidemiologic studies in which mortality is the end point and in which problems of compliance and cross-over have been uncontrollable.

Despite the uncertainties regarding the effects of exercise on progression of the atherosclerotic process, its benefits as an important component of cardiac rehabilitation in patients with established coronary heart disease are established. It increases aerobic work capacity and raises the threshold for angina. It promotes improved self image, enhances personal independence, and appears to reduce depression.

Although conclusive proof of the preventive role of exercise in coronary heart disease is not available, the evidence is sufficiently strong to support the recommendation of exercise as part of a program to decrease the risk of coronary heart disease and as part of the therapy for patients with coronary artery disease.

Literature Cited

1. *Health: United States 1981.* 1981. US Department of Health and Human Services. Hyattsville, Maryland, pp. 117–19
2. Froelicher, V. F., Oberman, A. 1972. Analysis of epidemiologic studies of physical inactivity as risk factor for coronary artery disease. *Prog. Cardiovasc. Dis.* 15:41–65
3. Froelicher, V. F. 1977. Does exercise conditioning delay progression of myocardial ischemia in coronary atherosclerotic heart disease? In *Cardiovascular Clinics,* ed. E. Corday, A. N. Brest, pp. 11–31. Philadelphia: Davis
4. Froelicher, V. F. 1978. Exercise and the prevention of coronary atherosclerotic heart disease. In *Cardiovascular Clinics,* ed. N. Wenger, A. N. Brest, pp. 13–23. Philadelphia: Davis
5. Froelicher, V., Battler, A., McKirnan, M. D. 1980. Physical activity and coronary heart disease. *Cardiology* 65: 153–90
6. Froelicher, V. F., Brown, P. 1981. Exercise and coronary heart disease. *J. Cardiac Rehabil.* 1:277–88
7. Fox, S. M., Haskell, W. T. 1968. Physical activity and the prevention of coronary heart disease. *Bull. NY Acad. Med.* 44:950–67
8. Fox, S. M., Naughton, J. P., Haskell, W. L. 1971. Physical activity and the prevention of coronary heart disease. *Ann. Clin. Res.* 3:404–32
9. Fox, S. M. 1976. Physical activity and coronary heart disease. In *Controversy in Cardiology,* ed. E. K. Chung, pp. 201–19. New York: Springer-Verlag
10. Leon, A. S., Blackburn, H. 1977. The relationship of physical activity to coronary heart disease and life expectancy. *Ann. NY Acad. Sci.* 301:561–78
11. Wyndham, C. H. 1979. The role of physical activity in the prevention of ischemic heart disease. *S. Afr. Med. J.* 56:7–13
12. Thomas, G. S., Lee, P. R., Franks, P., Paffenbarger, R. S. 1981. *Exercise and Health: The Evidence and the Implica-*

tions, pp. 23–54. Cambridge, Mass: Oelgeschlager, Gunn, & Hain
13. Taylor, H. L., Blackburn, H., Keys, A., Parlin, R. W., Vasquez, C., Puchner, T. 1970. Five-year follow-up of employees of selected U.S. railroad companies. *Circulation* 41(Suppl. I):20–39
14. Zukel, W. J., Lewis, R. H., Enterline, M. A., Painter, R. C., Ralston, L. S., Fawcett, R. M., Meredith, A. P., Peterson, B. 1959. A short-term community study of the epidemiology of coronary heart disease: a preliminary report on the North Dakota study. *Am. J. Public Health* 49:1630–39
15. Morris, J. N., Heady, J. A., Raffle, P. A. B., Roberts C. G., Parks, J. W. 1953. Coronary heart disease and physical activity of work. *Lancet* 2:1053–57, 1111–20
16. Morris, J. N., Heady, J. A., Raffle, P. A. B. 1956. Physique of London busmen: epidemiology of uniforms. *Lancet* 2:569–70
17. Morris, J. N., Kagan, A., Pattison, D. C., Gardner, M. J., Raffle, P. A. B. 1966. Incidence and prediction of ischemic heart disease in London busmen. *Lancet* 2:553–59
18. Oliver, R. M. 1967. Physique and serum lipids of young London busmen in relation to ischemic heart disease. *Br. J. Ind. Med.* 24:181–88
19. Morris, J. N. 1975. *Uses of Epidemiology.* pp. 163–65. New York: Churchill Livingstone. 3rd ed.
20. Kahn, H. A. 1963. The relationship of reported coronary heart disease mortality to physical activity of work. *Am. J. Public Health* 53:1058–67
21. Taylor, H. L., Klepetar, E., Keys, A., Parlin, W., Blackburn, H., Puchner, T. 1962. Death rates among physically active and sedentary employees of the railroad industry. *Am. J. Public Health* 52:1697–1707
22. Brown, R. G., Davidson, L. A. G., McKeown, T., Whitfield, A. G. W. 1957. Coronary artery disease: influences affecting its incidence in males in

the seventh decade. *Lancet* 2:1073–76
23. Brunner, D., Manelis, G. 1960. Myocardial infarction among members of communal settlements in Israel. *Lancet* 2:1049–50
24. Brunner, D., Manelis, G., Modan, M., Levin, S. 1974. Physical activity at work and the incidence of myocardial infarction, angina pectoris and death due to ischemic heart disease: an epidemiological study in Israeli collective settlements (Kibbutzim). *J. Chronic Dis.* 27:217–33
25. Adelstein, A. M. 1963. Some aspects of cardiovascular mortality in South Africa. *Br. J. Prev. Soc. Med.* 17:29–40
26. McDonough, J. R., Hames, C. G., Stulb, S. C., Garrison, G. E. 1965. Coronary heart disease among negroes and whites in Evans Country, Georgia. *J. Chronic Dis.* 18:443–68
27. Stamler, J., Lindberg, H. A., Berkson, M. D., Shaffer, A., Miller, W., Poindexter, A. 1960. Prevalence and incidence of coronary heart disease in strata of the labor force of a Chicago industrial corporation. *J. Chronic Dis.* 11:405–27
28. Karvonen, M. J., Rautaharju, P. M., Orma, E. 1961. Heart disease and employment: cardiovascular studies on lumberjacks. *J. Occup. Med.* 3:49–53
29. Shanoff, H. M., Little, J. A. 1961. Studies of male survivors of myocardial infarction due to "essential" atherosclerosis. I. Characteristics of the patients. *Can. Med. Assoc. J.* 84:519–29
30. Forssman, O., Lindegard, B. 1958. The post-coronary patient. A multidisciplinary investigation of middle-aged Swedish males. *J. Psychosom. Res.* 3: 89–125
31. Frank, C. W., Weinblatt, E., Shapiro, S., Sager, R. V. 1966. Physical inactivity as a lethal factor in myocardial infarction among men. *Circulation* 34: 1022–32
32. Shapiro, S., Weinblatt, E., Frank, C., Sager, R. V. 1969. Incidence of coronary heart disease in a population insured for medical care (HIP). *Am. J. Public Health* 59:1–101
33. Menotti, A., Puddu, V. 1976. Death rates among the Italian railroad employees, with special reference to coronary heart disease and physical activity at work. *Environ. Res.* 11:331–42
34. Chapman, J. M., Massey, F. J. 1964. The interrelationship of serum cholesterol hypertension, body weight, and risk of coronary disease. *J. Chronic Dis.* 17:933–49

35. Paul, O., Lepper, M. H., Phelan, W. H., Dupertain, G. W. 1963. A longitudinal study of coronary heart disease. *Circulation* 28:20–31
36. Cassel, J., Heyden, S., Bartel, A. C., Kaplan, B. H., Tyroler, H. A., Cornoni, J. C., Hames, C. G. 1971. Occupation and physical activity and coronary heart disease. *Arch. Intern. Med.* 128:920–28
37. Paffenbarger, R. S., Laughlin, M. E., Gima, A. S., Black, R. A. 1970. Work activity of longshoremen as related to death from coronary heart disease and stroke. *N. Engl. J. Med.* 282:1110–14
38. Paffenbarger, R. S., Hale, W. E. 1975. Work activity and coronary heart mortality. *N. Engl. J. Med.* 292:545–50
39. Paffenbarger, R. S., Hale, W. E., Brand, R. J., Hyde, R. T. 1977. Work-energy level, personal characteristics, and fatal heart attack: a birth-cohort effect. *Am. J. Epidemiol.* 105:200–13
40. Paffenbarger, R. S., Brand, R. J., Scholtz, R. I., Jung, D. L. 1978. Energy expenditure, cigarette smoking, and blood pressure level as related to death from specific diseases. *Am. J. Epidemiol.* 108:12–18
41. Brand, R. J., Paffenbarger, R. S., Sholtz, R. I., Kampert, J. B. 1979. Work activity and fatal heart attack studied by multiple logistic risk analysis. *Am. J. Epidemiol.* 110:52–62
42. Morris, J. N., Chave, S. P. W., Adam, C., Sirey, C., Epstein, L., Sheehan, D. J. 1973. Vigorous exercise in leisure time and the incidence of coronary heart disease. *Lancet* 1:333–39
43. Morris, J. N., Pollard, R., Everitt, M. G., Chave, S. P. W., Semmence, A. M. 1980. Vigorous exercise in leisure time: protection against coronary heart disease. *Lancet* 2:1207–10
44. Epstein, L., Miller, G. J., Stitt, F. W., Morris, J. N. 1976. Vigorous exercise in leisure time, coronary risk factors, and resting electrocardiogram in middle-aged civil servants. *Br. Heart J.* 38: 403–9
45. Kannel, W. B., Sorlie, P. 1979. Some health benefits of physical activity: the Framingham study. *Arch. Intern. Med.* 139:857–61
46. Salonen, J. T., Puska, P., Tuomilehto, J. 1982. Physical activity and risk of myocardial infarction, cerebral stroke and death. *Am. J. Epidemiol.* 115:526–37
47. Zeiner-Henriksen, T. 1976. Six-year mortality related to cardiorespiratory symptoms and environmental risk fac-

tors in a sample of the Norwegian population. *J. Chronic Dis.* 29:15–33

48. Paffenbarger, R. S., Wing, A. L., Hyde, R. T. 1978. Physical activity as an index of heart attack risk in college alumni. *Am. J. Epidemiol.* 108:161–75

49. Hammond, E. C., Garfinkel, L. 1969. Coronary heart disease, stroke, and aortic aneurysms: factors in the etiology. *Arch. Environ. Health* 19:167–82

50. Wilhelmsen, L., Tibblin, G., Aurell, M., Bjure, J., Ekstrom-Jodal, B., Grimby, G. 1976. Physical activity, physical fitness and risk of myocardial infarction. *Adv. Cardiol.* 18:217–30

51. Costas, R. Jr., Garcia-Palmieri, M. R., Nazario, E., Sorlie, P. D. 1978. Relation of lipids, weight, and physical activity to incidence of coronary heart disease: the Puerto Rico heart study. *Am. J. Cardiol.* 42:653–58

52. Blackburn, H., Taylor, H. L., Keyes, A. 1970. Coronary heart disease in seven countries. *Circulation* 41:154–95

53. Kannel, W. B. 1967. Habitual level of physical activity and risk of coronary heart disease: the Framingham study. *Can. Med. Assoc. J.* 96:811–12

54. Gordon, T., Kagan, A., Garcia-Palmieri, M., Kannel, W. B., Zukel, W. J., Tillotson, J., Sorlie, P., Hjortland, M. 1981. Diet and its relation to coronary heart disease and death in three populations. *Circulation* 63:500–15

55. Morris, J. N., Marr, J. W., Clayton, D. G. 1977. Diet and heart: a postscript. *Br. Med. J.* 2:1307–14

56. Ilmarinen, J., Fardy, P. S. 1977. Physical activity intervention for males with high risk of coronary heart disease: a three-year follow-up. *Prev. Med.* 6: 416–25

57. Taylor, H. L., Buskirk, E. R., Remington, R. D. 1973. Exercise in controlled trials of the prevention of coronary heart disease. *Fed. Proc.* 32:1623–27

58. Wilhelmsen, L., Sanne, H., Elmfeldt, D., Grimby, G., Tibblin, G., Wedel, H. 1975. A controlled trial of physical training after myocardial infarction. *Prev. Med.* 4:491–508

59. Shaw, L. 1981. Effects of a prescribed supervised program on mortality and cardiovascular morbidity in patients after a myocardiol infarction. *Am. J. Cardial.* 48:39–46

60. Shephard, R. J. 1980. Recurrence of myocardial infarction. Observation on patients participating in the Ontario Multicentre Exercise-Heart Trial. *Eur. J. Cardiol.* 11:147–57

61. Rechnitzer, P. A. 1979. The effects of training: reinfarction and death—an interim report. *Med. Sci. Sports* 11:322

62. Rechnitzer, P. A. 1979. Considerations in organizing a multicentre study to examine effects on exercise in mortality and reinfarction in postcoronary patients. *Med. Sci. Sports* 11:364–65

63. Palatsi, I. 1976. Feasibility of physical training after myocardial infarction and its effect on return to work, morbidity and mortality. *Acta Med. Scand. Suppl.* 599:1–84

64. Kallio, V., Hamalainnen, H., Hakkila, J., Luurila, O. 1979. Reduction in sudden deaths by a multifactorial intervention programme after acute myocardial infarction. *Lancet* 1:1091–94

65. Thomas, G. S. 1981. See Ref. 12, pp. 39–40

66. The Coronary Drug Project Research Group. 1975. Clofibrate and niacin in coronary heart disease. *J. Am. Med. Assoc.* 231:360–81

67. Bruce, R. S. 1973. Maximal oxygen intake and normographic assessment of functional aerobic impairment in cardiovascular disease. *Am. Heart J.* 85: 546–62

68. Amsterdam, E. A., Mason, D. T. 1977. Exercise testing and indirect assessment of myocardial oxygen consumption in evaluation of angina pectoris. *Cardiology* 62:174–89

69. Sarre, H. 1973. Exercise tolerance and physical training of non-selected patients after myocardial infarction. *Acta Med. Scand. Suppl.* 551:1–124

70. Kellerman, J. J., Ben-Ari, E., Chayet, M., Lapidot, C., Drory, Y., Fisman, E. 1977. Cardiocirculatory response to different types of training in patients with angina pectoris. *Cardiology* 62: 218–31

71. Letac, B., Cribier, A., Desplanches, J. F. 1977. A study of left ventricular function in coronary patients before and after physical training. *Circulation* 56:375–78

72. Franklin, B. A., Besseghini, I., Golden, L. H. 1978. Low intensity physical conditioning: effects on patients with coronary artery disease. *Arch. Phys. Med. Rehabil.* 59:276–80

73. Ehsani, A. A., Biello, D. R., Bloomfield, S. A., Holloszy, J. O. 1982. Exercise training improves intrinsic left ventricular performance in ischemic heart disease. *Clin. Res.* 30:480A (Abstr.)

74. Patterson, D. N., Shephard, R. J., Cunningham, D., Jones, N. L., Andrew, G. 1979. Effects of physical training on car-

diovascular function following myocardial infarction. *J. Appl. Physiol.* 47: 482–89

75. Ressl, J., Jandova, R., Stolz, I., Widimsky, J. 1977. Effects of physical training on central hemodynamics and working capacity in myocardial infarction. *Cardiology* 62:102 (Abstr.)

76. Detry, J.-M. R., Rousseau, M., Vandenbrouche, G., Kusumi, F., Brasseur, L. A., Bruce, R. A. 1971. Increased arteriovenous oxygen difference after physical training in coronary heart disease. *Circulation* 44:109–18

77. Rousseau, M. F., Brasseur, L. A., Detry, J.-M. R. 1973. Hemodynamic determinants of maximal oxygen intake in patients with healed myocardial infarction: influence of physical training. *Circulation* 48:943–49

78. Bjernulf, A. 1973. Haemodynamic effects of physical training after myocardial infarction. *Acta Med. Scand. Suppl.* 548:1–49

79. Eshani, A. A., Heath, G. W., Hagberg, J. M., Holloszy, J. O. 1979. Influence of exercise training on ischemic ST segment response in patients with coronary artery disease. *Circulation* 59,60(Suppl. II):22 (Abstr.)

80. Charuzi, Y., Vyden, J., Berman, D., Freeman, M., Cloobeck, S., Waxman, A., Mickle, E., Forrester, J. 1979. Myocardial perfusion by thalium-201 scintigraphy before and after cardiac rehabilitation. *Clin. Res.* 27:158A (Abstr.)

81. Gutschker, A., Schaller, K., Geissfer, W. 1977. Results of physical conditioning in patients with acute myocardial infarction over 65 years of age. *Cardiology* 62:135 (Abstr.)

82. Lee, S. J. K., McNulty, M., Hernandez, J. 1977. Effects of exercise training in patients with angina. *Cardiology* 62:84 (Abstr.)

83. Pratt, C. M., Welton, D. E., Squires, W. G. Jr., Kirby, T. E., Hartung, G. U., Miller, R. R. 1981. Demonstration of training effect during chronic beta-adrenergic blockade in patients with coronary artery disease. *Circulation* 64:1125–29

84. Frick, M. H., Katila, M. 1968. Hemodynamic consequences of physical training after myocardial infarction. *Circulation* 37:192–202

85. Froelicher, V., Jensen, D., Atwood, J. E., McKirnan, M. D., Gerger, K., Slutsky, R., Battler, A., Ashburn, W., Ross, J. 1980. Cardiac rehabilitation: evidence for improvement in myocardial perfusion and function. *Arch. Phys. Med. Rehabil.* 61:517–22

86. Verani, M. S., Hartung, G. H., Hoepfel-Harris, J., Welton, D. E., Pratt, C. M., Miller, R. R. 1981. Effects of exercise training on left ventricular performance and myocardial perfusion in patients with coronary artery disease. *Am. J. Cardiol.* 47:797–803

87. Nolewajka, A. J., Kostuck, W. J., Reshnitzer, P. A., Cunningham, D. A. 1979. Exercise and human collateralization: an angiographic and scintigraphic assessment. *Circulation* 60:114–21

88. Lee, A. P., Ice, R., Blessey, R., Sanmarco, M. E. 1979. Long-term effects of physical training on coronary patients with impaired ventricular function. *Circulation* 60:1519–26

89. Jensen, D., Atwood, J. E., Froelicher, V., McKirnan, M. D., Battler, A., Ashburn, W., Ross, J. 1980. Improvement in ventricular function during exercise studied with radionuclide ventriculography after cardiac rehabilitation. *Am. J. Cardiol.* 46:770–77

90. Battler, A., Froelicher, V. F., Mutsky, R., Watanabe, K., McKernan, M. D., Strong, M., Ashburn, L. J. 1982. Does exercise training improve left ventricular function in coronary artery disease patients? *Clin. Res.* 30:158A (Abstr.)

91. Detry, J.-M., Bruce, R. A. 1971. Effects of physical training on exertional ST-segment depression in coronary heart disease. *Circulation* 44:390–96

92. Redwood, D. R., Rosing, D. R., Epstein, S. E. 1972. Circulatory and symptomatic effects of physical training in patients with coronary artery disease and angina pectoris. *N. Engl. J. Med.* 286:959–65

93. Sim, D. N., Neill, W. A. 1974. Investigation of the physiological basis for increased exercise threshold for angina pectoris after physical conditioning. *J. Clin. Invest.* 54:763–70

94. Kattus, A. A., Jorgensen, C. R., Wocken, R. E., Alvaco, A. B. 1972. ST segment depression with near-maximal exercise: its modification by physical conditioning. *Chest* 62:678–83

95. Cooksey, J. D., Reilly, P., Brown, S., Bomze, H., Cryer, P. E. 1978. Exercise training and plasma catecholamines in patients with ischemic heart disease. *Am. J. Cardiol.* 42:372–76

96. Naughton, J. 1978. The National Exercise and Heart Disease Project. The prerandomization exercise program. Report Number 2. *Cardiology* 63:352–67

97. Kavanagh, T., Shephard, R. J., Tuck, J. A., Aureshi, S. 1977. Depression following myocardial infarction: The effects of distance running. *Ann. NY Acad. Sci.* 301:1028–38

98. Naughton, J., Buihn, J. G., Lategola, M. T. 1968. Effects of physical training on psychological and behavioral characteristics of cardiac patients. *Arch. Phys. Med. Rehabil.* 49:131–37

99. Carr, D. B., Bullen, B. A., Skriner, G. S., Arnold, M. A., Rosenblatt, M., Beitins, I. Z., Martin, J. B., McArthur, J. W. 1981. Physical conditioning facilitates the exercise-induced secretion of beta-endorphin and beta-lipotropin in women. *N. Engl. J. Med.* 305:560–63

100. Hartung, G. H., Rangel, R. 1981. Exercise training in post-myocardial infarction patients: comparison of results with high risk coronary and post-bypass patients. *Arch. Phys. Med. Rehabil.* 62:147–50

101. Oldridge, N. B., Nagle, F. J., Balke, B., Corliss, R. J., Kahn, D. R. 1978. Aortocoronary bypass surgery: effects of surgery and 32 months of physical conditioning on treadmill performance. *Arch. Phys. Med. Rehabil.* 59:268–75

102. Soloff, P. H. 1978–1979. Medically and surgically treated coronary patients in cardiovascular rehabilitation: a comparative study. *Int. J. Psychiatry Med.* 19:93–106

103. Morris, J. N., Crawford, M. D. 1958. Coronary heart disease and physical activity of work: evidence of a national necropsy survey. *Br. Med. J.* 2:1485–87

104. Spain, D. M., Bradess, V. A. 1960. Occupational physical activity and the degree of coronary atherosclerosis in "normal" men: a post-mortem study. *Circulation* 22:239–42

105. Kramsch, D. M., Aspen, A. J., Abramowitz, B. M., Kreimendahl, T., Hood, W. B. 1981. Reduction of coronary atherosclerosis by moderate conditioning exercise in monkeys on an atherogenic diet. *N. Engl. J. Med.* 305:1483–89

106. Froelicher, V. F. 1972. Animal studies of effect of chronic exercise on the heart and atherosclerosis: a review. *Am. Heart J.* 84:496–506

107. Williams, R. S., Logue, E. E., Lewis, J. L., Barton, T., Stead, N. W., Wallace, A. G., Pizzo, S. V. 1980. Physical conditioning augments the fibrinolytic response to venous occlusion in healthy adults. *N. Engl. J. Med.* 302:897–991

108. Butler, J., O'Brien, M., O'Malley, K., Kelly, J. G. 1982. Relationship of beta-adrenoreceptor density to fitness in athletes. *Nature* 298:60–62

109. Hickey, N., Mulcahy, R., Bourke, G. J., Graham, J., Wilson-Davis, K. 1975. Study of coronary risk factors related to physical activity in 15,171 men. *Br. Med. J.* 3:507–9

110. Cooper, K. H., Pollock, M. L., Martin, R. P., White, S. R., Linnerud, A. L., Jackson, A. 1976. Physical fitness levels vs selected coronary risk factors. A cross-sectional study. *J. Am. Med. Assoc.* 236:166–69

111. Hartung, G. H., Foreyt, J. P., Mitchell, R. E., Vlasek, I., Gotto, A. M. 1980. Relation of diet to high-density-lipoprotein cholesterol in middle-aged marathon runners, joggers, and inactive men. *N. Engl. J. Med.* 302:357–61

112. Thomas, G. S. 1981. See Ref. 12, pp. 56–57

113. Adner, M. M., Castelli, W. P. 1980. Elevated high-density lipoprotein levels in marathon runners. *J. Am. Med. Assoc.* 243:534–36

114. Wood, P. D., Haskell, W., Klein, H., Lewis, S., Stern, M. P., Farquhar, J. W. 1976. The distribution of plasma lipoproteins in middle-aged male runners. *Metabolism* 25:1249–57

115. Gordon, D. J., Witztum, J., Hunninghake, D., Gates, S., Glueck, C. J. 1982. Habitual physical activity and high density lipoprotein cholesterol in men with primary hypercholesterolemia: the Lipid Research Clinics coronary primary prevention trial. *Clin. Res.* 30:237A (Abstr.)

116. Brownell, K. D., Bachorik, P. S., Ayerle, R. S. 1982. Changes in plasma lipid and lipoprotein levels in men and women after a program of moderate exercise. *Circulation* 65:477–83

117. Lopez, A., Vial, R., Balart, L., Arroyave, G. 1974. Effects of exercise and physical fitness on serum lipids and lipoproteins. *Atherosclerosis* 20:1–9

118. Altekruse, E. G., Wilmore, J. H. 1973. Changes in blood chemistries following a controlled exercise program. *J. Occup. Med.* 15:110–13

119. Lampman, R. M., Santinga, J. T., Bassett, D. R., Mercer, N. M., Block, W. D., Flora, J. D., Foss, M. L., Thorland, W. G. 1977. Effectiveness of unsupervised and supervised high intensity physical training in normalizing serum lipids in men with type IV hyperlipoproteinemia. *Circulation* 57:172–80

120. Bonnano, J. A., Lies, J. E. 1974. Effects of physical training on coronary risk factors. *Am. J. Cardiol.* 33:760–64

121. Huttenen, J. K., Lansimies, E., Vouti-lainen, E., Ehnholm, C., Hietanen, E., Penttila, I., Shtonen, O., Rauramaa, R. 1979. Effect of moderate physical exercise on serum lipoproteins. *Circulation* 60:1220–29

122. Leon, A. S., Conrad, J., Hunninghake, D. B., Serfass, R. 1979. Effects of a vigorous walking program on body composition and carbohydrate and lipid metabolism of obese young men. *Am. J. Clin. Nutr.* 32:1776–82

123. Ballantyne, D., Clark, A., Dyker, G. S., Gillis, C. R., Hawthorne, V. M., Henry, D. A., Hole, D. S., Murdock, R. M., Semple, T., Stewart G. M. 1978. Prescribing exercise for the healthy: assessment of compliance and effects on plasma lipids and lipoproteins. *Health Bull.* 32:169–75

124. Gordon, T., Castelli, W. P., Hjortland, M. C., Kannel, W. B., Dawber, T. R. 1977. High density lipoprotein as a protective factor against coronary heart disease: the Framingham study. *Am. J. Med.* 62:707–14

125. Rotkis, T. C., Cote, R., Coyle, E., Wilmore, J. H. 1982. Relationship between high density lipoprotein cholesterol and weekly running mileage. *J. Cardiac Rehab.* 2:109–12

126. Lewis, S., Haskell, W. L., Wood, P. D., Manoogian, N., Bailey, J. E., Pereira, M. 1976. Effects of physical activity on weight reduction in obese middle-aged women. *Am. J. Clin. Nutr.* 30:716–24

127. Lampman, R. M., Santinga, J. T., Hodge, M. F., Block, W. D., Flora, J. D., Bassett, D. R. 1977. Comparative effects of physical training and diet in normalizing serum lipids in men with type IV hyperlipoproteinemia. *Circulation* 55:652–59

128. Scheuer, J., Tipton, C. M. 1977. Cardiovascular adaptations to physical training. *Ann. Rev. Physiol.* 39:221–51

129. Black, H. R. 1979. Nonpharmacologic therapy for hypertension. *Am. J. Med.* 66:837–42

130. Boyer, J. L., Kasch, F. W. 1970. Exercise therapy in hypertensive men. *J. Am. Med. Assoc.* 211:1668–71

131. Choquette, G., Ferguson, R. J. 1973. Blood pressure reduction in "borderline" hypertensives following physical training. *Can. Med. Assoc. J.* 108:699–703

132. Hypertension Detection and Follow-up Program Cooperative Group. 1979. Five-year findings of the hypertension detection and follow-up program: I. Reduction in mortality of persons with high blood pressure, including mild hypertension. *J. Am. Med. Assoc.* 242:2562–71

133. Vranic, M., Berger, M. 1979. Exercise and diabetes mellitus. *Diabetes* 28:147–67

134. Pederson, O., Beck-Nielsen, H., Heding, L. 1980. Increased insulin receptors after exercise in patients with insulin-dependent diabetes mellitus. *N. Engl. J. Med.* 302:886–92

135. Erkelens, D. W., Albers, J. J., Hazzard, W. R., Frederich, R. C., Bierman, E. L. 1979. High-density lipoprotein-cholesterol in survivors of myocardial infarction. *J. Am. Med. Assoc.* 242:2185–89

136. Hartung, H., Squires, W. G., Gotto, A. M. Jr. 1981. Effect of exercise training on plasma high-density lipoprotein cholesterol in coronary disease patients. *Am. Heart J.* 101:181–84

137. Woodhouse, S. P., Hathirat, S., Jensen, E., Johnson, A. L., Klassen, G. 1976. Effect of physical training on haemodynamic performance following myocardial infarction: a controlled study. *Can. Med. Assoc. J.* 115:238–44

138. Broustet, J. P., Boisseau, M., Bouloumie, J., Emerian, J. P., Series, E., Bricaud, U. 1978. The effects of acute exercise and physical training on platelet function in patients with coronary artery disease. *J. Cardiac Rehabil.* 9:28–31

139. Shephard, R. J. 1979. Cardiac rehabilitation in prospect. In *Heart Disease and Rehabilitation,* ed. M. L. Pollock, D. H. Schmidt. pp. 521–47. New York: Wiley

140. Schlesinger, Z., Barziloy, J. 1980. Prolonged rehabilitation of patients after acute myocardial infarction and its effects on a complex of physiological variables. *Heart Lung* 9:1038–43

141. Franklin, B. A., Besseghini, I., Golden, L. H. 1978. Low intensive physical conditioning: effects on patients with coronary artery disease. *Arch. Phys. Med. Rehabil.* 59:276–80

142. Shephard, R. J. 1980. Post-coronary rehabilitation, body composition and recurrent infarction. An analysis of data from the Ontario Exercise-Heart Collaborative Study. *Nutr. Metab.* 24:383–95

Ann. Rev. Med. 1983. 34:413–27

ANTIBIOTIC TREATMENT OF INFECTIVE ENDOCARDITIS

W. R. Wilson, M.D., and J. E. Geraci, M.D.

Departments of Infectious Disease and Internal Medicine, Mayo Clinic, Rochester, Minnesota 55901

ABSTRACT

At least 85% of patients with infective endocarditis can be cured with effective therapy. Streptococci or staphylococci cause 75% of cases of endocarditis. Patients with penicillin-sensitive viridans or nonenterococcal group D streptococcal endocarditis may be treated successfully with aqueous penicillin G alone for four weeks or with combined penicillin and streptomycin for two weeks. Enterococcal endocarditis should be treated for four to six weeks with a combination of aqueous penicillin G together with either streptomycin or gentamicin. Patients with endocarditis caused by *Staphylococcus aureus* should receive antimicrobial therapy for four to six weeks with a semisynthetic penicillin (nafcillin or oxacillin) or a cephalosporin such as cephalothin or cefazolin. In urgent cases where empiric antimicrobial therapy is necessary before the causative organism is identified, a combination of aqueous penicillin G, nafcillin, and gentamicin is effective therapy.

Introduction

During the preantibiotic era, the mortality of patients with infective endocarditis (IE) was 100%. Currently, at least 85% of patients can be cured. Host defense mechanisms play little role in the control of IE. In no other infectious disease does cure seem to be so dependent upon the administration of appropriate bactericidal antimicrobial agents. Valvular vegetations are composed of dense networks of avascular fibrin-platelet matrices that protect microorganisms buried within from phagocytes and other host defense mechanisms.

413

0066-4219/83/0401-0413$02.00

The role of the microbiology laboratory in the selection of appropriate antimicrobial therapy is probably more important in patients with IE than in patients with any other infection. The use of bactericidal antibiotics and advances in the technology of cardiac valve replacement significantly improved the outcome of patients with IE. Other factors that influence survival are the promptness of diagnosis and treatment, age, underlying condition of the patient, presence of intravascular valves or other prostheses, and the microbiologic etiology.

Microbiologic Spectrum of Infective Endocarditis

Virtually any microorganism is capable of causing IE (1–5). Table 1 lists the microbiologic causes of IE in 393 patients seen at Mayo Clinic during a 10-year period (1970–1979). At least 75% of cases of IE are caused by streptococci or staphylococci (2–4). The frequency of "culture-negative" endocarditis at Mayo Clinic has declined from 8% during the 1950s to 3% during the 1970s (1).

The Microbiology Laboratory in Diagnosis

In patients with suspected IE, the most important laboratory finding is the isolation of bacteria or fungi from at least two or more blood cultures obtained at intervals during a 48-hour period. Because bacteremias associated with IE are usually continuous, the timing of blood cultures is not critical, and if any blood cultures are positive most of the other cultures drawn will also be positive (6–8). In patients who have not received antibiotic treatment during the preceding two weeks, streptococci may be isolated from 96% from the first blood culture and 98% from one of the first two blood cultures (7). In this same study, staphylococci were isolated from the

Table 1   Microbiologic etiology of infective endocarditis at Mayo Clinic from 1970 through 1979

Microorganism		Number of patients		Percentage
Viridans streptococci		149		38
Group D streptococci		79		20
Enterococci	53		13	
Streptococcus bovis	26		7	
Staphylococcus aureus		72		18
Gram-negative bacilli		35		9
Staphylococcus epidermidis		16		4
Other microorganisms		29		7
Negative blood cultures		13		3
TOTAL		393		100

first blood culture in 90% and from one of the first two blood cultures in 100% of patients. In cases of IE caused by microorganisms other than streptococci or staphylococci, the causative agent was isolated from 82% of cases in the first blood culture and from 100% in one of the first two blood cultures (7). Antibiotic treatment given within two weeks before blood cultures were obtained reduced the positive cultures in 178 cases of streptococcal endocarditis from 97 to 91% ($P < 0.02$) (7). Based on the above data, it is rarely necessary to obtain more than three separate sets of blood cultures within a 24-hour period on two consecutive days in patients suspected of having IE.

Blood culture bottles are inoculated so that a $1:10$ ratio of blood to medium is achieved; this usually means an inoculum of 10 ml of blood per culture. Each blood culture set should incubate at least one bottle anaerobically. Blood cultures should be incubated for at least two weeks before being discarded as negative. If fastidious microorganisms are suspected, a longer incubation period may be required. If after 48–72 hours of incubation the initial blood culture remains negative, additional blood cultures should be obtained. These latter blood cultures may be helpful in patients who have received antibiotics. The role of the microbiology laboratory in performing susceptibility tests on the causative agent is discussed below.

Management

Recommending a single regimen for the management of all patients with IE is impossible. Therapy should be individualized for each patient. Several general principles, however, are universally applicable.

ESTABLISH MICROBIOLOGIC DIAGNOSIS   It is critically important to establish the microbiologic diagnosis, if possible, before starting antimicrobial therapy. In the subacute form of IE, most patients have been ill for weeks and in some cases for nine months or longer, and there is usually no great urgency to initiate antimicrobial therapy. Failure to establish the microbiologic cause of IE may result in prolonged hospitalization and increased cost, multiple iatrogenic complications related to the use of inappropriate therapy, progressive cardiac valvular damage with development of heart failure, and possible relapse of infection. In contrast, in patients with acute septic IE the use of antimicrobial agents should not be delayed until the results of blood cultures or other laboratory studies are known. Therapy should be begun promptly after blood has been obtained for the initial set of blood cultures.

USE EMPIRIC REGIMEN IN URGENT CASES   In urgent cases in which empiric antimicrobial therapy is necessary before the causative agent is identified, the regimen should include a combination of antibiotics effective against penicillin-sensitive streptococci, enterococci, and penicillinase-producing staphylococci. An effective regimen for these patients is a combination of aqueous penicillin G, nafcillin, and gentamicin. In patients allergic to penicillin, a combination of vancomycin and gentamicin may be used. In patients with acute prosthetic valve endocarditis, an empiric regimen should include agents effective against *Staphylococcus epidermidis,* Corynebacteria, *Staphylococcus aureus,* and streptococci. A combination of vancomycin, rifampin, and gentamicin is suggested for these patients (9).

USE BACTERICIDAL THERAPY   Once the identification or gram's stain and morphology of the organism isolated from blood cultures are determined, bactericidal antibiotic therapy should be initiated promptly. The potential toxicity of antimicrobials chosen must be considered and the least toxic, most effective regimen should be selected. The results of susceptibility tests may dictate changes in the antimicrobial regimen. The most widely used susceptibility test and the simplest to perform is the minimum inhibitory concentration (MIC)—the lowest concentration of antibiotics that will inhibit the growth of the causative bacteria. The MIC may be determined by disc diffusion (Kirby-Bauer), agar dilution, or broth dilution methods (10). The minimum bactericidal concentration (MBC)—the lowest concentration of antibiotic that will kill $\geq 99.9\%$ of the inoculum—is also helpful in determining optimal therapy (10). The MBC should be determined in most cases of IE to ensure that the antibiotic treatment is bactericidal. The peak serum concentration of the antibiotic administered should exceed the MBC of the bacteria isolated from blood culture.

The serum bactericidal titer (SBT) should be determined on the second day of antimicrobial therapy (10). The SBT measures the killing activity of the antimicrobial therapy in the patient's serum. The results are expressed as the lowest dilution of patient's serum that kills $\geq 99.9\%$ of the inoculum. Serum samples should be obtained at the anticipated peak serum antimicrobial concentration, usually one hour after administration of the antibiotic. Antibiotic therapy should be adjusted to achieve a peak serum concentration of antimicrobials that results in a SBT of $\geq 1:8$ (11–14). It is desirable to measure serum concentrations of antibiotics from the same serum specimen used to determine SBT. The serum concentrations assist in the interpretation of the SBT. A low SBT may be related to a simultaneously low serum concentration of antimicrobials rather than to a lack of bactericidal effect, and this suggests that the dosage should be increased. Serum concentrations should be measured periodically throughout the course of antimicrobial therapy to ensure adequate therapeutic levels in excess of the MBC and to avoid accumulation in the serum of potentially toxic concentrations of antibiotics.

Occasionally tests of synergy between antimicrobial combinations may be desirable. These tests are most helpful in patients with enterococcal IE or with endocarditis caused by unusual microorganisms or those resistant to multiple antibiotics, or as a guide for determining optimal combinations of antimicrobial agents.

ADMINISTER ANTIBIOTICS PARENTERALLY   In general, antimicrobial therapy should be administered parenterally rather than orally. Absorption from the gastrointestinal tract of orally administered antimicrobial agents may be unpredictable.

REPEAT BLOOD CULTURES AFTER ANTIMICROBIAL THERAPY IS STARTED   Within 48 hours after initiation of specific antimicrobial therapy, blood cultures should be obtained to ensure the efficacy of treatment. Persistently positive blood cultures in spite of apparently appropriate therapy could indicate myocardial, aortic root, or distal abscess, tolerance of bacteria to antimicrobial agents, or error in administration or dosage of antibiotics.

CONSULT CARDIAC SURGEON   It is preferable to treat patients with IE in facilities where emergency cardiac valve replacement may be performed if necessary. Patients with aortic valve IE may experience acute aortic insufficiency and immediate cardiac valve replacement may offer the only hope of survival. Patients with severe heart failure that is unresponsive to medical therapy should be considered candidates for prompt cardiac valve replacement irrespective of the duration of antimicrobial therapy preoperatively (15, 16). Procrastination in an attempt to complete a course of antimicrobial therapy preoperatively usually increases the risk of surgical mortality. The hemodynamic status of the patient is the most important factor in determining the need and the timing of cardiac valve replacement (17, 18).

PERFORM DAILY PHYSICAL EXAMINATION DURING TREATMENT   Subtle changes in body weight, blood pressure, cardiac auscultatory findings, and jugular venous pressure may presage abrupt hemodynamic decompensation.

ELIMINATE PORTAL OF ENTRY   Careful attention should be directed to the appropriate treatment and, if possible, elimination of the portal of entry, such as poor oral hygiene or urinary tract infection with or without stones. Dentulous patients who are not critically ill should have dental roentgenograms and an oral-surgery consultation so that necessary dental work may be performed while the patient is receiving antimicrobial therapy. Because of the association of inflammatory bowel disease and carcinoma of the colon, patients with IE caused by *Streptococcus bovis* should have a proctoscopic examination and colon roentgenogram while receiving antimicrobial therapy.

INSTRUCT IN PROPHYLAXIS   Before dismissal from the hospital, patients and their families should receive adequate instruction in prophylactic measures for IE.

OBTAIN FOLLOW-UP BLOOD CULTURES   Follow-up blood cultures should be obtained at one- and two-month intervals after completion of antimicrobial therapy. Relapses, if they occur, are most often within the first two months after completion of therapy.

DO NOT COMPROMISE   Physicians should respect the seriousness of IE and should resist the temptation to compromise in the duration and means of administration of therapy or to switch to less effective antimicrobial agents. After initiation of treatment, some patients, especially those with penicillin-sensitive streptococcal endocarditis, will experience a dramatic improvement and disappearance of fever. These improvements should not be interpreted as an indication that the antimicrobials may be switched to orally administered agents or that the length of therapy may be shortened. If hypersensitivity reactions occur during treatment, in most instances control of symptoms should be attempted before replacement with an alternative form of therapy. If major hypersensitivity reactions or other complications necessitate a change of antimicrobial treatment, physicians should use only those accepted forms of alternative therapy discussed below or as presented in standard reference sources.

Specific Antimicrobial Regimens

PENICILLIN-SENSITIVE STREPTOCOCCI   The regimens widely accepted as effective antimicrobial therapy for the treatment of patients with penicillin-sensitive (MIC $\leqslant 0.2$ μg/ml) streptococcal IE are listed in Table 2. The large majority of viridans streptococci and nonenterococcal group D streptococci (e.g. *S. bovis*) are exquisitely susceptible to penicillin, and patients with IE caused by these microorganisms can be treated successfully with aqueous penicillin G alone for four weeks. Penicillin and streptomycin act synergistically against viridans streptococci and this combination is equally effective in the treatment of these patients, as is penicillin alone. The relapse rate is approximately 1% for each of the three regimens suggested for the

Table 2 Treatment of penicillin-sensitive streptococcal (MIC ≤ 0.2 μg/ml) endocarditis

Organism	Regimens of choice	Duration of treatment (weeks)	Alternative regimens	Duration of treatment (weeks)
Viridans or nonenterococcal group D streptococci	Aqueous penicillin G 20 × 10⁶ U IV daily	4	Vancomycin[a] 7.5 mg/kg IV q6h or 15 mg/kg IV q12h daily	4
	or		or	
	procaine penicillin 1.2 × 10⁶ U IM q6h daily or aqueous penicillin G10–20 × 10⁶ U IV daily	2	cephalothin[b] 1.5 gm IV q4h daily	4
	plus			
	streptomycin[a] 7.5 mg/kg IM q12h daily	2		
	or			
	aqueous penicillin G 10–20 × 10⁶ U IV daily	4		
	plus			
	streptomycin[a] 7.5 mg/kg IM q12h daily	2		
Other groups; e.g. A, B, C, F, H, *S. pneumoniae*	Aqueous penicillin G 10–20 × 10⁶ U IV daily	4	Vancomycin or cephalothin as above	4
Relative penicillin-resistance (MIC > 0.2 μg/ml); nutritionally variant viridans streptococci	Aqueous penicillin G 10–20 × 10⁶ U IV daily	4	Vancomycin[a] 7.5 mg/kg IV q6h or 15 mg/kg IV q12h daily	4
	plus		plus	
	streptomycin[a] 7.5 mg/kg IM q6h daily		streptomycin[a] 7.5 mg/kg IM q6h daily	

[a] Dosages of streptomycin should not exceed 500 mg/dose; dosages of vancomycin should not exceed 500 mg q6 hours or 1 gm q12 hours. Dosages of streptomycin and vancomycin should be reduced in patients with abnormal renal function.
[b] Other cephalosporin may be used in equivalent dosage if organism is susceptible in vitro.

treatment of viridans or nonenterococcal group D streptococcal endocarditis (12, 19–21). Of the three, the two-week regimen is the most cost-effective. The two-week regimen should not be administered to patients with symptoms of IE greater than three months in duration or to patients with suspected mycotic aneurysm, cerebritis, or shock. Because of the risk of streptomycin-associated vestibular toxicity (approximately 2% of patients), the use of aqueous penicillin G alone is preferred in patients more than 65 years old or in those with impaired eighth cranial nerve function or abnormal renal function.

In our experience, the relapse rate is higher among patients with IE caused by nutritionally variant viridans streptococci (8%) than among patients with infections caused by viridans streptococci with normal growth requirements (1%). The former group of patients should be treated with penicillin together with streptomycin for at least four weeks. Nutritionally variant viridans streptococcal IE is associated with the formation of large friable valvular vegetations, and such patients are at risk of major arterial embolic events.

ENTEROCOCCI Enterococci are inhibited but not killed by penicillin alone; the successful treatment of patients with enterococcal endocarditis requires the use of penicillin plus an aminoglycoside. The synergistic activity of the two antibiotics results in a bactericidal effect. Approximately one third of enterococci are resistant to a high concentration of streptomycin (MIC $>$ 2000 μg/ml). Patients with infections caused by streptomycin-resistant enterococci should be treated with a combination of penicillin and gentamicin; patients with endocarditis caused by streptomycin-susceptible enterococci may be treated successfully with penicillin and streptomycin (Table 3) (22, 23). In our experience, the relapse rate among patients with streptomycin-susceptible enterococcal endocarditis is lower (8%) than that for patients with streptomycin-resistant enterococcal endocarditis (25%). The major risk factor for relapse is symptoms of infection for more than three months prior to the initiation of appropriate antimicrobial therapy. These patients should receive at least six weeks of combined penicillin-aminoglycoside therapy.

The use of streptomycin for four weeks in patients with enterococcal endocarditis results in vestibular toxicity in approximately 20% of patients. The dosage of gentamicin in patients with normal renal function should not exceed 3 mg/kg/day. In our experience, dosages of gentamicin in excess of this amount resulted in gentamicin-associated nephrotoxicity in 100% of patients with streptomycin-resistant enterococcal endocarditis.

Patients who are allergic to penicillin should be treated with vancomycin together with either streptomycin or gentamicin. Cephalosporins should not be used to treat patients with enterococcal endocarditis.

Table 3 Treatment of enterococcal endocarditis

Streptomycin susceptibility	Duration of symptoms of illness	Regimen of choice	Duration of treatment (weeks)	Alternative regimen	Duration of treatment (weeks)
MIC < 2000 μg/ml	< 3 months[c]	Aqueous penicillin G 20–40 × 10^6 U IV daily plus Streptomycin[a] 7.5 mg/kg IM q12h daily	4	Vancomycin[a] 7.5 mg/kg q6h or 15 mg/kg q12h IV daily plus Streptomycin[a] 7.5 mg/kg IM q12h daily or gentamicin[b] 1 mg/kg IV q8h daily	4
MIC > 2000 μg/ml	< 3 months[c]	Aqueous penicillin G 20–40 × 10^6 U IV daily plus Gentamicin[b] 1 mg/kg IV q8h daily	4	Vancomycin[a] *plus* gentamicin[b] as above	4

[a] Dosage of streptomycin should not exceed 500 mg/dose; dosage of vancomycin should not exceed 500 mg q6 hours or 1 gm q12 hours. Dosages of streptomycin and vancomycin should be reduced in patients with abnormal renal function.
[b] Dosage of gentamicin should be reduced in patients with abnormal renal function.
[c] Patients who have symptoms of illness greater than three months in duration should receive at least six weeks of treatment with aqueous penicillin G together with either streptomycin or gentamicin.

STAPHYLOCOCCI   A penicillinase-resistant penicillin should be used initially in the treatment of *S. aureus* endocarditis. If the strain does not produce penicillinase and is susceptible to penicillin (MIC ⩽ 0.1 μg/ml) patients may be treated successfully with aqueous penicillin G (Table 4). Vancomycin or cephalosporin may be used alternatively in patients who are allergic to penicillin. In most instances clindamycin is not bactericidal and is not optimal therapy for patients with staphylococcal endocarditis. The use of methicillin is not recommended because of the risk of methicillin-associated nephritis. The use of oxacillin and nafcillin may be associated with neutropenia or hepatitis.

IE caused by *S. epidermidis* is usually associated with cardiac valve prostheses or intracardiac foreign bodies. Most strains of *S. epidermidis* isolated from these patients are resistant to penicillin and methicillin, and the majority of strains contain subpopulations of microorganisms that are resistant to cephalosporins. The combination of vancomycin and rifampin is suggested for the treatment of patients with methicillin-resistant strains. Some authorities advocate the addition of gentamicin to vancomycin-rifampin therapy (9).

GRAM-NEGATIVE BACILLI   The great majority of *Hemophilus* sp., *Cardiobacterium hominis,* and *Actinobacillus actinomycetemcomitans* are highly susceptible to ampicillin. In our experience, patients infected by these bacilli may be treated successfully with ampicillin administered intravenously for three weeks (Table 5) (24, 25). Endocarditis caused by these fastidious slow-growing microorganisms is frequently associated with the formation of large cardiac valve vegetations, and systemic embolization is not uncommon.

Tricuspid valve endocarditis associated with intravenous drug abuse is often caused by *Pseudomonas aeruginosa.* These microorganisms are highly resistant to antimicrobial therapy, and cardiac valve replacement or excision is often necessary. The selection of antimicrobial therapy for the treatment of endocarditis caused by other gram-negative bacilli depends upon the results of antimicrobial susceptibility testing. A combination of antimicrobial agents is often required and should be administered for at least four weeks.

Miscellaneous Bacterial Causes of Endocarditis

NEISSERIA SP.   Endocarditis caused by either gonococci or meningococci should be treated with aqueous penicillin G. *Neisseria gonorrhoeae* should be tested for penicillinase production.

Table 4 Treatment of staphylococcal endocarditis

Microorganism	Regimen of choice	Duration of treatment (weeks)	Alternative regimens	Duration of treatment (weeks)
Penicillin-sensitive (MIC ≤ 0.1 μg/ml) *S. aureus* or *S. epidermidis*	Aqueous penicillin G 20 × 10^6 U IV daily	4–6	Vancomycin[a] 7.5 mg/kg q6h or 15 mg/kg q12h IV daily or cephalothin[b] 2 gm IV q4h daily	4–6
Penicillin-resistant (MIC > 0.1 μg/ml) methicillin-susceptible *S. aureus* or *S. epidermidis*	Oxacillin or nafcillin 2 gm IV q4h daily	4–6	Vancomycin or cephalothin as above	4–6
Methicillin-resistant *S. epidermidis*	Vancomycin[a] 7.5 mg/kg q6h or 15 mg/kg q12h IV daily plus Rifampin 600 mg orally daily (single dose)	4–6	Cephalothin[b] 2 gm IV q4h daily plus Rifampin 600 mg orally daily (single dose)	4–6

[a] Dosage of vancomycin should not exceed 500 mg q6 hours or 1 gm q12 hours. Dosage should be reduced in patients with abnormal renal function.

[b] Other cephalosporin may be used in equivalent dosage if organism is susceptible in vitro.

Table 5 Treatment of gram-negative bacillary endocarditis

Microorganism	Regimen of choice	Duration of treatment (weeks)	Alternative regimens	Duration of treatment (weeks)
Hemophilus sp. Cardiobacterium hominis Actinobacillus actinomy- cetemcomitans	Ampicillin 2 gm IV q4h daily	3	Penicillin allergy— desensitize patient and treat with ampicillin	3
Pseudomonas aeruginosa	Ureidopenicillin[a] in appropriate dose plus Amikacin[b] 5 mg/kg q8h IV daily	6		
Other gram- negative bacilli	See text	4–6		

[a] Ureidopenicillins include carbenicillin, ticarcillin, mezlocillin, piperacillin, etc.
[b] Dosage of amikacin should be reduced in patients with abnormal renal function.

CORYNEBACTERIUM SP.   These microorganisms are relatively common causes of prosthetic valve endocarditis, especially that occurring during the first two months after cardiac surgery. Corynebacteria that are susceptible to gentamicin may be treated with a combination of penicillin and gentamicin (Table 6). Corynebacteria resistant to gentamicin (MIC > 4 μg/ml) can be treated with vancomycin.

CANDIDA ENDOCARDITIS   Endocarditis caused by candida is usually associated with intravenous drug abuse or with recent cardiac valve replacement. Antifungal therapy should be administered with a combination of amphotericin B and 5-fluorocytosine (provided that the isolate is susceptible to 5-fluorocytosine in vitro). After seven to ten days of therapy the infected valve should be excised. Postoperative therapy with antifungal agents should be continued for at least four weeks.

CULTURE-NEGATIVE ENDOCARDITIS   The most common cause of "culture negative" endocarditis is the recent administration of antimicrobial agents. Rarely, culture-negative cases may be caused by *Brucella* sp., *Coxiella burnetii,* Aspergillus, and fastidious gram-negative bacilli (e.g. *Hemophilus* sp.). Unless clinical epidemiologic or serologic data suggest otherwise, patients with culture-negative IE should be treated with regimens outlined for enterococcal endocarditis plus the addition of oxacillin and nafcillin. Noninfectious conditions mimicking culture-negative en-

Table 6 Treatment of miscellaneous causes of endocarditis

Microorganism	Regimen of choice	Duration of treatment (weeks)	Alternative regimens	Duration of treatment (weeks)
Neisseria sp.	Aqueous penicillin G 20 × 10^6 U IV daily	4	Penicillin allergy—desensitize patient and treat with penicillin	4
Corynebacterium sp. gentamicin MIC < 4 μg/ml	Aqueous penicillin G 20 × 10^6 U IV daily plus gentamicin[a] 1 mg/kg q8h IV daily	4–6	Vancomycin[a] 7.5 mg/kg q6h or 15 mg/kg q12h IV daily	4–6
gentamicin MIC ≥ 4 μg/ml	Vancomycin[a] 7.5 mg/kg q6h or 15 mg/kg q12h IV daily	4–6		
Candida sp.	Amphotericin B 0.7–1.0 mg/kg IV daily, plus flucytosine 150 mg/kg/day orally in divided doses, *plus* cardiac valve replacement	6–8	None	
Culture-negative endocarditis	See text			

[a] Dosage of gentamicin and vancomycin should be reduced in patients with abnormal renal function. Dosages of vancomycin should not exceed 500 mg q6 hours or 1 gm q12 hours.

docarditis include acute rheumatic fever, marantic endocarditis, atrial myxoma, carcinoid syndrome, and systemic lupus erythematous.

Prosthetic Valve Endocarditis

The antimicrobial therapy for patients with prosthetic valve endocarditis is the same as that outlined above except that all patients should receive a minimum of four weeks of antimicrobial therapy. Early surgical intervention in patients with prosthetic valve endocarditis is suggested in selected patients with one or more of the following complications: (*a*) most cases of endocarditis caused by staphylococci, (*b*) congestive heart failure caused by valve dysfunction, (*c*) valve dehiscence, and (*d*) recurrent relapse after appropriate antimicrobial therapy (26). Patients with prosthetic valve endocarditis who require the use of anticoagulants are cautiously maintained on warfarin sodium (coumadin) with prothrombin times of 1–1½ times the control value. If central nervous system emboli occur in these patients, anticoagulants should be discontinued, and the patient observed; if no additional emboli occur and there is no progression of central nervous system disease, anticoagulant therapy may be reinstituted cautiously (27).

Literature Cited

1. Wilson, W. R., Washington, J. A. II. 1977. Infective endocarditis—a changing spectrum? (editorial). *Mayo Clin. Proc.* 52:254–55
2. Kaye, D. 1976. *Infective Endocarditis,* p. 47. Baltimore: Univ. Park
3. Lerner, P. I., Weinstein, L. 1966. Infective endocarditis in the antibiotic era. *N. Engl. J. Med.* 274:199–206, 259–66, 323–31, 388–93
4. Tompsett, R. 1967. Bacterial endocarditis: changes in the clinical spectrum. *Arch. Intern. Med.* 119:329–32
5. Shinebourne, E. A., Cripps, C. M., Hayward, G. W., Shooter, R. A. 1969. Bacterial endocarditis 1956–1965: analysis of clinical features and treatment in relation to prognosis and mortality. *Br. Heart J.* 31:536–42
6. Beeson, P. B., Brannon, E. S., Warren, J. V. 1945. Observations on the sites of removal of bacteria from the blood in patients with bacterial endocarditis. *J. Exp. Med.* 81:9–23
7. Werner, A. S., Cobbs, C. G., Kaye, D., Hook, E. W. 1967. Studies on the bacteremia of bacterial endocarditis. *J. Am. Med. Assoc.* 202:199–203
8. Belli, F., Waisbren, B. A. 1956. The number of blood cultures necessary to diagnose most cases of bacterial endocarditis. *Am. J. Med. Sci.* 232:284–88

9. Karchmer, A. W., Dismukes, W. E., Johnson, W. D. Jr., Wilson, W. R., Archer, G. L., Sande, M. A. 1980. Staphylococcus epidermidis prosthetic valve endocarditis. In *Current Chemotherapy and Infectious Disease: Proc. 11th Int. Congr. Chemother., 19th Intersci. Conf. Antimicrob. Agents Chemother.,* ed. J. D. Nelson, C. Grassi, 2:904–6. Washington DC: Am. Soc. for Microbiol.
10. Washington, J. A. II. 1981. Bactericidal tests. In *Laboratory Procedures in Clinical Microbiology,* ed. J. A. Washington II, pp. 715–28 New York: Springer-Verlag
11. Wilson, W. R., Geraci, J. E., Wilkowske, C. J., Washington, J. A. II. 1978. Short-term intramuscular therapy with procaine penicillin plus streptomycin for infective endocarditis due to viridans streptococci. *Circulation* 57:1158–61
12. Wilson, W. R., Thompson, R. L., Wilkowske, C. J., Washington, J. A. II, Giuliani, E. R., Geraci, J. E. 1981. Short-term therapy for streptococcal infective endocarditis: combined intramuscular administration of penicillin and streptomycin. *J. Am. Med. Assoc.* 245:360–63
13. Wilson, W. R., Giuliani, E. R., Danielson, G. K., Geraci, J. E. 1982. General considerations in the diagnosis and

treatment of infective endocarditis. *Mayo Clin. Proc.* 57:31–35

14. Hook, E. W., Guerrant, R. L. 1976. Therapy of infective endocarditis. See Ref. 2, p. 167

15. Wilson, W. R., Danielson, G. K., Giuliani, E. R., Washington, J. A. II, Jaumin, P. M., Geraci, J. E. 1978. Valve replacement in patients with active infective endocarditis. *Circulation* 58:585–88

16. Wallace, A. G., Young, W. G. Jr., Osterhout, S. 1965. Treatment of acute bacterial endocarditis by valve excision and replacement. *Circulation* 31:450–53

17. Wilson, W. R., Danielson, G. K., Giuliani, E. R., Washington, J. A. II., Jaumin, P. M. Geraci, J. E. 1979. Cardiac valve replacement in congestive heart failure due to infective endocarditis. *Mayo Clin. Proc.* 54:223–26

18. Mills, J., Utley, J., Abbott, J. 1974. Heart failure in infective endocarditis: predisposing factors, course, and treatment. *Chest* 66:151–57

19. Karchmer, A. W., Moellering, R. C. Jr., Maki, D. G., Swartz, M. N. 1979. Single-antibiotic therapy for streptococcal endocarditis. *J. Am. Med. Assoc.* 241:1801–6

20. Hoppes, W. L. 1977. Treatment of bacterial endocarditis caused by penicillin-sensitive streptococci (editorial). *Arch. Intern. Med.* 137:1122–23

21. Wolfe, J. C., Johnson, W. D. Jr. 1974. Penicillin-sensitive streptococcal endocarditis: in vitro and clinical observations on penicillin-streptomycin therapy. *Ann. Intern. Med.* 81:178–81

22. Serra, P., Brandimarte, C., Martino, P., Carlone, S., Giunchi, G. 1977. Synergistic treatment of enterococcal endocarditis: in vitro and in vivo studies. *Arch. Intern. Med.* 137:1562–67

23. Wilson, W. R., Wilkowske, C. J., Thompson, R. L., Geraci, J. E. 1979. Treatment of streptomycin-resistant enterococcal (SRE) infective endocarditis (IE) (Abstr.) Presented at 11th Int. Congr. Chemother., 19th Intersci. Conf. Antimicrob. Agents Chemother., Boston, October 1–5

24. Geraci, J. E., Greipp, P. R., Wilkowske, C. J., Wilson, W. R., Washington, J. A. II. 1978. *Cardiobacterium hominis* endocarditis: four cases with clinical and laboratory observations. *Mayo Clin. Proc.* 53:49–53

25. Geraci, J. E., Wilson, W. R., Washington, J. A. II. 1980. Ineffective endocarditis caused by *Actinobacillus actinomycetemcomitans:* report of four cases. *Mayo Clin. Proc.* 55:415–19

26. Karchmer, A. W., Dismukes, W. E., Buckley, M. J., Austen, W. G. 1978. Late prosthetic valve endocarditis: clinical features influencing therapy. *Am. J. Med.* 64:199–206

27. Wilson, W. R., Geraci, J. E., Danielson, G. K., Thompson, R. L., Spittell, J. A. Jr., Washington, J. A. II, Giuliani, E. R. 1978. Anticoagulant therapy and central nervous system complications in patients with prosthetic valve endocarditis. *Circulation* 57:1004–7

Ann. Rev. Med. 1983. 34:429–52

SWEATING AND ITS DISORDERS

Paul M. Quinton, Ph.D.

Division of Biomedical Sciences, University of California, Riverside, California
92521; and Department of Physiology, University of California, Los Angeles,
California 90024

ABSTRACT

Eccrine sweat is produced by millions of miniscule glands buried in the skin.
Eccrine sweating from the general body surface is an extremely important
function in human thermoregulation; disturbances either in the control of
sweating activity or in the glands themselves can result in problems ranging
from minor social embarrassment to fatal hyperpyrexia. A general review
of the function and control of normal sweating precedes an overview of
sweating abnormalities.

INTRODUCTION

The term sweating unfortunately refers to several distinct phenomena.
Sweating may refer to the passive loss of water through the skin, frequently
referred to as "insensitive" sweating. More usually, the term is used to
describe the active secretion of a watery fluid onto the body surface from
either eccrine or apocrine sweat glands. The apocrine glands are of minor
physiological importance. Their structure is described in much greater
detail than their function (82, 125). Consequently, we limit our considerations here to eccrine sweating and its disorders.

In contrast to apocrine glands, the eccrine sweat glands play a clear and
vital role in our ability to survive heat stress and maintain remarkably
constant homeothermic conditions under thermal loads that would be lethal
for most other animals. In fact, it may be argued that of all animals, man
has developed his sweat glands and brain to the greatest level of evolutionary sophistication (153). Except for the oral, anal, and genital areas, the

429

0066-4219/83/0401-0429$02.00

eccrine sweat glands are found in all skin covering the body surface in densities ranging from about 60 per cm^2 on the thigh to 350 per cm^2 on the forehead (125). In normal individuals, from 2 to 4 million glands are capable of maximally secreting from 2 to 4 liters of markedly hypotonic fluid per hour. Evaporation of this volume of water requires more than 18 kcal per minute, which provides man with an ability to dissipate heat faster than any other animal for extended periods.

The control of heat dissipation is as impressive as its magnitude. It is well appreciated that body temperature is normally fixed very close to 37°C. In unacclimated individuals exposed acutely to heat stress, sweating usually begins before the temperature has risen more than 1°C. In conditioned subjects, sweating begins almost simultaneously with heat load (198). It should be appreciated that these strict limits of thermal homeostasis are regulated to a very large extent by the interplay between sweat rate and skin blood flow, both of which are delicately correlated to the heat load (129). The importance of these mechanisms to normal body function is emphasized by the intense discomfort and loss of exercise tolerance among those who cannot sweat (121) and the the social stigmas and embarrassment placed on those whose sweat too much (48).

In this review we first describe the normal structure, innervation, and function of the eccrine sweat gland. Then, where possible, we deal with etiology and treatment of the various abnormalities, which may be considered categorically as one of three functional disorders: too much sweating (hyperhidrosis), too little sweating (anhidrosis), and altered sweat composition.

FUNDAMENTALS OF NORMAL SWEATING

Structure

Sweat glands usually exist as single units embedded in the loose matrix of subdermal connective tissue. The eccrine sweat gland is uniquely simple in that it consists of a single unbranched tubule coiled into a bolus that varies considerably in size but approximates 300 μm in diameter. The body of the gland, or bolus, is usually found from 2 to 5 mm below the epidermis.

Several separate components of the tubule can be identified. The proximal half of the gland is composed of a blind-ended secretory tubule completely coiled within the bolus. The secretory coil gives rise through a small segment of transition tubule to the coiled reabsorptive duct, which is also found entirely within the bolus. The body of the gland is then connected directly to the epidermis via a straight segment of reabsorptive duct opening onto the skin surface. In the skin of the palms and soles of the feet, the terminal portion of the duct spirals through the epidermis to form the acrosyringium (102).

In the secretory tubule, the tissue responsible for forming the sweat volume is a simple epithelium surrounded by dispersed myoepithelial cells. The epithelium is composed of two recognizable cell types. Light cells, which are larger and located more peripherally, are thought to be primarily responsible for fluid secretion. Dark cells, which are smaller, located closer to the lumen, and highly basophilic, are thought primarily to secrete macromolecular components (34). The myoepithelial cells probably provide structural strength (167) and support to the enclosed epithelial layer, as hydrostatic pressures (> 500 mm Hg) may be generated during secretion (171).

The continuity of the barrier between the cells and the tubule lumen is maintained by a relatively complicated network of tight junctions. The junctions are composed of 6 to 9 parallel and anastomosing strands (19). The junction joins both light and dark cells at their apical ends at the border of the tubule lumen as well as along their lateral surfaces to form intercellular canaliculi that are continuous with the lumen. The canaliculus may serve some function as a channel for a standing osmotic gradient in secretion (38), but the absence of Na/K-ATPase associated with their mem-

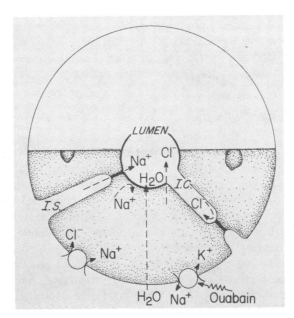

Figure 1   Components of the fluid secretion in the sweat gland. NaCl accumulates in the lumen as a function of the special properties of the epithelium. H_2O then moves passively to equilibrate iso-osmotically with the solutes trapped in the secretory lumen. See text for details. Dashed arrows indicate passive movements. Curved arrows indicate impermeable membranes or tight junctions. Zig-zag arrows indicate induced inhibition. (IS = intercellular space, IC = intercellular canaliculus.)

branes (155) leaves the exact role of these structures open to questions (Figure 1). The external perimeter of the tubule is defined by a thin layer of basement membrane consisting largely of elauin fibers (15).

The cytological organization of the coiled and straight portions of the reabsorptive duct is similar. However, as the duct approaches its opening through the epidermis, ductal epithelial cells become less differentiated and specialized. The coiled and straight portions of the reabsorptive duct are unique in being organized as two concentric layers of epithelial cells. The cells of these layers appear relatively homogeneous but differ somewhat: the apical membrane of the inner cells forms the lumen of the duct, whereas the basal membrane of the outer cells rests on the basement membrane, which completely surrounds the reabsorptive duct as it does in the secretory tubule. The apical surface of the cells of the inner layer are joined by tight junction structures similar to those found in the secretory tubule (19). As in frog skin (42), gap junctions are common between the epithelial cells of the duct. It seems likely that this organization serves as a functional syncytium (Figure 2).

Studies on dissected sweat glands revealed numerous enzymes associated with the tissue, including alkaline phosphatase, acid phosphatase, Na/K-ATPase, phosphatidic acid phosphatase, and lactic, malic, glucose-6-phosphate, isocitric, and succinic dehydrogenases (68) as well as monamine oxidase (185, 208) and acetyl cholinesterase (185, 195). Several detailed descriptions of the morphology of eccrine sweat glands are available (51, 81, 125).

Abnormalities of Structure

The numerous structural abnormalities associated with neoplasms of the sweat glands (74) are beyond the scope of this review, but several other classes of morphological alterations are known, some of which may be of diagnostic value. For example, in Lafora disease skin biopsy may provide an easily accessible tissue in diagnosis since the peripheral cells of the reabsorptive duct develop round, PAS-positive bodies of about the same size as the cell nucleus (27). The appearance of large cytoplasmic vacuoles in the cells of the acrosyringium and secretory coil may furnish distinguishing marks in the diagnosis of GM_1 gangliosidosis (43) and in genetic mucopolysaccharidoses (8). In hereditary amyloidosis (Finnish type), amyloid deposits in the region of the basal membrane create the impression of a great thickening of the basement membrane (29). In Anderson-Fabry disease, in which alpha galactosidase A is lacking, diminished sweating may be due to lipid accumulations in glands cells (65) as well as to degeneration of sympathetic nerves (25). Unmyelinated axons and axon terminals are absent in hereditary neuropathy type IV (congenital insensitivity to pain with anhidrosis) even though Schwann cell processes are present (104).

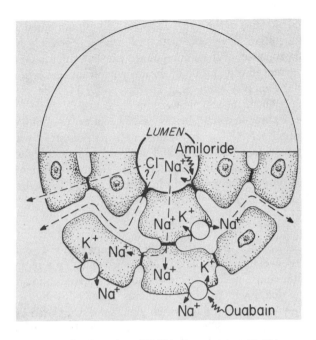

Figure 2 Components of reabsorption of NaCl in the sweat duct. NaCl is pumped out of the duct lumen by a ouabain inhibitable Na/K pump in the basal-lateral membranes of the bilayer epithelium of the duct. Na moves down its electrochemical gradient from the lumen into the cell passively via a pathway in the apical membrane, which can be blocked (curved arrow) by amiloride. Cl passively follows Na, but it is not known whether the Cl route out of the duct is through the cell or across the tight junction. Na, having crossed the apical membrane of the inner cell, can passively move between cells of both layers by diffusing through cell to cell contacts. Dashed arrows indicate passive movements. Zig-zag arrows indicate inhibition.

Although the change may not be an abnormality, Dobson noted increased numbers of vacuoles in the light cells of the secretory coil after profuse sweating episodes in subjects on low Na diets (40). In hypothyroidism, the light cells of the secretory coil frequently sequester small PAS-positive bodies that are resistant to diesterase (122).

Prolonged blockage of the sweat duct, whether by solid deposits or by proliferation of duct cells, leads to structural changes in the duct. Calcium deposits causing dilation of the duct may be a complication of hypercalcemia (71) or of idiopathic origin (57). Skin wounds, inflammation, neoplasms, and cysts are frequently accompanied by hyperplasia of the duct epithelial cells and dilation of the sweat duct (123). Similar changes may be expected from the numerous causes of miliaria, all of which seem to be related to blockage of the duct (41). Although epithelial hyperplasia is characteristic of duct dilation, in psoriatic skin, cell division in the sweat glands seems to be reduced by about 50% (66).

Intentional blocking of the sweat ducts with aluminum-based antiperspirants does not initiate detectable structural changes, possibly because the antibacterial properties of these compounds prevent miliaria type reactions (175). The current interpretation of the antiperspirant action of these compounds is that they physically plug the duct (147, 148), but it would not be surprising if chemical actions were involved also.

Extensive damage to sweat glands develops in areas of bulbous lesions found in a small percentage of comatose patients poisoned by agents such as carbon monoxide, barbiturates, and diazepam. The ducts show striking necrosis with vesiculation and degeneration. The reaction may be due to prolonged activity of the glands during drug-induced hyperthermia combined with ductal secretion of toxins (200).

Central Control

Afferent impulses are integrated in the hypothalamus to control thermoregulatory sweating. Stimulation of the preoptic area of the anterior hypothalamus elicits generalized sweating (181). Even though systemic excitation originating in the hypothalamus usually involves parasympathetic pathways and even though sweat glands are stimulated by parasympathetic agonists, central efferent discharges are carried via the sympathetic tracts (102). Roughly, spinal cord segments T2–T4 supply sweat glands on the head and neck, T2–T8 supply glands of the upper limbs, T6–T10 supply the trunk, and T11–L2 supply the lower extremities.

Central control is regulated as a function of afferent input from sensors for skin temperature and core temperature (181). Neuromuscular components may also affect hypothalamic output (198). Sweating rate is also modulated by physical parameters in the immediate vicinity of the sweat gland. Thus, decreases in the local skin temperature, in skin wettness (10, 26), and in blood flow all decrease local sweat activity (47, 133, 181). Systemic dehydration decreases overall sweat rates (62).

Gland Stimulation

The literature describing the innervation and stimulation of eccrine sweat glands is, at best, confusing. At present, however, although cholinergic fibers seem to be most prevalent, it is established that the gland receives dual innervation by both cholinergic and adrenergic fibers (195, 196). Corresponding to these findings, but with considerable variability in reports, sweat glands can be stimulated not only by cholinergic but also by α- and β-adrenergic agonists (162, 163, 167). Cholinergic stimulation generally provokes the largest response, while the response to β-adrenergic stimulation is usually weak (163, 189, 204). Cholinergic and α-adrenergic stimulation is dependent on extracellular calcium (144, 169). Sweating can also be elicited by elevating the extracellular calcium concentration (144) or by increasing the level of intracellular calcium by applying calcium ionophore A23187 (169). β-Adrenergic stimulation uniquely results in the intracellular accumulation of cAMP and does not require extracellular calcium (170).

Secretion

The biochemical events coupling stimulation by neurotransmitters to the secretion of fluid in the secretory coil are not well understood. However, the process almost certainly involves the active transport of electrolytes as a function of Na/K-ATPase located in the basal-lateral membranes of secretory cells (155). Secretion is blocked by the application of ouabain, a specific inhibitor of the enzyme (152, 168). No model for the secretory process coupling the movement of electrolytes to the energy provided by the enzyme has been proven for the sweat gland; the most probable scheme might be one similar to that put forward by Field (61), which may be applicable to fluid secretion in general. Some of the central elements of the proposed process in the context of the secretory cells of the sweat gland are shown in Figure 1. Here, energy from the Na/K pump (Na/K-ATPase) creates a substantial electrochemical gradient for Na movement into the cell. Cl is moved into the cell against its gradient by coupling its transport to the movement of Na into the cell via a neutral Na/Cl carrier. A Cl-permeable (Na-impermeable) apical membrane in the presence of a Cl-impermeable basal lateral membrane and paracellular shunt (tight junction pathway) permits Cl to leave the cell only by moving into the lumen. This transfer of negative charge to the lumen creates an electrochemical gradient that draws Na across the Cl-impermeable paracellular barrier (tight junction). Osmotic equilibrium is maintained by the isotonic movement of water (and other small, permeable solutes) into the lumen as well. The result of these net movements is an increase in hydrostatic pressure in the luminal compartment, which forces the precursor fluid (primary sweat) down the lumen and out of the gland through the reabsorptive duct. The rate of secretion may be controlled by regulating the Cl permeability of the apical membrane (61).

Although this model provides a role for the "outwardly" directed Na pump on the basal lateral membranes, it does not provide satisfactory insights into the role of the intracellular canaliculi. Likewise, the presumption of a Na-selective pathway through the tight junction does not seem to be wholly consonant with the observation (19) that the tight junction is composed of a relatively complicated network of junctional strands that are at least impermeable to lanthanum (80). Extracellular proteins are thought to be largely excluded from the primary sweat, and those macromolecules that are present are probably secreted by the dark cells of the secretory coil (81).

Maximal rates of secretion as high as 30 nl/min/gland have been observed with pharmacological stimulation in vivo or in vitro. However, the rate is highly variable among individuals and seems to be a function not only of sex and age but also of conditioning, season, and possibly diet (150).

Reabsorption

The function of the distal half of the sweat gland tubule is to reabsorb Na, Cl, HCO_3, and probably glucose and several other small solutes from the primary sweat so that water may be evaporated from the skin surface without a corresponding loss of essential solutes. This reabsorptive capacity of eccrine sweat glands is unique in primates and is probably most highly evolved in man (153). It imparts to man his superior advantage in coping with thermal stress. This advantage follows from the fact that conservation of the major solutes of the extracellular fluid compartment (ECF), which does not occur in lower animals, preserves the circulatory volume by mobilizing water from the larger intracellular fluid compartment (ICF) when water is lost during sweating. Hence, patients with cystic fibrosis who cannot effectively reabsorb sweat solutes are especially prone to heat prostration (39).

It is not known whether the ductal portion of the sweat duct is innervated or whether the reabsorptive process can be stimulated. Early microperfusion of single sweat glands (117, 118), suggested that some component in sweat was required to maintain reabsorption, but more recent observations on isolated segments of reabsorptive ducts (149, 152) show that reabsorption proceeds very well when such tissue is perfused with completely defined artificial medium and that, in fact, reabsorption rates were not different when osmotically adjusted human sweat was used as the perfusate. Hence, reabsorptive activity may be initiated simply by the presence of Na in the lumen of the duct.

As in the cells of the secretory coil, the concentration of Na in the reabsorptive duct cells is thought to be kept at a low level by the action of Na/K-ATPase in the cell membranes on the serosal surface (155). Figure 2 illustrates a possible model for reabsorption of electrolytes, which is notably similar to that proposed much earlier for frog skin (197). Here, the electronegativity of the cell interior coupled with the low cytoplasmic Na concentration creates a large driving force for the passive movement of Na out of the lumen into the cell via an amiloride-sensitive channel or carrier (152). An exchange of Na for protons at the apical membrane may play an important role in the absorption of HCO_3 (150, 151). The concentration of

K in sweat is slightly hypertonic possibly because K substitutes for protons in this exchange (180). The epithelial cells are connected by numerous gap junctions that may serve as intracellular pathways for the movement of reabsorbed solutes from the inner cells to the peripheral cells of the duct (Figure 2). It is not clear whether Cl moves intra- or paracellularly across the epithelial barrier, but the sweat duct is relatively impermeable to water (117).

HYPERHIDROSIS

Hyperhidrosis is a term applied to a variety of conditions in which an inappropriately large amount of sweat is produced. Hyperhidrosis may be either systemic, that is, generalized over the body surface, or localized to a very specific areas. It does not present a threat to health, but complaints arise from resulting discomfort and social embarrassment.

Localized Hyperhidrosis

Well-defined areas or regions that repetitively undergo hyperhidrosis are usually related to (*a*) emotional sweating, (*b*) gustatory sweating, or (*c*) neurological lesions.

EMOTIONAL SWEATING   Hyperhidrosis of the axillary, palmar, and/or plantar areas (areas that normally respond to emotional stress with sweat production) is almost always brought on by psychological stimuli (45). The condition is very rare among children and the elderly (96). The psychogenic component of stimulation of these glands and their lack of sensitivity to thermal stress (102) suggest that they are controlled more by cortical than by hypothalamic processes. There is some evidence that some of these patients may exhibit a lower overall ability to cope with stress (106).

Hyperhidrosis in the armpits is usually bilateral and commonly presents with the complaint of social embarrassment, even though no odor is usually associated with the condition (90). Bromohidrosis is absent because bacteria that act on the secretions of the apocrine glands are flushed away by the large volume of eccrine sweat. As much as 26 ml/hour of sweat from each armpit may be delivered (128).

It is characteristic that axillary hyperhidrosis is absent during sleep. Although thermal stimuli do not evoke the response, there is a subjective interpretation that warm environments exacerbate the problem. The condition usually develops equally among men and women during puberty, but women present more frequently than men (77, 96, 161).

The treatment of axillary hyperhidrosis involves interrupting the emotional stimulus, gland innervation, or the end organ. Lowering the level of anxiety with depressants (35) has its obvious problems. Conditioning and biofeedback may have some potential for control in some patients (44, 103). Direct treatment of the end organ surgically or pharmaceutically is a much more common form of therapy. Sympathectomy of the 2nd through the 4th thoracic ganglia is an effective, but complicated, control, which if successful completely abolishes sweat gland activity of the upper limbs (48, 77). Unfortunately, the procedure is not always certain to be complete, possibly because of anatomical variations in the sympathetic tract (72), and serious complications including death may arise (206). More conservative approaches involve subdermal ablation of the glands (77) or complete excision of the axillary skin by one of a number of techniques (11, 16, 17, 161). The application of aluminum chloride hexahydrate or zirconyl chloride reportedly gives excellent results if these chemicals are maintained in contact with the skin during a period of gland inactivity for several hours (50, 175). The use of local anesthetics (98) and topical application of propantheline (63) may give some relief, but pharmacological suppression is not uniformly successful (158).

The extent of hyperhidrosis of the palms may range from annoying, damp, and moist hands to sweat production that is so prolific that sweat drips continuously from the palms to the extent of being hazardous. Simultaneous plantar sweating occurs in about half of these patients, but axillary hyperhidrosis is usually not present. Excessive sweating elsewhere is almost always absent. Episodes generally appear to be initiated by psychological stress, but scratching and idiopathic causes may precipitate sweating also (28). The condition surfaces during childhood in perhaps 50% of known cases, usually goes unattended until adolescence when the problem is more likely to be a source of embarrassment (132), and resolves itself before the fourth decade of life (87).

Probably because of the thickness of the epidermis, the treatment of palmar and plantar hyperhidrosis with topical antiperspirants is usually not effective (2). The most permanent and effective treatment seems to be sympathectomy of the 2nd and 3rd thoracic ganglion (28, 132, 176). Although neurological explanations are not known, the procedure usually results in decreased plantar sweating as well (28). This observation plus the finding that patients with hyperhidrosis exhibit a reduced response to cholinomimetic stimulation that is reversed after T2-T3 gangliectomy suggest that these ganglia may play a more important role than previously recognized in modulating sudomotor control in thermoregulation (177). The procedure results in the loss of approximately one fifth of the thermoregulatory sweating surface of the body; the remaining surface adapts with increased compensatory sweating (176), which may lead to hyperhidrosis in some patients.

Iontophoresis of tap water is a less permanent, but generally effective, therapy (73, 107). Relief for 2 to 4 weeks may be obtained by passing a small direct current through the skin of the palms or soles of the feet for 20 to 30 minutes 2 to 3 times per week for a few weeks. Control of axillary hyperhidrosis with this method is ineffective (2, 73). It is widely believed that tap water iontophoresis inhibits sweating by inducing an abnormal keratinization that temporarily obstructs the sweat duct (173), but more recently Hill et al (86) were unable to find evidence of such a mechanism. It seems possible that the iontophoretic current, most of which is conducted through the sweat gland, may damage a neuroglandular component necessary for secretion. The iontophoresis of anticholinergic compounds such as poldine methosulfate (73), scopolamine (172), or glycopyrronium salts (2) provides relief much more rapidly, with fewer treatments, and for a longer period of time than tap water, but side-effects may prevent their use.

GUSTATORY SWEATING   Many people normally respond to highly irritating foods such as hot spices with detectable amounts of perspiration on the scalp and face (105). Rarely, otherwise normal persons respond idiosyncratically to specific foods such as cheese or chocolate, Claude Bernard, the 19th century French physiologist, being one of the most notable examples (83). The principal difference between normal and pathological gustatory sweating is that the latter usually, but not always, occurs asymmetrically and irrespective of the type of food being eaten (13, 83). Pathological gustatory sweating is most commonly associated with the face (69), but frequently involves the shoulder and side of the neck (6, 13). Rarely, other areas may be affected such as a small hyperhidrotic spot on the knee of an infant, which was stimulated by drinking milk (124).

In rare instances the condition may be hereditary (207), but almost without exception, the onset is subsequent to trauma to salivary gland innervation (79, 84) or to cervical-thoracic sympathetic ganglia (6, 13, 83). More recently, it has been appreciated that gustatory sweating may evolve as a complication of autonomic neuropathy (21, 186, 205).

Because of the extremely high probability that sweating over the temporal region of the head will follow parotidectomy (79, 179), the term "gustatory sweating" is frequently used synonymously with "auriculotemporal syndrome" or "Frey's Syndrome." The most widely accepted theory to explain Frey's syndrome holds that, after injury to innervation of the parotid, the parasympathetic terminals of the auriculotemporal nerve regenerate and aberrantly innervate the overlying sweat glands (69). The response can be acutely inhibited by anticholinergics (79, 83) or by nerve blocks to the optic ganglion (69), but the only long-lasting relief, which is not always successful, is through surgical intervention of the auriculotemporal or the chorda tympanic nerves (136). Unfortunately, symptoms may recur after several months, presumably owing to nerve regeneration (49, 69, 88).

Gustatory sweating of the upper parts of the body is a frequent complication of cervical and cervical-thoracic sympathectomy (6, 13, 83). The mechanism of the postoperative response is not well understood, but there is some evidence to suggest that it results from a regeneration and reorganization of the preganglionic fibers within the spinal chord after the axons of such fibers have been severed (6). There appears to be no highly acceptable treatment for these complications (21).

Gustatory sweating, when present in diabetic neuropathy, frequently affects the face and upper torso (186, 205). The phenomenon probably arises from abnormal resprouting of axons subsequent to nerve degeneration as the neuropathy progresses (21). Low doses of clonidine may be of possible benefit in suppressing the response (94).

Systemic Hyperhidrosis

Hyperhidrosis over the body surface is generally due to a disturbance in the autonomic nervous systems, a disorder in thermoregulation, or hypersensitivity to stimulation. Hyperhidrosis is always episodic. We have found no reports of continuous, permanent systemic hyperhidrosis.

Generalized hyperhidrosis is a symptom of several neuroendocrine disorders that may result from indirect effects on autonomic stimulation of sweating. Paroxyms of sweating are characteristic of pheochromocytoma and thyrotoxicosis. The former is the result of hypersecretion of catecholamines by adrenal tumors. Since local sweating can be blocked by hyoscine (146), it seems unlikely that the increased levels of circulating catecholamines stimulate sweating directly. Rather, sweating may be an appropriate physiological response to inappropriate thermogenesis stimulated by the excess of hormones (162).

Increased sweating in thyrotoxicosis may also be related to inappropriate heat production since the episodes are inhibited by β-adrenergic blockade (4). In acromegaly, the pituitary tumor releases an excess of growth hormone and prolactin. The relation between this abnormality and the associated sweating episodes is not understood, but the administration of bromocriptine, an ergot alkaloid, reportedly improves the general symptoms including cessation of inappropriate sweating (193).

The hyperhidrosis commonly experienced in hypotension and hypoglycemia is part of the autonomic response to systemic distress, but the reason, not to mention the mechanism, is not understood.

Disorders of thermoregulation leading to hyperhydrosis are not well documented, but sweating during post-menopausal "hot flushes," during "night sweats," and during defervescence may be examples of such phenomena. In each of these cases, the sweating appears to be part of the normal mechanism for acutely lowering the body temperature. A sudden increase in skin conductance and temperature immediately precedes the slight fall in core temperature that occurs during the sensation of hot flushes (191). Normally within 30 minutes after the onset of sleep, core temperature drops slightly less than 1°C, which is brought about by body sweating (67). Exaggerations of these normal mechanisms may be involved in the soaking night sweats associated with neuropathy in diabetes mellitus (70). In a case of diabetes insipidus, pitressin completely alleviated night sweats (157).

Excessive sweating experienced in some allergic diseases and in anxiety nervosa may arise because sweat glands are hypersensitive to stimulation. Sweat glands of patients with these conditions were found to be stimulated at lower doses of cholinergic agonist than were those of controls (93, 101, 203). It should be noted that the glands of subjects who sweat frequently generally exhibit lower stimulatory thresholds than those of people who do not. Thus, patients with conditions that result in frequent sweating may appear to be hypersensitive as compared to controls with less sweating activity. Hypersensitivity of sweat glands extends to familial dysautonomia, which is characterized by drenching sweats. Children with this autosomal recessive condition are hypersensitive to acetylcholine, which may result from poorly developed peripheral nerves (3, 22).

Finally, to illustrate some of the bizarre conditions of hyperhidrosis that may be encountered, we mention two sisters who sweated profusely from the back and chest when exposed to the cold (184).

ANHIDROSIS

Anhidrosis is the lack of sweat production in the presence of an appropriate stimulus such as heat or pharmacological agonists. Anhidrosis is rare, but it may be caused by a variety of insults and diseases. It may be systemic (where it is potentially fatal), segmental, or very localized. It may be acute or progressive, and it may originate peripherally or centrally. Since anhidrosis implies complete absence of sweating, some authors prefer the term hypohidrosis. We choose to use "anhidrosis" in a general sense for both terms.

Neural Lesions

Among central lesions, one of the most common and dangerous forms of anhidrosis occurs with heat stroke. Central control through the hypothalamus, brain stem, and spinal cord (24, 95, 126) fails due to the elevation of core temperature above 40–41°C. Loss of efferent input and systemic shut down of sweating initiates a vicious cycle between rising temperature and loss of cooling. The notion that anhidrosis in hyperpyrexia is due to direct damage of the sweat glands can probably be discarded in view of the fact that isolated sweat glands continue to secrete at temperatures in excess of 43°C (unpublished observations).

It is to be expected that tumors, injuries, or hemorrhages in the central nervous system may cause anhidrosis. Central lesions affecting sweating may also be observed in Parkinsonism and multiple sclerosis (131). Acute pandysautonomia produces acute loss of systemic sweating along with other losses of autonomic functions (209), which may be self-resolving (75). Anhidrosis is frequently associated with disturbances in the autonomic system that create orthostatic hypotension.

Spinal lesions are associated with anhidrosis below the level of the lesion. Consequently, high cervical lesions may predispose the patient to heat stroke (142), but lower cord injury patients usually thermoregulate relatively well even though the threshold for sweating is slightly higher than in normal subjects (190, 194). The magnitude of the deviation from the normal threshold seems to be related to the length of time since injury, but once sweating begins, the overall volume of sweat is only slightly less in paraplegics than in controls. Thus, normal evaporative cooling is maintained in spinal injury patients by increased compensatory sweating from sentient skin (89).

Damage to peripheral nerve tracts results in anhidrosis of a region closely paralleling that of the resulting parasthesia. The response of sweat glands differs markedly to pharmacological stimulation depending upon whether the injury is pre- or post-ganglionic. Post-ganglionic interruption results in the loss of secretory response to drugs within a few days to a few months after trauma, whereas the response is preserved after preganglionic injury (92, 115). Thus, progressive segmental anhydrosis noted with Holmes-Adie syndrome probably involves a peripheral neuronal defect since sweating cannot be induced by either systemic or local injection of acetylcholine or pilocarpine (113, 166). In contrast, idiopathic progressive segmental anhidrosis may occur as a preganglionic lesion (59). In the rare condition of congenital insensitivity to pain with anhidrosis (1, 188) the number of small myelinated nerves is greatly reduced and unmyelinated axons are almost completely lacking (119, 156) so that morphologically normal sweat glands are not innervated (104). It is puzzling that the glands, as might be expected from the postganglionic aberration, do not respond to cholinergic stimulants alone but apparently do respond to simultaneous stimulation with acetylcholine and adrenaline (201). Patients inheriting Anderson-Fabry disease are intolerant of heat due to generalized anhidrosis (202). It was previously assumed that this decrease in sweating was due to deterioration of the sympathetic pathways, but recent findings of pathological changes (cf the section on abnormalities of structure) in the sweat glands may complicate this interpretation (25, 65).

The symptoms expressed in some diabetes mellitus patients may involve the contradiction of hyperhidrosis of the face and shoulders and hands and heat intolerance due to anhidrosis of the extremities and lower body. Abnormalities in neural structure extend through the sympathetic pathways to the nerve fiber around the sweat glands (60). Anhidrosis may be a much more common expression and indication of autonomic neuropathy in diabetic patients than is generally recognized. Goodman (70) reports that 29 of 35 diabetic patients showed detectable anhidrosis.

Physical Damage

Sweat glands damaged physically by burns, scars, electron beam therapy, and skin infections lead to various conditions of anhidrosis. Deep burns and scars destroy sweat glands, which do not regenerate. The observed differences among post-burn subjects managing heat stress, some of whom have difficulty (165) and some of whom appear to manage normally (194), may simply be a function of individual conditioning and climatic conditions. Such subjects attempt to compensate for the loss of sweat glands by increasing the activity of remaining glands (121, 194). Following total body radiation during electron beam therapy, sweat gland function is decreased for several months, greatly increasing the risk of heat stroke. The mechanism of inhibition is not understood, but it probably involves destruction of germinal cells in the sweat duct. Normal sweating returns within six months (143).

Anhidrosis after exfoliating dermatitis was thought to be due to atrophy of the sweat duct (174); however, anhidrosis may develop sufficiently to cause heat intolerance even though sweat gland structure appears normal (30).

Some dermatological disorders may create occlusion of the sweat ducts to such an extent that sweating is substantially, if not completely, inhibited. Common examples are psoriasis and miliaria. Stripping off the stratum corneum in psoriasis increases sweat rates, but not to normal levels (97). The several forms of "prickly heat" or miliaria are all due to occlusion of the sweat duct and subsequent formation of vesicles in the skin (112), but the duct must be blocked for at least 48 hours for miliaria to develop (187), which may be an additional reason that miliaria does not commonly develop from the continual use of antiperspirants. Usually, the anhidrosis resulting from these conditions is local and not of thermoregulatory significance; however, episodes of miliaria may progressively involve more glands to the extent of severe intolerance to heat (174).

Congenital Abnormalities

Anhidrotic ectodermal dysplasia (AED) is a genodermatosis affecting structures developing embryologically from the ectoderm including a paucity or absence of sweat glands. It is classically thought to be inherited as a sex-linked recessive trait (159), but the variety of expressions and the expressions in females creates confusion and debate over classification and mode of inheritance (14, 141). Anhidrosis due to the complete lack of sweat glands may also occur without any of the other traits discernible in AED (98).

The inability to cope with heat stress due to the lack of sweat glands in AED is complicated by the simultaneous inability to regulate cutaneous vasodilation. This finding (18) may explain why AED subjects appear to be even more heat intolerant than cord injury subjects (194). In spite of these limitations, some patients learn to adopt behavioral patterns in thermoregulation that allow them to lead reasonably normal lives (160). The potential for hyperpyrexia in AED may be a precipitating factor in apparent sudden infant death syndrome (12).

Lack of sweating and heat intolerance may be present in several congenital ichthyosiform syndromes (37), but sweat glands are not always absent (199). Complete anhidrosis with a greatly reduced number of sweat glands occurs in rare forms of congenital poikiloderma (139).

COMPOSITION OF SWEAT

Normal Composition

An exact composition of sweat cannot be given and a "normal" range can be defined only for a few solutes. It is well established that the composition of normal sweat, at least with respect to inorganic and small organic solutes, varies greatly as a function of secretory rate. This variation of composition with rate can be explained in an oversimplified manner by assuming that transport processes in the duct tend toward saturation as the secretory load (volume) increases. Thus, in general, as sweat rate increases there is an increase in concentration of those solutes that are reabsorbed and a decrease in the concentration of those solutes that are secreted by the duct. Interpretation of this complex behavior is confounded by the facts that contaminants accumulated in the keritinized layer cannot be excluded easily from collected sweat, that there is significant variation among individuals, that hormones exert dramatic effects on certain constituents, and that undoubtedly there are numerous unrecognized factors also affecting the function of sweat glands.

With the exception of H and K, most electrolytes in sweat appear at concentrations below those in the extracellular fluid (ECF). Usually, the concentration of the major solute, NaCl, in sweat does not exceed 50 mM (39) and in well-acclimatized subjects it may be less than 15 meq/liter (31). HCO_3 decreases rapidly with falling sweat rates from more or less isotonic concentrations to less than 1.0 mM (53, 100, 150). Urea is generally present at levels corresponding to ECF concentrations and not determined by secretory rates (23). K is normally slightly higher in sweat than in the ECF, but as the sweat rate becomes very low, K may exceed 50 mM (55, 151). At low rates, the pH may fall below 5.0 (53). Similarly, Ca^{2+} is usually between 1 and 2 mM but rises exponentially at low sweat rates (54). The concentrations of Mg and PO_4 are in the submillimolar range (138, 145), but there is no data on the variation of these solutes with sweat rate.

Glucose concentration is reported to be usually between 0 and 6.0 mg/100 ml and independent of sweat rate (54, 112). The concentration of lactate ranges from 10 to 30 mM, but seems not to be a function of sweat rate (56, 99). Most amino acids have been detected in sweat at least in micromolar concentrations. Serine is in the highest concentration at about 1.0 mM while proline appears only in sweat from women (109, 110). The concentrations of amino acids in sweat appear to decrease as a function of conditioning (108).

The concentration of total protein in sweat ranges from about 30 to 110 mg per 100 ml. Major protein components are α-globulin, albumin, and a protein electrophoretically similar to, if not, γ-globulin. The presence of the immunoglobulins and specific antibodies to such antigens as tetanus and hepatitis B are assumed to play a protective role against invasion of the gland by external pathogens (20, 134). Like the small amounts of prostaglandin-like substances found in sweat (64), these agents may also play a role in the development of dermatological problems related to hypersensitivity. Small amounts of mucopolysaccharides are also present (135).

Several enzymes are found in sweat, including β-glucuronidase (58); a renin-like substance (52); α-amylase (130); cholinesterase and carboxyesterase, but no lipase (85). The renin-like substance is present at concentrations 30 times that found in the serum, which suggests that it is secreted by the gland for the production of angiotensin whose role, though provocative, is not known.

Not all substances found in sweat are necessarily secreted by the secretory coil. Both K and H are probably secreted by the reabsorptive duct, which, like the proximal tubule, is also capable of secreting certain organic compounds. For example, neutral red and methylene blue are secreted into the lumen of the isolated microperfused duct (151; unpublished observations).

Sweat glands are capable of secreting a variety of dye compounds in vivo
(91) which may be a ductal function.

Elevated NaCl Concentration

Alterations in the NaCl concentration of sweat are the most commonly
identified disorders in sweat composition. Most of these disorders appear
as an increase in NaCl. By far the best known and most intensively studied
abnormality in sweat composition of any type is that associated with the
fatal genetic disease cystic fibrosis (CF). In this disease, which affects the
exocrine glands in general, the concentrations of Na and Cl are almost
without exception above 60 mM (36, 39). While there is considerable overlap between normal and CF sweat, K is about twice as high in the latter
at high secretory rates (150), the residual anion ($Na^+ + K^+ - Cl^-$) also appears to be characteristically low (151). No differences in sweat rate between normal and CF glands have been noted (39, 54, 178).

The defect is reportedly due to the presence of a substance in CF sweat
that inhibits the reabsorptive transport of NaCl in the duct. Perfusion of
normal sweat ducts with CF sweat resulted in a decrease in the uptake of
NaCl (99, 118). The effect has not been observed uniformly (149).

The electrical potential difference between the extracellular fluid and
sweat at the opening of the sweat duct is about twice as negative in CF
glands (–60 mV) as in normal glands (–30 mV) (154). This finding, coupled
with the facts that in CF ducts overall NaCl reabsorption is inhibited and
Na is reabsorbed more rapidly than Cl (150), indicates that the Cl permeability in CF sweat ducts may be significantly lower than in normals. Hence,
independent of whether NaCl reabsorption in the CF duct is blocked by an
inhibitory factor or is due to an inherent defect of the ductal epithelium,
the NaCl transport process seems to be limited by the inability of Cl to move
passively out of the duct in following the active transport of Na (Figure 3).
Since Na cannot be transported without a co-ion without violating the
requirements of electroneutrality, the concentration of NaCl must remain
high in CF sweat (150, 154).

The stimulatory effects of aldosterone on hypertonic Na transport processes are well recognized (31–33). Consequently, any condition that de-
presses levels of aldosterone, such as Addison's disease or panhypopi-
tuitarism, or that blocks the effects of aldosterone, such as spironolactone
treatment, may raise the concentration of sweat NaCl to approach or exceed
100 mM (31). Similarly, Na may be high because the sweat glands are
refractory to the steroid (5).

The relation between pancreatitis, both calcifying and noncalcifying, and
elevated NaCl is more mystifying (7, 76). Although there is considerable
spread in the NaCl concentration values from these patients, more than half

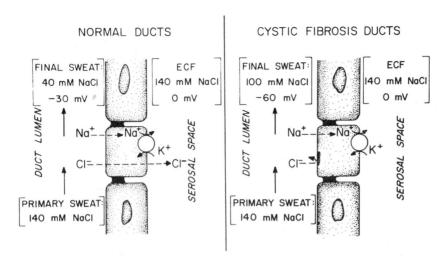

NORMAL DUCTS   CYSTIC FIBROSIS DUCTS

Figure 3 Parameters of NaCl reabsorption in the normal duct (*left*) are compared to those of the cystic fibrosis duct (*right*). The structure of the duct epithelium and the compositions of the primary and final sweat are simplified for illustrative purposes. The inability of Cl to permeate the epithelium of the CF duct (*curved arrow, right panel*) decreases the net transport of Na, resulting in a much higher final sweat concentration of NaCl. Since the Na/K pump continues to "try" to absorb the cation without its anion, the defect also results in an increased separation in charge reflected by a significantly increased electronegative potential across the duct. It is not known whether Cl normally moves through or between ductal cells (cf Figure 2).

have concentrations above 60 mM and half of these are above 90 mM (7). The combined, simultaneous abnormalities in the sweat gland and the pancreas hint of incomplete penetrance of cystic fibrosis, but the findings may also point to a common component in the ductal function in both glands.

Somewhat elevated NaCl concentrations (50–60 mM) have been attributed to nephrogenic diabetes insipidus. The relation is unexplained and vasopressin does not lower the sweat Na concentration (192), but treatment with a thiazide diuretic may (111).

Malnutrition may be a complicating agent in false-positive sweat tests for cystic fibrosis (114, 164), but these results are not without dispute (120).

Several disorders involving carbohydrate metabolism seem to be related to an increase in NaCl in the sweat. In hypothyroidism (myxedema), in which mucopolysaccharides accumulate in subcutaneous tissues, sweat chloride dropped from about 70 mM to less than 40 mM after thyroid extract was administered (116). Na concentrations approaching 200 mM in this disease have been reported (127). Such hypertonic concentrations must indicate either an abnormality in something other than in the reabsorptive process or an error due to evaporation in the collection technique. Elevated NaCl is not a uniformly consistent finding in glucose-6-phosphatase deficiency (glycogen storage disease Type I), but the NaCl in the sweat from a majority of these patients is reported to be above 50 mM (78). In contrast to results in these diseases, the sweat Na is normal in the mucopolysaccharidoses of Hunter's syndrome and Hurler's syndrome (8, 9).

Low NaCl Concentration

Whether or not it is possible to view the NaCl content of sweat as being abnormally low may be a matter of subjective interpretation since it is not uncommon for persons well acclimated to hot environments or strenuous exercise, particularly if the diet is not replete with Na, to lower the sweat NaCl to less than 15 mM (31). In any case, NaCl concentrations below this level are characteristic of the overproduction of corticosteroids in Cushing's syndrome, primary aldosteronism, and congenital aldosteronism (32). In this regard, the enhanced production of aldosterone secondary to cardiac failure, cirrhosis, nephropathies, and other diseases that decrease the effective arterial volume should not be ignored.

Other Abnormalities in Composition

Certain mental illnesses have interesting but unexplained expressions in the composition of sweat. Schizophrenics are reported to present a peculiar odor (182) due to a substance in their sweat identified as methyl hexenoic acid (183), but because of the method of sweat collection it is not clear whether the substance is produced by eccrine, apocrine, or sebaceous glands or is washed out from the skin. Extremely high levels of Na and K in palmar sweat reportedly correspond to the manic phase of manic-depressive illness (137). However, the very hypertonic values (Na = 244 mM; K = 82 mM) in these studies also raise suspicion about technical errors in collection. While speaking of problems related to mental state, we might mention that ethyl alcohol is secreted in sweat in concentrations that approximate its concentration in blood (23). Consequently, certain "induced" abnormalities in mental states are paralleled by abnormalities in sweat composition. Seizing upon this opportunity, it is suggested that a simple ethanol sweat-patch test be used to reveal the "truth" in drinking behavior (140).

Even though Na, Cl and K were not statistically different in sweat from controls and patients on renal dialysis, the concentrations of Ca, Mg, PO_4, and skin resistance are significantly elevated in the sweat from these patients (145). The etiology is not understood, but higher levels of Mg and SO_4 are also observed in parotid saliva from dialysis patients, which may indicate a generalized dysfunction of divalent ion metabolism or a compensatory mechanism expressed in exocrine glands in nephropathy patients (46).

Literature Cited

1. Abbruzzese, M., Gatti, R., Ratto, S., Bugiani, O. 1978. *Acta Neurol. (Napoli)* 33(5):413–18
2. Abell, E., Morgan, K. 1974. *Br. J. Dermatol.* 91:87–91
3. Aguoyo, A. J., Nair, C. P. V., Bray, G. M. 1971. *Arch. Neurol.* 24:106–16
4. Allen, J. A., Roddie, I. C. 1972. *J. Physiol.* 227:801–14
5. Anand, S. K., Froberg, L., Northway, J. D., Weinberger, M., Wright, J. C. 1976. *Pediatr. Res.* 10:677–82
6. Ashby, W. B. 1960. *Br. J. Surg.* 47:406–10
7. Bank, S., Marks, I. N., Novis, B. 1978. *Dig. Dis.* 23:178–81
8. Belcher, R. W. 1972. *Arch. Pathol.* 94:511–18
9. Belcher, R. W. 1973. *Arch. Pathol.* 96:339–41
10. Berglund, L. G., McNall, P. E. Jr. 1973. *J. Appl. Physiol.* 35(5):714–18
11. Bergvist, L., Engevik, L. 1979. *Br. J. Surg.* 66:482–84
12. Bernstein, R., Hatchuel, I., Jenkins, T. 1980. *Lancet* 2:1024
13. Bloor, K. 1969. *Brain* 92:137–46
14. Bocian, M., Rimoin, D. L. 1979. *Birth Defects: Orig. Artic. Ser.* XV(5B):239–51
15. Bock, P. 1979. *Separatum Exp.* 35:538–39
16. Borges, A. F. 1981. *Va. Med.* 108:550–52
17. Breach, N. M. 1979. *Ann. R. Coll. Surg. Engl.* 61:295–97
18. Brengelmann, G. L., Freund, P. R., Rowell, L. B., Olerud, J. E., Kraning, K. K. 1981. *Am. J. Physiol.* 240:H571–75
19. Briggman, J. V., Bank, H. L., Bigelow, J. B., Graves, J. S., Spicer, S. S. 1981. *Am. J. Anat.* 162:357–68
20. Brodersen, M., Wirth, M. 1976. *Acta Hepato-Gastroenterol.* 23(3):193–202
21. Bronshvag, M. M. 1978. *Am. J. Clin. Nutr.* 31:307–9
22. Brunt, P. W., McKusick, V. A. 1970. *Medicine* 49:343–74
23. Brusilow, S. W., Gordes, E. H. 1965. *Am. J. Physiol.* 209(6):1213–18
24. Cabanac, M. 1975. *Ann. Rev. Physiol.* 37:415–439
25. Cable, W. J., Kolodny, E. H., Adams, R. D. 1982. *Neurology* 32(5):498–502
26. Candas, V., Libert, J. P., Vogt, J. J. 1979. *J. Appl. Physiol.* 46(3):522–28
27. Carpenter, S., Karpati, G. 1981. *Neurology* 31(12):1564–68
28. Cloward, R. B. 1969. *J. Neurosurg.* 30:545–50

29. Collan, Y., Meretoja, J. 1978. *Ann. Clin. Res.* 10:43–47
30. Commens, C. A., Greaves, M. W. 1978. *Clin. Exp. Dermatol.* 3:99–101
31. Conn, J. W. 1963. *J. Am. Med. Assoc.* 183:775–81
32. Conn, J. W. 1963. *J. Am. Med. Assoc.* 183:871–78
33. Conn, J. W. 1949. *Arch. Intern. Med.* 83:416–28
34. Constantine, V. S., Mowry, R. W. 1966. *J. Invest. Dermatol.* 46(6):536–41
35. Cullen, S. I. 1972. *Postgrad. Med.* 52:77
36. Davis, P. B., Hubbard, V. S., di Sant'Agnese, P. A. 1980. *Am. J. Med.* 69:643–46
37. Der Kaloustian, V. M., Kurban, A. K. 1979. *Genetic Diseases of the Skin.* Berlin: Springer-Verlag
38. Diamond, J. M., Bossert, W. H. 1968. *J. Gen. Physiol.* 50:2061–83
39. di Sant'Agnese, P. A., Powell, G. F. 1962. *Ann. NY Acad. Sci.* 93:555–99
40. Dobson, R. L. 1962. *Advances in Biology of the Skin, Vol. III, Eccrine Sweat Glands and Eccrine Sweating,* ed. W. Montagna, R. A. Ellis, A. F. Silver, pp. 54–75. Oxford: Pergamon. 266 pp.
41. Dobson, R. L., Lobitz, W. C. Jr. 1957. *Arch. Dermatol.* 75:653–66
42. Dorge, A., Rick, R., Gehring, K., Thurau, K. 1978. *Pfluegers Arch.* 373:85–97
43. Drut, R. 1978. *J. Cutaneous Pathol.* 5:35–36
44. Duller, P., Gentry, W. D. 1980. *Br. J. Dermatol.* 103:143–46
45. Dunbar, H. F. 1935. *Emotions and Bodily Changes.* New York: Columbia Univ. Press
46. Earlbaum, A. M., Quinton, P. M. 1981. *Nephron* 28:58–61
47. Elizondo, R. S. 1973. *Fed. Proc.* 32(5):1583–87
48. Ellis, H. 1979. *Am. Surg.* 45(9):546–51
49. Ellis, H. 1972. *Br. J. Hosp. Med.* May, pp. 641–44
50. Ellis, H., Scurr, J. H. 1979. *Postgrad. Med. J.* 55:868–69
51. Ellis, R. A. 1962. See Ref. 40, pp. 30–53
52. Emrich, H. M., Dahlheim, H. 1977. *Klin. Wochenschr.* 55:291–92
53. Emrich, H. M., Oelert, H. 1966. *Pfluegers Arch.* 290:311–14
54. Emrich, H. M., Stoll, E., Friolet, B., Colombo, J. P., Richterich, R., Rossi, E. 1968. *Pediatr. Res.* 2:464–78
55. Emrich, H. M., Ullrich, K. J. 1966. *Pfluegers Arch. Gesamte Physiol. Menschen Tiere* 290:298–310
56. Emrich, H. M., Zweibel, R. K. H. 1966. *Pfluegers Arch.* 290:315–19

57. Eng, A. M., Mandrea, E. 1981. *J. Cutaneous Pathol.* 8:247–50
58. Evans, B. W., Kelsch, R. C., Howatt, W. F. 1974. *Am. J. Dis. Child.* 127:660–62
59. Faden, A. I., Chan, P., Mendoza, E. 1982. *Arch. Neurol.* 39:172–75
60. Faerman, I., Faccio, E., Calb, I., Razumny, J., Franco, N., Dominguez, A., Podesta, H. A. 1982. *Diabetologia* 22:96–99
61. Field, M. 1982. *Fluid and Electrolyte Abnormalities in Exocrine Glands in Cystic Fibrosis,* ed. P. M. Quinton, J. R. Martinez, U. Hopfer, pp. 227–39. San Francisco: San Francisco Press
62. Fortney, S. M., Nadel, E. R., Wenger, C. B., Bove, J. R. 1981. *J. Appl. Physiol.* 51(6)1594–1600
63. Frankland, J. C., Seville, R. H. 1971. *Br. J. Dermatol.* 85:578–81
64. Frewin, D. B., Eakins, K. E., Downey, J. A., Bhattacherjee, P. 1973. *Aust. J. Exp. Biol. Med. Sci.* 51:701–2
65. Fukuhara, N., Suzuki, M., Fujita, N., Tsubaki, T. 1975. *Acta Neuropatho.l (Berl.)* 33:9–21
66. Galosi, A., Pullmann, H., Steigleder, G. K. 1980. *Arch. Dermatol. Res.* 268:257-60
67. Geschickter, E. H., Andrews, P. A., Bullard, R. W. 1966. *J. Appl. Physiol.* 21:623–30
68. Gibbs, G. E. 1967. *Modern Problems in Pediatrics Cystic Fibrosis: Physiology and Pathophysiology of Serous Secretion, Clinical Investigations and Therapy,* ed. E. Rossi, E. Stoll, 10:95–99. Basel: Karger. 404 pp.
69. Glaister, D. H., Hearnshaw, J. R., Heffron, P. F., Peck, A. W. 1958. *Br. Med. J.* 2:942–46
70. Goodman, J. I. 1966. *Am. J. Med.* 41:831–35
71. Greenebaum, E. 1980. *Human Pathol.* 2(3):287–89
72. Greenhalgh, R. M., Rosengarten, D. S., Martin, P. 1971. *Br. Med. J.* 1:332–34
73. Grice, K., Sattar, H., Baker, H. 1972. *Br. J. Dermatol.* 86:72–78
74. Grice, K., Verbov, J. 1977. *Recent Advances in Dermatology,* ed. A. Rook, pp. 155–98. Edinburgh: Churchill Livingston
75. Guidi, L., Zeppilli, P., Sassara, M., Ghirlanda, G. 1981. *G. Ital. Cardiol.* 11:1151–59
76. Hanawa, M., Takebe, T., Takahashi, S., Koizumi, M., Endo, K. 1978. *Tohoku J. Exp. Med.* 125:59–69
77. Harahap, M. 1979. *J. Dermatol. Surg. Oncol.* 5:223–25
78. Harris, R. C., Cohen, H. I. 1963. *Pediatrics* 31:1044–46
79. Harrison, K., Donaldson, I. 1979. *J. R. Soc. Med.* 72:503–8
80. Hashimoto, K. 1971. *Ultrastructure Res.* 36:249–62
81. Hashimoto, K. 1978. *The Physiology and Pathophysiology of the Skin,* ed. A. Jarret, 5:1544–74. London: Academic. 326 pp.
82. Hashimoto, K. 1978. See Ref. 81, 5:1575–96
83. Haxton, H. A. 1948. *Brain* 71:16–25
84. Hays, L. L. 1978. *Laryngoscope* 88:1796–1824
85. Herrmann, W. P., Habbig, J. 1976. *Br. J. Dermatol.* 95:67–70
86. Hill, A. C., Baker, G. F., Jansen, G. T. 1981. *Cutis* 28(1):69–72
87. Hill, B. H. R. 1976. *Aust. J. Dermatol.* 17:92–93
88. Holloway, R. M., Singleton, G. T. 1967. *Eye, Ear, Nose Throat Mon.* 46:316–24
89. Huckaba, C. E., Frewin, D. B., Downey, J. A., Tam, H. S., Darling, R. C., Cheh, H. Y. 1976. *Arch. Phys. Med. Rehabil.* 57:268–74
90. Hurley, H. J., Shelley, W. F. 1966. *Br. J. Dermatol.* 78:127–40
91. Hurley, H. J., Witkowski, J. 1961. *J. Invest. Dermatol.* 36:259–72
92. Hyndman, O. R., Wolkin, J. 1941. *Arch. Neurol. Psychiatry* 45:446–67
93. Iskandar, S., Bradshaw, C. M., Szabadi, E. 1980. *Br. J. Clin. Pharmacol.* 10:303–5
94. Janka, H. U., Standl, E., Mehnert, H. 1979. *Ann. Intern. Med.* 91(1):130
95. Jarrett, A., Morimoto, T. 1978. See Ref. 81, 5:1597–1610
96. Jebson, R. P., Harris, J. D. 1976. *Australas. J. Dermatol.* 17:90–91
97. Johnson, C., Shuster, S. 1969. *Br. J. Dermatol.* 81:119–24
98. Juhlin, L., Evers, H., Broberg, F. 1979. *Acta Derm. Venereol.* 59:556–59
99. Kaiser, D., Drack, E., Rossi, E. 1970. *Lancet* 1:1003
100. Kaiser, D., Songo-Williams, R., Drack, E. 1974. *Pfluegers Arch.* 349:63–72
101. Kaliner, M. 1976. *J. Allergy Clin. Immunol.* 58(2):308–15
102. Kuno, Y. 1956. *Human Perspiration,* ed. R. F. Pitts. Springfield, Ill: Thomas
103. Kuypers, B. R. M., Cotton, D. W. K. 1972. *Br. J. Dermatol.* 87:154–60
104. Langer, J., Goebel, H. H., Veit, S. 1981. *Acta Neuropathol. (Berl.)* 54:199–202
105. Lee, T. S. 1954. *J. Physiol. (Lond.)* 124:528–42
106. Lerer, B., Jacobowitz, J., Wahba, A.

1980. *Intl. J. Psychiatry Med.* 10(1): 59–67
107. Levit, F. 1980. *Cutis* 26:192–94
108. Liappis, N., Janssen, E., Kesseler, K., Hildenbrand, G. 1980. *Eur. J. Appl. Physiol.* 45:63–67
109. Liappis, N., Jakel, A. 1975. *Arch. Dermatol. Res.* 254:185–203
110. Liappis, N., Kochbeck, E., Eckhardt, G., Hahne, H., Kesseler, K., Bantzer, P. 1980. *Arch. Dermatol. Res.* 269:311–23
111. Lobeck, C. C., Barta, R. A., Mangos, J. A. 1963. *J. Pediatr.* 62:868–75
112. Lobitz, W. C. Jr., Osterberg, A. E. 1947. *Arch. Dermatol. Syphilol.* 56: 827–33
113. Lucy, D. D., Van Allen, M. W., Thompson, H. S. 1967. *Neurology* 17(1):763–69
114. Mace, J. W., Schanberger, J. E. 1971. *Clin. Pediatr.* 10:285–86
115. MacMillan, A. L., Spalding, J. M. K. 1969. *J. Neurol. Neurosurg. Psychiatry* 32:155–60
116. Madoff, L. 1968. *J. Pediatr.* 73:244–46
117. Mangos, J. 1973. *Am. J. Physiol.* 224: 1235–40
118. Mangos, J. A. 1973. *Tex. Rep. Biol. Med.* 31:651–63
119. Matsuo, M., Kurokawa, T., Goya, N., Ohta, M. 1981. *Neurology* 31:1190–92
120. McCance, R. A., Rutishauser, I. H. E., Knight, H. C. 1968. *Lancet* 1:663–65
121. McGibbon, B., van Beaumont, W., Strand, J., Paletta, F. X. 1973. *Plast. Reconstr. Surg.* 52(2):164–70
122. Means, M. A., Dobson, R. L. 1963. *J. Am. Med. Assoc.* 186:113–15
123. Mehregan, A. H. 1981. *Am. J. Dermatopathol.* 3(1):27–31
124. Mellinkoff, S. M., Mellinkoff, J. 1950. *J. Am. Med. Assoc.* 142:901–2
125. Montagna, W., Parakkal, P. F. 1974. *The Structure and Function of Skin.* New York: Academic
126. Morgan, L. O., Vonderahe, A. R. 1939. *Arch. Neurol. Psychiatry* 42:83–91
127. Morse, W. I., Cochrane, W. A., Landrigan, P. L. 1971. *N. Engl. J. Med.* 264:1021–26
128. Munro, D. D., Julian, L. V., O'Gorman, D. J., Du Vivier, A. 1974. *Br. J. Dermatol.* 90:325–29
129. Nadel, E. R. 1979. *Med. Sci. Sports,* 11(1):31–35
130. Nikolajek, W. P., Emrich, H. M. 1976. *Eur. J. Pediatr.* 122:289–91
131. Noronha, M. J., Vas, C. J., Aziz, H. 1968. *J. Neurol. Neurosurg. Psychiatry* 31:19–22
132. O'Donoghue, G., Finn, D., Brady, M. P. 1980. *J. Pediatr. Surg.* 15(2):172–74

133. Ogawa, T. 1970. *J. Appl. Physiol.* 28(1): 18–22
134. Page, C. O. Jr., Remington, J. S. 1967. *J. Lab. Clin. Med.* 69(4):634–50
135. Pallavicini, J. C., Gabriel, O., di Sant-'Agnese, P. A., Buskirk, E. R. 1963. *NY Acad. Sci. Ann.* 106:330–38
136. Parisier, S. C., Binder, W. J., Blitzer, A., Friedman, W. H., Marowitz, W. F. 1978. *Ear Nose Throat J.* 57:51–73/213–25
137. Paschalis, C., Jenner, F. A., Lee, C. R., Hill, S. E., Jennings, G., Triccas, G. 1977. *Lancet* 1:502
138. Paunier, L., Girardin, E., Sizonenko, P. C., Wyss, M., Megevand, A. 1973. *Pediatrics* 52:446–48
139. Person, J. R., Perry, H. O. 1979. *Acta Derm. Venereol.* 59:347–51
140. Phillips, M., McAloon, M. H. 1980. *Alcoholism Clin Exp. Res.* 4:391–95
141. Pinheiro, M., Freire-Maia, N. 1982. *Arch. Dermatol.* 118:215–16
142. Pledger, H. G. 1962. *J. Bone Jt. Surg.* 44B:110–13
143. Price, N. M. 1979. *Arch. Dermatol.* 115:1068–70
144. Prompt, C. A., Quinton, P. M. 1978. *Nature* 272(5649):171–72
145. Prompt, C. A., Quinton, P. M., Kleeman, C. R. 1978. *Nephron* 20:4–9
146. Prout, B. J., Wardell, W. M. 1969. *Clin. Sci.* 36:109–17
147. Quatrale, R. P., Coble, D. W., Stoner, K. L., Felger, C. B. 1981. *J. Soc. Cosmet. Chem.* 32:107–36
148. Quatrale, R. P., Waldman, A. H., Rogers, J. G., Felger, C. B. 1981. *J. Soc. Cosmet. Chem.* 32:67–73
149. Quinton, P. M. 1982. *Cystic Fibrosis Club Abstr. 23rd Ann. Meet.* 23:77. Rockville, Md: Cystic Fibrosis Found.
150. Quinton, P. M. 1982. See Ref. 61, pp. 53–76
151. Quinton, P. M. 1982. *Pediatr. Res.* 16:533–37
152. Quinton, P. M. 1981. *Pfluegers Arch.* 391:309–13
153. Quinton, P. M. 1979. *Comparative Animal Nutrition: Nitrogen, Electrolytes, Water and Energy Metabolism,* ed. M. Rechcigl, 3:100–231. Basel: Karger
154. Quinton, P. M., Bijman, J. 1982. *Physiologist* 25(4):335
155. Quinton, P. M., Tormey, J. M. 1976. *J. Membr. Biol.* 29:383–99
156. Rafel, E., Alberca, R., Bautista, J., Navarrete, M., Lazo, J. 1980. *Muscle Nerve* 3:216–20
157. Raff, S. B., Gershberg, H. 1975. *J. Am. Med. Assoc.* 234(12):1252–53

158. Rayner, C. R. W., Ritchie, I. D., Stark, G. P. 1980. *Br. Med. J.* 280:1168
159. Reed, W. B., Lopez, D. A., Landing, B. 1970. *Arch. Dermatol.* 102:134–43
160. Rietschel, R. L. 1979. *Int. J. Dermatol.* 18(5):370–81
161. Rigg, B. M. 1977. *Plast. Reconstr. Surg.* 59(3):334–42
162. Robertshaw, D. 1979. *Med. Hypotheses* 5:317–22
163. Robertshaw, D. 1977. *J. Invest. Dermatol.* 69:121–29
164. Rosenfeld, R., Spigelblatt, L., Chicoine, R. 1979. *J. Pediatr.* 94(2):240–42
165. Roskind, J. L., Petrofsky, J., Lind, A. R., Paletta, F. X. 1978. *Ann. Plast. Surg.* 1(2):172–76
166. Ross, A. T. 1958. *Neurology* 8:809–17
167. Sato, K. 1977. *Rev. Physiol. Biochem. Pharmacol.* 79:52–97
168. Sato, K., Dobson, R. L. 1970. *J. Invest. Dermatol.* 55:53–56
169. Sato, K., Sato, F. 1981. *Am. J. Physiol.* 241(Cell Physiol. 10):C133–20
170. Sato, K., Sato, F. 1981. *Pfluegers Arch.* 390:49–53
171. Schulz, I. J. 1969. *J. Clin. Invest.* 48(8):1470–77
172. Shelley, W. B., Horvath, P. M. 1951. *J. Invest. Dermatol.* 16:267–74
173. Shelley, W., Horvath, P., Weidman, F., et al. 1948. *J. Invest. Dermatol.* 11:275
174. Shelley, W. B., Horvath, P. N., Pillsbury, D. M. 1950. *Medicine* 29:195–224
175. Shelly, W. B., Hurley, H. J. Jr. 1975. *Acta Derm. Venereol.* 55:241–60
176. Shih, C. J., Lin, M. T. 1979. *J. Neurosurg.* 50:88–94
177. Shih, C. J., Lin, M. T. 1980. *J. Neurosurg.* 53:684–89
178. Sibinga, M. S., Barbero, G. J. 1963. *J. Appl. Physiol.* 18(6):1226–30
179. Singleton, G. T., Cassisi, N. J. 1980. *Laryngoscope* 90:1636–39
180. Slegers, J. F. G. 1964. *Research on Pathogenesis of Cystic Fibrosis of the Pancreas (Mucoviscidosis)*, ed. P. A. di Sant'Agnese, pp. 119–28. Bethesda: NIH. 365 pp.
181. Smiles, K. A., Elizondo, R. S., Barney, C. C. 1976. *J. Appl. Physiol.* 40(5):653–57
182. Smith, K., Sines, J. 1960. *Arch. Gen. Psychiatry* 2:184
183. Smith, K., Thompson, G. F., Koster, H. D. 1969. *Science* 166:398–99
184. Sohar, E., Shoenfeld, U., Udassin, R., Magazanik, A., Revach, M. 1978. *Lancet* 2:1073–74
185. Sokolov, V. E., Shabadash, S. A.,

Zelikina, T. I. 1980. Transl. from *Izv. Akad. Nauk SSSR, Ser. Biol.* No. 5, Sept.-Oct. pp. 655–70
186. Stuart, D. D. 1978. *Ann. Intern. Med.* 89:223–24
187. Sulzberger, M. B., Griffin, T. B. 1969. *Arch. Dermatol.* 99:145–51
188. Swanson, A. G. 1963. *Arch. Neurol.* 8:299–306
189. Szabadi, E., Gaszner, P., Bradshaw, C. M. 1980. *Br. J. Clin. Pharmacol.* 10:301–3
190. Tam, H. S., Darling, R. C., Chen, H. Y., Downey, J. A. 1978. *Can. J. Physiol. Pharmacol.* 56:976–83
191. Tataryn, I. V., Lomax, P., Bajorek, J. G., Chesarek, W., Meldrum, D. R., Judd, H. L. 1980. *Maturitas* 2:101–7
192. Taussig, L. M., Braunstein, G. D. 1973. *J. Invest. Dermatol.* 60(4):197–202
193. Thorner, M. O., Chait, A., Aitken, M., Benker, G., Bloom, S. R., Mortimer, C. H., Sanders, P., Stuart Mason, A., Besser, G. M. 1975. *Br. Med. J.* 1:299–303
194. Totel, G. L. 1974. *J. Appl. Physiol.* 37(3):346–52
195. Uno, H. 1977. *J. Invest. Dermatol.* 69:112–20
196. Uno, H., Montagna, W. 1975. *Cell Tissue Res.* 158:1–13
197. Ussing, H. H., Zerahn, K. 1951. *Acta Phys. Scand.* 23:110–27
198. van Beaumont, W., Bullard, R. W. 1963. *Science* 141:643–46
199. van Everdingen, J. J. E., Rampen, R. H. J., van der Schaar, W. W. 1982. *Acta Derm. Venereol.* 62:76–78
200. Varma, A. J., Fisher, B. K., Sarin, M. K. 1977. *Arch. Intern. Med.* 137:1207–10
201. Vassella, F., Emrich, H. M., Kraus-Ruppert, R., Aufdermaur, F., Tonz, O. 1968. *Arch. Dis. Child.* 43:124–30
202. Wallace, H. J. 1973. *Br. J. Dermatol.* 88:1–23
203. Warndorff, J. A. 1970. *Br. J. Dermatol.* 83:306–11
204. Warndorff, J. A. 1971. *Br. J. Dermatol.* 86:282–85
205. Watkins, P. J. 1973. *Br. Med. J.* 1:583–87
206. Weaver, P. C., Copeman, P. W. M. 1971. *Proc. R. Soc. Med.* 64:607
207. Werde, C., Busch, F. 1909. *J. Am. Med. Assoc.* 53:207
208. Yasuda, K., Montagna, W. 1960. *J. Histochem. Cytochem.* 8:356–66
209. Young, K., Asbury, A. K., Adams, R. D., Corbett, J. L. 1969. *Trans. Am. Neurol.* 94:355

Ann. Rev. Med. 1983. 34:453–71

THE NATURAL HISTORY
OF FEBRILE SEIZURES[1]

Deborah G. Hirtz, M.D., and Karin B. Nelson, M.D.

Developmental Neurology Branch, National Institute of Neurological and
Communicative Disorders and Stroke

ABSTRACT

Febrile seizures are a common occurrence in early childhood and most
children who experience them do well. This article reviews the clinical
characteristics of febrile seizures, and summarizes the relevant clinical and
laboratory research. The natural history of febrile seizures, the recurrence
rate, and frequency of later epilepsy or intellectual handicap is presented,
and controversies in evaluation and treatment are discussed.

"A febrile seizure is an event in infancy or childhood, usually occurring between three
months and five years of age, associated with fever but without evidence of intracranial
infection or defined cause. Seizures with fever in children who have suffered a previous
nonfebrile seizure are excluded. Febrile seizures are to be distinguished from epilepsy,
which is characterized by recurrent nonfebrile seizures." (1)

The above definition was offered by a recent National Institutes of Health
(NIH) consensus conference on the management of febrile seizures. Young
children may experience seizures with fever that do not fit this definition.
Both convulsions and fever may occur together in such disorders as meningitis, hypernatremic dehydration, and toxic encephalopathy. Since these
illnesses may damage the brain even if no seizures occur, it is important to
exclude seizures that occur in clinical settings such as these when considering the natural history and prognosis of febrile seizures.

Estimated prevalence of febrile seizures ranges from 2 to 5% of young
children in the United States, making it the most common convulsive
disorder of early childhood (2–5). Almost two thirds of all young children
who experience a seizure have febrile seizures only (5).

[1]The US Government has the right to retain a nonexclusive royalty-free license in and to
any copyright covering this paper.

453

CLINICAL CHARACTERISTICS

Febrile seizures usually occur in children who are apparently normal, but they may also occur in children with neurologic abnormalities. Febrile seizures may be of any type, but most often they are generalized motor or, less commonly, focal motor; they are usually brief and self-limited.

The majority of febrile seizures begin by age three years (6) and the average age of onset is 18–22 months (7). The male:female ratio has been reported to range from 1.1:1 to 4:1 (4, 6).

Febrile seizures usually occur in the presence of a clinically recognizable infection, with central nervous system (CNS) infections excluded by definition. Among the most commonly associated illnesses are upper respiratory infections, otitis media, gastrointestinal infections, and roseola infantum. Lewis and others (8) recently documented viral infection in 87% of children admitted to hospital for a first febrile seizure. In addition to infection, any environmental factor such as an immunization that can lead to elevated temperature in a young child can trigger a seizure. Some and perhaps most of those seizures occurring soon after immunization may have the same mechanism as febrile seizures, as they are similar with regard to elevated temperature, age, family and personal history of febrile convulsions, and long-term outcome (9).

In two large population-based studies there was a slightly higher incidence in blacks than in whites, but the excess was not statistically significant (3, 4). Febrile seizures are reported to be about twice as common in certain Asian countries as in Western communities, and the recurrence rates are also higher. Ascertainment may be better in these countries because of high housing density with greater opportunity for observing a sleeping child. Also, rate and type of infectious diseases as well as genetic susceptibility may be different in different geographic areas (10).

GENETICS

It is generally agreed that there is a genetic predisposition to febrile convulsions (11–15). The exact pattern of heredity is unknown. A dominant mode of inheritance with reduced penetrance (16) or polygenic inheritance (17) appears most likely. Data from Rochester, Minnesota, shows siblings and offspring of patients with febrile convulsions to have a two- to threefold increase in risk (16). The prevalence of epilepsy in relatives of probands with febrile convulsions was no higher than in the general population in two large studies (15, 18). Others report some increase in frequency of nonfebrile seizures among siblings of febrile seizure probands (11, 19).

Electroencephalographic (EEG) evidence for genetic factors was reported by Metrakos & Metrakos (11), who found a high prevalence (47%)

of centrencephalic EEG recordings (3 per second spike/wave) in their sample of febrile seizure patients, and a relatively high prevalence of this EEG abnormality in parents and siblings. More support for the role of genetic factors in susceptibility to febrile convulsions was offered by Tay (20), who found an increase in dermatoglyphic abnormalities in children with febrile convulsions and in their parents.

PATHOPHYSIOLOGY

Neither experimental nor clinical experience has revealed a definitive mechanism for febrile convulsions. Circulating toxins, immune reactions (21), viral and bacterial invasion (8), relative lack of myelination and increased oxygen consumption in the immature febrile brain (6) have all been implicated in the pathogenesis. Early animal experiments by Wegman (21) led to the hypothesis that the height of the temperature and the rapidity of its rise were important factors. More recently, others have stressed immaturity of thermoregulatory mechanisms (22) and limited capacity of young animals to increase cellular energy metabolism at elevated temperatures (23). Yet another investigator suggests the hormone arginine vasopressin may play a role as a neuromodulator in the pathogenesis of febrile seizures (24). Whether it is a rapid rise of fever, the height of body temperature attained, or associated factors that trigger the seizure remains unknown.

Stephenson (25) proposed and clinically tested the hypothesis that vagally mediated asystole causes some febrile seizures. Another clinical study found in some febrile seizure patients a decrease in serum levels of immunoglobulin A, which may have led to frequent infectious illnesses (26).

Cerebrospinal Fluid Biochemical Findings

Spinal fluid has been examined for biochemical abnormalities in children with febrile convulsions. Neurotransmitter metabolites 5-hydroxyindoleacetic acid and homovanillic acid were not altered in febrile seizure patients (27). In cerebrospinal fluid (CSF) obtained within two hours after febrile convulsions, decreased levels of gamma-aminobutyric acid may have represented a pre-existing impairment of neurotransmission or may have been secondary to the convulsion (28). Biochemical signs of cerebral hypoxia were examined through lactate and pyruvate concentrations in 29 children 3–22 hours after febrile convulsions of less than 30 minutes duration (29). Alterations in CSF findings were seen in only two of the patients, one of whom had had brief repeated convulsions. The authors concluded hypoxic damage was unlikely to result from febrile convulsions of short duration. Investigators who looked at CSF and serum proteins in children within a short time after a febrile convulsion found no evidence of a disturbance of the blood brain barrier (30, 31). They therefore felt that cerebral inflammation was unlikely to be the cause of febrile seizures.

Effects of Experimental Febrile Seizures

The effects of experimental febrile convulsions on the developing brain have been studied in animal models. Both Wegman (21) and Lennox et al (32) found neuronal damage after experimental febrile convulsions, but could not distinguish the pathological changes from those caused by hyperthermia alone. Neuronal alterations typical of ischemic cell changes were seen in young baboons after prolonged seizures that were accompanied by hyperpyrexia, acidosis, hypoxia, and hypotension (33). Vannucci (34) pointed out that, in these animal models of febrile convulsions, one must induce temperatures well above those seen in the clinical setting, and that neuropathological changes are related to superimposed acidosis, hypoxemia, and hypotension as well as to hyperthermia.

McCaughran & Schechter (22) reported that rat pups who had infantile febrile convulsions were more susceptible to effects of a convulsant drug; they also found reductions in cholinergic receptor sites and synthetic enzymes in brains of adult rats subjected to experimental febrile convulsions as infants. Nealis and co-workers (35) showed later deficits in maze learning ability in rats subjected as neonates to a single experimental hyperthermic convulsion. In contrast, Werboff & Havlena (36) could find no lasting effect on body weight, learning ability, or audiogenic seizure susceptibility in rats who convulsed with fever in the neonatal period. In these animal studies, the temperature elevations required to produce seizures were extreme. Vannucci (37) concluded that we do not have a good experimental model of febrile seizures, and thus that extrapolations to the clinical situation are of uncertain validity.

NATURAL HISTORY

The natural history of febrile convulsions has been widely discussed. At issue are the recurrence of febrile seizures, the likelihood of subsequent nonfebrile seizures or epilepsy, the question of partial complex seizures as specific sequelae, and the later neurologic and intellectual outcome of children with febrile convulsions.

Recurrences

Although relatively few children who experience a febrile seizure ever develop nonfebrile seizures or epilepsy (see below), many experience recurrences of febrile seizures. In the Collaborative Perinatal Project (NCPP) of the National Institute of Neurological and Communicative Disorders and

Stroke, about a third of children had at least one recurrence: of those, half had two or more (3), and 9% had three or more recurrences of febrile seizure. Three fourths of recurrences took place within one year of the first febrile seizure, and 90% within two years. Van den Berg & Yerushalmy (4) found a similar recurrence rate.

The only consistent important factor in predicting likelihood of recurrence was early age of onset. The younger the child at his first attack, the more likely he was to have another febrile seizure. In the NCPP, convulsions that were complex (i.e. focal, lasting longer than 15 minutes, followed by transient or persistent neurologic deficit, or multiple in one day) were not more often followed by recurrences (3). The risk of a prolonged recurrence was quite small. After an initial brief seizure, only 1.4% of recurrences lasted thirty minutes or more, and none of these children went on to have nonfebrile seizures.

The total number of febrile seizures a child experiences appears little related to the eventual outcome. Ellenberg & Nelson found that recurrences had no effect on intelligence testing at age seven (38). With regard to epilepsy, children who have febrile seizure recurrences remain at relatively low risk. In two large studies, antecedent risk factors played a more important role in the prediction of later epilepsy than did number of febrile seizures (3, 4). Among all children with febrile seizures in the NCPP, the rate of nonfebrile seizures was less than 5% whether or not there were recurrences (Figure 1). A full discussion of the impact of recurrences on outcome in children with febrile seizures can be found in a recent review (39).

Epilepsy

Opinions regarding the likelihood of epilepsy following febrile seizures have varied considerably depending on the population studied. The older literature generally dealt with highly selected populations of hospitalized children or those from specialty referral centers, and most were retrospective (13, 14, 40–44). Such studies showed a great deal of variation in frequency of unfavorable outcome, from 2.6 to 76.9% (45). The report from the British National Child Development Study further emphasizes this difference in outcome based on sample selection: of 202 febrile seizure patients seen by general practitioners in England, 0.5% had subsequent nonfebrile seizures. In contrast, 19 of 164 (12%) admitted to hospitals or referred to specialists had subsequent nonfebrile seizures (46).

Livingston found an extremely high rate of epilepsy (93%) in children with prolonged febrile seizures, abnormal EEGs, age over six years, or with focal febrile seizures. He called these convulsions "epileptic seizures precipitated by fever" (47). Later investigators failed to confirm this high rate of

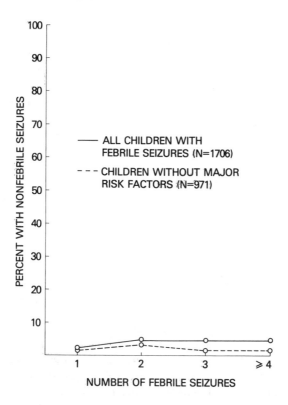

Figure 1 Percentage of children who developed nonfebrile seizures by age 7 years of 1706 children in the NCPP with febrile seizures, according to the number of febrile seizures experienced. The major risk factors were history of nonfebrile seizures in the immediate family, suspect or abnormal status prior to the first febrile seizure, and complex first febrile seizure.

epilepsy, but established that there is some increase in risk for later epilepsy among children with some of the risk factors Livingston stressed. For example, Nelson and Ellenberg delineated the following as risk factors: suspect or abnormal neurologic development prior to the first febrile seizure, a history of nonfebrile seizures in a parent or sibling, and a complex first febrile seizure, that is, one that is focal, lasts over 15 minutes, or is multiple in one day.

The rate of epilepsy is considerably lower in population-based studies: 1.5–4.6% (45). Of the 60% of children in the NCPP with febrile convulsions with none of the above risk factors, about 1% had at least one nonfebrile seizure by age seven; this rate was no different from the population as a whole. Of the 34% of children with febrile convulsions with one risk factor, 3% experienced at least one nonfebrile seizure. The highest rate of nonfebrile seizures, 13%, occurred in the 6% of children in the cohort with two or more risk factors (Figure 2). While onset of febrile seizures in the first year, and especially in the first six months of life, was associated with a higher risk of epilepsy (7), once the major risk factors of prior abnormal development, positive family history, and complex features were considered in the analysis, age of onset did not add significant additional predictive power (3). Van den Berg & Yerushalmy (4) reported a rate of nonfebrile seizures following febrile seizures of 3.1% in a five-year follow-up, which was three times the rate of controls. Hauser & Kurland (48) reported a 3% rate of later nonfebrile seizures.

Although the risk of epilepsy following febrile seizures is increased in identifiable groups, most who go on to develop epilepsy do not have any risk factors. Perhaps in the future other factors will be identified that place specific children at higher risk. In an interesting recent report, cytomegalovirus was found in the urine of children who developed nonfebrile seizures after febrile about twice as often as in children who did not develop nonfebrile seizures (49).

If nonfebrile seizures do develop, they usually have their onset relatively soon: 75% began within the first three years after the initial febrile seizure in a study with follow-up to age seven (7). The Rochester, Minnesota, cohort was followed to age 20, and, although the risk of epilepsy was quite low as in other population-based studies, it was increased over controls on into the third decade (18).

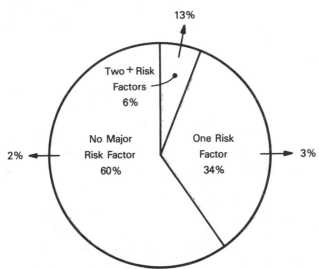

Figure 2   Nonfebrile seizures by age 7 years in children with febrile seizures, based on results from the NCPP on the outcomes of 1706 children. The risk factors were history of nonfebrile seizures in the immediate family, suspect or abnormal status prior to the first febrile seizure, and complex first febrile seizure. [From Ellenberg & Nelson (78), with permission.]

Thus, although the absolute risk of nonfebrile seizures following febrile is quite low, it is increased in children with febrile seizures relative to those who have none, but the increased rate of later epilepsy is confined to a subgroup of children with identifiable risk factors.

Partial Complex Seizures

It has been proposed that febrile seizures may increase the risk for partial complex seizures (temporal lobe or psychomotor epilepsy). Falconer (50) reported his experience with patients undergoing temporal lobectomy for intractable temporal lobe seizures. He found a history of prolonged febrile convulsions more often in those patients who demonstrated mesial temporal sclerosis than in those without that lesion. These patients were a highly selected referral group, and the definition of febrile convulsions employed by Falconer did not exclude acute neurologic illness at the time of the convulsion. In another surgical series of patients with focal epilepsy, Rasmussen (51) pointed out that when isolated febrile convulsions preceded complex partial seizures, they were usually due to an infectious agent or neurologic disease predating the febrile convulsions.

In nonsurgical series, Ounsted et al (52) found that 32% of 100 temporal lobe epilepsy patients had a history of prolonged febrile seizures. This series was retrospective, uncontrolled, and, like Falconer's, did not exclude seizures with fever and acute CNS infection. In prospective but highly selected referral or hospital populations (42, 43) the proportion of children who later developed complex partial seizures was higher than in unselected studies. Lee, Diaz & Melchior (53a) studied 362 unselected children with febrile convulsions (excluding convulsions accompanying CNS infection). They found the proportion of temporal lobe epilepsy in those 2% with epilepsy in adulthood to be the same as in a random population of epileptics.

Prospective population-based studies (7, 48) do not show an excess of complex partial epilepsy after febrile seizures. The NCPP did, however, show that children with febrile seizures were four times as likely to have later atypical absence or complex partial seizures as those with no prior seizures. Only 14% of the children in the NCPP with atypical absence attacks had had febrile seizures (7).

It is unlikely that one or a few brief febrile seizures will damage selected vulnerable neurons and lead to later complex seizures. Children who have febrile seizures are at increased risk of complex partial seizures compared to the general population, but a causal relationship is unproven. There is no documentation that increased risk is limited to children who have prolonged febrile convulsions. In the NCPP, no child had a prolonged febrile convulsion after a brief febrile convulsion and later complex partial seizures.

Levitan & Cowan (53b) propose three theories to account for a possible association: the febrile seizure could cause the increase in risk of complex partial seizures, the febrile seizure could be the first manifestation of a seizure disorder, or separate but associated risk factors could exist for both disorders.

Intellectual Outcome

The effect of febrile seizures on cognitive function has been debated. Although some reports in selected populations cited later intellectual dysfunction, no new permanent neurologic deficits were found in prospective cohorts with follow-up of all febrile seizure patients.

Some series (54–56) found a significant incidence of mental retardation in febrile seizure patients, but children with prior abnormalities and acute CNS infection at the time of the seizure were not excluded in these studies. Schiottz-Christiansen & Bruhn (54) showed more neurologic soft signs and an IQ score lowered by an average of 7 points in the one twin of a monozygous pair who had febrile seizures. These differences were unrelated to birth factors or features of the seizure. However, neurologic examinations before the seizures took place were not available (54). Smith & Wallace (57) recently reported lowered developmental quotients in children with recurrences versus those with single febrile seizures; but in that series the initial groups were not comparable with regard to expectation for intellectual outcome.

In the NCPP, febrile seizure patients were compared with their normal siblings on IQ testing with the Wechsler Intelligence Scales for Children. There was no effect on IQ or academic performance at age seven in those children free of definite or suspect abnormality prior to the first febrile seizure and in those with no subsequent nonfebrile seizures. Neither febrile seizure recurrence nor length of seizure over 30 minutes was associated with a deficit. Deficits were found in children who developed later nonfebrile seizures, particularly those with minor motor epilepsy; many of these children were abnormal prior to any seizure (38). These results were similar to the National Child Development Study in Great Britain, where children with febrile convulsions (and no nonfebrile seizures) did as well as the remainder of the population in school performance at seven years and eleven years (46).

Motor Handicap

Some studies observed motor handicap following febrile seizures, but these reports did not distinguish children with meningitis, pre-existing abnormalities, or specific neurologic diseases from those who meet the definition of febrile seizures employed here. In prospective studies of defined populations using the current definition, no new persisting hemipareses or other motor deficits have appeared with febrile seizures (3, 4). However, transient unilateral weakness (Todd's paresis) occurred after almost 0.5% of febrile seizures in the NCPP (3).

MANAGEMENT

In most cases a child with a febrile seizure is brought to medical attention after the seizure has ended. But an actively convulsing febrile child who presents to an emergency room or a doctor's office clearly should be treated as any other convulsing child: the airway must be kept clear, proper oxygenation maintained, and medication given to stop the convulsion. Diazepam, 3 mg/kg at a maximum rate of 1 mg per minute, is often administered intravenously. It must be used with care because of potential respiratory depression, especially in the presence of prior anticonvulsants. Fever should be reduced by sponging and antipyretics.

Sometimes it is not entirely clear whether a convulsion has occurred. A febrile convulsion is generally marked by rhythmic clonic movements, stiffening or limpness, is associated with loss of consciousness, and is followed by postictal unresponsiveness. Febrile seizures may be confused with breathholding spells, during which a febrile child may turn blue or show a few jerking movements. High fevers may cause toxic delirium or tremors, which may be difficult to distinguish from a seizure on the basis of parental report.

If a convulsion has indeed occurred, the physician must first identify whether there is an underlying illness that requires prompt and specific treatment. The most urgent diagnostic decision for the physician caring for the child with a convulsion with fever is whether a lumbar puncture need be done to rule out meningitis. Except in the young infant, children with meningitis will usually show specific clinical signs. Reports of clinically unsuspected meningitis in cases of convulsion with fever are extremely rare. According to Kudrjavcev (58), the yield from lumbar puncture of meningitis unsuspected on clinical grounds is between 0 and 1%, and between 0 and 0.3% for bacterial meningitis. Rutter & Smales (59) reported the results of lumbar puncture in 318 patients with febrile convulsions who had no clinical evidence of meningitis. The CSF showed infection in four, of whom two had bacterial meningitis. Two children with negative lumbar punctures developed meningitis within one to two days. Early in the course of meningitis an infected spinal fluid may not yet exhibit pleocytosis or changes in protein or sugar content, so that false reassurance can be derived from a lumbar puncture. Therefore performance of a lumbar puncture in a highly febrile young infant does not eliminate the need for careful follow-up.

Some authors have suggested guidelines for conditions mandating a spinal tap after a febrile convulsion. Wolf (60) and Ouellette (61) recommend spinal tap if a child is less than two years old, or after first febrile convulsion. Another opinion is that any febrile convulsion that is not brief and generalized should call for a lumbar puncture (62). Clearly, spinal fluid must be evaluated if any clinical suspicion of meningitis (such as prolonged lethargy) is present, regardless of whether this is the first febrile seizure of the child's life or whether a family history is positive for febrile seizures.

Most authors do not feel that routine skull x rays are useful. Nealis et al (63) reported no useful findings from a review of x rays in 489 cases of febrile convulsions. Computerized cranial tomography has not been proposed or studied as a routine investigation in febrile seizures.

Many physicians evaluate electrolytes, glucose, blood urea nitrogen, calcium, and phosphorus, but the yield from these procedures when performed routinely has been very small (64), and it seems wise to limit their use to circumstances in which there is specific clinical suspicion of abnormality. Brief, single, self-limited febrile seizures from which the child fully awakens are seldom due to conditions otherwise clinically inapparent such as hypoglycemia or toxins. The need for blood cultures, blood count, and urinalysis can be judged on the basis of potential utility in diagnosing the cause of the fever.

Of 260 responses to a questionnaire by Asnes et al (65), 24% of pediatricians routinely hospitalized children with a first febrile convulsion. Benefits of hospitalization include reassurance to overwrought parents, and close observation if meningitis is questioned. However, in some cases hospitalization may unnecessarily reinforce the idea that the child is now abnormal. Perhaps the optimal alternative is admission to a short-term observation unit, which allows the physician the opportunity to watch the child rouse and to discuss the situation with less agitated parents (66).

Parents are in great need of reassurance: 30% of parents who witnessed their child's febrile seizure thought the child was dying or dead (67). Other common parental fears that need to be addressed are questions of possible meningitis and epilepsy. Physicians can feel comfortable in reassuring parents that children do not die because of febrile convulsions; large cohort studies have not reported any deaths (3, 48). Earlier studies that reported deaths among hospitalized children with febrile convulsions included cases of meningitis, severe pre-existing handicap, and major electrolyte disturbances.

The value of the EEG in children with febrile convulsions, despite the frequency of abnormalities soon after the event, is uncertain at best. The EEG done within a week of a febrile convulsion will be abnormal in one third or more children (68, 69). The most frequent abnormality is occipital slowing, often asymmetrical. Fever alone can produce such a tracing. Abnormalities are more severe and frequent if convulsions are longer or focal, if there is prior brain abnormality, or if the fever is particularly high. The incidence of paroxysmal EEG abnormalities, most commonly 3 per second spike/wave, increases with age. Taistra et al (70) found 4–6 per second slow waves three or four times more often in children with febrile convulsions than in controls. Kajitani et al (71) noted an increase in rolandic spikes of the type associated with benign focal epilepsy of childhood. Spike/wave tracings are found in 40% or more of children with past febrile seizures if follow-up is continued for several years (10).

Some reports suggested that the EEG was useful in estimating risk of later epilepsy (40, 72–74). Other reports have indicated that even focal spikes or prolonged or focal slowing do not predict either epilepsy or febrile seizure recurrence (69, 75). Thus there is reasonable doubt that the EEG is of general value in the management of febrile convulsions. The major role of the EEG in management of children with febrile seizures is to help rule out underlying structural pathology in the child who has experienced a focal or lengthy seizure.

Treatment with Anticonvulsants

Those who advocate anticonvulsant therapy in the management of the child with a febrile convulsion argue that recurrences may increase the risk of having a severe or prolonged convulsion (76, 77). However, there is no evidence that the sequence of "febrile convulsion—severe recurrent febrile convulsion—epilepsy" occurs with any significant frequency. In order to prove that treatment to prevent recurrences might reduce the risk of epilepsy, an extremely large controlled and randomized trial would be needed, and none has been done to date (78). On the other hand, there has been no demonstration that anticonvulsant therapy does *not* lessen the likelihood of eventual epilepsy.

The more recent trend has been away from treating all children with febrile seizures with long-term anticonvulsants (79). Most recommendations for treatment include children with one or two of the risk factors. These are age less than 12–18 months, positive family history for nonfebrile seizures, and a seizure that is prolonged, focal, or multiple in one day (80–83). Although studies have not documented predictive value of EEG, some physicians treat based on EEG criteria, and Doose (84) treats all children with focal slowing on EEG in the first hours after convulsion and all those with persistent EEG abnormalities.

Most physicians tend to treat with increasing numbers of recurrences and when there is a high level of parental anxiety (85). Those who advocate chronic anticonvulsant treatment of selected children with febrile seizures are including from one to two thirds of all children with febrile seizures (86). If the ultimate goal of treatment is the prevention of recurrences, then the most rational course might be treatment only of children whose initial seizure occurred at an early age, as early age of onset is the only well-established predictor of recurrence.

Phenobarbital has been the treatment of choice in the prophylaxis of febrile seizures, but, as discussed below, other drugs have recently come under investigation. Although many physicians recommend oral phenobarbital at the time of feverish illness only, this approach is probably more useful in reassuring parents and physicians than in preventing recurrences. One report (87) that found phenobarbital minimally effective in reducing recurrences when given only during febrile episodes was retrospective, observational, and uncontrolled. Since the half-life of phenobarbital is 24–100 hours and it takes at least five half-lives to achieve a steady-state blood level, an acute dose, unless so large as to risk oversedation and respiratory depression in an ill child, would not be prophylactic (88). Nevertheless, a 1975 questionnaire revealed that over 50% of responding pediatricians regularly prescribed intermittent phenobarbital therapy during febrile episodes only (65).

Studies have confirmed the effectiveness of daily phenobarbital in reducing the risk of recurrent febrile seizures (75, 89–91). Three to five milligrams per kilogram per day in one or two doses are sufficient to achieve a steady-state blood level. Most advocate therapeutic levels ranging from 15 to 18 μg/ml (88–94). The dose required to achieve therapeutic blood levels of phenobarbital is age-dependent, since clearance mechanisms are faster for younger children.

Most authors continue treatment for 1½ to 2 years, or to a minimum age of 4 to 5 years, whichever is later (77, 80, 82, 89, 91, 99). When the medication is discontinued it must be gradually tapered over 1–2 months to avoid the possibility of withdrawal seizures.

Even with strong efforts on the part of the physician to encourage regular administration of medication, compliance is a serious problem. Studies of daily administration of phenobarbital in children with febrile seizures report noncompliance rates as high as 48% (75). One reason for poor cooperation may be that once the parent sees the child is back to normal, anxiety is decreased about the possibility of recurrence. A substantial share of poor compliance may be related to changes in behavior the child may exhibit while on phenobarbital (89, 91, 95). Some parents express anxiety about the possibility of addiction to barbiturate, and many simply forget to give the medication regularly.

Reported side-effects of daily phenobarbital in the young child are common, generally behavioral, and consist of irritability, sleep disturbances, and hyperactivity. These side-effects occur with a frequency as high as about 40% (95). Some of these effects are transient even if the drug is continued. None is known to persist once the drug is decreased or stopped (89, 96). Although unproven in a clinical trial, evidence suggesting the possibility of immediate and long-term effects of chronic phenobarbital on cognitive development in young children is troublesome. A study of epileptic subjects taking phenobarbital showed impairment of short-term memory (97), and phenobarbital given to normal adult volunteers impaired performance on learning tasks and vigilance (98). Other disturbing evidence is the reduction in brain growth and levels of protein, DNA, and RNA in phenobarbital-treated rat pups (99), and the reduction of enzyme markers of neuronal development in tissue culture (100).

A child's development is progressing rapidly but unevenly at the age of susceptibility to febrile seizures. The measurement of drug effect on learning and memory requires different instruments depending on the age at testing. Serious methodological problems hamper the determination of the risks versus benefits of phenobarbital used to prevent febrile seizure recurrences, and no convincing trial to compare risks and benefits has yet been completed.

Another rarer side-effect of phenobarbital is skin rash, with occasional progression to exfoliative dermatitis. Phenobarbital may also be involved in drug interactions of clinical significance with drugs such as cortisol, dexamethasone, vitamin D, and diazepam (101). Because the use of phenobarbital may alter the metabolism of acetaminophen, Wilson (102) suggests further study is needed of anticonvulsant and antipyretic interaction in the febrile child.

Sodium valproate is effective for prevention of febrile seizure recurrence, in a total daily dose of between 20 and 40 mg/kg (103). Behavioral changes are apparently less common than with phenobarbital, but the rare life-threatening occurrence of pancreatitis and acute liver failure make caution advisable in prescribing this drug for widespread use (84). Lesser complications include gastrointestinal dysfunction, weight gain, platelet dysfunction, and hair loss (101). Given to young animals, valproate was reported to inhibit brain growth (104).

Ideally, it would be preferable to limit drug exposure to the period when a child is actually at risk for a febrile seizure recurrence, which is in the early hours of an acute febrile illness. Diazepam is rapidly absorbed and can produce therapeutic anticonvulsant levels within minutes (105). Thorn (96) compared rectal administration of diazepam at the onset of illness with continuous treatment with phenobarbital to prevent recurrent febrile seizures. Overall, recurrences were less with diazepam than phenobarbital because of compliance failures with phenobarbital, even though parents sometimes did not recognize that illness was present until the seizure occurred. Knudsen (106) used rectal diazepam successfully, but cautioned that because of the sedative side-effects, the possibility exists of delaying a diagnosis of meningitis. Another investigator suggested that diazepam given orally at the onset of fever can prevent febrile seizures (107). Some European authorities now recommend the prescription of rectal diazepam for administration by parents in the home, which should enable the early treatment of any seizure that occurs and prevent lengthy convulsions (108).

Phenytoin and carbamazepine have not been proven effective in preventing febrile seizure recurrences at usual doses (109–111).

The question has been raised whether antipyretics alone could effectively reduce febrile seizure recurrences. One study (112) found that counselling parents about antipyretic therapy was less effective than chronic administration of phenobarbital. However, there was no measurement of the compliance with the antipyretic regimen, so evaluation of this possibility is still needed. Antipyretic agents given in a combination with 30 mg of phenobarbital as soon as fever was noted also did not protect against febrile seizures (113). Nevertheless, most clinicians would seek to keep body temperature below 102°F with a combination of antipyretics and tepid sponging.

CONCLUSION

Febrile seizures are seizures in young children with fever not due to central nervous system infection or illness. They tend to run in families, and most are generalized and brief. While febrile seizures can be frightening to the observer, their outcome generally is quite good and, even if they recur, the long-term outlook with regard to intellect and neurologic function is usually not altered. In the vast majority of children with later neurologic deficits the problems can be attributed to conditions predating the febrile seizures.

The risks following seizures may have been overemphasized in the past, and the disadvantages of chronic anticonvulsant medication in young children are not clearly delineated. Many physicians advise treatment of selected children who are at increased risk of future epilepsy, even though most of these children will never develop nonfebrile seizures. A reliable evaluation of the risks versus the benefits of chronic anticonvulsant therapy in febrile seizures is not yet available. Alternatives to chronic phenobarbital prophylaxis are being investigated. New therapies must first be proven safe and efficacious, but they show promise of offering a wider range of solutions to the dilemma of febrile seizure management.

Literature Cited

1. Consensus Statement. 1980. Febrile seizures: long-term management of children with fever-associated seizures. *Pediatrics* 66:1009–12
2. Leviton, A., Cowan, L. D. 1982. Epidemiology of seizure disorders in children. *Neuroepidemiology* 1:40–83
3. Nelson, K. B., Ellenberg, J. H. 1978. Prognosis in children with febrile seizures. *Pediatrics* 61:720–27
4. van den Berg, B. J., Yerushalmy, J. 1969. Studies on convulsive disorders in young children. I. Incidence of febrile and nonfebrile convulsions by age and other factors. *Pediatr. Res.* 3:298–304
5. Nelson, K. B. 1980. Febrile seizures. In *Pediatrics Update*, ed. A. J. Moss, pp. 380–87. New York: Elsevier
6. Ouellette, E. M. 1974. The child who convulses with fever. *Pediatr. Clin. North Am.* 21:467–81
7. Nelson, K. B., Ellenberg, J. H. 1976. Predictors of epilepsy in children who have experienced febrile seizures. *N. Engl. J. Med.* 295:1029–33
8. Lewis, H. M., Parry, J. V., Parry, R. P., Davies, H. A., Sanderson, P. J., Tyrrell, D. A. J., Valman, H. B. 1979. Role of viruses in febrile convulsions. *Arch. Dis. Child.* 54:869–76
9. Hirtz, D. G., Nelson, K. B., Ellenberg, J. H. 1983. Seizures Following Childhood Immunization. *J. Pediatr.* 102:14–18
10. Hauser, W. A. 1981. The natural history of febrile seizures. In *Febrile Seizures*, ed. K. B. Nelson, J. H. Ellenberg, pp. 5–17. New York: Raven
11. Metrakos, J. D., Metrakos, K. 1970. Genetic factors in epilepsy. *Epilepsy Mod. Probl. Pharmacopsychiatry* 4:71–86
12. Jennings, M. T., Bird, T. D. 1981. Genetic influences in the epilepsies. *Am. J. Dis. Child.* 135:450–57
13. Livingston, S., Bridge, E. M., Kajdi, L. 1947. Febrile convulsions: a clinical study with special reference to heredity and prognosis. *J. Pediatr.* 31:509–12
14. Lennox, W. G. 1953. Significance of febrile convulsions. *Pediatrics* 11:341–57
15. Frantzen, E., Lennox-Buchthal, M., Nygaard, A., Stene, J. 1970. A genetic study of febrile convulsions. *Neurology* 20:909–17
16. Annegers, J. F., Hauser, W. A., Anderson, V. E., Kurland, L. T. 1982. The risks of seizure disorders among relatives of patients with childhood onset epilepsy. *Neurology* 32:174–79

17. Tsuboi, T. 1977. Genetic aspects of febrile convulsions. *Hum. Genet.* 38:169–73
18. Annegers, J. F., Hauser, W. A., Elveback, L. R., Kurland, L. T. 1979. The risk of epilepsy following febrile convulsions. *Neurology* 29:297–303
19. van den Berg, B. J. 1974. Studies on convulsive disorders in young children. IV. Incidence of convulsions among siblings. *Dev. Med. Child Neurol.* 16:457–64
20. Tay, J. S. H. 1979. Dermatoglyphics in children with febrile convulsions. *Br. Med. J.* 1:660–62
21. Wegman, M. E. 1939. Factors influencing the relation of convulsions and hyperthermia. *J. Pediatr.* 14:190–202
22. McCaughran, J. A. Jr., Schechter, N. 1982. Experimental febrile convulsions: long-term effects of hyperthermia-induced convulsions in the developing rat. *Epilepsia* 23:173–83
23. Holtzman, D., Obana, K., Olson, J. 1981. Hyperthermia-induced seizures in the rat pup: a model for febrile convulsions in children. *Science* 213:1034–36
24. Kasting, N. W., Veale, W. L., Cooper, K. E., Lederis, K. 1981. Vasopressin may mediate febrile convulsions. *Brain Res.* 213:327–33
25. Stephenson, J. B. P. 1978. Two types of febrile seizure: anoxic (syncopal) and epileptic mechanisms differentiated by oculocardiac reflex. *Br. Med. J.* 2:726–28
26. Nihei, K., Nakajima, S., Yamamoto, A., Nagayama, E. 1979. Febrile convulsion and IgA. *Brain Dev.* 1:242
27. Habel, A., Yates, C. M., McQueen, J. K., Blackwood, D., Elton, R. A. 1981. Homovanillic acid and 5-hydroxyindoleacetic acid in lumbar cerebrospinal fluid in children with afebrile and febrile convulsions. *Neurology* 31:488–91
28. Loscher, W., Rating, D., Siemes, H. 1981. GABA in cerebrospinal fluid of children with febrile convulsions. *Epilepsia* 22:697–702
29. Simpson, H., Habel, A. H., George, E. L. 1977. Cerebrospinal fluid acid-base status and lactate and pyruvate concentrations after short (< 30 minutes) first febrile convulsions in children. *Arch. Dis. Child.* 52:836–43
30. Siemes, H., Siegert, M., Hanefeld, F. 1978. Febrile convulsions and blood-cerebrospinal fluid barrier. *Epilepsia* 19:57–66
31. Eeg-Olofsson, O., Wigertz, A. 1982. Immunoglobulin abnormalities in cere-

brospinal fluid and blood in children with febrile seizures. *Neuropediatrics* 13:39–41

32. Lennox, U. A., Sibley, W. A., Zimmerman, H. M. 1954. Fever and febrile convulsions in kittens. A clinical, electroencephalographic, and histopathologic study. *J. Pediatr.* 45:179–90

33. Meldrum, B. S., Horton, R. W. 1973. Physiology of status epilepticus in primates. *Arch. Neurol.* 28:1–9

34. Vannucci, R. C. 1981. Metabolic and pathological consequences of experimental febrile seizures and status epilepticus. See Ref. 10, pp. 43–57

35. Nealis, J. G. T., Rosman, N. P., DePiero, T. J., Ouellette, E. M. 1978. Neurologic sequelae of experimental febrile convulsions. *Neurology* 28:246–50

36. Werboff, J., Havlena, J. 1963. Febrile convulsions in infant rats, and later behavior. *Science* 142:684–85

37. Vannucci, R. C. 1981. Section discussion. See Ref. 10, p. 79

38. Ellenberg, J. H., Nelson, K. B. 1978. Febrile seizures and later intellectual performance. *Arch. Neurol.* 35:17–21

39. Nelson, K. B., Ellenberg, J. H. 1981. The role of recurrences in determining outcome in children with febrile seizures. See Ref. 10, pp. 19–25

40. Tsuboi, T., Endo, S. 1977. Febrile convulsions followed by nonfebrile convulsions. A clinical, electroencephalographic and follow-up study. *Neuropädiatrie* 8:209–23

41. Millichap, J. G. 1968. Occurrence of spontaneous seizures. In *Febrile Convulsions*, pp. 92–97. New York: Macmillan

42. Wallace, S. J. 1977. Spontaneous fits after convulsions with fever. *Arch. Dis. Child.* 52:192–96

43. Chevrie, J. J., Aicardi, J. 1979. Convulsive disorders in the first year of life: persistence of epileptic seizures. *Epilepsia* 20:643–49

44. Chang, M.-H., Shen, Y.-Z. 1978. Simple febrile convulsions in children. A retrospective clinical and follow-up study. *Acta Paediatr. Sin.* 19:16–25

45. Ellenberg, J. H., Nelson, K. B. 1980. Sample selection and the natural history of disease. Studies of febrile seizures. *J. Am. Med. Assoc.* 243:1337–40

46. Ross, E. M., Peckham, C. S., West, P. B., Butler, N. R. 1980. Epilepsy in childhood: findings from the National Child Development Study. *Br. Med. J.*, Jan. 26, pp. 207–10

47. Livingston, S. 1958. Convulsive disorders in infants and children. *Adv. Pediatr.* 10:1113–19

48. Hauser, W. A., Kurland L. T. 1975. The epidemiology of epilepsy in Rochester, Minnesota, 1935 through 1967. *Epilepsia* 16:1–66

49. Iannetti, P., Fiorilli, M., Sirianni, M. C., Pana, A., Aiuti, F. 1982. Nonfebrile seizures after febrile convulsions: possible role of chronic cytomegalovirus infection. *J. Pediatr.* 101:27–31

50. Falconer, M. A. 1971. Genetic and related aetiological factors in temporal lobe epilepsy. *Epilepsia* 12:13–31

51. Rasmussen, T. 1979. Relative significance of isolated infantile convulsions as a primary cause of focal epilepsy. *Epilepsia* 20:395–401

52. Ounsted, C., Lindsay, J., Norman, R. 1966. Biological factors in temporal lobe epilepsy. *Clin. Dev. Med.,* Vol. 22

53a. Lee, K., Diaz, M., Melchior, J. C. 1981. Temporal lobe epilepsy—not a consequence of childhood febrile convulsions in Denmark. *Acta Neurol. Scand.* 63:231–36

53b. Leviton, A., Cowan, L. D. 1981. Do febrile seizures increase the risk of complex partial seizures? An epidemiologic assessment. See Ref. 10, pp. 65–74

54. Schiottz-Christensen, E., Bruhn, P. 1973. Intelligence, behavior and scholastic achievement subsequent to febrile convulsions: an analysis of discordant twin-pairs. *Dev. Med. Child Neurol.* 15:565–75

55. Aicardi, J., Chevrie, J. 1976. Febrile convulsions: neurological sequelae and mental retardation. In *Brain Dysfunction in Infantile Febrile Convulsions*, ed. M. A. B. Brazier, F. Coceani, pp. 247–57. New York: Raven

56. Sofijanov, N. G. 1982. Clinical evolution and prognosis of childhood epilepsies. *Epilepsia* 23:61–69

57. Smith, J. A., Wallace, S. J. 1982. Febrile convulsions: intellectual progress in relation to anticonvulsant therapy and to recurrence of fits. *Arch. Dis. Child.* 57:104–7

58. Kudrjavcev, T. 1981. Skull X-rays and lumbar puncture in a young child presenting with a seizure and fever. See Ref. 10, pp. 221–29

59. Rutter, N., Smales, O. R. C. 1977. Role of routine investigations in children presenting with their first febrile convulsion. *Arch. Dis. Child.* 52:188–91

60. Wolf, S. M. 1978. Laboratory evaluation of the child with a febrile convulsion. *Pediatrics* 62:1074–76

61. Ouellette, E. M. 1977. Managing febrile seizures. *Drug Ther.* 2:37–39
62. Jaffe, M., Bar-Joseph, G., Tirosh, E. 1981. Fever and convulsions—indications for laboratory investigations. *Pediatrics* 67:729–31
63. Nealis, J. G. T., McFadden, S. W., Asnes, R. A., Ouellette, E. M. 1977. Routine skull roentgenograms in the management of simple febrile seizures. *J. Pediatr.* 90:595–96
64. Gerber, M. A., Berliner, B. C. 1981. The child with a "simple" febrile seizure. Appropriate diagnostic evaluation. *Am. J. Dis. Child.* 135:431–33
65. Asnes, R. S., Novick, L. F., Nealis, J., Nguyen, M. 1975. The first febrile seizure: a study of current pediatric practice. *J. Pediatr.* 87:485–88
66. Camfield, P. 1981. Section discussion. See Ref. 10, p. 148
67. Rutter, N., Metcalfe, D. H. 1978. Febrile convulsions—what do parents do? *Br. Med. J.* 2:1345–46
68. Lennox-Buchthal, M. A. 1973. Febrile convulsions: a reappraisal. *Electroenceph. Clin. Neurophysiol. Suppl.* 32: 77–87
69. Frantzen, E., Lennox-Buchthal, M., Nygaard, A. 1968. Longitudinal EEG and clinical study of children with febrile convulsions. *Electroenceph. Clin. Neurophysiol.* 24:197–212
70. Taistra, R., Gerken, H., Doose, H. 1976. EEG spectral analysis in children with febrile convulsions. *Eur. Neurol.* 14:1–10
71. Kajitani, T., Ueoka, K., Nakamura, M., Kumanomidou, Y. 1981. Febrile convulsions and rolandic discharges. *Brain Dev.* 3:351–59
72. Lennox, M. A. 1949. Febrile convulsions in childhood. A clinical and electroencephalographic study. *Am. J. Dis. Child.* 78:868–82
73. Wallace, S. J. 1976. Neurological and intellectual deficits: convulsions with fever viewed as acute indications of lifelong developmental defects. See Ref. 55, pp. 259–77
74. Livingston, S. 1968. Infantile febrile convulsions. *Dev. Med. Child Neurol.* 10:374–76
75. Thorn, I. 1975. A controlled study of prophylactic long-term treatment of febrile convulsions with phenobarbital. *Acta. Neurol. Scand. Suppl.* 60:67–73
76. Hammill, J. F., Carter, S. 1966. Febrile convulsions. *N. Engl. J. Med.* 274: 563–64
77. Pollack, M. A. 1978. Continuous phenobarbital treatment after a "simple febrile convulsion." *Am. J. Dis. Child.* 132:87–89
78. Ellenberg, J. H., Nelson, K. B. Long-term clinical trials on the use of prophylaxis for prevention of recurrences of febrile seizures and epilepsy. See Ref. 10, pp. 267–78
79. Brown, J. K. 1982. Editorial: benign prognosis for a malignant condition. *Dev. Med. Child Neurol.* 24:279–80
80. Oberman, J. W. 1980. Therapy after two febrile convulsions. *Am. Family Physician* 21:21
81. Wallace, S. J. 1976. Treatment of convulsions with fever. See Ref. 55, pp. 301–5
82. Fishman, M. A. 1979. Febrile seizures: the treatment controversy. *J. Pediatr.* 94:177–84
83. Wolf, S. M. 1979. Controversies in the treatment of febrile convulsions. *Neurology* 29:287–290
84. Doose, H. 1981. Febrile convulsions: to treat or not to treat! *Neuropediatrics* 12:95–96
85. Addy, D. P. 1981. Prophylaxis and febrile convulsions. *Arch. Dis. Child.* 56:81–83
86. Nelson, K. B. Can treatment of febrile seizures prevent subsequent epilepsy? See Ref. 10, pp. 267–78
87. van den Berg, B. J., Yerushalmy, J. 1971. Studies on convulsive disorders in young children. II. Intermittent phenobarbital prophylaxis and recurrence of febrile convulsions. *J. Pediatr.* 78: 1004–12
88. Porter, R. 1981. Pharmacokinetic basis of intermittent and chronic anticonvulsant drug therapy in febrile seizures. See Ref. 10, pp. 107–18
89. Wolf, S. M., Carr, A., Davis, D. C., Davidson, S., Dale, E. P., Forsythe, A., Gondenberg, E. D., Hanson, R., Lulejian, G. A., Nelson, M. A., Treitman, P., Weinstein A. 1977. The value of phenobarbital in the child who has had a single febrile seizure: a controlled prospective study. *Pediatrics* 59:378–85
90. Pilgaard, S., Hansen, F. J., Paerregaard, P. 1981. Prophylaxis against febrile convulsions with phenobarbital. *Acta Paediatr. Scand.* 70:67–71
91. Camfield, C. S., Chaplin, S., Doyle, A. B., Shapiro, S. H., Cummings, C., Camfield, P. R. 1979. Side effects of phenobarbital in toddlers; behavioral and cognitive aspects. *J. Pediatr.* 95:361–65
92. Hojo, H., Nakano, S., Kataoka, K. 1979. Serum levels of phenobarbital and carbamazepine in children with convulsive disorders, with reference to thera-

peutic levels of phenobarbital to prevent recurrence of febrile and afebrile convulsions. *Brain Dev.* 11:502–9

93. Faer, O., Kastrup, K. W., Nielsen, E. L., Melchior, J. C., Thorn, I. 1972. Successful prophylaxis of febrile convulsions with phenobarbital. *Epilepsia* 13:279–85

94. Freeman, J. M. 1978. Febrile seizures: an end to confusion. *Pediatrics* 61: 806–8

95. Hirtz, D. G. 1981. Effects of treatment for prevention of febrile seizure recurrence on behavioral and cognitive function. See Ref. 10, pp. 193–202

96. Thorn, I. 1981. Prevention of recurrent febrile seizures: intermittent prophylaxis with diazepam compared with continuous treatment with phenobarbital. See Ref. 10, pp. 119–26

97. MacLeod, C. M., Dekaban, A. S., Hunt, E. 1978. Memory impairment in epileptic patients: selective effects of phenobarbital concentration. *Science* 202: 1102–4

98. Hutt, S. J., Jackson, P. M., Belsham, A., Higgins, G. 1968. Perceptual motor behaviour in relation to blood phenobarbitone level: a preliminary report. *Dev. Med. Child Neurol.* 10:626–32

99. Diaz, J., Schain, R. J. 1978. Phenobarbital: effects of long-term administration on behavior and brain of artificially reared rats. *Science* 199:90–91

100. Bergey, G. K., Swaiman, K. F., Schrier, B. K., Fitzgerald, S., Nelson, P. G. 1981. Adverse effects of phenobarbital on morphological and biochemical development of fetal mouse spinal cord neurons in culture. *Ann. Neurol.* 9: 584–89

101. Wilson, J. T. 1981. Observed and potential risks of anticonvulsant medications in children. See Ref. 10, pp. 153–67

102. Wilson, J. T. 1981. Antipyretic management of febrile seizures. See Ref. 10, pp. 231–39

103. Cavazzuti, G. B. 1975. Prevention of febrile convulsions with dipropylacetate. *Epilepsia* 16:647

104. Diaz, J., Shields, W. D. 1981. Effects of dipropylacetate on brain development. *Ann. Neurol.* 10:465–68

105. Dhillon, S. Ngwane, E., Richens, A. 1982. Rectal absorption of diazepam in epileptic children. *Arch. Dis. Child.* 57:264–67

106. Knudsen, F. U. 1979. Rectal administration of diazepam in solution in the acute treatment of convulsions in infants and children. *Arch. Dis. Child.* 54:855–57

107. Dianese, G. 1979. Prophylactic diazepam in febrile convulsions. *Arch. Dis. Child.* 54:244–45

108. Deonna, T. 1982. Traitement des convulsions febriles: nouvelles donnees et nouvelles options. *Helv. Paediatr. Acta* 37:7–10

109. Melchior, J. C., Buchthal, F., Lennox-Buchthal, M. 1971. The ineffectiveness of diphenylhydantoin in preventing febrile convulsions in the age of greatest risk, under three years. *Epilepsia* 12: 55–62

110. Monaco, F., Sechi, G. P., Mutani, R., Meloni, T., Mela, M. G., Masia, G., Tondi, M. 1980. Lack of efficacy of carbamazepine in preventing the recurrence of febrile convulsions. In *Antiepileptic Therapy: Advances in Drug Monitoring,* ed. S. I. Johannessen, et al, pp. 75–79. New York: Raven

111. Camfield, P. R., Camfield, C. S., Tibbles, J. A. R. 1982. Carbamazepine does not prevent febrile seizures in phenobarbital failures. *Neurology* 32:288–89

112. Camfield, P. R., Camfield, C., Shapiro, S., Cummings, C. 1980. The first febrile seizure-antipyretic instruction plus either phenobarbital or placebo to prevent a recurrence. *J. Pediatr.* 97:16–21

113. Mackintosh, T. F. 1970. Studies on prophylactic treatment of febrile convulsions in children. Is it feasible to inhibit attacks by giving drugs at the first sign of fever or infection? *Clin. Pediatr.* 9:283–86

Ann. Rev. Med. 1983. 34:473–89

SENSORY EVOKED POTENTIALS:

Clinical Applications in Medicine

Leslie J. Dorfman, M.D.

Department of Neurology, Stanford University School of Medicine, Stanford,
California 94305

Introduction

An evoked potential (EP) is the transient electrical response of the nervous
system to a stimulus. In the normal course of events, the human nervous
system is constantly generating EPs in response to a barrage of internal and
external sensory stimuli. In order to record EPs for diagnostic purposes, it
is necessary (*a*) to generate a controlled, discrete, and usually brief sensory
stimulus; (*b*) to record electrical responses from the appropriate portions
of the nervous system; and (*c*) to eliminate competing or interfering electrical signals, which tend to obscure the minute EPs. In theory, there are
as many different kinds of EP as there are modalities of sensation. In
practice, three major modalities have come to be widely applied: visual
(VEP), auditory (BAEP), and tactile or somatosensory (SEP) evoked potentials.

RECORDING CONSIDERATIONS EPs are usually recorded with the
same type of electrodes employed for electroencephalography (EEG),
namely, metal discs applied on the scalp with electrolyte paste. The electrode locations are determined by the anatomy of the sensory system under
study. For SEP recordings, electrodes are sometimes placed also over the
spinal cord and proximal segments of peripheral nerves. The electrical
signals are amplified and displayed on an oscilloscope, then either photo-
graphed or plotted in *x*-*y* format for a permanent record.

SIGNAL AVERAGING The EP signals are generally quite small in relation to other bioelectrical phenomena such as EEG, electrocardiogram, and
electro-oculogram; and are also subject to contamination from external
electrical noises such as those emanating from power lines and fluorescent

473

0066-4219/83/0401-0473$02.00

lights, and the intrinsic noise of the recording/amplifying devices. In order to enhance the definition of the EP (the "signal") relative to these various "noises," a special signal processing technique known as "averaging" is routinely employed. In this technique, time segments, or epochs, of recorded electrical activity containing the EP of interest are summed together. Prior to summation, the epochs are aligned according to the known time of stimulus occurrence. In the process of summing together many occurrences of the stimulus and EP, the various background noises, which are random with respect to stimulus delivery, tend to be diminished by a factor proportional to $1/\sqrt{N}$, where N is the number of epochs summed. The EP, on the other hand, which always occurs at a fixed interval following the stimulus, repeatedly superimposes upon itself in the summation or averaging process and becomes progressively better defined. An example of signal averaging is shown in Figure 1.

In contemporary technology, the signal averaging process for extraction of EPs is usually performed digitally, i.e. the electrical signals are discretely sampled prior to processing. One advantage of digital processing is that the numerical magnitudes of the EP latencies and amplitudes are readily determined from the sampled waveform using, for example, a cursor on the oscilloscope screen, rather than by hand measurement.

NOMENCLATURE   The wave components of an EP complex are usually designated according to their electrical polarity (positive or negative), and either their location in the wave sequence (1, 2, 3, etc) or their approximate post-stimulus latency in milliseconds (ms). Both systems of nomenclature tend to break down in the presence of disease, where there may be more or fewer components than normal, and their latencies may be markedly altered.

Visual Evoked Potentials

VEPs were the first modality of EP to gain widespread clinical application. This probably reflects many factors, including the importance of vision, the relative ease of presenting a controlled visual stimulus, and the clear definition of the neuroanatomical substrate of vision. Early studies made extensive use of stroboscopic light flash as the visual stimulus (1). During the past decade it has become clear that more consistent responses which lend themselves more readily to clinical application are obtained when the visual stimulus is complex. This probably reflects in part the preferential activation of visual cortical neurons by complex stimuli. Accordingly, most clinical laboratories now employ pattern stimuli rather than flash to elicit VEPs. The most widely used stimulus is a checkerboard pattern of light and dark squares that reverses itself (the light squares become dark and vice versa)

NUMBER
OF RESPONSES
AVERAGED

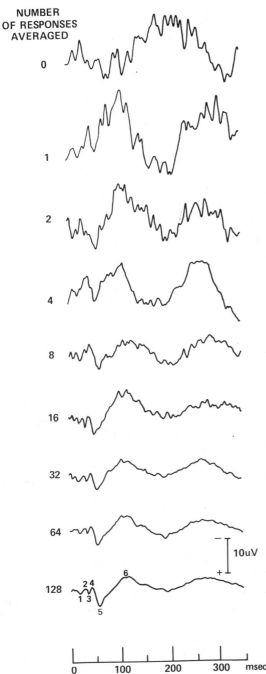

Figure 1 Extraction of a somatosensory evoked potential from background EEG activity, illustrating the principle of signal averaging. The stimulus, delivered to the median nerve at the wrist, occurs at time = 0. Note that a single 350-ms epoch of EEG containing the evoked potential (1) cannot be distinguished from a similar epoch without a response (0), because the response is very small in relation to the ongoing background EEG. As more and more response-containing epochs are averaged together (2 through 128), the evoked potential becomes progressively better defined by reduction of the nonstimulus-related EEG noise. In the bottom tracing, the first six waves of the SEP are numbered sequentially. (From 90, courtesy of C. V. Mosby Co.)

at a predetermined frequency. The patient must cooperate by attending to the pattern stimulus. In those situations where patient cooperation cannot be obtained, the flash stimulus may be preferred.

ANATOMY   Visual stimulation excites the rod and cone receptors of the retina and generates a local receptor potential known as the electroretinogram (ERG). This is sometimes of diagnostic importance in ophthalmology, and is best recorded with electrodes pasted on the skin close to the eye, or with a contact lens electrode mounted on the cornea (2). When anterior components of the VEP are studied, there may be contamination from ERG. With the pattern-reversal stimulus described above, there is no net change in total luminous flux, and almost no measurable ERG is generated.

The rod and cone signals traverse the bipolar and ganglion cell layers of the retina, where they undergo considerable processing, then are conducted via the nerve fiber layer to the optic nerve. In the optic chiasm, the fibers from the left and right hemiretinae, respectively, segregate and project along the ipsilateral optic tracts. The tract fibers synapse in the lateral geniculate nucleus of the thalamus, and the axons of the geniculate neurons constitute the optic radiations which then converge upon visual cortical neurons in the calcarine cortex. Intracortical connections link the primary visual cortex with the so-called visual association areas in the occipito-parietal and occipito-temporal regions.

NORMAL VEP   When the entire visual field of one eye is stimulated with checkerboard pattern reversal, the VEP is dominated by a large V-shaped positivity with peak latency of approximately 100 ms (P100; Figure 2). Earlier and later components are also present in many cases but these are of limited diagnostic import. The latency, and to a lesser extent the amplitude, of P100 vary in a systematic way with the brightness, contrast, and focus of the checkerboard pattern; with the frequency of stimulation; and with the visual acuity, pupil size, and age of the subject (3–9). When stimulus and subject parameters are held constant, the latency of P100 shows relatively small variation across normal individuals (standard deviation of the mean is on the order of 5 ms in most laboratories), and there is usually not more than about a 10-ms difference in the latency of P100 between the two eyes of a normal subject (10, 11). The amplitude of P100 is maximal in the midline occipital region and falls off fairly symmetrically about the midline.

Most of P100 is generated from the central portion of the visual field, with the lower part of the field contributing more than the upper part (12). When the left or right hemi-field of one eye is stimulated, the VEP

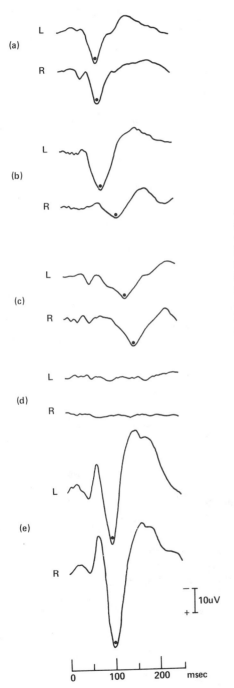

Figure 2 Examples of normal and abnormal pattern-reversal visual evoked potentials. (*A*) Normal tracings; the dots indicate the P100 wave peaks. (*B*) Small, delayed VEP from the right eye in a case of unilateral optic neuritis. (*C*) Bilateral delayed VEPs in postinfectious acute disseminated encephalomyelitis. (*D*) Absent VEPs in cerebro-retinal degeneration. (*E*) Unusually large VEPs in a patient with myoclonic epilepsy. (From 90, courtesy of C. V. Mosby Co.)

exhibits complex topographic distribution on the scalp, with the apparent paradox of earlier components on the side ipsilateral to the stimulated field (13–15).

ABNORMAL VEP   Lesions of the cornea, lens, or optic media may produce abnormalities of the VEP by diminishing the effective stimulus intensity reaching the retina. In cases where the optic media are completely opacified, and it is vital to determine retinal integrity, a method has been described for eliciting a VEP by stimulating the retina electrically, using a contact lens electrode mounted on the cornea (16). In the absence of ocular pathology, abnormality of the VEP is most often encountered in disorders affecting the anterior portion of the visual pathway, i.e. the optic nerve and chiasm. In general, two types of VEP abnormality may be distinguished, corresponding to two categories of pathophysiologic process. Demyelinative lesions such as optic neuritis tend to prolong VEP latency but to preserve the general configuration of the response, particularly of P100 (10–12, 17, 18; Figure 2b, 2c). Compressive, destructive, or degenerative lesions that interrupt axons, on the other hand, tend to diminish the amplitude and alter the configuration of the VEP, with or without lesser degrees of latency prolongation (15, 19–23; Figure 2d).

Retrochiasmal lesions of the visual pathway tend to produce abnormalities that are best appreciated on hemi-field stimulation (15, 17, 24, 25). In rare conditions, such as some forms of myoclonic epilepsy, abnormally large VEPs may be seen (Figure 2e).

Somatosensory Evoked Potentials

Unlike vision and audition, somesthesis is not a unitary sense; it is made up of multiple modalities, including the sensations of touch, vibration, joint position, pinprick, deep pain, temperature, and possibly others. While special experimental protocols have permitted the generation of EPs more or less limited to one or another of these modalities (26, 27), such specificity is beyond the capability of most clinical EP laboratories. SEPs are ordinarily generated using percutaneous pulse electrical stimulation of a mixed peripheral nerve, such as the median or ulnar nerve in the arm, or the peroneal or posterior tibial nerve in the leg. This type of stimulus activates peripheral sensory axons without regard to their functional specificity. A variety of clinical and experimental studies confirmed, however, that the familiar SEP recorded with scalp electrodes is mediated almost entirely by the posterior column-medial lemniscal system, which is believed to subserve the sensations of vibration, joint position, and possibly discriminative touch (28–30).

ANATOMY   The somatosensory system spans the length and breadth of the human body. The distance from the site of stimulation on the wrist or ankle, or on a digit, to the recording site on the scalp is usually more than one meter in adults, and is sometimes closer to two. A lesion at any point along the conduction pathway may give rise to abnormality of the SEP. Hence, it is frequently helpful to record from multiple sites along the conduction path in order to localize the lesion by identifying the segment of pathway in which conduction fails (see below).

The cell bodies of the primary somatosensory neurons are located in the dorsal root ganglia of the spinal cord. Afferent impulses traverse the peripheral nerves and plexuses, then enter the spinal cord via the dorsal roots and ascend in the ipsilateral posterior column to synapse in the gracile or cuneate nucleus at the cervico-medullary junction. The second-order sensory neurons ascend through the brain stem in the medial lemniscus, decussate, and synapse in the contralateral ventral posterior lateral nucleus of the thalamus. The thalamo-cortical projections terminate primarily in the primary somatosensory (postrolandic) region, in the well-known "homunculus" topography. In keeping with the attitude of the homunculus, SEPs from the leg are best recorded from the vertex of the scalp, near the interhemispheric fissure, whereas responses from the arm are maximal somewhat more laterally and inferiorly.

The trigeminal nerve and its various nuclear connections constitute the somatosensory system of the cranial nerves. Special techniques have been described for measuring SEPs to electrical and painful stimulation in the territory of the trigeminal nerve (31, 32).

NORMAL SEP   When an upper limb nerve is stimulated, the earliest potential of cerebral origin is a small negativity with a peak latency of approximately 20 ms (so-called N1 or N20; wave "2" in the lower trace of Figure 1) (33). When a leg nerve is stimulated, the initial negativity is often not seen, possibly because of a different geometric orientation of the generator neurons. Instead, there is usually onset of a large positivity at approximately 35 ms, with the longer latency representing in large part the increased conduction distance (30, 34–37). There is usually not more than a 2-ms side-to-side asymmetry.

With electrodes located close to the spine and neck, and using high-order signal averaging, one may identify very small early potentials that probably correspond to transit of the impulse volley through the spinal roots and cauda equina, along the spinal cord, and quite likely through the brain stem as well (26, 33, 38–42). Whether one records "near-field" cortical potentials or "far-field" subcortical or spinal potentials depends not only on the location of the recording electrodes but also on the gain and bandpass of the amplification system and on the number of responses averaged.

ABNORMAL SEP   The diagnostically important early components of SEP, being much smaller in amplitude than the VEP, for example, are relatively less robust in the face of disease. Thus, in relatively mild demyelinating lesions, the early elements of the SEP sequence may be recognizable but delayed. However, in many pathological circumstances, the disturbance of impulse conduction results in loss of recognizable early components; this can be a sensitive indicator of pathology, but it lacks specificity.

When multiple recording sites are used simultaneously, the location of a lesion may often be identified. Hence, in spinal cord lesions involving the lower cervical, thoracic, or lumbar segments, it may be possible to record the lower limb peripheral nerve volley, the lumbar root/cauda equina potential, and possibly some propagating spinal SEP, but not the cervical or thalamo-cortical components of the scalp responses (35, 36, 40–42); the integrity of the cervical cord and more rostral structures may be verified by measuring the SEP from the upper limb (30). Infarcts, tumors, and other destructive lesions are associated with abnormal SEPs if the lemniscal pathway is involved (43–50). Lesions altering only the spinothalamic pathway, such as the Wallenberg medullary infarct, usually spare the SEP (50, 51). In situations of dissociated sensory loss, as in syringomyelia, anterior spinal artery infarction, and some cerebral lesions, the SEP abnormality is almost invariably limited to those body parts with impaired joint position sense (28, 30, 50).

Brainstem Auditory Evoked Potentials

Unlike visual and somatosensory EPs, auditory EPs do not show the anticipated localization to the auditory (i.e. superior temporal) cortex, but instead are widely distributed over the scalp with amplitude maximum near the vertex. These intermediate and late responses have been studied in a number of contexts, including several studies describing apparent interhemispheric asymmetries to meaningful word stimuli, presumably related to hemispheric dominance for language (52, 53). For neurodiagnostic purposes, attention has focused on the very earliest elements of the AEP, which were shown in human and animal studies to arise from brainstem structures (54, 55), and hence are called brainstem AEPs, or BAEPs. Broad-band click stimuli are optimal for eliciting these early potentials; unfortunately, tones are much less effective, which makes BAEP recording inappropriate for pure tone audiometry.

ANATOMY   Auditory receptors are located in association with hair cells along the basilar membrane of the cochlea, and impulses arising here are conducted along the auditory (VIIIth cranial) nerve to the cochlear nucleus located in the rostral medulla. From here impulses ascend a complex, bilaterally represented pathway involving the superior olivary complex, trapezoid body, nuclei of the lateral lemniscus, inferior colliculus, and thence to the medial geniculate nuclei of the thalamus, and ultimately to superior temporal cortex. As shown in Figure 3, the first five wave peaks of the BAEP are considered to be associated with specific structures along the auditory pathway from the rostral medulla to the inferior colliculus in the lower midbrain. The relationship of subsequent waves to the more rostral parts of the auditory pathway is still undetermined.

NORMAL BAEP   As shown in Figure 3, the normal BAEP consists of a sequence of five (or more) waves occurring within the first 10 ms after the stimulus. They are ordinarily displayed with a positive-up polarity convention, and numbered I through V. While the configuration of the wave sequence tends to be relatively constant for a given recording configuration in a specific individual, there is a certain amount of inter-individual variability, particularly in the configuration of the IV-V complex (56–58). Under pathological conditions, the negativity after wave V is often useful as a marker of that event. Since wave I is generated in the auditory nerve, its latency is a measure of peripheral auditory function, whereas the latency difference between wave I and the subsequent waves, particularly III and V, may be taken as measures of conduction along the auditory pathways intrinsic to the brainstem. The latencies of all wave peaks are inversely related to stimulus intensity. Above approximately 45 dB HL, further increases in the stimulus intensity cause all the wave peaks to shift in synchrony, so that the interpeak latency differences do not change. This is of prime importance in distinguishing peripheral from central auditory disorders.

ABNORMAL BAEP   Lesions at any point along the auditory pathway from the ear to the inferior colliculus may produce abnormalities of the BAEP. Lesions of the cochlea and the distal segment of the auditory nerve produce abnormalities that involve wave I, as well as subsequent waves. If the lesion is at or rostral to the cochlear nucleus, then wave I is normal but subsequent waves are delayed, and the V-I latency difference may be prolonged. Demyelinative, compressive, and destructive lesions involving the brainstem all tend to prolong the interpeak latency differences, and if severe may cause later waves of the EP to be lost (59–69).

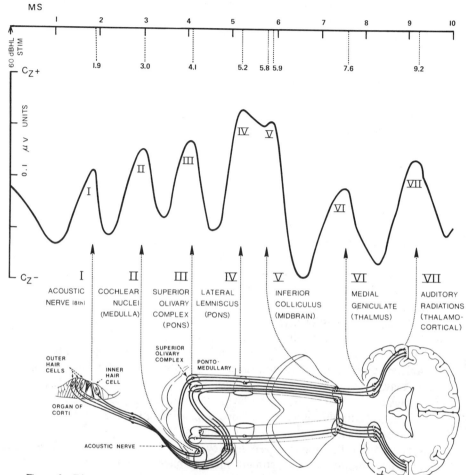

Figure 3 Diagram of normal latencies for vertex-positive brainstem auditory potentials (waves I through VII) evoked by clicks 60 dB above normal hearing threshold at a rate of 10 per second. Lesions at different levels of the auditory pathway tend to produce response abnormalities beginning with indicated components, although this does not specify the precise generators of the response; the relative contribution of axonal and synaptic activity to the response are as yet unknown. (From Stockard, J. J., Stockard, J. E., Sharbrough, F. W. 1977. *Mayo Clin. Proc.* 52:761–66; courtesy of E. Grass.)

BAEPs are of particular utility in ruling out brainstem injury in the patient with coma of unknown cause. BAEPs are usually normal in coma due to metabolic disorders, intoxications, and bihemispheric cerebral dysfunction. A number of studies demonstrated that BAEPs are preserved even during the deepest stages of surgical anesthesia, when the spontaneous EEG is abolished, as long as the brainstem is structurally intact (60, 70, 71).

Specific Clinical Applications

SENSORY IMPAIRMENT   When a patient complains of sensory disturbance, it is frequently difficult to verify the degree of sensory dysfunction through the clinical examination without relying heavily on the patient's subjective report of perceptual experiences. Analysis of sensory EPs provides a quantifiable and objective measure of sensory dysfunction, and offers the opportunity to repeat the measurement serially in order to determine either the progress of a disease or response to therapy. In the visual and auditory domains, it is possible simultaneously to test function of the sensory receptors and of the central conduction pathways, and thus to determine whether a complaint of visual or hearing impairment is related to dysfunction in the sense organ or in the central nervous system. Sensory receptor function is more difficult to measure electrically in the somatosensory domain; here, the properties of conduction in the peripheral sensory nerves provide a baseline against which the characteristics of central conduction may be compared. Interestingly, in the presence of peripheral nerve disease it is sometimes easier to identify components of the cerebral SEP than to measure the compound peripheral nerve action potential, which leads to the concept of central "amplification" of the peripheral somatosensory volley (72).

LOCALIZATION OF CNS LESIONS   In each of the major EP modalities, some degree of localization of dysfunction can be accomplished with electrophysiologic testing. In the visual domain, it is the whole field/half field characteristics of the response that indicate whether the lesion is pre- or post-chiasmal (13–15, 17, 24, 25). When the SEP is recorded with multiple electrodes at different points along the somatosensory pathway, it is frequently possible to identify the point at which conduction fails or deteriorates, corresponding to a localized lesion (30, 35–37, 39–42, 44–50). In BAEP recordings, the presence or absence of specific wave breaks may indicate the rostral/caudal location of the brainstem disturbance (59–69).

MULTIPLE SCLEROSIS   EP recording is a valuable adjunct in the diagnosis of multiple sclerosis (MS; 8, 10–12, 18, 35–37, 39, 40, 59, 65, 72–76). The demyelinative nature of the lesions in this disorder interferes with impulse propagation along the affected axons (73). A vital element in the clinical diagnosis of MS is the demonstration of multiple lesions affecting white matter of the central nervous system. The clinical strategy for using EPs is to examine sensory systems *not* obviously involved clinically; if conduction abnormalities can be demonstrated in sensory pathways remote from the region(s) of clinical involvement, this is interpreted as evidence of multifocal involvement. Examples would include the finding of a delayed VEP in a patient with transverse myelitis, or an abnormal BAEP in a patient with optic neuritis. Numerous investigations have demonstrated abnormalities of all three modalities of EP in patients with MS (74, 75); the incidence and magnitude of abnormality correlates in a general way with the duration and severity of the disease, and with other diagnostic tests (76). In general, the VEP shows the highest incidence of abnormality, with the SEP next lower, and the BAEP shows the lowest incidence of abnormality (possibly reflecting the small volume of brain tissue being examined).

HYSTERIA   EP analysis can be exceedingly helpful in the evaluation of patients with sensory symptoms that may be psychophysiologic in nature (i.e. hysteria or conversion reaction) or that may represent frank malingering. It must be noted that normal EPs do not necessarily mean that there can be no coexistent dysfunction in the tested sensory system. However, in many cases of nonorganic sensory disturbance, the EPs from the affected part may be completely normal and indistinguishable from those generated in asymptomatic body parts. Hence, one may encounter perfectly normal VEPs in patients with hysterical blindness, and normal symmetrical SEPs in an individual with hysterical hemi-anesthesia. While EP evaluation should not be the sole criterion for determining whether a symptom may be psychophysiologic in nature, it is often very helpful when the electrophysiologic studies confirm the clinical impression.

COMA   EP recordings are of assistance in evaluating the integrity of the central nervous system in the comatose patient. The SEP and BAEP, in particular, are valuable indicators of brainstem function when coma is thought to be a reflection of cerebral bihemispheric dysfunction (60, 70, 71, 77). EP recordings have also been proposed as adjunctive electrophysiological criteria of brain death (78–80).

TRAUMA   EP analysis has been shown to have value in determining the localization and severity of injuries to both the peripheral and central nervous systems, particularly the plexuses, spinal cord, and brainstem, which are otherwise not readily evaluated in a functional sense except by clinical examination (30, 48, 49, 70, 71, 80–83). Some reports claim prognostic value for EP studies in cases of severe head injury (84).

INTRAOPERATIVE MONITORING   There is growing interest in using EP monitoring during neurosurgical procedures in order to prevent injury to vital structures. Reports have described the use of VEP monitoring during surgery in the orbit, near the optic nerve, and adjacent to the optic chiasm as in removal of pituitary tumors or intracranial aneurysms (85–87). BAEP monitoring has found greatest application in surgery for removal of acoustic neuromas (88). SEP monitoring has been advocated during surgery to remove intraspinal tumors, and during scoliosis surgery (89). Special stimulating and recording techniques must be employed because of the constraints imposed by the surgical procedure, and the electrically noisy environment of the operating suite. While the reports to date are only preliminary, it seems likely that there will be increasing interest in this type of electrophysiologic monitoring during critical neurosurgical operations.

PEDIATRICS   The use of EP technology as applied to the special neurological, sensory and developmental problems of childhood is the subject of a recent review (90).

PERCEPTUAL AND COGNITIVE DISORDERS   There exists an extensive body of literature on the analysis of intermediate and late wave components of EPs (i.e. components occurring 100 ms after the stimulus, or later) in relation to psychological processes such as perception, cognition, decision-making, reasoning, and motivation (see, for example, 91). In general, these so-called event-related potentials have yet to find substantive application in clinical medicine.

Additional Readings

In addition to the specific bibliographic citations, the interested reader is referred to several recent reviews and compendia that address many technical and clinical aspects of EP technology (92–97).

Literature Cited

1. Kooi, K. A. 1979. *Visual Evoked Potentials in Central Disorders of the Visual System.* Hagerstown, Pa: Harper & Row. 161 pp.
2. Ikeda, H., Tremain, K. E., Sanders, M. D. 1978. Neurophysiological investigation in optic nerve disease: combined assessment of the visual evoked response and electroretinogram. *Br. J. Ophthalmol.* 62:227–39
3. Halliday, A. M., McDonald, W. I., Mushin, J. 1973. Delayed pattern-evoked responses in optic neuritis in relation to visual acuity. *Trans. Ophthalmol. Soc. UK* 93:315–24
4. Hawkes, C. H., Stow, B. 1981. Pupil size and the pattern evoked visual re-

sponse. *J. Neurol. Neurosurg. Psychiatry* 44:90–91
5. Sokol, S., Moskowitz, A. 1981. Effect of retinal blur on the peak latency of the pattern evoked potential. *Vision Res.* 21:1279–86
6. Collins, D. W. K., Carroll, W. M., Black, J. L., Walsh, M. 1979. Effect of refractive error on the visual evoked response. *Br. Med. J.* 1:231–32
7. Harter, M. R., White, C. T. 1968. Effects of contour sharpness and check-size on visually evoked cortical potentials. *Vision Res.* 8:701–11
8. Hennerici, M., Wenzel, D., Freund, H. J. 1977. The comparison of small-size rectangle and checkerboard stimulation for the evaluation of delayed visual

evoked responses in patients suspected of multiple sclerosis. *Brain* 100:119–36

9. Sokol, S., Moskowitz, A., Towle, V. L. 1981. Age-related changes in the latency of the visual evoked potential: influence of check size. *Electroencephalogr. Clin. Neurophysiol.* 51:559–62

10. Halliday, A. M., McDonald, W. F., Mushin, J. 1973. Visual evoked response in the diagnosis of multiple sclerosis. *Br. Med. J.* 4:661–64

11. Shahroki, F., Chiappa, K. H., Young, R. R. 1978. Pattern shift visual evoked responses: two hundred patients with optic neuritis and/or multiple sclerosis. *Arch. Neurol.* 35:65–71

12. Asselman, P., Chadwick, D. W., Marsden, C. D. 1975. Visual evoked responses in the diagnosis and management of patients suspected of multiple sclerosis. *Brain* 98:261–82

13. Blumhardt, L. D., Barrett, G., Halliday, A. M., Kriss, A. 1978. The effect of experimental "scotomata" on the ipsilateral and contralateral responses to pattern-reversal in one half-field. *Electroencephalogr. Clin. Neurophysiol.* 45:376–92

14. Blumhardt, L. D., Halliday, A. M. 1979. Hemisphere contributions to the composition of the pattern-evoked potential waveform. *Exp. Brain Res.* 36:53–69

15. Haimovic, I. C., Pedley, T. A. 1982. Hemi-field pattern reversal visual evoked potentials. *Electroencephalogr. Clin. Neurophysiol.* 54:111–31

16. Potts, A. M., Inoue, J., Buffum, D. 1968. The electrically evoked response of the visual system (EER). *Invest. Ophthalmol.* 7:269–78

17. Blumhardt, L. D., Barrett, G., Halliday, A. M. 1977. The asymmetrical visual evoked potential to pattern reversal in one half field and its significance for the analysis of visual field defects. *Br. J. Ophthalmol.* 61:454–61

18. Wilson, W. B. 1978. Visual-evoked response differentiation of ischemic optic neuritis from the optic neuritis of multiple sclerosis. *Am. J. Ophthalmol.* 86:530–35

19. Carroll, W. M., Mastaglia, F. L. 1979. Leber's optic neuropathy: a clinical and visual evoked potential study of affected and asymptomatic members of a six-generation family. *Brain* 102:559–80

20. Dorfman, L. J., Nikoskelainen, E., Rosenthal, A. R., Sogg, R. L. 1977. Visual evoked potentials in Leber's hereditary optic neuropathy. *Ann. Neurol.* 1:565–68

21. Halliday, A. M., Halliday, E., Kriss, A., McDonald, W. I., Mushin, J. 1976. The pattern-evoked potential in compression of the anterior visual pathways. *Brain* 99:357–74

22. Carroll, W. M., Kriss, A., Baraitser, M., Barrett, G., Halliday, A. M. 1980. The incidence and nature of visual pathway involvement in Friedreich's ataxia: a clinical and visual evoked potential study of 22 patients. *Brain* 103:413–34

23. Livingstone, I. R., Mastaglia, F. L., Edis, R., Howe, J. W. 1981. Visual involvement in Friedreich's ataxia and hereditary spastic ataxia: a clinical and visual evoked response study. *Arch. Neurol.* 38:75–79

24. Kuroiwa, Y., Celesia, G. G. 1981. Visual evoked potentials with hemifield pattern stimulation: their use in the diagnosis of retrochiasmatic lesions. *Arch. Neurol.* 38:86–90

25. Streletz, L. J., Bae, S. H., Roeshman, R. M., Schatz, N. J., Savino, P. J. 1981. Visual evoked potentials in occipital lobe lesions. *Arch. Neurol.* 38:80–85

26. Pratt, H., Starr, A. 1981. Mechanically and electrically evoked somatosensory potentials in humans: scalp and neck distributions of short latency components. *Electroencephalogr. Clin. Neurophysiol.* 51:138–47

27. Starr, A., McKeon, B., Skuse, N., Burke, D. 1981. Cerebral potentials evoked by muscle stretch in man. *Brain* 104:149–66

28. Halliday, A. M. 1967. Changes in the form of cerebral evoked responses in man associated with various lesions of the nervous system. *Electroencephalogr. Clin. Neurophysiol. Suppl.* 25:178–86

29. Larson, S. J., Sances, A., Christenson, P. C. 1966. Evoked somatosensory potentials in man. *Arch. Neurol.* 15:88–95

30. Dorfman, L. J., Perkash, I., Bosley, T. M., Cummins, K. L. 1980. Use of cerebral evoked potentials to evaluate spinal somatosensory function in patients with traumatic and surgical myelopathies. *J. Neurosurg.* 52:654–60

31. Bennett, M. H., Jannetta, P. J. 1980. Trigeminal evoked potentials in humans. *Electroencephalogr. Clin. Neurophysiol.* 48:517–26

32. Stohr, M., Petruch, F., Scheglmann, K. 1971. Somatosensory evoked potentials following trigeminal nerve stimulation in trigeminal neuralgia. *Ann. Neurol.* 9:63–66

33. Desmedt, J. E., Cheron, G. 1980. Somatosensory evoked potentials to finger stimulation in healthy oc-

togenarians and in young adults: wave forms, scalp topography and transit times of parietal and frontal components. *Electroencephalogr. Clin. Neurophysiol.* 50:404–25

34. Dorfman, L. J. 1977. Indirect estimation of spinal cord conduction velocity in man. *Electroencephalogr. Clin. Neurophysiol.* 42:26–24

35. Dorfman, L. J., Bosley, T. M., Cummins, K. L. 1978. Electrophysiological localization of central somatosensory lesions in patients with multiple sclerosis. *Electroencephalogr. Clin. Neurophysiol.* 44:742–53

36. Eisen, A., Odusote, K. 1980. Central and peripheral conduction times in multiple sclerosis. *Electroencephalogr. Clin. Neurophysiol.* 48:253–65

37. Eisen, A., Nudleman, K. 1979. Cord to cortex conduction in multiple sclerosis. *Neurology (NY)* 29:189–93

38. Desmedt, J. E., Cheron, G. 1980. Central somatosensory conduction in man: neural generators and interpeak latencies of the far-field components recorded from neck and right or left scalp and earlobes. *Electroencephalogr. Clin. Neurophysiol.* 50:382–403

39. Eisen, A., Stewart, J., Nudleman, K., Cosgrove, J. B. R. 1979. Short-latency somatosensory responses in multiple sclerosis. *Neurology (NY)* 29:827–34

40. Anziska, B., Cracco, R. Q., Cook, A. W., Feld, E. W. 1978. Somatosensory far field potentials: studies in normal subjects and patients with multiple sclerosis. *Electroencephalogr. Clin. Neurophysiol.* 45:602–10

41. Cracco, R. Q. 1973. Spinal evoked response: peripheral nerve stimulation in man. *Electroencephalogr. Clin. Neurophysiol.* 35:379–86

42. Phillips, L. H., Daube, J. R. 1980. Lumbosacral spinal evoked potentials in humans. *Neurology (NY)* 30:1175–83

43. Tsumoto, T., Hirose, N., Nonaka, S., Takahashi, M. 1973. Cerebrovascular disease: changes in somatosensory evoked potentials associated with unilateral lesions. *Electroencephalogr. Clin. Neurophysiol.* 35:463–73

44. Ertekin, C., Mutlu, T., Sariva, Y., Uckardesler, L. 1980. Electrophysiological evaluation of the afferent spinal roots and nerves in patients with conus medullaris and cauda equina lesions. *J. Neurol. Sci.* 48:419–33

45. Ganes, T. 1980. Somatosensory conduction times and peripheral, cervical and cortical evoked potentials in patients with cervical spondylosis. *J. Neurol. Neurosurg. Psychiatry* 43:683–89

46. El Negamy, E., Sedgwick, E. M. 1979. Delayed cervical somatosensory potentials in cervical spondylosis. *J. Neurol. Neurosurg. Psychiatry* 42:238–41

47. Eisen, A., Elleker, B. 1980. Sensory nerve stimulation and evoked cerebral potentials. *Neurology (NY)* 30:1097–1105

48. Landi, A., Copeland, S. A., Wynn Parry, C. B., Jones, S. J. 1980. The role of somatosensory evoked potentials and nerve conduction studies in the surgical management of brachial plexus injuries. *J. Bone Joint Surg. Br. Vol.* 62:492–96

49. Jones, S. J. 1979. Investigation of brachial plexus traction lesions by peripheral and spinal somatosensory evoked potentials. *J. Neurol. Neurosurg. Psychiatry* 42:107–16

50. Noel, P., Desmedt, J. E. 1975. Somatosensory cerebral evoked potentials after vascular lesions of the brain-stem and diencephalon. *Brain* 98:113–28

51. Namerow, N. S. 1969. Somatosensory evoked responses following cervical cordotomy. *Bull. Los Angeles Neurol. Soc.* 34:184–87

52. Grabow, J. D., Aronson, A. E., Rose, D. E., Greene, K. L. 1980. Summated potentials evoked by speech sounds for determining cerebral dominance for language. *Electroencephalogr. Clin. Neurophysiol.* 49:38–47

53. Grabow, J. D., Aronson, A. E., Rose, D. E., Greene, K. L. 1980. Hemispheric potentials evoked by speech sounds during discrimination tasks. *Electroencephalogr. Clin. Neurophysiol.* 49:48–58

54. Jewett, D. L., Williston, J. S. 1971. Auditory evoked far field potentials averaged from the scalp of humans. *Brain* 94:681–93

55. Picton, T. W., Hillyard, S. A., Krausz, H. I., Galambos, R. 1974. Human auditory evoked potentials. I. Evaluation of components. *Electroencephalogr. Clin. Neurophysiol.* 36:179–90

56. Rowe, M. J. III. 1978. Normal variability of the brainstem auditory evoked response in young and old subjects. *Electroencephalogr. Clin. Neurophysiol.* 44:459–70

57. Chiappa, K. H., Gladstone, K. J., Young, R. R. 1979. Brain stem auditory evoked responses: studies of waveform variations in 50 normal human subjects. *Arch. Neurol.* 36:81–87

58. Stockard, J. E., Stockard, J. J., Westmoreland, B. F., Corfits, J. L. 1979. Brainstem auditory-evoked responses:

normal variation as a function of stimulus and subject characteristics. *Arch. Neurol.* 36:823–31

59. Chiappa, K. H., Harrison, J. L., Brooks, E. B., Young, R. R. 1980. Brainstem auditory evoked responses in 200 patients with multiple sclerosis. *Ann. Neurol.* 7:135–43

60. Starr, A., Archor, J. 1975. Auditory brain stem responses in neurological disease. *Arch. Neurol.* 32:761–8

61. Stockard, J. J., Rossiter, V. S. 1977. Clinical and pathologic correlates of brain stem auditory response abnormalities. *Neurology (Minneapolis)* 27:326–25

62. Starr, A., Hamilton, A. E. 1976. Correlation between confirmed sites of neurological lesions and abnormalities of far-field auditory brainstem responses. *Electroencephalogr. Clin. Neurophysiol.* 41:595–608

63. Selters, W. A., Brackmann, D. E. 1977. Acoustic tumor detection with brain stem electric audiometry. *Arch. Otolaryngol.* 103:181–87

64. Clemis, J. D., Mitchell, C. 1977. Electrocochleography and brain stem responses used in the diagnosis of acoustic tumors. *J. Otolaryngol.* 6:447–59

65. Robinson, K., Rudge, P. 1980. The use of the auditory evoked potential in the diagnosis of multiple sclerosis. *J. Neurol. Sci.* 45:235–44

66. Ochs, R., Markand, O. N., DeMyer, W. E. 1979. Brainstem auditory evoked responses in leukodystrophies. *Neurology (Minneapolis)* 29:1089–93

67. Gilroy, J., Lynn, G. E. 1978. Computerized tomography and auditory-evoked potentials: use in the diagnosis of olivopontocerebellar degeneration. *Arch. Neurol.* 35:143–47

68. Fujita, M., Hosoki, M., Miyazaki, M. 1981. Brainstem auditory evoked responses in spinocerebellar degeneration and Wilson disease. *Ann. Neurol.* 9:42–47

69. Satya-Murti, S., Cacace, A., Hanson, P. 1980. Auditory dysfunction in Friedreich ataxia: result of spiral ganglion degeneration. *Neurology (NY)* 30:1047–53

70. Tsubokawa, T., Nishimoto, H., Kitamura, M., Katayama, Y., Moriyasu, N. 1980. Assessment of brainstem damage by the auditory brainstem response in acute severe head injury. *J. Neurol Neurosurg. Psychiatry* 43:1005–11

71. Seales, D. M., Rossiter, V. S., Weinstein, M. E. 1979. Brainstem auditory evoked responses in patients comatose as a result of blunt head trauma. *J. Trauma* 19:347–52

72. Eisen, A., Purves, S., Hoirch, M. 1982. Central nervous system amplification: its potential in the early diagnosis of multiple sclerosis. *Neurology (NY)* 32:359–64

73. McDonald, W.I. 1974. Pathophysiology in multiple sclerosis. *Brain* 97:179–96

74. Chiappa, K. H. 1980. Pattern-shift visual, brainstem auditory, and short-latency somatosensory evoked potentials in multiple sclerosis. *Neurology (NY)* 30:110–23

75. Purves, S. J., Low, M. D., Galloway, L. L., Reeves, B. 1981. A comparison of visual, brainstem auditory, and somatosensory evoked potentials in multiple sclerosis. *Can. J. Neurol. Sci.* 8:15–20

76. Paty, D. W., Blume, W. T., Brown, W. F., Jaaroal, N., Kertesz, A., McFinnis, W. 1979. Chronic progressive myelopathy: investigation with CSF electrophoresis, evoked potentials and CT scan. *J. Neurol.* 6:419–24

77. Hume, A. L., Cant, B. R., Shaw, N. A. 1979. Central somatosensory conduction time in comatose patients. *Ann. Neurol.* 5:379–84

78. Goldie, W. D., Chiappa, K. H., Young, R. R., Brooks, E. B. 1981. Brainstem auditory and short latency somatosensory evoked responses in brain death. *Neurology (NY)* 31:248–56

79. Anziska, B. J., Cracco, R. Q. 1980. Short latency somatosensory evoked potentials in brain dead patients. *Arch. Neurol.* 27:222–25

80. Trojaborg, W., Jorgensen, E. O. 1973. Evoked cortical potentials in patients with "isoelectric" EEGs. *Electroencephalogr. Clin. Neurophysiol.* 35:301–9

81. Hume, A. L., Cant, B. R. 1981. Central somatosensory conduction after head injury. *Ann. Neurol.* 10:411–19

82. Rowe, M. J. III., Carlson, C. 1980. Brainstem auditory evoked potentials in postconcussion dizziness. *Arch. Neurol.* 37:679–83

83. Sedgwick, E. M., El-Negamy, E., Frankel, H. 1980. Spinal cord potentials in traumatic paraplegia and quadriplegia. *J. Neurol. Neurosurg. Psychiatry* 43:823–30

84. Greenberg, R. P., Becker, D. P., Miller, J. D., Mayer, D. J. 1977. Evaluation of brain function in severe human head trauma with multimodality evoked potentials. 2. Localization of brain dysfunction and correlation with post-

traumatic neurological conditions. *J. Neurosurg.* 47:163–77

85. Wright, J. E., Arden, G., Jones, B. R. 1973. Continuous monitoring of the visually evoked response during intraorbital surgery. *Trans. Ophthalmol. Soc. UK* 93:311–14

86. Wilson, W. B., Kirsch, W. M., Neville, H., Stears, J., Feinsod, M., Lehman, R. A. W. 1976. Monitoring of visual function during parasellar surgery. *Surg. Neurol.* 5:323–29

87. Feinsod, M., Selhorst, J. B., Hoyt, W. F., Wilson, C. B. 1976. Monitoring optic nerve function during craniotomy. *J. Neurosurg.* 44:29–31

88. Levine, R. A. 1979. Monitoring auditory evoked potentials during acoustic neuroma surgery. In *Neurological Surgery of the Ear,* ed. H. Silverstein, H. Norrell, 2:287–93. Birmingham: Aesculapius

89. McCallum, J. E., Bennett, M. H. 1975. Electrophysiologic monitoring of spinal cord functions during intraspinal surgery. *Surg. Forum.* 26:469–71

90. Mizrahi, E. M., Dorfman, L. J. 1980. Sensory evoked potentials: clinical applications in pediatrics. *J. Pediatr.* 97:1–10

91. Callaway, E., Tueting, P., Koslow, S. H., eds. 1978. *Event-Related Brain Potentials in Man.* New York: Academic. 626 pp.

92. Chiappa, K. H., Ropper, A. H. 1982. Evoked potentials in clinical medicine. *N. Engl. J. Med.* 306:1140–50, 1205–11

93. Starr, A. 1978. Sensory evoked potentials in clinical disorders of the nervous system. *Ann. Rev. Neurosci.* 1:103–27

94. Eisen, A. 1982. The somatosensory evoked potential. *Can. J. Neurol. Sci.* 9:65–77

95. Desmedt, J. E., ed. 1977. *Visual Evoked Potentials in Man: New Developments.* Oxford: Clarendon 556 pp.

96. Desmedt, J. E., ed. 1980. *Clinical Uses of Cerebral, Brainstem and Spinal Somatosensory Evoked Potentials.* Basel: Karger 347 pp.

97. Naunton, R. F., Fernandez, C., eds. 1978. *Evoked Electrical Activity in the Auditory Nervous System.* San Francisco: Academic 582 pp.

Ann. Rev. Med. 1983. 34:491–500

SUPERACTIVE GONADOTROPIN-RELEASING HORMONE AGONISTS

Ronald S. Swerdloff, M.D., and David Heber, M.D., Ph.D.

Department of Medicine, Harbor-UCLA Medical Center, University of
California at Los Angeles School of Medicine, Torrance, California 90509

ABSTRACT

Superactive GnRH agonists represent a new class of pharmacologic agents
that inhibit reproductive function in both men and women when administered chronically. These hormonal drugs are being tested extensively as
both male and female contraceptive agents, as a treatment for prostate
cancer, and as a new treatment for idiopathic precocious puberty. Other
potential uses include treatment for endometriosis, hirsutism, polycystic
ovarian disease, and severe intractable androgen-related acne. This chapter
reviews the effects of GnRH agonists on gonadotropin and steroid hormone
secretion in both men and women, and assesses the potential of these agents
in the varied clinical uses delineated above.

The isolation, structural characterization, and synthesis of gonadotropin-
releasing hormone (GnRH), the hypothalamic decapeptide controlling
pituitary gonadotropin secretion (1, 2), led to the synthesis of a number of
long-acting stimulatory analogs of GnRH (3, 4). It was hypothesized that
these agents could be used to treat hypogonadal patients with releasing
hormone deficiency (1), but it was soon discovered that chronic GnRH or
GnRH analog administration in animals and humans led to a paradoxical
inhibition of reproductive function. In males, chronic agonist administration inhibited gonadotropin secretion, testicular steroidogenesis, and spermatogenesis (5–11). In females, inhibition of gonadotropin secretion,
ovarian steroidogenesis, ovulation, and luteal function were reported (12–
16). These observations led to the clinical testing of GnRH agonists as a

491

hormonal treatment for precocious puberty (17) and steroid-sensitive tumors (e.g. prostate cancer) (18), as male and female contraceptive agents (19, 20), and as a treatment for other disorders where it would be desirable to suppress gonadal function.

The authentic decapeptide GnRH is synthesized in the hypothalamus and is released into the hypophyseal portal circulation. GnRH binds to its specific membrane receptor on the surface of the pituitary gonadotropin-secreting cell, and thereby stimulates the synthesis and secretion of both gonadotropic hormones, luteinizing hormone (LH) and follicle-stimulating hormone (FSH). Long-acting agonists also bind to this receptor (21) but lead to a prolonged release of gonadotropins compared to authentic GnRH. This prolonged stimulatory effect correlates with prolonged intrapituitary localization of agonist (22). Following continuous exposure to GnRH or its agonists, the pituitary gland becomes refractory to GnRH stimulation despite the presence of LH stores within the gonadotroph (23). Continuous intravenous infusions of GnRH lead to down-regulation of pituitary gonadotropin secretory responses in men and women (24–26). Current evidence from animal studies suggests that both decreased membrane receptors (due to both hormone occupancy and decreased receptor numbers) and an uncoupling of the GnRH receptor from the gonadotropin secretory mechanism contribute to GnRH-induced pituitary desensitization (27). Since GnRH agonists have a similar course of action in the human, it is likely that the same mechanisms observed in animals mediate the inhibition of gonadotropin secretion observed in both men and women.

Extrapituitary effects of GnRH agonist on gonadal steroidogenesis have also been demonstrated in animals. Two separate mechanisms for such effects have been proposed. First, Auclair et al (9) noted that, after seven days of GnRH agonist administration in male rats, testosterone secretion and gonadotropin receptors in the testis were suppressed. These authors subsequently proposed that a sustained increase in circulating LH levels observed secondary to agonist stimulation led to a secondary down-regulation of testicular gonadotropin receptors resulting in an inhibition of gonadal steroidogenesis (11). Second, membrane receptors for GnRH were localized in the Leydig cell compartment of the rat testis (27) and in ovarian homogenates (28), which leads to the hypothesis that GnRH agonists act directly on the gonad to inhibit steroidogenesis. There is extensive data on the ability of GnRH agonists to inhibit directly ovarian and testicular steroidogenesis in vitro (29–32). This effect requires prolonged exposure (2 days) of gonadal cells to GnRH agonists in vitro and thus differs from the stimulatory pituitary effects of GnRH. Short-term in vitro studies in the testis failed to demonstrate the inhibitory effects of GnRH agonist (33), and the exact mechanism of the direct inhibition of gonadal steroidogenesis by

GnRH agonist is not clear. In cultured granulosa cells, FSH-stimulated progesterone formation (3β-hydroxysteroid dehydrogenase) is inhibited and FSH-stimulated breakdown of progesterone to an inactive metabolite (200α-dehydroprogesterone) is enhanced by agonist treatment (34). In the testes obtained from rats treated in vivo with GnRH agonist, 17,20-desmolase and 17-hydroxylase activities are decreased, which decreases formation of androgen precursors of testosterone and increases progesterone and pregnenolone concentration relative to their 17-hydroxylated metabolites (35).

The data supporting direct gonadal effects of GnRH agonist in humans are more convincing for females than for males in our view. There is little question that GnRH agonists can inhibit progesterone production by the corpus luteum in the human (15, 16), but this effect can be counteracted by chorionic gonadotropin administration (16). Since placental production of chorionic gonadotropin could interfere with the luteolytic effects of agonist, this strategy for the development of a female contraceptive remains problematic. The direct gonadal effects of agonist on testicular steroidogenesis do not appear to mediate the inhibition of reproductive function noted either in the rhesus monkey (36) or the ram (37). Our own data in four patients with prostate cancer treated for 6 months with 1 mg daily injections of D-leu[6]desGly[10] GnRH ethylamide (Leuprolide) as part of the Tap Pharmaceutical–Abbott Prostatic Adenocarcinoma Clinical Trial demonstrate a primary inhibition of pituitary gonadotropin secretion secondary to chronic agonist treatment (Table 1).

Faure et al (38), using another agonist (Buserelin, Hoechst-Roussel) reported that, following chronic agonist treatment, circulating 17-hydroxyprogesterone and testosterone levels were lowered in the presence of normal pregnenolone and progesterone levels. These data were interpreted as evidence for 17,20-desmolase and 17-hydroxylase inhibition in the human. However, since in the human male, 17-hydroxyprogesterone (39) is primar-

Table 1   Effects of chronic agonist (D-leu[6]desGly[10] GnRH ethylamide) treatment on pituitary and gonadal hormones

Day of study	Basal LH (mIU/ml)	ΔLH (mIU/ml)	Basal FSH (mIU/ml)	ΔFSH (mIU/ml)	T (ng/dl)	ΔT (ng/dl)
1	12.5 ± 5.5	96 ± 20	11.5 ± 1.8	75 ± 26	384 ± 49	228 ± 79
5	30.4 ± 6.3	6.4 ± 2.6	14.7 ± 2.4	1.5 ± 0.9	652 ± 148	62.5 ± 41
56	$6.25 \pm .48$	2.8 ± 1.2	6.8 ± 0.8	2.1 ± 0.5	29 ± 2.45	7.3 ± 5.8
180	5.5 ± 0.9	2.2 ± 1.1	8.2 ± 1.1	$2.9 \pm .17$	31 ± 8.4	9.5 ± 3.8

ily secreted by the testes, while pregnenolone and progesterone also result from adrenal steroidogenesis, these data are also consistent with a selective gonadal effect mediated via pituitary actions of GnRH agonist. Recently, Huhtanieni & Clayton (40) were unable to identify GnRH receptors in a human testis at autopsy, while pituitary GnRH receptors were readily identified. These data, in our view, support the premise that the primary site of action of GnRH agonists in the human is the pituitary gland, with the exception of inhibition of corpus luteum function. Additional data are required to clarify this important question.

Studies of GnRH agonist as a male contraceptive demonstrated reversible suppression of spermatogenesis (19), but agonist treatment predictably led to androgen deficiency and had to be discontinued after six or seven weeks in five of eight subjects because of impotence. Libido and potency returned two weeks after stopping agonist therapy, but the appearance of these symptoms represented a significant drawback to the application of GnRH agonists alone as male contraceptive agents. Of three subjects who completed ten weeks of therapy, only one was azoospermic. Studies in our laboratories had anticipated the need for combined analog treatment and androgen replacement if these agonists were to be applied successfully as male contraceptives. In castrate rats, synergistic inhibition of gonadotropin secretion occurred when GnRH agonist and testosterone were combined (41); in intact rats, GnRH agonist and testosterone in combination enhanced suppression of spermatogenesis compared to either agent used alone (10). Recently, we treated four normal male volunteers with either 100 μg of a GnRH agonist (d[Nal$_2$]^{6}GnRH, Syntex Laboratories, Palo Alto, California) daily for 10 days or with this agonist regimen combined with a single dose of 200 mg of testosterone enanthate on day 1 of agonist treatment (42). As shown in Figure 1, combined treatment with GnRH agonist and testosterone enhanced the inhibition of gonadotropin secretion compared to treatment with GnRH agonist alone. Rabin et al (19) administered a GnRH agonist, DTrp^{6}Pro^{9}NEt GnRH (approximately equipotent to the agonist we have tested), both alone at a "low" dose of 50 μg daily subcutaneously and in combination with bimonthly 100-mg injections of testosterone enanthate. The degree of oligospermia observed in six subjects was similar to that reported following agonist treatment alone, and azoospermia was not achieved during a 20-week treatment period in any subject. It is likely that the GnRH agonist regimens tested to date by Rabin and his colleagues for their effects on spermatogenesis used too low a dose of agonist, studied in combination with a dose of testosterone that, by itself, clearly did not suppress spermatogenesis. Our ongoing trials of a four-fold higher dose of agonist combined with a dose of testosterone enanthate previously demonstrated by us to markedly, though not completely, sup-

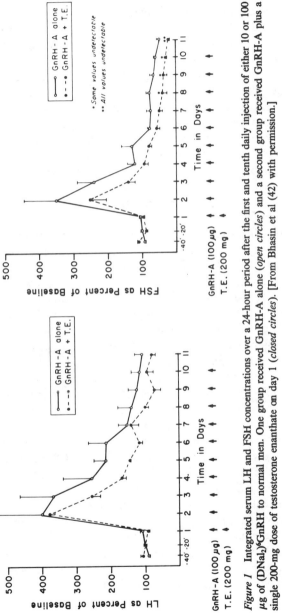

Figure 1 Integrated serum LH and FSH concentrations over a 24-hour period after the first and tenth daily injection of either 10 or 100 μg of (DNal₂)⁶GnRH to normal men. One group received GnRH-A alone (*open circles*) and a second group received GnRH-A plus a single 200-mg dose of testosterone enanthate on day 1 (*closed circles*). [From Bhasin et al (42) with permission.]

press spermatogenesis (43) should yield more effective suppression of spermatogenesis than that observed in any regimen of GnRH tested to date.

Major problems remain to be solved before GnRH agonists can be used as female contraceptive agents. When given daily, the GnRH agonist Buserlin (Hoechst-Roussel) inhibits ovarian steroidogenesis and ovulation (14). Complete inhibition of ovarian steroidogenesis would simulate the menopause, requiring replacement therapy with estrogen-progestins and thus negating the value of these agents as a new approach to female contraception. Partial suppression of the reproductive hormonal axis with the retention of estrogen secretion, but failure of ovulation, would require careful dose regulation in order to prevent various forms of dysfunctional uterine bleeding ranging from amenorrhea to unpredictable breakthrough bleeding. In addition, unopposed estrogen effects secondary to agonist treatment can result in endometrial hyperplasia (20) with increased risk of endometrial carcinoma (44). An alternative approach is selectively to induce defects in corpus luteum function with agonist treatment, thereby interfering with the implantation of a fertilized egg. In 15 patients, Sheehan & Yen (45) administered a GnRH agonist for one or two successive days during the luteal phase (i.e. after the LH peak). A fall in estrogen and progesterone significantly shortened the luteal phase in 26 of 27 treatment cycles when agonist was given from 6 to 9 days after the LH peak, but in only 3 of 13 cycles when given from 1 to 5 days after the LH peak. Corpus luteal dysfunction could also be induced by interfering with the FSH rise that normally occurs early in the follicular phase of a menstrual cycle. This approach would utilize agonist during the first few days after menstruation to impair follicular development and produce inadequate corpus luteum function on that basis. The degree of corpus luteum dysfunction induced must predictably prevent ovum implantation to be an effective contraceptive method, since these women would presumably still ovulate.

Studies of GnRH agonists in the treatment of prostate cancer are encouraging. In our own studies (48) and those reported by Warner, Santen & Max (49) as part of the Tap Pharmaceutical–Abbott Laboratories Prostatic Adenocarcinoma Clinical Trial, GnRH agonist suppressed serum testosterone into the castrate range following eight weeks of therapy. In our studies, this was accompanied by marked suppression of both LH and FSH, which implicates the pituitary gland as the primary site of agonist action in the human male with chronic administration. The ability to obtain a medical castration predictably should lead to response frequencies comparable to those obtained with diethylstilbestrol administration or orchiectomy and, in our view, GnRH agonists will soon be the hormonal treatment of choice in prostatic carcinoma.

Experience with the treatment of idiopathic precocious puberty is still limited. There is no other satisfactory hormonal treatment for these children who suffer the dual social disabilities of stunted growth and premature sexual function. It has been demonstrated clearly that hormonal abnormalities in these children can be reversed with agonist treatment and that reproductive hormonal function resumes after discontinuing therapy (17) (Figure 2). It remains to be demonstrated in longer-term trials that the beneficial effects expected on ultimate adult height are attained, and such studies are currently being carried out.

Superactive GnRH agonist therapy has been proposed as a treatment for a host of diseases that are dependent to some extent on gonadal steroid secretion, including polycystic ovarian disease, hirsutism, acne, and, most recently, endometriosis (50). In a small number of women with endometriosis, GnRH agonist treatment was shown to cause reversible medical castra-

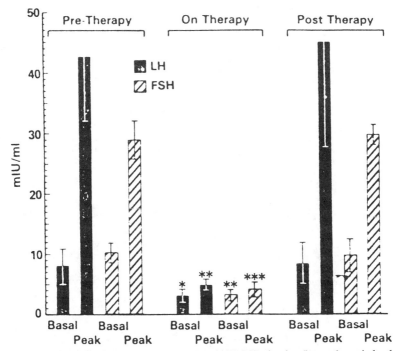

Figure 2 Effect of GnRH analog on basal and peak (GnRH-stimulated) gonadotropin levels in five girls with idiopathic precocious puberty. The basal LH and FSH values for each patient are means of 26 measurements. The peak values are the highest LH and FSH levels attained during the standard GnRH stimulation tests performed in each patient. The levels during therapy were measured during the eighth week of treatment. The post-therapy levels were measured eight weeks after discontinuation of GnRH-A treatment. Patients 4 and 5 continued to receive GnRH-A. [From Comite et al (17) with permission.]

tion, but a direct comparison of GnRH agonist and established treatment of endometriosis with progestational agents or oophorectomy remains to be performed to determine whether or not GnRH agonists will indeed form a new approach to treating endometriosis.

Superactive GnRH agonists were originally proposed as agents to treat GnRH deficiency states, but for such disorders as hypogonadotropic hypogonadism (46) and idiopathic infertility due to presumed hypothalamic dysfunction (47) the pulsatile administration of authentic GnRH by programmable portable infusion pumps will be the likely approach of the future. The incidental inhibitory effects of superactive GnRH agonists found in the course of investigating their use as GnRH replacement therapy should provide a powerful new class of hormonal therapeutic agents useful in the areas of male and female contraception, the therapy of hormone-dependent tumors (e.g. prostatic cancer), the therapy of idiopathic precocious puberty, and, perhaps, the therapy of endometriosis.

Literature Cited

1. Schally, A. V., Arimura, A., Kastin, A., Matsuo, H., Baba, Y., Redding, T., Nair, R., Debeljuk, L., White, W. 1971. Gonadotropin releasing hormone: one polypeptide regulates secretion of luteinizing and follicle stimulating hormones. *Science* 173:1036
2. Amoss, M., Burgus, R., Blackwell, R., Vale, W., Fellows, R., Guillemin, R. 1971. Purification, amino acid composition and *N*-terminus of the hypothalamic luteinizing hormone releasing factor of ovine origin. *Biochem. Biophys. Res. Commun.* 44:205
3. Vale, W., Rivier, C., Brown, M., Leppaluoto, J., Ling, N., Monahan, M., Rivier, J. 1976. Pharmacology of hypothalamic regulatory peptides. *Clin. Endocrinol.* (*Suppl.*) 5:2615
4. Sandow, J., König, W., Geiger, R., Uhmann, R., vonRechenberg, W. 1978. Structure-activity relationship in the LHRH molecule. In *Control of Ovulation*, ed. D. B. Crighton, G. R. Foxcroft, N. B. Haynes, p. 49. London: Butterworths
5. Swerdloff, R. S., Peterson, M., Vera, A., Batt, R. A. L., Heber, D., Bray, G. A. 1978. The hypothalamic-pituitary axis in genetically obese (ob/ob) mice: response to LHRH. *Endocrinology* 103: 542-47
6. Hetzel, W. D., Nicile, C. H., Pfeiffer, E. F. 1977. Analytical study on the effects of GnRH (DesGly^{10}D-Leu-6) ethylamide. *Acta Endocrinol.* (*Suppl.*) 208:35

7. Davies, T., Gomez-Pan, A., Watson, M. J., Mountjoy, C. Q., Hanber, J. P., Besser, G. M., Hall, R. 1977. Reduced gonadotropin response to releasing hormone after chronic administration to impotent men. *Clin. Endocrinol.* 6: 213-18
8. Sandow, J., Rechenberg, W. F., Jerzabek, G. 1977. Endocrine effects of chronic treatment with LHRH analog D-Ser(TBU)^{6}ethylamide. *Acta Endocrinol.* (*Suppl.*) 208:33
9. Auclair, C., Kelly, P. A., Coy, D. H., Schally, A. V., Labrie, F. 1977. Potent inhibitory activity of DLeu^{6}desGly^{10} LHRH ethylamide on LH/hCG and PRL testicular receptor levels in the rat. *Endocrinology* 101:1980
10. Heber, D., Swerdloff, R. S. 1981. Gonadotropin-releasing hormone analog and testosterone synergistically inhibit spermatogenesis. *Endocrinology* 108:2019-21
11. Labrie, F., Auclair, C., Cusan, L., Kelly, P. A., Pelletier, G., Ferland, F. 1978. Inhibitory effects of LHRH and its agonists on testicular gonadotropin receptors and spermatogenesis in the rat. *Int. J. Andrology* (*Suppl.*) 2:303-18
12. Bowers, C. Y., Folkers, K. 1976. Contraception and inhibition of ovulation by minipump infusion of the luteinizing hormone, active analogs and antagonists. *Biochem. Biophys. Res. Commun.* 72:1003
13. Rivier, C., Rivier, J., Vale, W. 1978. Chronic effects of (DTrp^{6}Pro^{9}NEt)

luteinizing hormone releasing factor on reproductive processes in the female rat. *Endocrinology* 103:2299

14. Bergquist, C., Nillius, S. J., Wide, L. 1979. Inhibition of ovulation in women by intranasal treatment with a luteinizing hormone releasing hormone agonist. *Contraception* 19:497

15. Bergquist, C., Nillius, S. J., Wide, L. 1980. Effects of luteinizing hormone-releasing hormone agonist on luteal function in women. *Contraception* 22:287

16. Casper, R. F., Sheehan, K. L., Yen, S. S. C. 1980. Chorionic gonadotropin prevents LRF-agonist-induced luteolysis in the human. *Contraception* 21:471

17. Comite, F., Cutler, G. B., Rivier, J., Vale, W., Loriaux, D. L., Crowley, W. F. 1981. Short-term treatment of idiopathic precocious puberty with a long-acting analogue of LHRH. *N. Engl. J. Med.* 305:1546–51

18. Faure, H., Lemay, A., Belanger, A., Labrie, F. 1982. Inhibition of testicular steroidogenesis by chronic administration of a potent LHRH agonist, HOE 766, to patients with cancer of the prostate. *J. Androl.* 3:43

19. Rabin, D., Linde, R., Doelle, G., Alexander, N. 1981. Experience with a potent GnRH agonist in normal men: an approach to the development of a male contraceptive. In *LHRH Peptides as Female and Male Contraceptives,* ed. G. Zatuchini, J. Shelton, J. Sciarra, pp. 296–306. Philadelphia: Harper & Row

20. Nillius, S. J., Bergquist, C., Wide, L. 1978. Inhibition of ovulation in women by chronic treatment with a stimulatory LRH analogue—a new approach to birth control. *Contraception* 17:537

21. Heber, D., Odell, W. D. 1978. Pituitary receptor binding activity of active, inactive, superactive and inhibitory analogs of gonadotropin-releasing hormone. *Biochem. Biophys. Res. Commun.* 82:67–73

22. Reeves, J. J., Tarnavsky, G. K., Becker, S. R., Coy, D. H., Schally, A. V. 1977. Uptake of iodinated LHRH analogs in the pituitary. *Endocrinology* 101:540

23. deKoning, J., Van Dieten, J. A. M. J., van Rees, G. P. 1978. Refractoriness of the pituitary gland after continuous exposure to luteinizing hormone releasing hormone. *J. Endocrinol.* 79:311

24. Heber, D., Swerdloff, R. S. 1981. Down-regulation of pituitary gonadotropin secretion in postmenopausal females by continuous gonadotropin re-

leasing hormone administration. *J. Clin. Endocrinol. Metab.* 52:171–72

25. McNeil, L. W., McKenna, T. J., Lacroix, A., Beneveniste, R., Rabin, D. 1979. Seventy-two hour infusions of LHRH into normal men: gonadotropin and testicular steroid response. *J. Clin. Endocrinol. Metab.* 49:149

26. Rabin, D., McNeil, L. W. 1980. Pituitary and gonadal desensitization after continuous luteinizing hormone-releasing hormone infusion in normal females. *J. Clin. Endocrinol. Metab.* 51:873

27. Clayton, R. N. 1982. Gonadotropin-releasing hormone modulation of its own pituitary receptors; evidence for biphasic regulation. *Endocrinology* 111:152–61

27a. Bourne, G. A., Regiani, S., Payne, A. H., Marshall, J. C. 1980. Testicular GnRH receptors—characterization and localization on interstitial tissue. *J. Clin. Endocrinol. Metab.* 51:407

28. Reeves, J. J., Seguin, C., Lefebvre, F. A., Kelly, P. A., Labrie, F. 1980. Similar luteinizing hormone-releasing hormone binding sites in rat anterior pituitary and ovary. *Proc. Natl. Acad. Sci. USA* 77:5567

29. Hsueh, A. J. W., Erickson, G. F. 1979. Extrapituitary action of gonadotropin-releasing hormone: direct inhibition of ovarian steroidogenesis. *Science* 204:854

30. Hsueh, A. J. W., Ling, N. C. 1979. Effect of an antagonistic analog of gonadotropin-releasing hormone upon ovarian granulosa cell function. *Life Sci.* 25:1223

31. Hsueh, A. J. W., Schreiber, J. R., Erickson, G. F. 1981. Inhibitory effect of gonadotropin releasing hormone upon cultured testicular cells. *Mol. Cell. Endocrinol.* 21:43

32. Clayton, R. N., Katikieni, M., Chan, V., Dufau, M. L., Catt, K. J. 1980. Direct inhibition of testicular function by gonadotropin-releasing hormone: mediation by specific gonadotropin-releasing hormone receptors in interstitial cells. *Proc. Natl. Acad. Sci. USA* 77:4459

33. Badger, T. M., Beitins, I. Z., Ostrea, T., Crisafulli, J. M., Little, R., Saidel, M. E. 1980. Luteinizing hormone-releasing hormone does not inhibit testosterone production in rat interstitial cells *in vitro. Endocrinology* 106:1149

34. Jones, P. B. C., Hsueh, A. J. W. 1981. Direct stimulation of ovarian progesterone metabolizing enzyme by gonadotro-

500   SWERDLOFF & HEBER

35. Belanger, A., Cusan, L., Auclair, C., Seguin, C., Caron, S., Labrie, F. 1980. Effect of an LHRH agonist and hCG on testicular steroidogenesis in the adult rat. *Biol. Reprod.* 22:1094–1102

36. Resko, J. A., Belanger, A., Labrie, F. 1982. Effects of chronic treatment with a potent luteinizing hormone-releasing hormone agonist on serum luteinizing hormone and steroid levels in the male rhesus monkey. *Biol. Reprod.* 26:378–84

37. Fraser, H. M., Lincoln, G. H. 1980. Effects of chronic treatment with an LHRH agonist on the secretion of LH, FSH and testosterone in the ram. *Biol. Reprod.* 22:269–76

38. Faure, N., Labrie, F., Lemay, A., Belanger, A., et al. 1982. Inhibition of serum androgen levels by chronic intranasal and subcutaneous administration of a potent luteinizing hormone-releasing hormone agonist in adult men. *Fertil. Steril.* 37:416–24

39. Lipsett, M. B. 1970. Steroid secretion by the human testis. In *The Human Testis*, ed. E. Rosemberg, C. A. Paulsen, p. 407. New York: Plenum (A Serono Foundation Symposium)

40. Huhtanieni, I. T., Clayton, R. N. 1982. Absence of gonadotrophin-releasing hormone receptors in human gonads. *Proc. Joint Br. Endocrinol. Soc. London Abstr.* 122

41. Heber, D., Swerdloff, R. S. 1980. Male contraception: synergism between superactive GnRH analog and testosterone in suppressing gonadotropin. *Science* 209:936

42. Bhasin, S., Heber, D., Steiner, B., Swerdloff, R. S. 1982. Enhanced inhibition of gonadotropin secretion in man by combined GnRH agonist and testosterone. *J. Clin. Endocrinol. Metab.* Submitted

43. Swerdloff, R. S., McClure, R. D., Palacios, A., Campfield, L. A., Brosman, S. A. 1978. Clinical evaluation of testosterone enanthate in the reversible suppression of spermatogenesis in the human male. Efficacy, mechanism of action and adverse effects. *Proc. Hormonal Control of Male Fertility, 1977,* ed. D. J. Patanelli, p. 41. Washington, DC: US Dept. Health, Educ. Welfare; Natl. Inst. Health

44. Lipsett, M. B. 1977. Estrogen use and cancer risk. *J. Am. Med. Assoc.* 237:1112–16

45. Sheehan, K. L., Yen, S. S. C. 1981. Clinical studies with LHRH agonists. In *LHRH Peptides as Female and Male Contraceptives*, ed. G. I. Zatuchini, J. D. Shelton, J. J. Sciarra, pp. 237–41. Philadelphia: Harper & Row

46. Crowley, W. F., Beitins, I. Z., Vale, W., et al 1980. The biologic activity of a potent analogue of gonadotropin-releasing hormone in normal and hypogonadotropic men. *N. Engl. J. Med.* 302:1052–57

47. Hammond, C. B., Wiebe, R. H., Harvey, A. F., et al. 1979. Ovulation induction with luteinizing hormone-releasing hormone in amenorrheic infertile women. *Am. J. Obstet. Gynecol.* 135:924–39

48. Heber, D., Swerdloff, R. S., Steiner, B., Rajfer, J. 1982. The pituitary gland: primary site of action of GnRH agonists in the human male. *J. Clin. Invest.* Submitted

49. Warner, B., Santen, R. J., Max, D. 1982. Successful "medical castration" with a superagonist analog of GnRH in treating prostatic carcinoma. *Clin. Res.* 30:493A

50. Meldrum, D. R., Chang, R. J., Lu, J., Vale, W., Rivier, J., Judd, H. L. 1982. "Medical oophorectomy" using a long-acting GnRH agonist—a possible new approach to the treatment of endometriosis. *J. Clin. Endocrinol. Metab.* 54:1081–83

Ann. Rev. Med. 1983. 34:501–17

EARLY DIAGNOSIS
OF COLORECTAL CANCER

Robert B. Fath, Jr., M.D., and Sidney J. Winawer, M.D.

Gastroenterology Service, Department of Medicine, Memorial Sloan-Kettering Cancer Center; and the Department of Medicine, Cornell University Medical College, New York, New York 10021

ABSTRACT

Screening of asymptomatic patients at risk is potentially the most effective means for detecting early colorectal carcinoma. Sensitive and specific tests are available for this purpose. However, an aggressive approach by the physician and compliance by the patient population are necessary for the proper implementation of this screening process.

INTRODUCTION

Colorectal carcinoma is the second most common malignancy in men and women in the United States, with approximately 120,000 new cases each year. Of major concern is the fact that survival following surgery has not been significantly altered over the past forty years. The five-year survival for this disease is 42%, a figure reflective of the advanced stage of the cancer in most patients at the time of initial diagnosis. However, if the diagnosis is established prior to the onset of symptoms, the large majority of patients will have localized disease, and the five-year survival approaches 90% (1). In view of our poor understanding of those factors contributing to the pathogenesis of colorectal carcinoma, the improved survival for the asymptomatic patient as compared to the symptomatic patient, the slow doubling time of this tumor, the limited benefit of chemotherapy for advanced disease, and the knowledge that certain lesions may antedate this malignancy, aggressive screening offers our best means of abating the impact of colorectal carcinoma.

501

0066-4219/83/0401-0501$02.00

Screening identifies asymptomatic individuals within a large population group who have signs suggestive of a particular disease. Essential to the establishment of a screening process are several fundamental principles (2):

1. The disease is of public significance.
2. The natural history of the disease is understood and can be effectively altered by the screening program.
3. Screening tests and more specific diagnostic modalities are available for the recognition of the disease in the asymptomatic patient.
4. Physicians are willing to utilize aggressively the proposed screening process.
5. The general public is both informed and motivated.
6. The cost of the screening process should fall within the framework of the public health expenditures.

Furthermore, the screening tests, as well as the confirmatory diagnostic modalities, must be scrutinized for their validity and predictiveness. Validity is a measure of both sensitivity and specificity. Sensitivity is the ability of a test to give a positive result when the patient has the disease in question. Specificity, on the other hand, is the ability of a test to give a negative result when the patient does not have the disease. Obviously, there is a fine balance between these two criteria, for one is often increased to the detriment of the other. In general, it is preferable to select the more sensitive test for the purpose of screening. This will essentially exclude the disease when the test is negative. However, if sensitivity is high at the expense of a low specificity, many false positives will occur and result in many unnecessary diagnostic workups. For the purpose of confirming the presence of the disease, the more specific test is best utilized. The predicability of a test is the probability that a disease is present or absent in the setting of a positive or negative test, respectively. This criterion depends upon both the validity of the test and the physician's pretest estimation of the likelihood of the disease. Certainly, a positive screening test is more meaningful for patients at risk for the disease. This last statement bears particular relevance to the screening process for colorectal cancer, for there are definite subpopulations at risk for this neoplasm. Therefore, the thoughtful application of valid screening and diagnostic tests to these groups at risk is necessary for the early detection of colorectal carcinoma.

The purpose of this discussion is to review the salient features of the screening process for colorectal carcinoma with emphasis on the identification of groups at risk, the available screening tests, confirmatory diagnostic modalities, and the overall approach to screening and diagnosis.

GROUPS AT RISK FOR COLORECTAL CANCER
Average Risk

AGE It is now well recognized that the risk for colorectal carcinoma significantly increases beyond the age of 40–45 years, and doubles in each succeeding decade to a peak at age 75 years (3). Men and women are essentially at equal risk (Table 1).

High Risk

HISTORY OF COLORECTAL ADENOMA The potential premalignancy of adenomatous polyps has been a controversial topic in past years. There is an increased risk of colorectal carcinoma in patients with adenomas. In a 15-year follow-up of 305 patients with adenomas documented by proctosigmoidoscopic examination, Prager and associates noted a doubling of the incidence of colorectal cancer in the general population (4). In one fourth to one third of resected colonic segments for large bowel cancer, solitary or multiple adenomas are present (5, 6). Recently, the adenoma-carcinoma sequence, as proposed by Hill et al (7), has gained wide acceptance. They suggest that most carcinomas arise in adenomatous tissue. This risk of malignant transformation is 40% for villous adenomas and 22% and 5% for tubulovillous and tubular adenomas, respectively (8). It is also evident that the greater the size of the polyp, the greater is the frequency of atypia and frank carcinoma. In a series by Ekelund & Lindstrom (9), 44% of adenomas less than 5 mm in size were either moderately or well differen-

Table 1 Groups at risk for colorectal cancer

Average risk	High risk
Age	Associated Disease
asymptomatic individuals over 40 years of age	ulcerative colitis
	granulomatous colitis
	Past History
	colorectal carcinoma and adenoma
	breast and genital carcinoma in women
	Family History
	adenomatous polyposis syndromes
	juvenile polyposis
	colorectal carcinoma and adenoma
	cancer family syndrome

tiated as opposed to only 27% of adenomas greater than 10 mm in size. Morson (10) reported that approximately 50% of adenomas greater than 2 cm in size contained invasive carcinoma. Therefore, it seems advisable to remove detected colorectal adenomas. The benefit of such prophylaxis is supported by the 25-year study of Gilbertsen and associates at the University of Minnesota (11). Proctosigmoidoscopic polypectomy, in more than 18,000 patients under surveillance, significantly reduced the predicted incidence of rectal carcinoma.

HISTORY OF COLORECTAL CARCINOMA   Patients with a history of colorectal carcinoma are at risk for the recurrence of large bowel cancer. Schottenfeld, Berg & Vitsky (12) reported on a series of 4771 patients at the Memorial Sloan-Kettering Cancer Center with colorectal carcinoma. A previous or synchronous colorectal carcinoma was noted in 5.5% of these patients. The subsequent annual incidence of multiple primary colorectal carcinomas was 0.35%, a risk three times greater than that in the general population. This risk increased six-fold if adenomas were detected in the operative specimen.

HISTORY OF BREAST OR GENITAL CARCINOMA   Epidemiologic studies indicate that women with a history of either breast or genital carcinoma are at increased risk for cancer of the large intestine. Schoenberg et al (13) found this risk to be 1½ times that of the general population. However, it is not clear if this group of patients is independent of that with the family cancer syndrome.

FAMILIAL POLYPOSIS SYNDROMES   Familial polyposis coli is the most common of the polyposis syndromes and is characterized by a myriad of small, mostly sessile, adenomatous polyps covering the colon and rectum. The disease is inherited as an autosomal dominant trait with approximately 90% penetrance. The polyps rarely appear before the age of ten years. Prophylactic colectomy is recommended at an early age because the risk of colorectal carcinoma progressively increases to 100% by the fifth decade.

Gardner's syndrome is also inherited as an autosomal dominant trait. It is characterized by large bowel polyposis in association with facial osteomas and various soft tissue tumors. Rarely, polyps may be found in the stomach and small intestine. There is a high incidence of colorectal carcinoma, and prophylactic colectomy is advisable.

Oldfield's and Turcot's syndromes are rare forms of adenomatous polyposis coli associated with sebaceous cysts and central nervous system tumors, respectively. These two syndromes may in fact represent variants of either familial polyposis coli or Gardner's syndrome.

Peutz-Jeghers syndrome is probably inherited as a single dominant pleio-trophic gene with a high degree of penetrance. Typically, gastrointestinal polyps and mucocutaneous melanin pigmentation are present. Although the polyps resemble adenomas, they are actually hamartomas. Associated gastrointestinal carcinoma is uncommon and is estimated to occur in 2–3% of all cases (14).

Generalized juvenile polyposis and juvenile polyposis coli are syndromes in which the colon and other portions of the gastrointestinal tract or the large bowel alone are carpeted with hamartomatous polyps. Associated congenital anomalies are common. Only one third of the cases are familial. The hamartomatous polyp was previously thought not to be premalignant. However, there have been recent reports of atypical juvenile polyposis in which adenomatous foci within the juvenile polyp and colorectal carcinoma were present (15). The frequency of such cases and therefore the need for surveillance remains to be determined. Of note is the occurrence of colorectal carcinoma in some family members of patients with juvenile polyposis. Carcinomas of the stomach, duodenum, and pancreas have also been described in the kindred of these patients.

FAMILIAL COLORECTAL CARCINOMA   Certain families have been identified in which there is a high incidence of colorectal carcinoma inherited as an autosomal dominant trait. Characteristically, members of such families develop colorectal cancer at a relatively early age and the majority of tumors occur in the proximal large bowel. There is a high frequency of solitary adenomatous polyps in these patients.

CANCER FAMILY SYNDROME   An increased risk of developing adeno-carcinoma at multiple sites, including the breast, ovary, and, more frequently, the endometrium and colon, has been documented in a few family aggregates. Like familial colorectal carcinoma, inheritance appears to be an autosomal dominant trait. Affected individuals are prone to developing adenocarcinoma in one of the above-described sites at an early age (16).

FAMILY HISTORY OF COLORECTAL CARCINOMA   Individuals who have first-degree relatives with colorectal carcinoma are at increased risk for developing the disease themselves. Studies by Woolf (17), Macklin (18), and Lovett (19) concur that the risk is approximately three-fold greater than that in the general population. Both Macklin and Lovett excluded families with familial polyposis from their studies.

INFLAMMATORY BOWEL DISEASE   Colorectal cancer occurs more often in patients with ulcerative colitis. Indeed, this incidence was reported to be 7–11 times that in the general population (20, 21). The longer the duration of the colitis, the progressively greater is the cumulative risk for carcinoma. However, some authors feel that the risk for colorectal cancer is exaggerated. At the St. Mark's Hospital in London, England, one of the largest referral centers for colitic diseases in Great Britain, only two cases per annum of carcinoma complicating ulcerative colitis have been recorded over the past 30 years (22). Besides duration of disease, particularly when greater than seven years, extent of colonic involvement significantly influences the risk for cancer (23). The incidence is greatest in the patient with universal colitis, less in the patient with left-sided colitis, and no greater than in the average-risk patient with proctitis. Severity of the first episode of colitis and the presence of chronic symptomatology may also have a minor bearing on the incidence (24). Age of onset of the disease is no longer felt to contribute to the risk for colorectal cancer. Screening is essential with this group of patients, for their carcinomas tend to be multiple, flat, infiltrative, and highly malignant.

There appears to be a slight increased risk for carcinoma of both the small and large intestines in patients with Crohn's disease (25–33); however, the risk is certainly not as great nor as well defined as in ulcerative colitis.

GENERAL SCREENING MEASURES

Digital Rectal Examination

The digital rectal examination is a simple, safe, and relatively painless means of evaluating the distal rectum and anal canal. Tumors within a distance of approximately 7.5 cm can effectively be palpated (34). Small lesions may be missed because of overlying stool and mucous.

Fecal Occult Blood Testing

With the introduction of the Hemoccult® slide[1] in 1967 by Greegor, testing for fecal occult blood has become an integral part of the screening process for the early detection of colorectal cancer (35). Many of the previously available tests for fecal occult blood, including the hematest and the benzidene test, were fraught with a high percentage of both false-positive and false-negative reactions (36). Comparatively, the Hemoccult slide is more sensitive and specific, particularly when the patient smears two different portions of a stool each day for three days while following a high-bulk, red-meat-free, and, ideally, a fresh-fruit- and vegetable-free diet. Peroxidases found in animal hemoglobin and bacteria as well as in fresh fruits and vegetables may cause a false-positive reaction. Reducing agents, such as

[1]From SmithKline Diagnostics, Sunnyvale, California.

Table 2 Hemoccult slide test characteristics

Test reagents	Filter paper impregnated guaiac; hydrogen peroxide and denatured alcohol
Analyte	Hemoglobin
Test rationale	Phenolic oxidation of guaiac in the presence of Hb
Known chemical interference	Compounds with peroxidase activity
Minimum sensitivity	1 g crystalline human Hb in aqueous solution 0.2 g Hb/100 g stool under simulated conditions[a]
Stability following specimen application	30 days if test is strongly positive (+4) on day 1; 4–5 days if test is weakly positive (+1) on day 1
Stability related to Hb concentration	Yes
Effect of rehydration on sensitivity	Increased sensitivity with increased rate of false-positive reactions
Effect of diet on sensitivity	Foods containing peroxidase activity should be avoided (particularly uncooked vegetables and fruit)

[a] Blood added to stool in vitro.

ascorbic acid, may interfere with the oxidation of the guaiac reagent and thus increase the false negativity. Bulk is included in the diet, presumably for tumor abrasion with the stimulation of bleeding. This point remains to be documented (Tables 2, 3).

Multiple studies support Greegor's observation that the Hemoccult test is a potentially useful screening tool for colorectal cancer (37–41) (Table 4). In 1974, a controlled study was instituted at the Strang Clinic in cooperation with the Memorial Sloan-Kettering Cancer Center (42). Thus far, over 22,000 patients have been entered into this trial. Between 1 and 3.7% of asymptomatic patients over the age of 40 years have had positive slides. In 50% of these patients, further workup revealed a neoplasm (38% adenomas and 12% carcinomas). Preliminary data suggest that the detected

Table 3 Recommended methodology for fecal occult blood testing

Dietary restriction	meat-free; high fiber; low peroxidase
Number of smears	6
Type of slides	impregnated guaiac, immunochemical
Rehydration	only if strict low peroxidase diet is used
Storage interval	4 days preferred
Quality control	window or lab assay

Table 4   Fecal occult blood test: clinical data

Patient compliance	
motivated groups	80%
unmotivated groups	15%
Rate of positive slides	
unhydrated	1–5%
hydrated	up to 20%
Predictive value for neoplasia	18–50%
Staging of detected cancers	
(% Dukes' A & B)	60–80%
False positivity	
unhydrated slide	2%
hydrated slide	up to 20%
False negativity for cancer	
hydrated slides	9%
unhydrated slides	10–20%
False negativity for adenomas	60–75%
Other	complements sigmoidoscopy minimal risk colonoscopy important in workup of (+) patients

carcinomas are less invasive than those generally found in the symptomatic individual (Figures 1, 2).

Rigid Proctosigmoidoscopy

Rigid proctosigmoidoscopy has long been a standard procedure used to detect rectosigmoid carcinomas. Its potential value is evident when one considers the fact that approximately 50% of all colorectal cancers are within its reach. At the Strang Clinic, 26,124 men and women between 1940 and 1954 underwent proctosigmoidoscopic examination (43), of whom 58 were found to have colorectal carcinoma. Of those patients followed over a subsequent 15-year period, there was a survival rate of 90%. Furthermore, this instrument is useful in detecting and removing rectosigmoid adenomas. The benefit of proctosigmoidoscopic polypectomy was suggested in the study of Gilbertsen and associates at the University of Minnesota, as previously mentioned (44).

Flexible Fiberoptic Sigmoidoscopy

The introduction of the 60-cm flexible fiberoptic sigmoidoscope makes possible a more proximal examination of the colon as compared to the rigid instrument. On the average, the 60-cm flexible endoscope can be inserted three times further than the rigid proctosigmoidoscope and, therefore, has

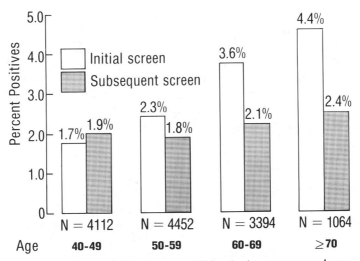

Figure 1   Rate of positive occult blood tests on initial and subsequent screens by age.

the potential of detecting three times as many adenomas and carcinomas. This advantage is certainly paramount when one considers that colon cancers are more often proximal than they were in the past. Biopsy as well as cytological studies can be simply and safely performed through the biopsy channel of the instrument. Perhaps the major drawback of the 60-cm flexible fiberoptic sigmoidoscope is the need for a well-trained endoscopist. This problem may be eliminated by the development of a shorter flexible instru-

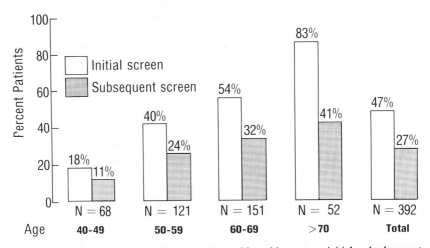

Figure 2   Rate of neoplastic findings in patients with positive tests on initial and subsequent screens by age.

ment. The Memorial Sloan-Kettering Cancer Center and the Strang Clinic initiated a multicenter evaluation of a 30-cm flexible sigmoidoscope (45). The technique of handling the instrument was easily learned by the nonendoscopist. When compared with the rigid proctosigmoidoscope, the flexible 30-cm instrument could be inserted to a greater depth with less patient discomfort. The cost effectiveness of this instrument is yet to be determined.

SPECIFIC CONFIRMATORY DIAGNOSTIC MODALITIES

Barium Enema

With the advent of colonoscopy, the limitations of the barium enema soon became apparent. The single column study can miss many polyps and small carcinomas. Though the sensitivity of the test can be amplified by using the air-contrast technique, smaller adenomas and flat carcinomas may not be visualized. However, the barium enema remains a useful diagnostic modality, particularly in conjunction with flexible fiberoptic sigmoidoscopy or as a complement to colonoscopy. In a small percentage of patients, endoscopic examination of the proximal portion of the colon may not be possible because of a fixed sigmoid loop or diverticular disease. Endoscopic blind areas can exist in the cecum, splenic flexure, and hepatic flexure. For these reasons, the barium enema is a useful adjunct to colonoscopy. It should be stressed that both a normal barium enema and flexible sigmoidoscopic examination are insufficient in clearing a patient with either a positive Hemoccult test or symptoms suggestive of a colorectal carcinoma.

Colonoscopy

Colonoscopy is the single best diagnostic test for the evaluation of the colon. It is an integral part of the diagnostic armamentarium for the investigation of positive screening tests and for the surveillance of high-risk groups. In 90% of all patients, the long colonoscope can be advanced to the cecum. Fixation of the sigmoid loop secondary to adhesions and diverticular disease rather than redundancy of the colon are the more common factors that prevent proximal inspection of the colon. Major advances in the design of the instrument and in the technique of colonoscopy have significantly improved patient tolerance and minimized the risk of complications. The superiority of colonoscopy as compared to barium enema is most evident in the detection of small neoplasms, in the differentiation of fecal residue from colorectal lesions, and in surveying anastomotic sites in patients following colonic resection for carcinoma. In addition, biopsy, polypectomy, and both lavage and brush cytologic studies can be conducted through the biopsy channel. These operations are of vital importance in the early detection of colorectal carcinoma and they underscore the diagnostic significance of colonoscopy.

Polypectomy

The malignant potential of adenomas is a generally accepted concept. With the introduction of colonoscopic polypectomy in 1969, the surgical resection of polyps has become an unusual necessity (46). The snare cautery technique facilitates total excision of colorectal polyps with a low complication rate. Polyps less than 5 mm in size can be sampled and coagulated with a hot biopsy forceps. Biopsy of colorectal polyps is generally contraindicated for it is nontherapeutic and it may be diagnostically misleading. Most pedunculated and small sessile polyps can be safely removed by colonoscopy. Select larger sessile adenomas may be carefully removed segmentally during one or two endoscopic sessions in experienced hands. Adenomas with foci of carcinoma can be safely excised as the total treatment if invasion of the stalk, vascular structures, or lymphatics is not evident. Subsequent colonoscopic surveillance is mandatory in all cases.

Biopsy

Endoscopic biopsy is perhaps best utilized in the surveillance of patients with long-standing ulcerative colitis. According to Morson & Pang (47), rectal biopsies demonstrating severe dysplasia are highly predictive of similar histologic changes elsewhere in the colon. Segmental biopsies in conjunction with lavage cytology throughout the length of the colon may optimize the detection of severe dysplasia and carcinoma in this group of patients. Of course, biopsy is necessary to confirm the diagnosis of suspicious lesions encountered during colonoscopy.

Cytology

Prerequisites for the application of cytological studies in the detection of colorectal dysplasia and carcinoma are the availability of an experienced cytologist and a well-prepared bowel, which eliminates the difficulty of analyzing specimens contaminated by stool. The two most commonly used cytologic methods are the lavage and brush techniques. Lavage cytology is optimally applied to those patients with diffuse premalignant diseases of the colon such as ulcerative colitis or familial polyposis. The area of interest is irrigated with a high-pressure stream of saline that is subsequently collected, fixed with alcohol, and analyzed.

For the experienced cytologist, false-positive interpretations are rare and may, in fact, signal imminent neoplastic transformation. With target cytology, a small brush is employed to expose and collect a high concentration of mucosal cells. Strictures and anastomotic sites can be brushed circumferentially. A combination of brushings and biopsies provide the best yield in the diagnosis of colorectal carcinoma. In some centers, the sensitivity of target cytology exceeds that of both endoscopic biopsy and lavage cytology.

Carcinoembryonic Antigen

The carcinoembryonic antigen (CEA) assay is of little value in screening for early colorectal carcinoma since the value is normal or only mildly elevated in the majority of patients (48). However, serial assays are helpful in monitoring patients for recurrent disease following resection of a colorectal carcinoma. A preoperatively elevated CEA level falls to normal after complete excision of the tumor (49). A subsequent rise in the value is highly indicative of a recurrent malignancy (50). In 40% of these patients, resectable localized disease is found during a second-look laparotomy (51).

APPROACH TO SCREENING AND DIAGNOSIS

Asymptomatic Patients at Standard Risk

All patients over the age of 40–45 years should undergo fecal occult blood testing yearly and proctosigmoidoscopy every 3–5 years (Figure 3). A positive screening test requires further investigation with both an air-contrast barium enema and colonoscopy. If this comprehensive workup is negative in the setting of positive fecal occult blood testing, evaluation of the upper gastrointestinal tract is advisable.

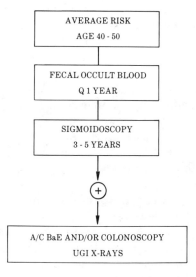

Figure 3   Proposed schedule for screening average-risk patients.

Asymptomatic Patients At High Risk

Patients with a history of colorectal carcinoma or adenomatous polyps are at greatest risk for metachronous lesions 3–5 five years after resection of the index lesion(s). Patients with colorectal carcinoma should undergo colonoscopy with brushings of the anastomotic site, six months postoperatively. One year after surgery, a barium enema, chest x ray, and an abdominal CT scan should be done. These same tests, with the possible exception of the barium enema, should again be repeated one year later. This will permit the physician to definitively clear the colon of synchronous lesions and the anastomotic site for the rare but potential recurrence of carcinoma. Thereafter, colonoscopy can be performed every three years with interval fecal occult blood testing (Figure 4). In addition, periodic liver function chemistries, CBC and CEA assay and liver scan should be obtained. Patients with a history of colorectal adenomas require colonoscopy one year after the initial resection of all adenomas from the colon. If no additional polyps are noted, subsequent examinations can then be performed at three-year intervals. Fecal occult blood testing should continue to be performed annually.

Patients at risk for an adenomatous polyposis syndrome rarely manifest the disease before the age of ten years. Beyond this age, biannual sigmoidoscopic examination is warranted. Since diffuse studding of the large bowel is characteristic of these syndromes, periodic distal colonic examination will allow detection of affected individuals. Once adenomas become evident, colectomy should be considered. If the rectosigmoid is surgically spared,

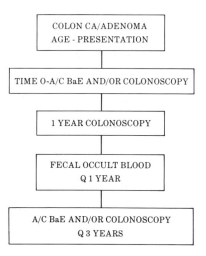

Figure 4 Proposed schedule for screening patients who have had a colon cancer or adenoma excised.

biannual sigmoidoscopy with lavage cytology is indicated. New adenomas can be endoscopically removed.

In members of families with the cancer syndrome or familial colorectal cancer, there is an extremely high incidence of colorectal carcinoma in view of the autosomal dominant mode of inheritance. Surveillance should begin at the age of twenty years and consist of fecal occult blood testing yearly and an air-contrast barium enema and/or colonoscopy every 3–5 years.

Patients with a history of genital or breast cancer or with a family history of colorectal carcinoma require annual fecal occult blood testing and sigmoidoscopy every 3–5 years (Figure 5). Surveillance should begin in the former groups when either the breast or genital adenocarcinoma is identified, and in the latter group in early adulthood.

Patients with ulcerative colitis of greater than seven years duration require yearly colonoscopy with segmental biopsies and lavage cytology. Optimally, interval flexible fiberoptic sigmoidoscopy with rectal biopsies can be performed. Patients must be surveyed during the quiescent phase of their disease, for the significance of dysplasia in the setting of acute or resolving inflammation is questionable. Patients with disease of less than seven years duration should undergo yearly sigmoidoscopy with rectal biopsies. At present, surveillance for patients with Crohn's disease is not indicated in view of the relatively small risk for colorectal carcinoma. However, with both the recent increased incidence of this disease and the improved survival of these patients, the risk for cancer may take on greater significance in the future and thus necessitate routine screening for these patients.

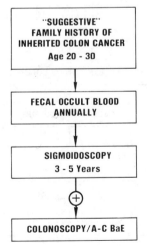

Figure 5   Proposed schedule for screening patients with "suggestive" family history of inherited colon cancer.

Symptomatic Patients

Patients with symptoms suggestive of colorectal carcinoma often delay medical evaluation. Many of these symptoms are so commonplace, including abdominal pain, constipation, diarrhea, and rectal bleeding, that there is little suspicion of an underlying neoplastic process (52). An aggressive workup is warranted when the patient presents with symptoms suggestive of colorectal carcinoma. Unfortunately, these individuals often have advanced disease.

SUMMARY

The factors responsible for the pathogenesis of colorectal carcinoma are poorly defined. Screening of those groups at risk is presently our best means of curtailing the mortality from this disease. Sensitive and specific tests are available for this purpose; however, the effectiveness of such a screening process is most contingent on the aggressiveness of the physician and the compliance of the patient. Unfortunately, only a minority of individuals in this country submit to routine medical checkups for preventive purposes. Therefore, a reorientation of the patient's understanding of proper health care as well as early cancer detection is necessary. With greater public awareness and participation in the screening process, the need for cost-effective programs becomes crucial.

Research is currently being directed toward the detection of more specific tumor markers that will help identify patients at risk or with colorectal cancer at an early stage. As more data become available from ongoing controlled trials, such as the National Polyp Study and the genetic high-risk registry programs, we will be better able to define the natural history of colorectal carcinoma and appropriately revise our concepts of screening for this disease.

Literature Cited

1. Miller, D. G. 1976. The early diagnosis of cancer. In *The Pathophysiology of Cancer,* ed. F. Homberger. Basel: Karger
2. Wilson, J. M. G., Jungner, G. 1968. Principles and practice of screening for disease. *Public Health Pap.* 34:26–39
3. Waterhouse, J., Muir, D., Corea, P., Powell, J., eds. 1976. *Cancer Incidence in Five Continents,* Vol. III. Lyon: Int. Agency for Res. on Cancer
4. Prager, E. C., Swinton, N. W., Young, J. L., et al. 1974. Followup study of patients with benign mucosal polyps discovered by proctosigmoidoscopy. *Dis. Colon Rect.* 17:322–24
5. Rider, J. A., Kirsner, J. B., Moeller, H. C. 1959. Polyps of the colon and rectum. *J. Am. Med. Assoc.* 170:633–38
6. Winawer, S. M., Sherlock, P., Schottenfeld, D., et al. 1976. Screening for colon cancer. *Gastroenterology* 70:783–89
7. Hill, M. J., Morson, B. C., Bussey, H. J. R. 1978. Aetiology of adenocarcinoma sequence in large bowel. *Lancet* 1:245–47
8. Morson, B. C. 1977. Polyps and cancer of the large bowel. In *International Academy of Pathology Monograph, The Gastrointestinal Tract,* ed. J. H. Yardley, B. C. Morson, M. R. Abell, pp. 101–8. Baltimore: Williams & Wilkins

9. Ekelund, G., Lindstrom, C. 1974. Histopathological analysis of benign polyps in patients with carcinoma of the colon and rectum. *Gut* 15:654–63
10. Morson, B. C. 1977. See Ref. 8, pp. 101–8
11. Gilbertsen, V. A. 1974. Proctosigmoidoscopy and polypectomy in reducing the incidence of rectal cancer. *Cancer* 94:936–39
12. Schottenfeld, D., Berg, J. W., Vitsky, B. 1969. Incidence of multiple primary cancers. II. Index cancers arising in the stomach and lower digestive system. *J. Natl. Cancer Inst.* 43:77–86
13. Schoenberg, B. J., Greenberg, R. A., Eisenberg, H. 1966. Occurrence of certain multiple primary carcinomas in females. *J. Natl. Cancer Inst.* 43:15–32
14. Schwabs, A. D., Klaus, K. J. 1980. Gastrointestinal polyposis. *Viewpoints Dig. Dis.,* Vol. 12, No. 1
15. Grigioni, W. F., Alampi, G., Martinelli, G., et al 1981. Atypical juvenile polyposis. *Histopathology* 5:361–76
16. Lynch, H. T., Harris, R. E., Lynch, P. M., et al. 1977. The role of heredity in multiple primary cancer. *Cancer* 40:1849–54
17. Woolf, C. M. 1958. A genetic study of carcinoma of the large intestine. *Am. J. Hum. Genet.* 10:42–52
18. Macklin, M. T. 1960. Inheritance of cancer of the stomach and large intestine in man. *J. Natl. Cancer Inst.* 24:551–71
19. Lovett, E. 1976. Family studies in cancer of the colon and rectum. *Br. J. Surg.* 63:13–18
20. Edwards, F. C., Truelove, S. C. 1964. The course and prognosis of ulcerative colitis. IV. Carcinoma of the colon. *Gut* 5:15–22
21. deDombal, F. T., Watts, J. M., Watkinson, G., et al 1966. Local complications of ulcerative colitis: strictures, pseudopolyps, and carcinoma of the colon and rectum. *Lancet* 1:1442–47
22. Butt, J. H., Lennard-Jones, J. E., Ritchie, J. K. 1980. A practical approach to the risk of cancer in inflammatory bowel disease. *Med. Clin. North Am.* 66:1203–20
23. Devroede, G. J., Taylor, W. F., Sauer, W. G., et al. 1971. Cancer risk and life expectancy of children with ulcerative colitis. *N. Engl. J. Med.* 258:17–21
24. Edwards, F. C. 1964. *Gut* 5:15–22
25. Beachley, M. C., Loebel, A., Lankan, C. A., et al. 1973. Carcinoma of the small intestine in chronic regional enteritis. *Am. J. Dig. Dis.* 18:1095–98
26. Ben Asher, H. 1971. Adenocarcinoma of the ileum complicating regional enteritis. *Am. J. Gastroenterol.* 55:391–98
27. Bruni, H., Lilly, J., Newman, W., et al. 1971. Carcinoma as a complication of regional enteritis. *South Med. J.* 64:577–80
28. Jones, J. H. 1969. Colonic cancer and Crohn's disease. *Gut* 10:651–54
29. Kipping, R. A. 1976. Crohn's disease of the colon with carcinoma of the rectum. *Proc. R. Soc. Med.* 63:753
30. Konig, H., Hermaneck, P., Rosch, W. 1976. Unusual course of chronic colitis. *Acta Hepato-Gastroenterol.* 23:227–31
31. Lightdale, C. J., Sternberg, S. S., Posner, G., et al 1975. Carcinoma complicating Crohn's disease. Report of seven cases and a review of the literature. *Am. J. Med.* 59:262–66
32. Perrett, A. D., Truelove, S. C., Massarella, G. R. 1968. Crohn's disease and carcinoma of the colon. *Br. Med. J.* 2:466–68
33. Sheil, F. O., Clark, C. G., Goligher, J. C. 1968. Adenocarcinoma associated with Crohn's disease. *Br. J. Surg.* 55:53–58
34. Goligher, J. C. 1975. *Surgery of the Anus, Rectum and Colon,* pp. 59–96. Springfield, Ill: Thomas. 3rd ed.
35. Greegor, D. H. 1967. Diagnosis of large-bowel cancer in the asymptomatic patient. *J. Am. Med. Assoc.* 201:943–45
36. Ostrow, J. D., Mulvaney, C. A., Hansel, J. R., et al 1973. Sensitivity and reproducibility of chemical tests for fecal occult blood with an emphasis on false-positive reactions. *Am. J. Dig. Dis.* 18:930–40
37. Bond, J. H., Gilbertsen, V. A. 1977. Early detection of colonic carcinoma by mass screening for occult stool blood: preliminary report. *Gastroenterology* 72(5):A-8/1031
38. Frühmorgen, P., Demling, L. 1978. First results of a prospective field study with a modified guaiac test for evidence of occult blood in the stool. In *Early Detection of Colorectal Cancer,* ed. K. Goerttler, Nurnberg: Wachholz
39. Glober, G. A., Peskoe, S. M. 1974. Outpatient screening for gastrointestinal lesions using guaiac-impregnated slides. *Am. J. Dig. Dis.* 19:399–403
40. Hastings, J. B. 1974. Mass screening for colorectal cancer. *Am. J. Surg.* 127:228–33
41. Miller, S. F., Knight, R. A. 1977. The early detection of colorectal cancer. *Cancer* 40:945–49

42. Winawer, S. J., Leidner, S. D., Miller, D. G., et al. 1977. Results of a screening program for the detection of early colon cancer and polyps using fecal occult blood testing. *Gastroenterology* 72(5): A-127/1150 (Abstr.)

43. Hertz, R. E., Deddish, M. R., Day, E. 1960. Value of periodic examination in detecting cancer of the rectum and colon. *Postgrad. Med.* 27:290–94

44. Gilbertsen, V. A. 1974. *Cancer* 94: 936–39

45. Weissman, G. S., Winawer, S. J., Sergi, M., et al. 1982. Preliminary results of a multicenter evaluation of a 30 cm flexible sigmoidoscope by non-endoscopists. *Gastrointest Endosc.* 28(2):150 (Abstr.)

46. Wolff, W.I., Shinya, H. 1973. A new approach to colonic polyps. *Ann. Surg.* 178:367–78

47. Morson, B. C., Pang, L. S. C. 1967. Rectal biopsy as an aid to cancer control. *Gut* 8:423–34

48. Chu, T. M., Murphy, G. P. 1978. Carcinoembryonic antigen: evaluation as a screening assay in non-cancer clinics. *NY State J. Med.* 78:794–99

49. Thomson, D. M. P., Krupey, J., Freedman, S. O., et al. 1969. The radioimmunoassay of circulating carcinoembryonic antigen of the human digestive system. *Proc. Natl. Acad. Sci. USA* 61:161

50. Sorokin, J. J., Sugarbaker, P. H., Zamcheck, N., et al. 1974. Serial CEA assays: use in detection of recurrence following resection of colon cancer. *J. Am. Med. Assoc.* 228:4953

51. Martin, E. W., James, K. J., Hurtubise, P. E., et al. 1977. The use of CEA as an early indicator for gastrointestinal tumor recurrence and second-look procedures. *Cancer* 39:440–46

52. Jones, I. S. C. 1976. An analysis of bowel habit and its significance in the diagnosis of carcinoma of the colon. *Am. J. Proctol.* 27:45–56

Ann. Rev. Med. 1983. 34:519–47

STRUCTURAL VARIANTS OF HUMAN GROWTH HORMONE: Biochemical, Genetic, and Clinical Aspects[1]

Rajender K. Chawla, Ph.D., John S. Parks, M.D., and Daniel Rudman, M.D.

Department of Medicine, Emory University School of Medicine, and the Clinical Research Facility, Emory University Hospital, 1364 Clifton Road N.E., Atlanta, Georgia 30322

ABSTRACT

Human growth hormone (hGH) is a mixture of peptides in which the major physiologic component is a single chain polypeptide of 191 residues with a molecular weight of 22,000 ("22K" form). The minor components differ from the 22K form in terms of *mass* (e.g. the 20K form, a single-chain peptide synthesized by deletion of residues 32–46 of the 22K isomer, and the 45K variant formed by aggregation of the 22K molecule), or of *charge* (e.g. the more acidic two-chain forms α_2 and α_3 which are generated by proteolytic deletion of residues 135–140 and 135–146 from the 22K variant). The minor components also differ from the 22K molecule in (*a*) their metabolic effects; (*b*) their capacity to bind to antiserum raised against the 22K form in a radioimmunoassay (RIA); and (*c*) their ability to bind to membrane receptors for the 22K hGH in a radioreceptor assay (RRA). Two genes, N and V, involved in the biosynthesis of hGH, are located on human chromosome 17. Heritable alterations of the N gene may cause deficiency of immunoreactive hGH and growth failure. A pathologic variant of hGH has also been identified which is indistinguishable from the 22K form on RIA, but which has low reactivity on hGH-RRA and low somatomedogenic activity. Several mechanisms to account for this bioinactive variant are discussed.

[1]Supported by USPHS Grants 1-R01-AM31149–01 and RR39 and March of Dimes Grant 6–309.

519

0066-4219/83/0401-0519$02.00

1. INTRODUCTION

1.1 Historical Background

Growth hormone (GH) has been in the forefront of endocrine research for almost one hundred years. Early research studied how hypophysectomy affected the body size of the rat, the frog, and the dog (1–5). In the young animal hypophysectomy stunted growth, and in the mature animal it caused weight loss and visceral atrophy. Exogenous administration of pituitary extracts reversed these effects. From these observations emerged the concept of a pituitary growth hormone or somatotropin.

Li and co-workers isolated GH from bovine pituitary glands in 1945 (6). Subsequent work by Li, as well as by Wilhelmi and others (7–11), established procedures for isolating human GH (hGH) in what was considered to be homogeneous form by the standards of the 1950s, e.g. ion-exchange resin and cellulose column chromatography, paper electrophoresis, and sedimentation analysis (12, 13). It was recognized that the hormone not only stimulated growth of skeletal and soft tissues, but also influenced protein, carbohydrate, and fat metabolism. GH was then purified from the pituitary glands of other animals. The GHs from different species were all simple, globulin-like proteins, but they differed in amino acid composition and structure (11). Human GH and GH from pig, cattle, and sheep shared regions of structural homology, but the somatotropins from the latter three species were inactive in man. The human pituitary dwarf responded only to human and monkey GH. The human, porcine, bovine, and ovine somatotropins, however, promoted growth of the hypophysectomized rat (11).

1.2 Biochemical and Physiologic Characteristics of hGH

The molecular weight of hGH is 22,000 and it consists of 191 residues with two loops formed by disulfide bridges (Figure 1). The molecule is predominantly α-helical in secondary structure (14).

Table 1 summarizes the biologic effects associated with hGH, and Table 2 describes laboratory assays used to determine its bioactivities (15). The primary function of the hormone is to promote proportionate growth of both soft and skeletal tissues. These anabolic effects are at least in part mediated by hGH-dependent growth factors called somatomedins (14, 16). The growth-promoting characteristic of hGH is measured by either (a) the weight gain test, in which the increase in body weight of the young hypophysectomized rat is monitored during 10 daily injections of the hormone, or (b) the tibia assay, in which the growth of the proximal epiphysis of the tibia of the young hypophysectomized rat is measured after 4 daily hGH injections. Other assays measure metabolic actions of the hormone on mus-

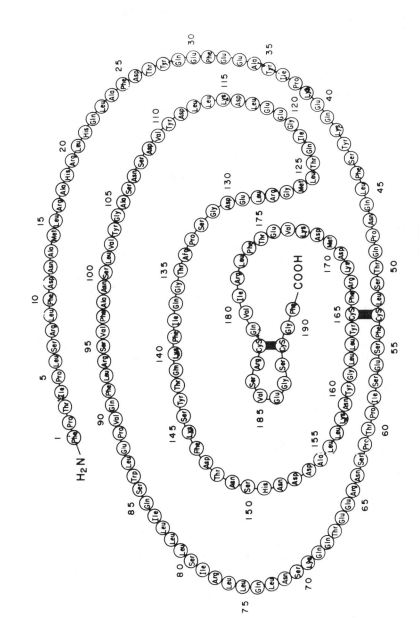

Figure 1 Covalent structure of hGH.

cle, adipose tissue, and mammary gland. The latter target organ reveals the lactogenic property of hGH.

Human GH binds to specific receptors on cultured human lymphocytes; on the plasma membrane fractions of leporine or rodent hepatocytes and of leporine mammary glands; and on human, canine, or rodent adipocytes (17–20). The specific binding of radiolabeled hormone to these cells reflects the bioactivity of hGH and provides the basis of radioreceptor assays (RRA), which are 10^6 times more sensitive than the weight gain and tibial assays mentioned above. Human GH can also be measured on the basis of its immunoreactivity by radioimmunoassay (RIA). While the sensitivity of the bioassays in Table 2 ranges from 10 to 100 μg, that of RRA and RIA is about 1–10 ng.

1.3 Heterogeneity of hGH

During the late 1950s and early 1960s, newly introduced techniques for analysis of peptides and proteins showed that even the purest preparations of hGH available at that time were heterogeneous (21–23). Starch block gel electrophoresis, polyacrylamide gel electrophoresis (PAGE), and isoelectric focusing of the available preparations of hGH showed 4 to 6 components (24–27). These techniques separated proteins or peptides on the basis of net molecular charge. Similarly, analysis of plasma hGH by gel filtration chromatography, which separated molecules on the basis of size, revealed 2 to 4 major components (28–31). The charge and mass variants of hGH revealed by these methods possessed different degrees of somatotropic bioactivity and immunoactivity.

Table 1 Effects of hGH

Metabolic	Stimulates amino acid transport
	Stimulates protein synthesis in most cell types
	Stimulates DNA/RNA synthesis in most cell types
	Stimulates polyamine synthesis
	Stimulates lipolysis
	Inhibits insulin action on glucose metabolism
Physiologic	Increases renal blood flow, glomerular filtration rate, and tubular reabsorption of PO_4
	Increases basal metabolic rate
	Stimulates new bone formation
	Stimulates erythropoiesis
	Expands extracellular fluid space
Anatomic	Accelerates linear growth
	Reduces adipose mass and enlarges lean body mass (muscle, liver, kidney, heart, GI tract, pancreas, skeleton, connective tissue)

Table 2 Bioassays for hGH

Assay number	Species	Type of assay	Experimental conditions	Response measured	Target organ	Process stimulated
1	rat	weight gain	in vivo; hypophysectomy	change in body weight	body	whole body growth
2	rat	tibia	in vivo hypophysectomy	growth of epiphysis	epiphyseal cartilage	skeletal growth
3	rat	thymidine incorporation	in vivo-in vitro; hypophysectomy	^{3}H thymidine incorporation into DNA	costal cartilage	DNA synthesis
4	rat	leucine incorporation	in vitro; hypophysectomy	^{3}H leucine incorporation into protein	diaphragm	protein synthesis
5	mouse	lactogenic prolactin	in vitro; culture	induction of N-acetyl lactosamine synthetase	mammary gland	enzyme induction
6	rat	AIB transport	in vitro; hypophysectomy	^{14}C AIB transport	diaphragm	amino acid transport
7	rat	3-0-methyl glucose transport	in vitro; hypophysectomy	3-0-methyl ^{14}C glucose transport	diaphragm	sugar transport
8	rat	^{14}C glucose utilization	in vitro; hypophysectomy	^{14}C glucose conversion to $^{14}CO_2$	epididymal fat body	glucose utilization
9	mouse	diabetogenic	in vivo; ob/ob hereditary obese	glucose tolerance		anti-insulin
10	rat	polyamine synthesis	in vivo	ornithine decarboxylase	liver	enzyme synthesis
11	rabbit, rat	radioreceptor assays	in vitro	specific binding of labeled hGH	membrane fractions of hepatocytes of rabbit or rat, membranes of rabbit mammary glands and rat hepatocytes	

These data led to the suggestion that hGH as secreted by the pituitary gland may not represent a unique molecular species, but may instead comprise a family of peptides. Although the major component of this family is the "22K" hormone with the covalent structure shown in Figure 1, variant forms also exist that may be of physiologic and clinical significance.

Additional evidence for heterogeneity of hGH came from recent discoveries about the molecular biology and pathology of this hormone. Studies on the enzymes and genes responsible for the biosynthesis of hGH identified mechanisms that could contribute to its molecular heterogeneity. It was demonstrated in 1976 that biosynthesis of GH proceeds by postribosomal proteolytic modification of a larger "pre-hGH" molecule (32). In 1980, Goodman et al (33) identified two different genes for hGH, one of which, designated hGH-N, has a sequence corresponding to that of the peptide structure of the 22K hormone, while the other or "variant" gene, designated hGH-V, has several sequence variations and omissions. The latter may have a low level of expression but nevertheless could contribute to the molecular heterogeneity of the hormone.

In addition, clinical studies during 1979–1982 identified a group of short-statured children whose pituitary glands secreted normal amounts of immunoreactive hGH, but who nevertheless appeared to be functionally GH deficient (15). In such children, the plasma may contain a variant type of hGH that retains the antigenic property but has lost the growth-promoting action. These children may represent a pathologic example of the molecular heterogeneity of hGH.

1.4 Scope of this Review

The object of this article is to review the several lines of evidence published in the literature that point to multiple forms of hGH: heterogeneity in net molecular charge of hypophyseal hGH, indicating "charge variants" in this location; heterogeneity in size of hypophyseal and plasma hGH, indicating "mass variants"; the existence of two genes for hGH biosynthesis; the physiologic occurrence of a "pre-hGH" as a special example of mass variant; and the evidence for a "bioinactive" pathologic variant of hGH associated with growth failure. Finally we speculate about the possible functions of physiologic variants of the hormone, and the mechanisms that could be responsible for the appearance of pathologic bioinactive variants.

2. CHARGE VARIANTS OF hGH

2.1 Charge Variants of hGH Extracted from the Pituitary Gland

The variants were isolated either from crude pituitary extracts, or from clinical or immunochemical grade hGH supplied by the National Institutes of Health (NIH) (10, 34). The former is used to treat GH-deficient children; the latter is more highly purified and serves as a reference standard and radioligand in the RIA.

2.1.1 STARCH BLOCK GEL ELECTROPHORETIC ANALYSIS OF PITUI-TARY hGH   Ferguson & Wallace (24) in 1961 resolved the contemporary NIH standard preparation of purified hGH by starch block gel electrophoresis into four major (readily stainable by nigrosin) and two minor (poorly stainable by nigrosin) bands. All components possessed tibial and lactogenic somatotropic activities. Soon thereafter, Barrett et al (35) confirmed the above observations, but reported that only the major bands had somatotropic activity. In 1966, Berson & Yalow suggested that deamidation of the native hormone could be responsible for the heterogeneous forms of pituitary and plasma hGH (36). Lewis & Cheever (37) proposed that all preparations of hGH may be contaminated with a proteinase that could contribute to heterogeneity.

2.1.2 PAGE ANALYSIS OF PITUITARY hGH: THE WORK OF CHRAM-BACH AND ASSOCIATES   In 1973, Chrambach and associates reported their analysis of several preparations of hGH (immunologic and clinical NIH grades) by a multiphasic PAGE system at several pHs (38–40). They isolated a family of variants or "isohormones," labeled B, C, D, and E, which were indistinguishable in molecular size (radius) but showed progressive increase in molecular net charge, i.e. lower isoelectric point, from B to E. Variant B was the major component; digestion with plasmin resulted in its conversion progressively to isohormones C, D, and E. Asparagine or glutamine residues were not deamidated during this process. In immunoactivity, these variants were indistinguishable from the standard hGH preparations. The more acidic isohormones D and E were of particular interest because their bioactivity, as measured by lactogenic assay, by rat tibia assay, and by capacity to raise plasma somatomedin level, was three to eight times greater than that of B (39, 40). In the weight gain assay, E was only about two times more potent than B. Baumann & Nissley (41) showed that plasmin converts B to D and E by a proteolytic cleavage in the large disulfide loop (Figure 1). Other studies confirm that the region 126–140 of this loop is very susceptible to proteolytic cleavage (11, 14, 42). The metabolic clearance rate of the cleaved hormones is significantly slower than that of isomer B; this factor may at least partially account for their enhanced biological activity (43).

2.1.3 PAGE ANALYSIS OF PITUITARY hGH: THE WORK OF LEWIS AND ASSOCIATES   The other noteworthy work in this area came from Lewis et al (44, 45), who isolated and characterized by PAGE four charge variants of hGH from saline extracts of human pituitary glands. These forms, labeled α_1, α_2, α_3, and β, appear to be similar to the isohormones studied by Chrambach et al in terms of their electrophoretic mobility, but this correspondence has not been formally established. Lewis and associates reported the biochemical characteristics of these forms. While insufficient quantities of α_1 were available for chemical characterization, α_2 and α_3 were shown to lack residues 135–140 and 135–146, respectively; the β variant was more extensively degraded and was not characterized. These isohormones, termed the two-chain forms of hGH, clearly arose by selective proteolytic cleavages and deletions of peptides from the large disulfide loop of the hormone. All modified forms were indistinguishable from the intact hormone by RIA. The proteolytically altered form had enhanced biological activity in the tibial and lactogenic assays; α_3 was most potent, being five times more active than native hGH on tibial assay and about ten times more active on lactogenic assay.

The potentiation of the activities of hGH by selective proteolytic modification suggests that this mechanism may also operate in vivo. Lewis et al (45, 46) proposed that the 22K hormone synthesized in the pituitary gland must be "activated" by plasmin or thrombin-like enzymes before it can cause the metabolic effects listed in Table 1. None of the charge variants has been detected in plasma or in pituitary granules. However, the more acidic variants appeared when a homogenate of a pituitary gland was kept at 5°C for 48 hr at pH 7.6 (47). Therefore, the pituitary charge variants either are experimental artifacts not occurring naturally, or else are formed physiologically only while or after the granules are secreted (U. J. Lewis, personal communication). Also see Section 2.2.

Three additional minor charge variants were observed by Lewis and co-workers in pituitary extracts. In 1980, they isolated a variant of hGH with N-acetylphenylalanine at the N-terminus; it was equipotent with native hGH in the tibial and lactogenic assays and in binding to hGH antibodies (47). In 1981, this group reported two desamido forms of hGH resulting from deamidation of the asparagine residue at 152 and of the glutamine residue at 137. Their bioactivities were not reported (48, 49).

2.1.4 ISOELECTRIC FOCUSING OF PITUITARY hGH   Two analyses of hGH by isoelectric focusing (IEF) deserve special mention. Hummel et al (27) wished to learn whether or not IEF could separate human prolactin from hGH in crude saline extracts of the pituitary gland. Their analyses of IEF fractions with specific RIAs for hGH and prolactin showed that the two hormones could be separated by this technique; pI of the major hGH component was 4.78 and that of prolactin was 6.00. Hummel et al also found that there were three additional minor components of hGH with pI

5.40, 5.05, and 4.58. Neither the physicochemical characteristics nor the physiologic effects of these forms were described. Similar charge heterogeneity was also noted when the clinical grade hGH used to treat GH-deficient children was analyzed by IEF.

Another study of this type was done recently by Lewis and his associates (47). These workers analyzed by IEF (pH gradient 4–6) a clinical grade hGH preparation that was free of all minor charge isomers described above (i.e. α and β forms) and of all minor mass variants to be described in the following section (i.e. disulfide dimer, 20K isomer, and 24K isomer). Contrary to their expectations, they noted that even this preparation was far from homogeneous in the IEF system and had two minor bands—one anodal and one cathodal—in addition to the major hGH band (22K molecule). No characterization of these minor components has been reported.

2.2 Charge Variants of Plasma hGH

We mentioned in Section 2.1 that none of the charge variants identified in the pituitary-derived hGH has been shown to exist in plasma. Even with a special RIA designed to detect two-chain forms of hGH, Lewis et al were not able to detect these forms in the blood stream. The physiologic significance of these isomers, therefore, is uncertain.

Nevertheless, two recent reports indicate that these variants may indeed be formed in vivo. The charge isomers of hGH were isolated from the tissue culture of a pituitary adenoma (50), and a peptide corresponding to the deletion peptide—residues 132–146 of hGH—has been detected in blood (U. J. Lewis, personal communication).

In summary, PAGE reveals at least four charge isomers in pituitary hGH: isomers B, C, D, and E of Chrambach, and α_1, α_2, α_3, and β of Lewis. These forms arise by proteolytic modification of the 22K hormone. They are more acidic and possess greater biological activity then the parent molecule. However, with currently available techniques, they cannot be detected in pituitary granules or in plasma.

3. MASS VARIANTS OF hGH

Interest in this subject began about 1965 and was triggered by two circumstances: (a) reports on size heterogeneity in plasma of other peptide hormones such as ACTH, insulin, parathyroid hormone, and gastrin (51–55), and (b) availability of gel permeation chromatography and a specific RIA (23, 36) to quantify immunoreactive hGH in the chromatographic effluent fractions. The mass variants are of two types: those resulting from aggregation, and those arising from deletion of certain amino acids in the structure of the 22K isomer (Figure 1).

3.1 Aggregates of hGH in the Pituitary Gland

On gel filtration (e.g. on a Sephadex® G-75 column), the immunoreactive hGH of pituitary extracts eluted in two regions—the first corresponding to molecular weight of about 45,000 (45K variant), and the second corresponding to molecular weight of about 22,000. Frohman et al (56) analyzed the freshly prepared crude extracts of human pituitary glands and found that the 45K hormone was an aggregate form of hGH responsible for about 1% of the GH immunoreactivity in the gland, and that almost 80% of this aggregate could be dissociated to the 22K size by treatment with guanidine. Beneveniste et al (57) and Gorden and associates (58) also reported similar forms of hGH in the pituitary-derived material. However, Beneveniste et al were able to convert all of the 45K variant to the smaller molecule only by treatment with mercaptoethanol and urea. They concluded that about 60% of the 45K hGH consisted of a dimer of two peptide chains connected by an unspecified number of disulfide bonds; the remaining aggregates were presumably held together by noncovalent bonds. The bioactivity of the dimer was not investigated by these workers.

Lewis and co-workers (59) confirmed the presence of this aggregate in their detailed study on the biochemical characteristics and physiologic effects of the 45K material isolated from "purified" hGH. They labeled it the interchain dimer. This form could be converted to the 22K variant by treatment with mercaptoethanol and, like hGH, had phenylalanine as its N-terminal amino acid. Compared to the 22K form, the dimer was about 10% as active in the weight gain assay and about 50% as active in the lactogenic assay. Its antibody-binding capacity was about 50% as great as that of the monomeric form. The physiologic significance of this variant is not clear; it could be a dimer formed during storage of pituitary glands, since hGH has a strong tendency to form aggregates (14).

The existence of another mass variant, "pre-GH," in the adenohypophysis was revealed by incubation with wheat germ extract of mRNA derived from cultured rat pituitary tumor. The conversion of pre-hGH to hGH involves removal of the so-called peptide (molecular weight about 2000) from the N-terminus of the molecule by a protease bound to the membrane of the rough endoplasmic reticulum. The extension peptide, also called the signal or leader peptide, is known to be present at the N-terminus of most nascent polypeptide hormones and has a key function in the synthesis and secretion of the fully active hormone (60). Also see Section 6.3.

3.2 Aggregates of hGH in Plasma

The aggregated forms of hGH observed in plasma are similar to those reported in the hypophysis. Gel filtration of serum revealed hGH immunoreactivity in several molecular weight regions. The larger forms, accounting for about 30% of the total immunoactivity, were detected in the regions 40K to 70K ("big" hGH) and > 100K ("big big" hGH) (61–63). Initially it was suggested that the immunoreactivity in the high-molecular-weight region represented hGH bound to a plasma carrier protein (64, 65). Subsequent work ruled out the existence of such a transport protein (61). Lewis et al (59), and Gorden and co-workers (58) showed that the "big" hGH had a molecular weight of 45,000 and was similar to the 45K disulfide dimer in the pituitary gland. Two types of "big" hGH were identified: urea stable, which did not deaggregate in 6 M urea, and urea labile, which dissociated to the 22K form. The urea labile form was presumably the noncovalent aggregate of monomeric hGH (47, 57).

The biologic and immunoactivities of "big" hGH have been compared to those of the monomeric or "little" form of the plasma hormone. The binding capacities to antibodies raised against 22K hGH were identical; this is in contrast to the lower binding capacity of the 45K material derived from the pituitary gland. The bioactivity of the plasma "big" hGH (as measured by an RRA using cultured human lymphocytes or rabbit hepatocyte membranes) was only 26–40% that of the monomeric form. Since sufficient quantities of the aggregate were not available, its biologic activity as measured by other procedures (e.g. tibia assay) could not be determined (66).

Ellis et al (67) reported another variant of hGH in plasma that is different from the "big" hGH mentioned above. Their interest grew out of earlier observations that there was a marked discrepancy in the hGH concentrations of plasma as measured by the tibia assay and by a specific RIA (68). Thus, the ratio between the tibial bioactivity and the RIA immunoactivity in plasma ranged from 50 to 200, as compared to 1 for 22K hGH. Ellis et al fractionated large amounts of plasma on a gel permeation column and identified an isomer with molecular weight of about 80,000 (the 80K isomer), for which the ratio of tibial bioactivity to immunoactivity was more than 100. This material had an isoelectric point of about 5, but no other physicochemical characteristics were reported.

Ellis et al could not detect any 80K material in the human pituitary gland. Earlier they had noted a high concentration of a similar isomer in rat plasma; the molecular weight and tibial bioactivity to immunoactivity ratio for the rat plasma isomer resembled those found for the human 80K variant (67). Although the rat pituitary gland had only a trace level of this isomer, its concentration in jugular plasma was about three times that in the aortic plasma. Therefore it was proposed that the 80K variant in human plasma might arise from an enzymatic modification of the 22K hormone synthesized in the hypophysis. However, there have been no other studies on the biochemical nature, physiologic significance, or origin of the 80K material since it was first reported in 1976. Additional work is needed to learn if this material is indeed a true variant of hGH or an artifact.

3.3 Nonaggregated Mass Variants of hGH in the Pituitary Gland

The most thoroughly investigated mass isomers of hGH are reported from the laboratory of Lewis and co-workers (47). Their studies on charge variants of hGH isolated from saline extracts of the pituitary gland were described in Section 2.1.3.

These workers first removed the charge variants from the major component of their hGH, in an attempt to obtain a homogeneous preparation of the hormone. Analysis of this preparation on SDS-PAGE by the method of Weber & Osborn (69) revealed 3 minor bands (molecular weight 45,000, 24,000, and 20,000) in addition to the major 22K band (59, 70). The 45K form was shown to be a disulfide dimer and was described in Section 3.2 (59). The 24K material was identical to 22K hGH except that the peptide chain was nicked between residues 139 and 140 without deletion of any amino acid. The break in the peptide chain within the large disulfide loop converted it to a two-chain form, altered its secondary structure, enlarged its molecular radius, and hence increased its apparent molecular weight. The 24K hGH may arise from a specific, post-translational proteolytic modification of the 22K form. 24K hGH was immunologically indistinguishable from the 22K isomer reference hGH. It was inactive in the tibia assay, but on lactogenic assay the material was more potent than the native 22K isomer. It may well be that the prolactin activity usually associated with hGH is not inherent in the parent molecule but resides instead in the modified 24K form (47).

The 20K form may be a direct gene product, which, unlike other hGH variants, does not result from postribosomal modification of the 22K molecule. It is a single polypeptide chain whose amino acid sequence differs from that of 22K hGH by the deletion of residues 32–46. In the pituitary gland, it accounts for 5–10% of the total hGH (47). Its tendency to dimerize may at least partially explain why it remained undetected in the high-molecular-weight region and was usually discarded (71).

On RIA for hGH, the 20K variant was only one third as active as the 22K form. In the body weight gain assay and in the tibial assay in hypophysectomized rats, and in the somatomedin-generating assay in man, the 20K variant was equipotent with the 22K form. In other bioassays, however, the shortening of the peptide chain by 15 residues in the N-terminal region caused noticeable changes (41, 47). Thus the variant did not have the early insulin-like properties of hGH (hypoglycemia and decrease in serum free fatty acids), and did not stimulate glucose uptake by the fat pad. In addition, in RRA using pregnant rat liver membranes as receptors, the 20K variant was only 3–20% as potent as hGH in displacing ^{125}I-labeled hGH. In RRA using mammary gland plasma membranes, the 20K form was

22–53% as effective as hGH. These data suggest that hGH and its 20K variant may not share the same binding sites in target cells; the 20K form could bind to its own specific receptors although none has yet been identified (73).

Since the amino acid sequence of the 20K variant is identical to that of the 22K variant except for deletion of the peptide corresponding to residues 32–46, Chapman et al (72) and Wallis (75) asked whether the 20K molecule is formed by a unique gene, or whether it is produced in some fashion from the same gene whose messenger RNA produces pre-22K hGH. Fiddes et al (74) reported the presence of an intron (an excised portion of a gene) in the hGH-N gene immediately following the DNA coding for residue 31 of hGH. Therefore, mRNA for 20K hGH might be produced by removal, from the hGH-N gene transcript, of this intron plus bases required for coding of the sequence 32–46. A specific gene for 20K hGH or its prehormone has not, however, been excluded.

3.4 Nonaggregated Mass Variants of hGH in Plasma

The 24K variant described by Lewis in the pituitary gland has not been detected in plasma, but the limiting factors could be its low concentration and the lack of a specific antibody directed against the 24K form. Recently, it was reported that about 5% of serum hGH is of the 20K variety, which is in line with its reported concentration in the pituitary gland (G. Baumann, personal communication).

In summary, within the pituitary gland, besides the predominant 22K hGH, three minor mass variants of the hormone have been identified: 45K, 24K, and 20K. A pre-hGH (molecular weight about 24,000 but not to be confused with the 24K variant studied by Lewis) is also present. The 45K isomer is an aggregate, which probably arises during storage of the 22K form. The 24K variant, formed by a specific proteolytic cleavage of the 22K molecule between residues 139 and 140, may be responsible for the lactogenic activity of hGH. The 20K variant may be a unique gene product or may be generated by a rearrangement of the mRNA responsible for the 22K form. The relative concentrations of the variants in pituitary extracts and plasma do not always correlate. For example, the 24K variant, present in minute quantities (exact level not specified) in the pituitary gland, is not detectable in plasma. The 20K variant makes up about 5% of total hGH both in pituitary gland and in plasma. The 45K variant accounts for about 1% of the hormone in the hypophysis, but its concentration in plasma is about 30% of the total. The 80K variant, on the other hand, accounts for more than 80% of the total tibial bioactivity of the plasma, but is not detectable in the pituitary gland.

4. GENETIC BASIS OF hGH SYNTHESIS

4.1 Structure of the hGH Genes

The DNA sequence that codes for pituitary pre-22K hGH was reported by Martial et al (74) and by Roskam & Rougeon (75) in 1979. These investigators constructed recombinant DNA copies of pre-hGH mRNA from human pituitary glands. The sequence was found to be 94% homologous with the sequence (76) coding for the closely related 191 amino acid placental hormone, human chorionic somatomammotropin (hCS). Recombinant cDNA probes for both hormones were used to detect hGH and hCS gene sequences in restriction enzyme digests of whole cellular DNA. Fiddes et al (77) found that there were two nonallelic copies of hGH genes and at least three copies of hCS genes in each hGH and hCS gene cluster. Although some physical linkage relationships have been established (33, 78, 79), the exact number and linear array of hGH and hCS genes are not known. This family of genes has been localized to the long arm of human chromosome 17 (80, 81), as shown in Figure 2 (*top*).

Several members of the hGH and hCS gene family have been cloned and sequenced. These include the normal pituitary hGH or hGH-N gene (82, 83), the nonallelic variant hGH or hGH-V gene (83), an hCS gene whose sequence differs slightly from that of the major component of hCS mRNA (83), and another hCS gene (N. Eberhardt, personal communication). There are remarkable similarities among the genes. Overall, the extent of sequence homology in noncoding as well as coding regions is 90–95%. The organization of the other genes corresponds closely to the organization of the hGH-N gene, which is shown in Figure 2 (*bottom*). There are five exons or coding sequences, designated I–V, which are separated by four introns or intervening sequences, designated A–D. The positions and lengths of the four introns are identical in the hGH-N, hGH-V, and hCS genes. Exon I contains some 5' untranslated nucleotides, trinucleotide codons −26 to −24 of the pre-hGH signal peptide, and the first nucleotide of codon −23. The second exon codes for the remainder of the signal peptide and amino acids 1 to 31 of hGH. Exons III, IV, and V code for amino acids 32 to 71, 72 to 126, and 127 to 191, respectively. Introns A, B, C, and D contain 256, 209, 93, and 253 base pairs. Each intron begins with a GH dinucleotide and ends with an AG. Coding sequences are spliced together at these junctions during the post-transcriptional processing of mRNA. The hGH-N gene contains an alternate splice point [designated B' in Figure 2 (*bottom*) preceding the codon for amino acid 47 (82, 83)]. As suggested by Wallis (84), the 20K hGH, which lacks amino acids 32 to 46 of 22K hGH (85), may arise from splicing of the pre-hGH messenger precursor RNA at this point.

Recent studies provide detailed information about the sequence of the hGH-V gene (83) and the properties of a peptide hormone which can be produced from the hormone in an artificial system (86). These studies (86, 87) do not answer the question of whether the gene is expressed in vivo and whether it accounts for some of the variant forms of hGH found in pituitary extracts, serum, or culture medium of explants of pituitary tumors (88). The hGH-V gene specifies a polypeptide that differs from hGH at 15 positions (83). Two of these differences are found in the 26 amino acid leader peptide and the remainder are found in the mature protein. As compared to normal hGH, the hGH-V peptide has lost two acidic amino acids and gained three basic ones. There is a predicted increase in the isoelectric point to pH 8.9. Gene fragments containing the hGH-N and hGH-V genes have been ligated to SV-40 DNA and expressed in monkey kidney cells (86). This system

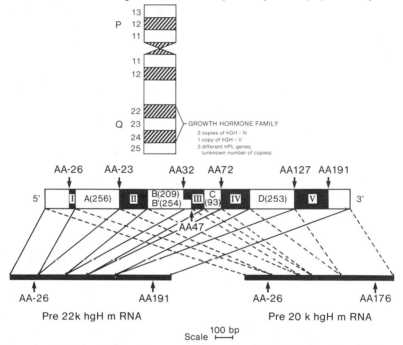

Figure 2   (*Top*) Map of human chromosome 17 (based on McKusick's *Mendelian Inheritance in Man*). This is a representation of the pattern of chromosome 17 under standard staining techniques. The dark and light bands are given numbers outward from the centromere to facilitate identification. The GH gene family is located on the long arm, designated q, somewhere within the region of bands 22–24. Found here are two identical copies of the hGH-N gene, one copy of the hGH-V gene, and an unknown number of copies of three different hPL genes. (*Bottom*) Theoretical representation of the hGH gene and the mRNA from it. The hGH gene contains three introns: intron A between amino acids (AA) 24, intron B between AA 31 and 32, and intron C between AA 71 and 72. These are excised out when the gene is transcribed into the mRNA for the hormone.

permits transcription of the genes, splicing of the mRNA, translation, removal of the signal peptide, and secretion of the mature hormones into the culture medium. Peptide products of the two genes have been characterized by gel filtration and their potencies have been compared with pituitary hGH, 20K hGH, and bacterially produced 192 amino acid methionyl hGH (89) in radioimmunoassays and radioreceptor assays (86, 87). On Sephadex G-100 gel filtration, a high molecular weight component of the hGH-V gene product eluted with the void volume and about 70% of the material eluted in a volume appropriate for little hGH. Antibodies to pituitary hGH cross react weakly with hGH-V. The displacement curves are non-parallel and give radioimmunoassay potency estimates 5–10% of that for hGH. In contrast, the potency of hGH-V in displacing radiolabelled hGH from human lymphocytic cell receptors is 50% and from pregnant rabbit liver membranes is 100% of that of standard hGH. From these results, it follows that the radioreceptor to radioimmunoassay potency ratio of hGH-V is >10 for human receptor and > 20 for lactogenic receptor systems. The RRA-to-RIA ratios of 20K hGH, methionyl hGH, and the hGH-N gene product produced in monkey kidney cells are all between 0.9 and 1.5 (87). If the hGH-V gene is expressed in vivo, it could account for molecules with high biological activity but low immunoreactivity in both 80K and 22K fractions. Further investigations of this interesting possibility will require development and application of radioimmunoassay systems with specificity for the hGH-V gene product.

4.2 Heritable Alterations of the hGH Genes

Recent studies of two types of hGH gene deletion provide information about the physiological significance of the hGH-N and hGH-V genes. In the first, homozygosity for a 7.5-kilobase (kb) pair deletion including the hGH-N gene results in a severe form of hGH deficiency (90). Affected children are somewhat small for gestational age and have seriously impaired postnatal growth (91). No hGH is detectable by radioimmunoassay. Treatment with pituitary hGH produces a transient improvement in growth, which is terminated by the development of high titers of antibodies to hGH. The phenotype suggests complete absence of immunoreactive and biologically active hGH. These findings suggest that the hGH-N gene is solely responsible for production of hGH and that the hGH-V gene does not provide a surrogate hormone. A second gene deletion disorder involves loss of the hGH-V gene and all of the hCS genes (92). The hGH-N gene and another gene, which has been termed "hGH-like," are retained. In this disorder, there is complete absence of immunoreactive hCS in maternal serum and in extracts of the fetal placenta (93), but prenatal and postnatal growth are normal (92). These findings indicate that the hGH-V gene product is not required for growth.

Molecular genetic techniques have also been applied to more common forms of autosomal recessive deficiency of growth hormone in which there is generally some hGH detectable by immunoassay. Theoretically, this type of disorder might be due to a mutation within the hGH-N gene. Through analysis of the transmission of certain common polymorphic variations of restriction sites within the hGH and hCS gene cluster, it was possible to show that about half of the examples of this disorder were not linked to the hGH gene (94). Similar types of analysis may be applied to patients with the syndrome of bioinactive hGH to determine whether this condition involves a defect in the hGH-N gene.

5. BIOINACTIVE hGH

Short statured children are usually defined as those below the third percentile for chronologic age. Thus the prevalence is 30 per 1000. Until 1960, the diagnosis of GH deficiency as the cause of short stature in a particular child was not possible, unless other signs of pituitary diseases were present, because there was no way to measure endogenous hGH in serum. With the introduction of the RIA method (95) and provocative agents for GH release (96), it became possible to identify the GH-deficient child. Peak serum GH < 4 ng/ml was defined as total GH deficiency, and 4–8 ng/ml as partial deficiency (97).

The prevalence of hGH deficiency in the general population is about 1 in 5000 (98, 99). Thus, less than 1% of short stature in the general population can be attributed to deficiency of immunoreactive hGH. Besides proportionate growth retardation, the hGH-deficient child shows retarded bone age, low plasma somatomedin C (SmC) concentration, and, frequently, ACTH or TSH deficiency. The low SmC and growth velocity are promptly corrected by hGH at doses of 6–12 units per week (100, 101).

During the 1960s, hGH treatment was tried in several types of dwarfism not caused by hGH deficiency: Turner syndrome, low-birth-weight dwarfism, and idiopathic short stature (102, 103). Little or no growth acceleration was observed. It was concluded that among short-statured children only the 1% with hGH deficiency could benefit from conventional doses of hGH.

This conclusion may need to be modified by the introduction of two new methods for evaluating the hGH/Sm axis: measurement of serum hGH by RRA (104) as well as by RIA (95), and measurement of plasma SmC, usually by RIA (105). Specifically, the concept has been introduced that some children's growth failure is caused by a *functional* hGH deficiency resulting from pituitary secretion of a structurally abnormal hGH with substantial immunoreactivity but little or no bioactivity.

The "bioinactive hGH" concept was introduced by Kowarski et al in 1978 (106). These workers described two male dwarfs, both 3 years old, with delayed bone age and normal serum immunoreactive hGH response to insulin hypoglycemia. Serum hGH was measured not only by RIA, but also by RRA (pregnant rabbit liver membrane). The RRA/RIA ratio was subnormal. Growth velocities were 2 and 4.5 cm/yr; hGH at 0.1 U/kg/12 hr for 48 hr normalized the Sm level in both patients. During treatment with 6 units hGH weekly for 8–12 months, growth rates increased 6-fold and 2-fold. Kowarski et al concluded that in these two children, the dwarfism was caused by a bioinactive endogenous hGH with subnormal RRA/RIA ratio.

In 1978 Hayek et al (107) reached the same conclusion about a 3-yr-old girl with growth retardation and retarded bone age. Plasma immunoreactive GH rose to over 100 ng/ml after dopa, arginine, and glucagon were administered. SmC was increased from 0.19 to 0.73 units/ml by hGH, and growth velocity improved.

Frazer et al in 1980 (108) described 5 prepubertal children with growth failure, subnormal plasma Sm, and abnormally low RRA/RIA ratio for serum GH. The low Sm value was corrected in all 5 children by hGH, and growth velocity was improved in 3 children.

In 1981 Rudman et al (109) described 9 children (7 boys and 2 girls) who appeared to have growth retardation caused by a bioinactive hGH. Ages ranged between 8 and 11 years. Bone age was retarded by 2–4 years. Both during sleep and in response to insulin hypoglycemia, serum immunoreactive GH response was normal (average peak values 23–25 ng/ml), but the RRA (pregnant rabbit liver membrane)/RIA ratio was subnormal (average 0.4 compared to normal 0.8–1.2). Plasma SmC, measured by RIA, was subnormal (average 0.24 compared to normal 0.4–2.0). Growth velocity in these 9 children averaged only 1.7 cm/yr (normal range for this age group is 4–8 cm/yr). When these children were treated with 9–12 units hGH/wk, SmC rose into the normal range, and growth velocity accelerated 4.5-fold. From these three studies, the present criteria for bioinactive GH listed in Table 4 emerged.

The children in the four published reports present one or more pathologic variants of hGH with subnormal bioactivity/immunoreactivity ratio. Whether these "clinical" variants correspond to any of the "laboratory" variants with reduced bioactivity, listed in Table 3, is presently unknown, because the serum GH in the bioinactive children has not yet been characterized in terms of size, charge, and profile of bioactivities. Some of the major unanswered questions about bioinactive GH syndrome are (a) Is there only one or are there several types of bioinactive GH? (b) For (each type of) bioinactive GH, what is the structure, charge, and molecular weight? Are all somatotropic bioactivities uniformly depressed? Is the immunoreactivity of each, per unit mass, normal? (c) How does (each type of) bioinactive hGH arise? By the expression of a gene other than GH gene N? By abnormal processing of the messenger of gene N? By abnormality at a postribosomal step, such as the pre-hGH to hGH conversion? (*d*) How is (each type of) bioinactive GH inherited? (*e*) For (each type of) bioinactive GH, what is the prevalence in the general population and in the short population?

6. IMPLICATIONS AND CONCLUSIONS

6.1 Summary

Table 3 summarizes the known variants of hGH and their characteristics. The physiologic significance of the pituitary charge variants with enhanced bioactivity is still uncertain, but the existence in plasma of hGH variants with differing bioactivity to immunoactivity ratios seems established (i.e. Ellis' 80K variant and the 20K and 45K isomers). It is of interest that similar data are reported for another pituitary hormone, human prolactin (hPRL). This peptide exists in at least two molecular sizes (110, 111); the large isomer is apparently a dimer and accounts for about 8% of the pituitary and for about 25% of the plasma hPRL. In hypothyroid patients, the plasma level of this hormone, as measured by RIA, is invariably elevated (112). In these patients, however, the RRA to RIA ratio for plasma hPRL is significantly lower than in normals (1.0 vs 4.0). Thus, the phenomenon of pathologic variants of pituitary hormones with depressed bioactivity to immunoactivity ratios may not be confined to hGH.

If we assume that all the hGH variants in Table 3 circulate in vivo, then the scheme shown in Figure 3 can be proposed.

6.2 Physiologic Functions of the Variants

The rationale for the existence of a family of peptides with hGH-like metabolic effects was discussed by Lewis et al (47). Such a family may indeed be required to account for the large and sometimes contradictory profile of the physiologic activities associated with this hormone. Thus each peptide in the group could conceivably represent a unique hormone with specific receptors and physiologic functions. The parent 22K molecule might have only limited metabolic functions. Activation processes involving specific structural modifications and aggregations might be necessary so that some somatotropic properties could be enhanced and other activities could appear. Supporting this postulate are the potentiated somatomedin-generating activity and tibial growth activity of the charge variants and the 80K variant, and the enhanced lactogenic activity of the 24K variant.

Table 3 Major charge and mass variants of hGH profile of physiochemical and biologic characteristics

Variant	How identified	Occurrence	Biochemical characteristics	Bioactivity as compared to 22K hGH[a]	Immunoreactivity as compared to 22K hGH
A. Charge variants					
1. B	PAGE analysis of NIH grade hGH	1. Pituitary extracts.	1. Exact structures not known.	1. Prolactin assay. $\dfrac{B = 1.0}{C, D, \text{ and } E = 3.0}$ 2. Tibia assay. $\dfrac{B = 1.0}{C, D, \text{ and } E = 3.0}$	All forms = 1.0
C		2. Not detected in plasma or pituitary granules.	2. B is the most predominant form; C, D, and E are more acidic than B and arise due to its proteolysis.	3. Somatomedin assay. $\dfrac{B = 1.0}{C, D, \text{ and } E = 3.0}$ 4. Weight gain assay. $\dfrac{B = 1.0}{\begin{array}{l}C, D = 3.0 \\ E = 2.0\end{array}}$.	
D					
E					
2. α_1	PAGE analysis of saline extracts of pituitary.	1. Pituitary extracts.	1. α_1 – not studied Insufficient quantities.	1. Tibia assay. $\dfrac{\alpha_1, \alpha_2 = 1.2}{\begin{array}{l}\alpha_3 = 5.0 \\ \beta = 1.1\end{array}}$	All forms = 1.0
α_2		2. Not detected in plasma and pituitary granules.	2. α_2 – two chain form with deletion of residue 135–140.	2. Prolactin assay. $\dfrac{\alpha_1, \alpha_2 = 5.5}{\begin{array}{l}\alpha_3 = 10.0 \\ \beta = 4.5\end{array}}$	
α_3			3. α_2 – two chain form with deletion of residue 135–146.		
β			4. β – not studied. Extensively degraded.		
3. Two desamido variants	PAGE analysis of saline extracts of pituitary	1. Pituitary extracts. 2. Plasma or pituitary granules not analyzed for these variants.	First isomer: $Asn_{152} \rightarrow Asp$ Second isomer: $gln_{137} \rightarrow glu$	Not reported	Not reported

4. Blocked N-terminal variant	PAGE analysis of saline extracts of pituitary	1. Pituitary extracts. 2. Plasma or pituitary granules not analyzed for these variants.	N-terminal phenylalanine acetylated at the free amino group	Tibia assay = 1.0 Lactogenic assay = 1.0	1.0
B. Mass variants					
1. 80K variant	Gel filtration of plasma	Plasma		1. Tibia assay = 100–200	0.01
2. 45K variant	Gel filtration of pituitary extracts and plasma	Pituitary and plasma.	1. Molecular weight differences. 2. Aggregated 22K; can be dissociated to monomeric material with urea and mercaptoethanol.	Pituitary material 1. Lactogenic assay = 0.5 2. Weight gain assay = 0.1 Plasma Material RRA = 0.26	0.3
3. 24K variant	SDS-PAGE analysis of pituitary extract free of charge variants.	Pituitary extracts.	1. Proteolytic cleavage between residues 139 and 140. 2. Apparent molecular weight increased due to conformational change.	1. Tibia assay. 0.0 to 0.1 2. Lactogenic assay. 1.8	1.0
4. 20K variant	SDS-PAGE analysis of pituitary extract free of charge variants.	Accounts for 5–10% of total GH in pituitary and plasma.	One chain peptide similar to 22K with the residues 32–46.	1. Tibia assay. 1.0 2. Body weight assay. 1.0 3. Somatomedin generative assay. 1.0 4. Early insulin like activity. 0.0 5. RRA. 0.03 to 0.5	0.3
5. pre hGH	Incubation of mRNA from pituitary cultures with wheat germ extract.	Pituitary cultures.	1. Not isolated 2. May have an N-terminal peptide (mol wt 2000) which is cleaved to give rise to 22K hormone.	Not reported	Not reported

[a] Bio- and immunoactivities of 22K hGH are taken to be 1.0.

Table 4 Diagnostic criteria for bioinactive hGH in short children (References 91–93)

1. Peak GH (RIA) after provocative tests and during sleep > 12 ng/ml.
2. Current height < 3rd percentile.
3. Bone age/chronologic age < 0.8.
4. Growth velocity below normal for chronologic age by two standard deviations (2 SD) or more.
5. Plasma SmC (average of three estimates) below normal average for chronologic age by 2 SD or more.
6. RRA/RIA ratio for serum GH below normal average by 2 SD or more.
7. Normalization of SmC after 10 days' hGH at 0.08 units/kg/day.
8. Normalization of growth velocity and serum SmC during 6 months treatment with hGH at 0.08 units/kg/day.
9. Growth velocity and SmC decline to subnormal rates within 2 months and within 10 days, respectively, after long-term hGH treatment is stopped.

6.3 The Origin of Bioinactive hGH

An aberrant form of hGH, which is metabolically inert but immunologically active, could arise from genetic errors in the biosynthesis of pre-hGH, or from postribosomal errors in processing this molecule, or its product 22K form, with resultant inactivation or failure of activation.

Numerous possible genetic disorders in the biosynthesis of hGH are listed in Table 5. Five types of error are mentioned here: (*a*) The 22K hGH gene, hGH-N, could be present but not fully expressed. Instead, the chromosome-linked hGH-V gene could be expressed with formation of a bioinactive peptide chain. (*b*) In addition to the two different hGH genes, chromosome 17 also has three different genes for hPL, as shown in Figure 2. The

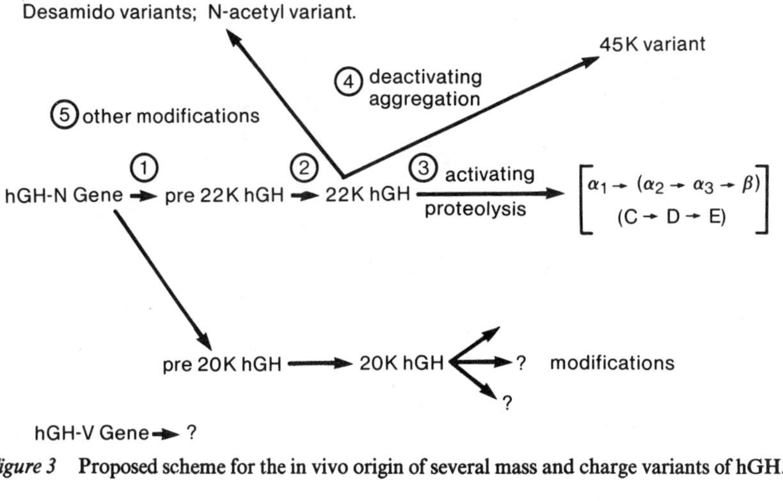

Figure 3 Proposed scheme for the in vivo origin of several mass and charge variants of hGH.

homologies in the amino acid sequences as well as the immuno-cross-reactivities of the two hormones were mentioned in Section 4.2. If an hPL gene were expressed instead of the hGH-N gene, the result might be secretion of an immunoreactive "hGH" with low somatotropic bioactivity. (c) There could be intragenic deletions, insertions, or substitutions of bases within the hGH-N gene; the result might be a peptide chain with omissions or substitutions of key residues causing retention of the antigenic site but not of the bioactive site. (d) Another source of genetic error in the biosynthesis of hGH could be in the conversion of the pre-22K hGH to the 22K hormone (step 2 in Figure 3). Human GH, like most other polypeptide hormones, is synthesized as a precursor molecule that contains an N-terminal extension of about 20 amino acid residues. This leader or signal sequence is necessary in order for the nascent peptide to attach to a specific receptor on the membrane bilayer of the rough endoplasmic reticulum, and to be transferred across the membrane. The leader sequence is subsequently cleaved by a membrane-bound protease. The mature form of the hormone can then be stored or secreted. A defect or aberration in the proteolytic cleavage of the leader sequence could give rise to an hGH variant that is biologically inert but antigenically active. (e) Lewis et al (47) postulated that an activation of the 22K hormone may be essential for a complete expression of its biologic effects. If this is true, then the bioactivity of the plasma hGH will depend on the relative activities of step 3 in Figure 3. If the activating step is predominant, then a completely active molecule may be generated. However, if the deactivating step 4 dominates, then the resulting molecule will lack bioactivity. It can be postulated that a dysfunction or irregularity in the modification steps could seriously alter the function of the endogenous hGH/Sm axis.

To identify the cause and nature of bioinactive hGH, two approaches are necessary. The first involves analysis of the patient's nuclear DNA by restriction endonucleases (94). Aliquots of nuclear DNA prepared from normal controls and from individuals suspected to have bioinactive hGH can be digested with various restriction endonucleases, analyzed by electrophoresis on agarose gels, hybridized to labeled hGH probes, and then autoradiographed. A comparison of the different patterns could reveal gene abnormalities responsible for an aberrant hGH.

The second approach is to characterize the patient's plasma GH by physical, immunochemical, and bioassay techniques. The bioinactive hGH could differ from normal 22K hGH in net molecular charge and/or apparent molecular weight. Analysis of the patient's plasma hGH by recently available techniques could identify such differences. The immunoreactive hGH in an aliquot of plasma can be extracted by specific affinity chromatography, and analyzed by a gel permeation, an ion-exchange or an absorption

Table 5 Possible mistakes from the hGH–N gene to 22K hGH, any of which could lead to production of a bioinactive hGH instead of normal 22K hGH

Level of expression of defect	Effect on patient's 22K hGH
The whole gene	
Expression of "hGH–V" or hPL gene instead of hGH–N gene (all three genes are located in the same region of chromosome 17)	22K form absent; related protein present
Duplication	overproduced
Deletion, translocation, inversion	absent or shortened
Intragenic	
Base substitution	normal except for substitution
Base deletion, insertion	too short
mRNA	
Unstable; abnormal synthesis; shortened life span	absent or shortened
Transport defect	absent
Abnormal processing enzymes	absent, shortened, or lengthened
tRNA	
Unstable, abnormal synthesis	absent or shortened
Unstable binding; enzymes, factors	absent or shortened
Ribosomes	
Unstable, abnormal synthesis	absent
Unstable binding	absent or shortened
Postribosomal processing	
Absence or abnormality of protease that releases the leader sequence	replaced by 24K pre-hGH

column on high performance liquid chromatography; the immunoreactive hGH content of the fractions can then be determined (36, 113, 114). These experiments should establish any major deviations from normal in molecular size or charge. In addition, plasma aliquots can be analyzed by IEF, PAGE, and SDS-PAGE, and each gel can then be sliced and assayed for its hGH content by RIA. Two-dimensional electrophoretic techniques (e.g. IEF in the first dimension and SDS-PAGE in the second dimension) could also be useful in this regard (27, 69, 115).

ACKNOWLEDGMENT

We are grateful to Drs. G. Baumann, U. J. Lewis, C. H. Li, J. B. Mills, and A. E. Wilhelmi for their help and suggestions for this review. We also wish to thank all investigators who made available to us their data before publication. Special thanks are due to Ms. Carol J. Berry for her valuable help during preparation of this manuscript.

Literature Cited

1. Crowe, S. J., Cushing, H., Homans, J. 1910. Experimental hypophysectomy. *Bull. Johns Hopkins Hosp.* 21:126–69
2. Bell, W. B. 1917. Experimental operations on the pituitary. *Q. J. Exp. Physiol.* 11:77–126
3. Evans, H. M., Long, J. A. 1921. The effect of the anterior lobe administered intraperitoneally upon growth, maturity, and oestrus cycles of the rat. *Anat. Rec.* 21:62
4. Smith, P. E. 1927. The disabilities caused by hypophysectomy and their repair. *J. Am. Med. Assoc.* 88:158–61
5. Smith, P. E. 1930. Hypophysectomy and a replacement therapy in the rat. *Am. J. Anat.* 45:205–56 (and references cited therein)
6. Li, C. H., Evans, H. M., Simpson, M. E. 1945. Isolation and properties of the anterior hypophysial growth hormone. *J. Biol. Chem.* 159:353–66
7. Li, C. H., Liu, W. K. 1964. Human pituitary growth hormone. *Experentia* 20:169–78 (and references cited therein)
8. Wilhelmi, A. E., Fishman, J. B., Russell, J. A. 1948. A new preparation of crystalline growth hormone. *J. Biol. Chem.* 176:735–42
9. Raben, M. S., Westermayer, V. W. 1951. Recovery of growth hormone in purification of corticotropin. *Proc. Soc. Exp. Biol. Med.* 78:550–51
10. Reisfeld, R. A., Mucilli, A. S., Williams, D. E., Steelman, S. L. 1962. Human growth hormone: preparation from acetone powder. *Endocrinology* 71:559–63
11. Wilhelmi, A. E. 1975. Chemistry of growth hormone. In *Handbook of Physiology,* ed. R. O. Greep, E. B. Astwood, Sect. 7, Vol. 4, pp. 59–78. Washington, DC: Am. Physiol. Soc.
12. Smith, E. L., Brown, D. M., Fishman, J. B., Wilhelmi, A. E. 1949. Sedimentation diffusion and molecular weight of crystalline pituitary growth hormone. *J. Biol. Chem.* 177:305–10
13. Li, C. H. 1956. Hormone of the anterior pituitary gland. Part I. Growth and adrenocorticotropic hormones. *Adv. Protein Chem.* 11:102–90
14. Wilhelmi, A. E. 1982. Structure and functions of growth hormone. In *Hormone Drugs, Proc. FDA/USP Workshop on Drug Ref. Stand. for Insulins, Somatotropins, and Thyroid Hormones.* Rockville, MD: US Pharm. Conv.
15. Rudman, D. 1981. Potential clinical indications for human growth hormone. In *Insulins, Growth Hormone, and Recombinant DNA Technology,* ed. J. L. Gueriguian, pp. 161–75. New York: Raven
16. Phillips, L. S., Vassilopoulou-Sellin, R. 1980. Somatomedins. *N. Engl. J. Med.* 302:438–46
17. Lesniak, M. A., Roth, J., Gorden, P., Gavin, J. R. 1973. Human growth hormone radioreceptor assay using cultured human lymphocytes. *Nature New Biol.* 241:20
18. Freisen, H. G. 1979. Prolactin and growth hormone receptors: regulation and characterization. *Fed. Proc.* 38:2610 (and references cited therein)
19. Moore, W. V., Jin, D. 1978. Polymeric and monomeric human growth hormone binding to rat liver plasma membranes. *J. Clin. Endocrinol. Metab.* 46:374–79
20. Fagin, K. D., Lackey, S. L., Reagan, C. R., DiGirolamo, M. 1980. Specific binding of growth hormone by rat adipocytes. *Endocrinology* 107:608–15
21. Smithies, O. 1955. Zone electrophoresis in starch gels: group variations in the serum proteins of normal human adults. *Biochem. J.* 61:629–41
22. Ornstein, L., David, B. J. 1962. *Disc Electrophoresis.* Rochester, NY: Distillation Products Industries
23. Porath, J., Flodin, P. 1959. Gel filtration: a method for desalting and group separation. *Nature* 183:1657–59
24. Ferguson, K. A., Wallace, A. L. C. 1961. Prolactin activity of human growth hormone. *Nature* 190:632–33
25. Cheever, E. V., Lewis, U. J. 1969. Estimation of the molecular weights of multiple components of growth hormone and prolactin. *Endocrinology* 85:465–73
26. Chrambach, A., Yadley, R. A., Ben-David, M., Rodbard, D. 1973. Isohormones of human growth hormone. *Endocrinology* 93:848–57
27. Hummel, B. C. W., Brown, G. M., Hwang, P., Friesen, H. G. 1975. Human and monkey prolactin and growth

hormone: separation of polymorphic forms by isoelectric focusing. *Endocrinology* 97:855–67

28. Touber, J. L., Mainguy, P. 1963. Heterogeneity of human growth hormone. Its influence on a radioimmunoassay of the hormone in serum. *Lancet* 1:1403–5

29. Irie, M., Barrett, R. J. 1962. Immunologic studies of human growth hormone. *Endocrinology* 71:277–87

30. Hunter, W. M. 1965. Homogeneity studies on human growth hormone. *Biochem. J.* 97:199–208

31. Lewis, U. J., Dunn, J. T., Bonewald, L. F., Seavey, B. K., Vanderlaan, W. P. 1978. A naturally occurring structural variant of human growth hormone. *J. Biol. Chem.* 253:2679–87

32. Sussman, P. M., Tushinski, R. J., Bancroft, F. C. 1976. Pregrowth hormone: product of the translation in vitro of messenger RNA coding growth hormone. *Proc. Natl. Acad. Sci. USA* 73:29–33

33. Goodman, H. M., DeNoto, F., Fiddes, J. C., Hallewell, R. A., Page, G. S., Smith, S., Tischer, E. 1980. Structure and evolution of growth hormone related genes. In *Mobilization and Reassembly of Genetic Information, Miami Winter Symp,* ed. W. A. Scott, R. Werner, D. R. Joseph, J. Schultz, pp. 15–179. New York: Academic

34. Raben, M. S. 1959. Human growth hormone. *Recent Prog. Horm. Res.* 15:71–105 (and references cited therein)

35. Barrett, R. J., Friesen, H., Astwood, E. B. 1962. Characterization of pituitary and peptide hormones by electrophoresis in starch gel. *J. Biol. Chem.* 237:432–39

36. Berson, S. A., Yalow, R. S. 1966. State of human growth hormone in plasma and changes in stored solutions of pituitary growth hormone. *J. Biol. Chem.* 241:5745–49

37. Lewis, U. J., Cheever, E. V. 1965. Evidence for two types of conversion reactions for prolactin and growth hormone. *J. Biol. Chem.* 240:247–52

38. Chrambach, A., Yadley, R. A., Ben-David, M., Rodbard, D. 1973. Isohormones of human growth hormone. I. Characterization by electrophoresis and isoelectric focusing in polyacrylamide gel. *Endocrinology* 93:848–57

39. Yadley, R. A., Chrambach, A. 1973. Isohormones of human growth hormone. II. Plasmin-catalyzed transformation and increase in prolactin biological activity. *Endocrinology* 93:858–65

40. Yadley, R. A., Rodbard, D., Chrambach, A. 1973. Isohormones of human growth hormone. III. Isolation by preparative polyacrylamide gel electrophoresis and characterization. *Endocrinology* 93:866–73

41. Baumann, G., Nissley, S. P. 1979. Somatomedin generation in response to activated and nonactivated isohormones of human growth hormone. *J. Clin. Endocrinol. Metab.* 48:246–50

42. Kostyo, J. L. 1974. The search for the active core of pituitary growth hormone. *Metabolism* 23:885–99

43. Baumann, G. 1979. Metabolic clearance rates of isohormones of human growth in man. *J. Clin. Endocrinol. Metab.* 49:495–99

44. Singh, R. N. P., Seavey, B. K., Rice, V. P., Lindsey, T. T., Lewis, U. J. 1974. Modified forms of human growth hormone with increased biological activities. *Endocrinology* 94:883–91

45. Lewis, U. J., Singh, R. N. P., Peterson, S. M., Vanderlaan, W. P. 1976. Human growth hormone: a family of proteins. In *Growth Hormone and Related Peptides,* ed. A. Pecile, E. E. Muller, pp. 64–74. New York: Elsevier

46. Lewis, U. J. 1965. In *Human Pituitary Growth Hormone, Rep. 54th Ross Conf. Pediatr. Res.,* ed. R. M. Blizzard, pp. 76–79. Columbus, Ohio: Ross Labs

47. Lewis, U. J., Singh, R. N. P., Tutwiler, G. F., Sigel, M. B., Vanderlaan, E. F., Vanderlaan, W. P. 1980. Human growth hormone: a complex of proteins. *Recent Prog. Horm. Res.* 36:477–508

48. Lewis, U. J., Singh, R. N. P., Bonewald, L. F., Seavey, B. K. 1981. Altered proteolytic cleavage of human growth hormone as a result of deamidation. *J. Biol. Chem.* 256:11645–50

49. Deleted in proof

50. Kohler, P. O., Bridson, W. E., Chrambach, A. 1971. Human growth hormone produced in tissue culture: characterization by polyacrylamide gel electrophoresis. *J. Clin. Endocrinol.* 32:70–76

51. Steiner, D. F., Cunningham, D., Spigelman, L., Aten, B. 1967. Insulin biosynthesis; evidence for a precursor. *Science* 157:697–700

52. Roth, J., Gorden, P., Pastan, I. 1968. "Big insulin." A new component of plasma insulin detected by immunoassay. *Proc. Natl. Acad. Sci. USA* 61:138–45

53. Yalow, R. S., Berson, S. A. 1971. Size heterogeneity of immunoreactive human ACTH in plasma and in extracts of pituitary glands and ACTH producing

thyoma. *Biochem. Biophys. Res. Commun.* 44:439–45

54. Berson, S. A., Yalow, R. S. 1968. Immunochemical heterogeneity of parathyroid hormone in plasma. *J. Clin. Endocrinol. Metab.* 28:1037–47

55. Yalow, R. S., Berson, S. A. 1970. Size and charge distinctions between endogenous human plasma gastrin in peripheral blood and heptadecapeptide gastrins. *Gastroenterology* 58:609–15

56. Frohman, L. A., Burek, L., Stachura, M. E. 1972. Characterization of growth hormone different molecular weights in rat, dog, and human pituitaries. *Endocrinology* 91:262–69

57. Beneveniste, R., Stachura, M. E., Scabo, M., Frohman, L. A. 1975. Big growth hormone (GH): conversion to small GH without peptide cleavage. *J. Clin. Endocrinol. Metab.* 41:422–25

58. Gorden, P., Hendricks, C. M., Roth, J. 1973. Evidence for "big" and "little" components of human plasma and pituitary growth hormone. *J. Clin. Endocrinol. Metab.* 36:178–84

59. Lewis, U. J., Peterson, S. M., Bonewald, L. F., Seavey, B. K., Vanderlaan, W. P. 1977. An interchain disulfide dimer of human growth hormone. *J. Biol. Chem.* 252:3697–3702

60. Lingappa, V. R., Blobel, G. 1980. Early events in the biosynthesis of secretory and membrane proteins: the signal hypothesis. *Recent Prog. Horm. Res.* 36:451–75

61. Goodman, A. D., Tanenbaum, R., Rabinowitz, D. 1972. Existence of two forms of immunoreactive growth hormone in human plasma. *J. Clin. Endocrinol. Metab.* 35:868–78

62. Wright, D. R., Goodman, A. D., Trimble, K. D. 1974. Studies on "big" growth hormone from human plasma and pituitary. *J. Clin. Invest.* 54:1064–73

63. Benker, G., Sandman, K., Thrandt, L., Hackenberg, K., Reinwein, D. 1979. Gel filtration studies of serum growth hormone in acromegaly following bromocriptin administration. *Horm. Res.* 11:151–60

64. Hadden, D. R., Pront, T. E. 1964. A growth hormone binding protein in normal human serum. *Nature* 202:1342–43

65. MacMillan, D. R., Schmid, J. M., Eash, S. A., Read, C. H. 1967. Studies on the heterogeneity and serum binding of human growth hormone. *J. Clin. Endocrinol.* 27:1090–94

66. Soman, V., Goodman, A. D. 1977. Studies of the composition and radi-

oreceptor activity of "big" and "little" human growth hormone. *J. Clin. Endocrinol. Metab.* 44:569–81

67. Ellis, S., Vodian, M. A., Grindeland, R. D. 1978. Studies on bioassayable growth hormone-like activity of plasma. *Recent Prog. Horm. Res.* 34:213–38

68. Ellis, S., Grindeland, R. E., Reilly, T. J., Yang, S. H. 1976. Studies on the nature of plasma growth hormone. See Ref. 45, pp. 75–83

69. Weber, K., Osborn, M. 1969. The reliability of molecular weight determination by dodecyl sulfate-polyacrylamide. *J. Biol. Chem.* 244:4406–12

70. Singh, R. N. P., Seavey, B. K., Lewis, U. J. 1974. Heterogeneity of human growth hormone. *Endocrinol. Res. Commun.* 1:449–64

71. Lewis, U. J., Dunn, J. T., Bonewald, L. F., Seavey, B. K., Vanderlaan, W. P. 1978. A naturally occurring structural variant of human growth hormone. *J. Biol. Chem.* 253:2679–87

72. Chapman, G. E., Rogers, K. M., Brittain, T., Bradshaw, R. A., Bates, O. J., Turner, C., Cary, P. D., Crane-Robinson, C. 1981. The 20,000 molecular weight variant of human growth hormone. *J. Biol. Chem.* 256:2395–2401

73. Sigel, M. B., Thorpe, N. A., Kobrin, M. S., Lewis, U. J., Vanderlaan, W. P. 1981. Binding characteristics of a biologically active variant of human growth hormone (20 K) to growth hormone and lactogen receptors. *Endocrinology* 108:1600–3

74. Martial, J. A., Hallewell, R. A., Baxter, J. D., Goodman, H. M. 1979. Human growth hormone: complementary DNA cloning and expression in bacteria. *Science* 205:602–7

75. Roskam, W. G., Rougeon, F. 1979. Molecular cloning and nucleotide sequence of the human growth hormone structural gene. *Nucleic Acids Res.* 7:305–20

76. Shine, J., Seeburg, P. H., Martial, J. A., Baxter, J. D., Goodman, H. M. 1977. Construction and analysis of recombinant DNA for human chorionic somatomammotropin. *Nature* 270:494–99

77. Fiddes, J. C., Seeburg, P. H., DeNoto, F. M., Hallewell, R. A., Baxter, J. D., Goodman, H. M. 1979. Structure of genes for human growth hormone and chorionic somatomammotropin. *Proc. Natl. Acad. Sci. USA* 76:4294–98

78. Seeburg, P. H. 1980. Structure and regulation of pituitary hormone genes. In

Polypeptide Hormones, ed. R. F. Beers, E. G. Bassett, pp. 19–31. New York: Raven

79. Moore, D. D., Walker, M. D., Diamond, D. J., Conkling, M. A., Goodman, H. M. 1982. Structure, expression and evolution of growth hormone genes. *Rec. Prog. Hormone Res.* 38: 197–225

80. Owerbach, D., Rutter, W. J., Martial, J. A., Baxter, J. D., Shows, T. B. 1980. Genes for growth hormone, chorionic somatomammotropin and growth hormone-like gene on chromosome 17 in humans. *Science* 209:289–92

81. George, D. L., Phillips, J. A., Franeke, U., Seeburg, P. H. 1981. The genes for growth hormone and chorionic somatomammotropin are on the long arm of human chromosome 17 in regions q21→qter. *Hum. Genet.* 57:138–41

82. DeNoto, F. M., Moore, D. D., Goodman, H. M. 1981. Human growth hormone DNA sequence and mRNA structure: possible alternative splicing. *Nucleic Acids Res.* 9:3719–30

83. Seeburg, P. H. 1982. The human growth hormone gene family: Nucleotide sequences show recent divergence and predict a new polypeptide hormone. *DNA* 1:239–49

84. Wallis, M. 1980. Growth hormone: deletion in the protein and introns in the gene. *Nature* 284:512–13

85. Lewis, U. J., Bonewald, L. F., Lewis, L. J. 1980. The 20,000-dalton variant of human growth hormone: location of the amino acid deletions. *Biochem. Biophys. Res. Commun.* 92:511–16

86. Pavlakis, G. N., Hizuka, N., Gorden, P., Seeburg, P., Hamer, D. H. 1981. Expression of two human growth hormone genes in monkey cells infected by simian virus 40 recombinant. *Proc. Natl. Acad. Sci. USA* 78:7398–7402

87. Hizuka, N., Hendricks, C. M., Pavlakis, G. N., Hamer, D. N., Gorden, P. 1982. Properties of human growth hormone polypeptides: purified from pituitary extracts and synthesized in monkey kidney cells and bacteria. *J. Clin. Endocrinol. Metab.* 55:545–50

88. Talamantes, F., Lopez, J., Lewis, U. J., Wilson, C. B. 1981. Multiple forms of growth hormone: detection in medium from cultured pituitary explants. *Acta Endocrinol.* 98:8–13

89. Goeddel, D. V., Heynecker, H. L., Hozumi, T., Arentzen, R., Itakura, K., Yansura, D. G., Ross, M. J., Miozarri, G., Crea, R., Seeburg, P. H. 1979. Direct expression in *Escherichia coli* of a DNA sequence coding for human growth hormone. *Nature* 281:544–48

90. Phillips, J. A. III, Hjelle, B. L., Seeburg, P. H., Zachman, M. 1981. Molecular basis for familial isolated growth hormone deficiency. *Proc. Natl. Acad. Sci. USA* 78:6372–75

91. Illig, R. 1970. Growth hormone antibodies in patients treated with different preparations of human growth hormone. *J. Clin. Endocrinol. Metab.* 31:679–88

92. Wurzel, J. M., Parks, J. S., Herd, J. E., Nielsen, P. V. 1982. A gene deletion is responsible for absence of human chorionic somatomammotropin. *DNA* 1:251–57

93. Nielsen, P. V., Pederson, H., Kampmann, E. M. 1979. Absence of human placental lactogen in an otherwise uneventful pregnancy. *Am. J. Obstet. Gynecol.* 135:322–26

94. Phillips, J. A. III, Parks, J. S., Hjelle, B. L., Herd, J. E., Plotnick, L. P., Migeon, C. J., Seeburg, P. H. 1982. Genetic analysis of familial isolated growth hormone deficiency type I. *J. Clin. Invest.* 70:489–95

95. Schalch, D. S., Parker, M. L. 1964. A sensitive double antibody immunoassay for human growth hormone in plasma. *Nature* 203:1141–42

96. Frasier, S. D. 1974. A review of growth hormone stimulation tests in children. *Pediatrics* 53:929–37

97. Joss, E. E. 1975. Growth hormone deficiency in childhood. *Mongr. Pediatr.* 5:1–42

98. Lacey, K. A., Parkin, J. M. 1974. A community study of children in New Castle Upon Tyne. *Lancet* 1:42–46

99. Vimpani, G. V., Vimpani, A. F., Lindgard, G. P., Cameron, E. M. H., Farquhar, J. W. 1977. Prevalence of severe growth hormone deficiency. *Br. Med. J.* 2:427–30

100. Henneman, P. H. 1968. The effect of human growth hormone on growth of patients with hypopituitarism. *J. Am. Med. Assoc.* 205:828–36

101. Copeland, K. C., Underwood, L. E., Van Wyck, J. J. 1980. Induction of immunoreactive somatomedin C in human serum by growth hormone: dose-response relationships and effects on chromatographic profiles. *J. Clin. Endocrinol. Metab.* 50:690–97

102. Tanner, J. M., Whitehouse, R. H. 1967. Growth response of 26 children with short stature given human growth hormone. *Br. Med. J.* 2:69–75

103. Tanner, J. M., Whitehouse, R. H., Hughes, P. C. R., Vince, F. P. 1971. Effect of human growth hormone treatment for 1 to 7 years on growth of 100 children, with growth hormone deficiency, low birth weight, inherited smallness, Turner's syndrome and other complaints. *Arch. Dis. Child.* 46:745–82

104. Herington, A. C., Jacobs, L. S., Daughaday, W. J. 1974. Radioreceptor and radioimmunoassay quantitation of human growth hormone in acromegalic serum: overestimation by immunoassay and systematic differences between antisera. *J. Clin. Endocrinol. Metab.* 39:257–62

105. Furlaneho, R. W., Underwood, L. E., Van Wyk, J. J., D'Ercole, A. J. 1977. Estimation of somatomedin C levels in normals and patients with pituitary disease by radioimmunoassay. *J. Clin. Invest.* 60:648–57

106. Kowarski, A. A., Schneider, J., Ben Galim, E., Weldon, V. V., Daughaday, W. H. 1978. Growth failure with normal serum RIA-GH and low somatomedin activity: somatomedin restoration and growth acceleration after exogenous GH. *J. Clin. Endocrinol. Metab.* 47:461–64

107. Hayek, A., Peake, G. T., Greenberg, R. E. 1978. A new syndrome of short stature due to biologically inactive but immunoactive growth hormone. *Pediatr. Res.* 12:413

108. Frazer, T. E., Gavin, J. R., Daughaday, W. H., Hillman, R. E., Weldon, V. V. 1980. Growth hormone dependent growth failure. *Pediatr. Res.* 14:478

109. Rudman, D., Kutner, M. H., Blackston, R. D., Cushman, R. A., Bain, R. P., Patterson, J. H. 1981. Children with normal-variant short stature: treatment with human growth hormone for six months. *N. Engl. J. Med.* 305:123–31

110. Suh, M. K., Frantz, A. G. 1974. Size heterogeneity of human prolactin in plasma and pituitary extracts. *J. Clin. Endocrinol. Metab.* 39:928–35

111. Farkouh, N. M., Packer, M. G. Frantz, A. G. 1979. Large molecular size prolactin with reduced receptor activity in human serum: high proportion in basal state and reduction after thyrotropin-releasing hormone. *J. Clin. Endocrinol. Metab.* 48:1026–32

112. Silverman, A. Y., Schwartz, S. L., Steger, R. W. 1982. A quantitative difference between immunologically and biologically active prolactin in hyperthyroid patients. *J. Clin. Endocrinol. Metab.* 44:272–75

113. Vinik, A., Kaplan, S. L., Grumbach, M. M. 1973. Purification, characterization and comparison of immunological properties of monkey chorionic somatomammotropin with human and monkey growth hormones, human chorionic somatomammotropin and ovine prolactin. *Endocrinology* 92:1051–64

114. Hancock, W. S., Sparrow, J. T. 1981. Used of mixed mode high-performance liquid chromatography for separation of peptide and protein mixtures. *J. Chromatogr.* 206:71–82

115. Catsimpoolas, N. 1976. Isoelectric focussing. In *Hormones in Human Blood,* Ed. M. N. Antoniades, pp. 551–62. Cambridge, Mass: Harvard Univ. Press

SUBJECT INDEX

A

Acetaminophen
   interactions with
      phenobarbital, 466
Acetylcholinesterase
   in sweat glands, 432
Acetylcysteine
   and kidney stone dissolution,
      364, 366
N-Acetyl-(L-cysteine
      (Mucomyst®)
   in kidney stone dissolution,
      364
Acetylsalicylic acid
   and glucose-induced insulin
      secretion, 8–10
Acne
   androgen-related
      hormonal treatment of,
         491, 497
Acquired immunodeficiency
      syndrome (AIDS)
   and dermatologic infections,
      211
Acromegaly
   and pituitary hormones, 283,
      287–90, 292
ACTH
   see Adrenocorticotrophin
      hormone
Acute lymphocytic leukemia
      (ALL)
   and antibody treatment, 110,
      112, 114
Acute myocardial infarction
   see Myocardial infarction
Acyclovir
   and dermatologic infections
      in compromised host,
         211–12
Addison's disease
   and abnormal sweating, 446
Adenine arabinoside
   in infection therapy
      for compromised hosts,
         212
Adenoma
   colorectal
      and cancer risk, 503–4,
         509, 513–14
Adenosine triphosphate (ATP)
   and pseudohypopara-
      thyroidism, 259, 261
Adenylate cyclase
   in Graves' disease, 271
   role in cAMP synthesis
      and pseudohypopara-
         thyroidism, 259–61

Adolescence
   depressive disorder in, 232,
      236
   iron deficiency in, 63
Adrenal steroids
   as chemotherapeutic agents
      and cognitive defects,
         39–40
   and renin release
      in congestive heart failure,
         171
Adrenocorticotrophin hormone
      (ACTH)
   and angiotensin system
      in congestive heart failure,
         171
   and growth hormone
      deficiency, 535
   and onset of Graves' disease,
      278
   and pituitary tumor
      management, 284,
         291–92
Adriamycin
   side effects of, 40
Albright's hereditary
      osteodystrophy
   and pseudohypopara-
      thyroidism, 259–64
Alcohol
   interactions with cannabis,
      256
Alcohol consumption
   and coronary heart disease,
      189
Alcoholism risk
   and depressive disorder, 237
Aldosterone
   and angiotension
      in congestive heart failure,
         171, 173, 175
   role in sweating disorders,
      446–47
Allergic diseases
   and sweating disorders, 441
Alloantibody diseases
   and plasma exchange
      therapy, 80, 83–84
Amenorrhea
   and prolactin-secreting
      tumors, 285
Amino acids
   in sweat composition, 445
Amino acid sequence
   of human growth hormone,
      521
γ-Aminobutyric acid (GABA)
   role in febrile seizures, 455
Aminoglycoside

   in infection therapy
      for compromised hosts,
         213
Amodiaquine
   and drug-resistant malaria,
      325
Amotivation
   and cannabis use, 251
Amoxicillin
   in gonorrhea treatment,
      342–43, 353
Amphetamines
   and cannabis interactions,
      256
Ampicillin
   in endocarditis treatment,
      422
   in gonorrhea treatment,
      342–43, 353
Amyloidosis
   and sweat gland
      abnormalities, 432
Anderson-Fabry disease
   and sweat gland
      abnormalities, 432,
         442–43
Anemia
   and iron absorption, 62
   in renal therapy, 29
   transfusion-dependent
      and hemapheresis, 72–73
Aneurysms
   surgical removal of
      and evoked potential use,
         485
   surgical treatment of
      see Subarachnoid
         hemorrhage
Angiotensin II
   role in congestive heart
      failure
      see Congestive heart
         failure
Anhidrosis
   treatment of, 441–44
      congenital abnormalities,
         444
      neural lesions, 441–43
      physical damage, 443–44
Anhidrotic ectodermal
      dysplasia
   and sweating disorders, 444
Animal studies
   of insulin resistance, 153–54
Antibiotic resistance
   and urethral infection
      treatment, 338–39
Antibiotics
   in malaria treatment, 328–30

Heparin
    as anticoagulant, 94, 101–2
Hepatic enzyme metabolism
    and cannabis inhibition, 256
Heritability
    of diabetes mellitus type I,
        13–18
    of febrile seizures, 454–55
    of pseudohypopara-
        thyroidism, 259–64
Herpes simplex virus
    and dysuria in women, 351
    and infection risk
        for compromised hosts,
            211
Hexamethylmelamine
    side effects of, 40
Hirsutism
    hormonal treatment of, 491,
        497
Histamine release
    and products of complement
        activation, 48
Histocompatibility antigens
    and kidney transplants,
        133–38
    see also HLA
HLA antigens (Human
    leukocyte antigens, group
    A)
    in kidney transplant survival,
        133–37, 142
    and suitable kidney donors,
        26
HLA-B27
    and susceptibility to sexually
        acquired arthritis, 346
HLA-DR antigens
    as cell markers, 119, 122
HLA-linked gene
    and iron absorption, 55,
        65–66
HLA tissue typing
    and predisposition to diabetes
        mellitus, 13–17
Hodgkin's disease
    and dermatologic infection
        risk, 212
Hookworm infestation
    and iron deficiency, 64
Hormonal antagonists
    of insulin action
        and insulin resistance,
            151–52
Hormonal interactions
    as cause of diabetes mellitus,
        1
Hormones
    and glandular tumors
        see Pituitary tumors
    superactive agonists

    see Gonadotropin-releasing
        hormone agonists
    variants of growth hormone
        see Growth hormone
Hospitals
    spread of respiratory
        syncytial virus in,
            311–18
Hot flushes
    and hyperhidrosis, 440–41
Human chorionic
    somatomammotropin
    and growth hormone gene
        structure, 532
Human leukocyte antigen
    (HLA) DRW-3
    in Graves' disease, 270–71,
        274, 277
    see also HLA
Human leukocyte interferon
    in infection therapy
        for compromised hosts,
            212
Human lymphocyte antigen
    (HLA)
    and insulin-dependent
        diabetes, 297–98
    see also HLA
Hunter's syndrome
    and sweating disorders, 448
Hurler's syndrome
    and sweating disorders, 448
Hybridomas
    lymphocyte
        see Tumor therapy
Hydration
    and renal failure in children,
        22
Hydrocephalus
    following subarachnoid
        hemorrhage, 372–73
5-Hydroxytryptamine
    see Serotonin
Hyperandrogenism
    and insulin resistance, 158
Hypercalcemia
    and delirium
        in cancer, 44
Hypercholesterolemia
    as coronary risk factor
        and exercise, 393, 397–98,
            404–6
    in diabetics, 162
Hypereosinophilic syndromes
    use of leukapheresis in, 76
Hyperglycemia
    chronic
        and diabetes diagnosis and
            classification, 295–96,
                298
    and heart failure in diabetics,
        166
    role of prostaglandins in, 6, 9

Hyperhidrosis
    see Sweating
Hyperinsulinemia
    and insulin resistance studies,
        153–54
Hyperlipidemia
    role of diet in
        see Atherosclerosis
Hyperparathyroidism
    prophylaxis against
        in renal failure therapy,
            22, 24, 28
    and pseudohypopara-
        thyroidism, 263
Hyperphosphatemia
    in pseudohypopara-
        thyroidism, 260
    treatment of
        in renal failure therapy, 24
Hyperprolactinemia
    treatment of, 283, 285, 288
Hypertension
    and aneurysm therapy, 371
    as coronary risk factor
        and exercise, 393, 397,
            402, 404–6
    in diabetics, 162
Hyperthermia
    drug-induced
        and sweat gland damage,
            434
Hyperthyroidism
    pathogenesis of, 267–78
        autoimmunity, 268–69
        basis for altered immunity,
            277–78
        genetic predisposition,
            269–71
        Graves' hyperthyroidism,
            271–72
        human thyroid-stimulating
            activity, 272–77
Hyperviscosity syndrome
    and plasma exchange
        therapy, 79, 81
Hypnosedatives
    and cognitive deficits in
        cancer, 41
Hypocalcemia
    in pseudohypopara-
        thyroidism, 260, 262,
            264
Hypocomplementemia
    and infections
        see Complement system
Hypogammaglobulinemia
    and inherited absence of C3,
        50
Hypoglycemia
    and childhood depressive
        disorder, 238

and insulin receptor studies,
149, 157
role of prostaglandins in, 7
Hypogonadotropic
hypogonadism
hormonal treatment of, 498
Hypothalamic disturbance
and aneurysm therapy, 372
Hypothyroidism
and sweating disorders, 447
Hysteria
and evoked potential
analysis, 484

I

Iatrogenic complications
in endocarditis, 415
see also Dermatologic
infections; Cognitive
defects; Respiratory
syncytial virus
IBM 2997
and hemapheretic
technology, 71
Ibuprofen
and glucose-induced insulin
secretion, 8
Ig
see Antibodies; Antigens;
Immunoglobulin
Imipramine
in childhood depression
treatment, 240–42
Immune complexes
and plasma exchange
therapy, 80, 84–85
Immune reactions
and febrile seizures, 455
Immune response
in bowel disease, 195–201
Immunization
of children
and febrile seizures, 454
Immunoactivity
of growth hormone, 529,
541–42
Immunodeficiency diseases
and dermatologic infection,
211–12
Immunofluorescence
in cell marker identification,
121–22
Immunoglobulin antibodies
(IgG)
in infection defense, 49, 51
in tumor therapy, 108
Immunoglobulin antibodies
(IgM)
in tumor therapy, 108
Immunoglobulins (Ig)
and cell markers

in leukemia and
lymphoma, 118–19,
123, 126
in complement system, 49
of Graves' disease patients
and hyperthyroidism,
267–78
in inflammatory bowel
disease, 197, 199–201
Immunological events
leading to diabetes mellitus
type I, 13–18
cell-mediated immune
mechanisms, 15–16
gut endocrine related
antibodies, 17
humoral autoimmune
responses, 14–15
other endocrine glands and
pathogenesis, 16–17
prolonged latency, 16
Immunological factors
in kidney transplants
see Kidney transplant
survival
Immunology
and compromised host
see Dermatologic
infections
Immunophenotypes
of lymphoid leukemias,
121–24
Immunoreactivity
of growth hormone, 536–37
Immunoregulation
in bowel disease
see Inflammatory bowel
disease
Immunosuppression
as cannabis effect, 255
induction by
lymphocytapheresis, 76,
79
Immunosuppressive therapy
and dermatologic infection,
207–16
see Dermatologic
infections
in kidney transplants, 25,
27–28, 31–32, 133–34
and plasma exchange
therapy, 79, 85
and risk of nosocomial RSV,
317–18
Impaired glucose tolerance
and diabetes classification
and diagnosis
see Diabetes
Indomethacin
and glucose homeostasis,
4–6, 8
Infants
iron deficiency in, 63

rate of gastric emptying and
metabolism, 224
respiratory syncytial virus in
nosocomial spread, 312–18
Infection control
and nosocomial spread of
RSV, 317–18
see Respiratory syncytial
virus
Infections
damage to vessels
and postphlebitic
syndrome, 97
during cancer
and cognitive defects, 39,
41
and hypocomplementemia
see Complement system
recurrent
and complement
measurement, 51–52
see also Dermatologic
infections; Respiratory
syncytial virus; Urethral
infections; and specific
pathogens
Infertility
idiopathic
hormonal treatment of,
498
Inflammatory bowel disease
and endocarditis, 418
immunoregulation in,
195–201
antilymphocyte antibodies,
197
cell-mediated immunity,
197–98
etiology and pathogenesis,
196
humoral immunity, 197
immunologic observations,
196–97
intestinal mucosal
mononuclear cells,
199–201
peripheral blood studies,
198
and risk of colorectal cancer,
505–6
Insulin
and diabetes classification
and diagnosis, 296–97
see also Diabetes; Diabetes
mellitus
Insulin-dependent diabetes
mellitus (IDDM)
diagnosis and classification,
299, 303
Insulin hypoglycemia
and growth hormone
immune reaction, 536

Substance abuse
see Cannabis
Sucrose
and dietary fat
in coronary heart disease,
182
Suicide
thoughts of
and depressive mood
assessment, 236
Sulfisoxazole
in gonorrhea treatment,
344–45
Sulfonamide-pyrimethamine
combinations
in malaria treatment, 322,
325–26
Sulfonamides
in urethritis treatment, 347
Suppressor cell function
in immunoregulation in
bowel disease, 198
Surgery
use of evoked potentials
during, 484–85
see Subarachnoid
hemorrhage
Surgical dressings
and dermatologic infection
risk, 216
Sweating, 429–48
anhidrosis, 441–44
central control, 434
composition of sweat, 44–48
congenital abnormalities, 444
emotional, 437–39
gland stimulation, 434–35
gustatory, 439–40
hyperhidrosis, 437–41
neural lesions, 441–43
normal, 430–42
physical damage, 443
reabsorption, 436–37
secretion, 435–36
structural abnormalities,
432–34
Systemic lupus erythematosus
and C5 deficiency, 51
and Graves' disease, 268
and plasma exchange
therapy, 76, 80, 84–85

T

Tannins
role in iron absorption, 59
Tartaric acid
role in iron absorption, 59
Tea
and reduction of iron
absorption, 59
Temperature control
and sweating, 430, 434,
440–41, 444

Teprotide
in congestive heart failure
treatment, 174–75
Teratogenicity
of marijuana, 255
Testosterone secretion
and hormone agonists,
492–95
Tetracyclines
in gonorrhea treatment,
342–43, 347, 353
in malaria treatment, 325,
328–29
δ-9-Tetrahydrocannabinol
(THC)
see Cannabis
Thalassemia major
and iron absorption, 64
THAM-E
in kidney stone dissolution,
359, 363–64, 366
THC
see Cannabis
Thermoregulation
disorders of
see Sweating
Thiazide diuretics
in heart failure
and diabetes, 166
Thinking disorders
assessment of, 42
in cancer patients
see Cognitive defects
Thoracic duct drainage
as antirejection therapy
in kidney transplants,
31–32
Thought disorder
cannabis-induced, 250–51
Thrombophlebitis
see Postphlebitic syndrome
Thromboxane
in diabetes mellitus, 2–3
in postphlebitic syndrome,
97
Thrombocytopenic purpura
and plasma exchange
therapy, 72, 79, 82 85
Thyroid
see Hyperthyroidism;
Pseudo-
hypoparathyroidism
Thyroid-stimulating hormone
(TSH)
deficiency
and growth hormone
deficiency, 535
and hyperthyroidism,
267–68, 271–73, 276–78
and tumor management, 284
Thyrotoxicosis
antibody analysis in, 15–17
Thyrotropin
resistance to

and pseudohypopara-
thyroidism, 261
Thyrotropin-binding inhibitory
immunoglobulin (TBII)
and autoimmunity in
hyperthyroidism, 268,
272
Thyrotropin-releasing hormone
(TRH)
in Graves' disease, 271
and pituitary tumor
management, 284–85
Tissue typing
and transplant donation, 30
see HLA
Toxins
and plasma exchange
therapy, 80–81
Training effect
of exercise
and coronary heart
disease, 392, 399,
401–2, 404
Transferrin
and iron absorption, 62–63
Transfusion therapy
in renal therapy for children,
30–31
Transplant
renal
see Renal transplant
survival
see Kidney transplant
survival
Trauma
assessment of
by evoked potential
studies, 484
Tricyclic antidepressants
in cancer
and cognitive deficits, 41
Triglycerides
and gastric emptying rates,
226
Trimethoprim-sulfamethoxazole
in urethritis treatment, 347,
353
Tumors
steroid-sensitive
see Prostate cancer
Tumor therapy
with antibodies, 107–15
antigenic modulation, 111
antiidiotype antibody, 113
bone marrow transplants,
113–14
clinical studies, 108–9
future prospects, 114–15
mouse monoclonal
antibodies, 110–11
problems encountered in,
108–9, 114
therapeutic effects, 111–12
toxicity, 110

CUMULATIVE INDEXES

CONTRIBUTING AUTHORS, VOLUMES 30–34

CHAPTER TITLES, VOLUMES 30–34

571

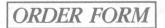

ORDER FORM

NEW BOOKS
FROM
ANNUAL REVIEWS INC.

NOW YOU CAN
CHARGE THEM
TO

VISA   MasterCard

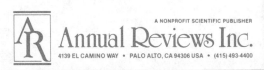

A NONPROFIT SCIENTIFIC PUBLISHER
Annual Reviews Inc.
4139 EL CAMINO WAY • PALO ALTO, CA 94306 USA • (415) 493-4400

Please list the volumes you wish to order by volume number. If you wish a standing order (the latest volume sent to you automatically each year), indicate volume number to begin order. Volumes not yet published will be shipped in month and year indicated. All prices subject to change without notice.

ANNUAL REVIEW SERIES

Annual Review of **ANTHROPOLOGY**		Prices Postpaid per volume USA/elsewhere	Regular Order Please send: Vol. number	Standing Order Begin with: Vol. number
Vols. 1-10	(1972-1981)	$20.00/$21.00		
Vol. 11	(1982)	$22.00/$25.00		
Vol. 12	(avail. Oct. 1983)	$27.00/$30.00	Vol(s). _____	Vol. _____

Annual Review of **ASTRONOMY AND ASTROPHYSICS**

Vols. 1-19	(1963-1981)	$20.00/$21.00		
Vol. 20	(1982)	$22.00/$25.00		
Vol. 21	(avail. Sept. 1983)	$44.00/$47.00	Vol(s). _____	Vol. _____

Annual Review of **BIOCHEMISTRY**

[Vols. 28-48 $18.00/$18.50
Price effective through 12/31/82]

Vols. 28-50	(1959-1981)	$21.00/$22.00		
Vol. 51	(1982)	$23.00/$26.00		
Vol. 52	(avail. July 1983)	$29.00/$32.00	Vol(s). _____	Vol. _____

Annual Review of **BIOPHYSICS AND BIOENGINEERING**

Vols. 1-10	(1972-1981)	$20.00/$21.00		
Vol. 11	(1982)	$22.00/$25.00		
Vol. 12	(avail. June 1983)	$47.00/$50.00	Vol(s). _____	Vol. _____

Annual Review of **EARTH AND PLANETARY SCIENCES**

Vols. 1-9	(1973-1981)	$20.00/$21.00		
Vol. 10	(1982)	$22.00/$25.00		
Vol. 11	(avail. May 1983)	$44.00/$47.00	Vol(s). _____	Vol. _____

Annual Review of **ECOLOGY AND SYSTEMATICS**

Vols. 1-12	(1970-1981)	$20.00/$21.00		
Vol. 13	(1982)	$22.00/$25.00		
Vol. 14	(avail. Nov. 1983)	$27.00/$30.00	Vol(s). _____	Vol. _____

SEE ORDERING INFORMATION ON PAGE 4.

Annual Review of **ENERGY**		Prices Postpaid per volume USA/elsewhere	Regular Order Please send: Vol. number	Standing Order Begin with: Vol. number
Vols. 1-6	(1976-1981)	$20.00/$21.00		
Vol. 7	(1982)	$22.00/$25.00		
Vol. 8	(avail. Oct. 1983)	$56.00/$59.00	Vol(s). _____	Vol. _____

Annual Review of **ENTOMOLOGY**

Vols. 7-26	(1962-1981)	$20.00/$21.00		
Vol. 27	(1982)	$22.00/$25.00		
Vol. 28	(avail. Jan. 1983)	$27.00/$30.00	Vol(s). _____	Vol. _____

Annual Review of **FLUID MECHANICS**

Vols. 1-13	(1969-1981)	$20.00/$21.00		
Vol. 14	(1982)	$22.00/$25.00		
Vol. 15	(avail. Jan. 1983)	$28.00/$31.00	Vol(s). _____	Vol. _____

Annual Review of **GENETICS**

Vols. 1-15	(1967-1981)	$20.00/$21.00		
Vol. 16	(1982)	$22.00/$25.00		
Vol. 17	(avail. Dec. 1983)	$27.00/$30.00	Vol(s). _____	Vol. _____

Annual Review of **IMMUNOLOGY — New Series 1983**

Vol. 1	(avail. April 1983)	$27.00/$30.00	Vol(s). _____	Vol. _____

Annual Review of **MATERIALS SCIENCE**

Vols. 1-11	(1971-1981)	$20.00/$21.00		
Vol. 12	(1982)	$22.00/$25.00		
Vol. 13	(avail. Aug. 1983)	$64.00/$67.00	Vol(s). _____	Vol. _____

Annual Review of **MEDICINE: Selected Topics in the Clinical Sciences**

Vols. 1-3, 5-15	(1950-1952; 1954-1964)	$20.00/$21.00		
Vols. 17-32	(1966-1981)	$20.00/$21.00		
Vol. 33	(1982)	$22.00/$25.00		
Vol. 34	(avail. April 1983)	$27.00/$30.00	Vol(s). _____	Vol. _____

Annual Review of **MICROBIOLOGY**

Vols. 15-35	(1961-1981)	$20.00/$21.00		
Vol. 36	(1982)	$22.00/$25.00		
Vol. 37	(avail. Oct. 1983)	$27.00/$30.00	Vol(s). _____	Vol. _____

Annual Review of **NEUROSCIENCE**

Vols. 1-4	(1978-1981)	$20.00/$21.00		
Vol. 5	(1982)	$22.00/$25.00		
Vol. 6	(avail. March 1983)	$27.00/$30.00	Vol(s). _____	Vol. _____

2

SEE ORDERING INFORMATION ON PAGE 4.